黄帝针灸甲乙經

The Systematic Classic
of
Acupuncture & Moxibustion

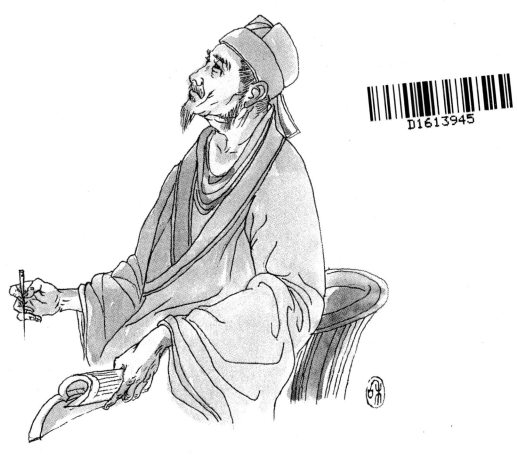

by Huang-fu Mi

Translated by

Yang Shou-zhong and Charles Chace

Published by:
BLUE POPPY PRESS
A Division of Blue Poppy Enterprises, Inc.
5441 Western Ave., Suite 2
Boulder, CO 80301
www.bluepoppy.com

First Edition, July 1994
Second printing, April 2004

ISBN 0-936185-29-5
LC #91-72854

DISCLAIMER: The information in this book is given in good faith. However, the author and the publishers cannot be held responsible for any error or omission. The publishers will not accept liabilities for any injuries or damages caused to the reader that may result from the reader's acting upon or using the content contained in this book. The publishers make this information available to English language readers for research and scholarly purposes only.

The publishers do not advocate nor endorse self-medication by laypersons. Chinese medicine is a professional medicine. Laypersons interested in availing themselves of the treatments described in this book should seek out a qualified professional practitioner of Chinese medicine.

COMP Designation: This work is a connotative translation using a standard translational terminology.

Cover & Page design: Eric J. Brearton

COMP Designation: Original work

10 9 8 7 6 5 4 3 2 1

Printed at NetPub Corporation, Poughkeepsie, N.Y.

TRANSLATORS' PREFACE

The ancient classics of acupuncture and moxibustion are not what one would consider user friendly. While source materials such as the *Su Wen (Basic Questions)*, *Ling Shu (Spiritual Pivot)*, and the *Nan Jing (Classic of Difficulties)* are the bedrock upon which nearly every style of acupuncture is based, these texts are not teaching texts per se, nor are they clinical manuals. Anyone who has perused the *Nei Jing (Inner Classic)* in Chinese or examined any of its piecemeal translations in English will most likely have been struck by its internal contradictions and the difficulty of finding what one is looking for. During the late Han dynasty, Huang–fu Mi undertook the task of organizing the existing acupuncture literature in a systematic manner. The *Zhen Jiu Jia Yi Jing (Systematic Classic of Acupuncture and Moxibustion,* 针灸甲乙经）was the result of this effort and was the first book of its kind. Huang–fu Mi's *magnum opus* consists of twelve books containing a total of One hundred twenty-eight chapters. The first six books deal with the basic theories of acupuncture and moxibustion, while the last six deal with acupuncture and moxibustion therapeutics. In this work, we find the first systematic exposition of the basic theories of Chinese medicine, the acupoints, channels and connecting vessels, needling techniques, and the clinical application of acupuncture and moxibustion. It also contains an analysis of the various patterns of disease in the areas of internal medicine (*nei ke*), external medicine (*wai ke*), pediatrics (*er ke*), and gynecology (*fu ke*). Huang–fu Mi initiated a new system in cataloguing acupoints. On the limbs the points are grouped according to channels, but on the trunk he introduced regional divisions. Because of the convenience of this approach, Huang–fu Mi's system of arranging materials pertaining to therapeutics is preserved today in many acupuncture textbooks.

The Systematic Classic is based on three classics: the *Su Wen*, *Ling Shu* and *Ming Tang Zhen Jiu Zhi Yao (The Acupuncture and Moxibustion Treatment Essentials of the Enlightening Hall)* or *Ming Tang (Enlightening Hall)* for short. The last, as its name suggests, was a book specifically on acupuncture and moxibustion. It was held in high regard in ancient times but was lost long ago. Huang–fu Mi is responsible for the preservation of much of the material in the *Ming Tang* book because so much of it was incorporated into the *Jia Yi Jing*. It is not unreasonable to say that Huang–fu Mi's work defined acupuncture as we know it today.

The *Ling Shu* is another of the sources used to compile the *Jia Yi Jing*. Even hundreds of years ago, the *Ling Shu* had become so garbled over the long course of its transmission that many parts of it were unreadable. Scholars through the centuries have devoted themselves to the collation and rectification of the *Ling Shu* in an attempt to restore it to its original appearance. These efforts would have been impossible without reference to the *Jia Yi Jing*. The *Ling Shu* as we know it today quite simply would not exist without the *Jia Yi Jing*.

The *Jia Yi Jing* is important not just because it helped preserve other ancient acupuncture and moxibustion texts. The *Jia Yi Jing* itself enriched and expanded the theories expounded in the *Ling Shu* and *Ming Tang*. It then provided them with clinical applications in acupuncture and moxibustion, the locations of the acupoints, the determination and detailed description of the channels and connecting vessels, instructions on needling technique, and illustrations of the indications of the acupoints.

The *Su Wen* records only one hundred sixty acupoints, and these are for the most part mentioned without reference to their locations, indications, or clinical applications. The *Jia Yi Jing* adds one hundred eighty–nine points to this list, increasing the total number to three hundred forty–nine points. While the expositions on pathogenesis, diagnosis, and the pathophysiology of disease in the *Ling Shu* and *Su Wen* are indeed instructive these books are not oriented toward clinical practice and most often do not contain therapies for specific, clinically encountered problems. The *Jia Yi Jing*, on the other hand, is a clinically oriented manual arranged in a manner that a student or practitioner can easily access. It presents the reader with the signs and symptoms of a given disease, and then provides us with acupuncture moxibustion treatment choices. Having made these choices, the *Jia Yi Jing* then provides us with a clear description of what to expect from its formulas and their relevant points, the depths of needle insertion, the number of cones allowed in moxibustion, and the manipulation of the needles, etc.

Throughout the history of acupuncture no other work has challenged the predominance of the *Jia Yi Jing*. It has been cited and referred to as an authority in countless books on Chinese Medicine throughout the centuries. Without the *Jia Yi Jing*, these texts would not exist in the state they do today. During the Tang Dynasty, the *Wai Tai Mi Yao Fang (The Secret Essentials of a Provincial Governor)* by Wang Tao, the *Bei Ji Qian Jin Fang (Prescriptions Worth a Thousand Taels of Gold)* by Sun Si–miao, and the *Zhu Bing Yuan Hou Lun (Treatise on the Origin and Symptoms of Various Diseases)* by Chao Yuan–fang all borrowed something from the *Jia Yi Jing*. The most important medical works during the Song dynasty, included the *Tong Ren Shu Xue Zhen Jiu Tu Jing (The Classic of the Atlas of Acupoints on the Bronze Statue)* by Wang Wei–yi and the *Zhen Jiu Zi Sheng Jing (The Classic of Nourishing Life with Acupuncture Moxibustion)* by Wang Zhi–zhong and it is widely acknowledged that these are based upon the *Jia Yi Jing*. During the Ming dynasty, such time–honored acupuncture books as the *Zhen Jiu Ju Ying (A Gathering of Outstanding Acupuncture and Moxibustion Works)* by Gao Wu and the *Zhen Jiu Da Cheng (The Great Compendium of Acupuncture and Moxibustion)* by Yang Ji–zhou are also believed to be based on the *Jia Yi Jing*. This is also true of the *Zhen Jiu Ji Cheng (The Collection of [Writings on] Acupuncture and Moxibustion)* by Liao Ren–hong of the Qing dynasty, probably the most worthy acupuncture/moxibustion book of its time.

From even a cursory review of the medical literature from the Song dynasty onward, it is evident that no writing on acupuncture and moxibustion has surpassed the preeminence of the *Jia Yi Jing*. Texts on classical Chinese acupuncture and moxibustion published in the fifteen hundred years since Huang–fu Mi's death have added only twelve channel points to the number contained in the *Jia Yi Jing*. Moreover, most of these books borrow materials from the *Jia Yi Jing* and use it as their blueprint and basis.

While the *Su Wen* and *Ling Shu* laid the foundation for acupuncture and moxibustion, it was the *Jia Yi Jing* that made it a scientific system. In this light, Huang–fu Mi is indeed a true pioneer of medicine as opposed to a mere collator. Over the centuries since its creation, the *Jia Yi Jing* has been recognized as an authority on acupuncture and moxibustion by governments as well as physicians. During the Tang Dynasty, one of the most prosperous periods in Chinese history, students at the Imperial Medical College were assigned only the *Su Wen* and *Ling Shu*, the *Jia Yi Jing*. No student could graduate as a doctor unless he had passed an examination on these books. In the Song dynasty, emperors often took personal responsibility for organizing the collation and rectification of the medical classics and the *Jia Yi Jing* was one of the books on which they focused their attentions.

Subsequent to the Tang Dynasty, neighboring countries such as Japan and Korea introduced similar imperial medical institutions where the prescribed textbooks were also the *Su Wen, Ling Shu,* and *Jia Yi Jing.* The definitive ancient version of the *Jia Yi Jing* was found not in China but was reintroduced to this country from Japan.

Over the centuries, *The Systematic Classic* has had wide variety of titles including *"Huang Di Jia Yi Jing (The Yellow Emperor's Classic of Acupuncture and Moxibustion), Zhen Jiu Jia Yi Jing (The Systematic Classic of Acupuncture and Moxibustion), Zhen Jiu Jing (The Acupuncture and Moxibustion Classic), Huang Di Zhen Jiu Jia Yi Jing (The Yellow Emperor's Systematic Classic of Acupuncture and Moxibustion),* and *Huang Di San Bu Zhen Jiu Jia Yi Jing (The Yellow Emperor's Classic of Acupuncture and Moxibustion based on the Three Books).* Since the author himself claimed his book was based on works of the Yellow Emperor, it is not surprising to see the Yellow Emperor's name in the title. Nor should the words *"San Bu"* in the title confuse the reader. *San* means three, while *bu* means works. This is understandable since this classic was derived from three other books, the *Su Wen, Ling Shu,* and the *Ming Tang.*

There is some question as to why Huang–fu Mi chose the words *Jia Yi* for the title of his tome. These are the first two of the ten heavenly stems. It was a common practice in ancient China to arrange materials in order of the ten heavenly stems or twelve earthly branches rather than numbering them. This would be similar to using A, B, C to order a sequence of information in English and this system of categorization is in common use in Chinese publications even today. This explanation raises the question as to why the author preferred the ten heavenly stems to the twelve earthly branches. After all, the number of earthly branches correlates nicely with the number of books in this classic and they are an equally valid numbering system. This has been a controversial question for a long time and so far no consensus has been reached. One might conjecture that the author believed that heaven is superior to earth in terms of the values inherent in ancient Chinese philosophy and, therefore, the heavenly stems are more suitable for the title of a book which might "bring happiness, harmony, and peace to the whole land and benefit infinite generations to come" as Huang–fu Mi hoped. This supposition is supported by the fact that the heavenly stems were and are used today to denote degrees of importance or quality, and the earthly branches have seldom been used in this way. In a Chinese schoolboy's report card, grades are often recorded as *jia* or *yi.* It may also be used as a superlative. For instance, a description of the scenery in Hang–zhou might be described as *jia* under heaven. Here the word means first, the highest, the best. Another interpretation is that *jia* and *yi* were and are frequently used in juxtaposition to represent the two sides involved in an interaction, such as a project, a contract, or in an interlocution. This is germane to the fact that the material in the *Jia Yi Jing* is arranged as a series of questions and answers between the Yellow Emperor and Qi Bo, Bo Gao and other interlocutors. This usage is also confirmed in the Chinese etymological dictionary, *Ci Yuan (The Origin of Words),* which contains an entry defining *jia yi* as two interlocutors.

There is another hypothesis which, upon initial consideration, sounds equally plausible and has attracted a fair amount of support in the research community. According to this line of reasoning, the original number of books or volumes in this classic was not twelve but ten, and thus correlate to the number of the heavenly stems. The two additional chapters were extracted or separated out from the rest of the book by later editors. However, the preface written by Huang–fu Mi himself indicates that this classic consists of twelve books and there is no convincing evidence to support the ten book hypothesis. Supporters of this thesis remain undaunted by Huang–fu Mi's statement, arguing that it was quite natural and easy for subsequent editors to make the necessary alterations in Huang's preface to bring it into accord with the rest of the book.

On Huang–fu Mi's biography

Huang–fu Mi's style name was Shi–an, his infant name was Jing, and his self–called name was Xuan Yan (Occult Composure). He was born in 215 and died in 282 CE. Brought up in the remote area of then An Ding county (presently Ling Tai County, Gansu Province), he lived in poverty during his childhood and was adopted by one of his uncles. As a boy, he was not very industrious and was apparently so dull that he was often made fun of and called a fool by his friends. He remained largely idle until he was twenty, when he suddenly developed an appreciation for the importance of scholarship. Once he applied himself to his studies, he proved himself to be quite diligent. His poor family could not afford tutor's fees for him, textbooks, or time away from work, but he managed to overcome all these obstacles in his pursuit of an education. He never went anywhere without the books he had borrowed from his neighbors and he read them during breaks at work or while tending the cattle in the fields. It was not long before he was considered an eminent scholar with wide-ranging interests. He is said to have had a perfect mastery of the doctrines of the correct academic schools and to have been possessed of remarkable talents, especially in the area of literature. Huang–fu Mi composed many works over the course of his life which were widely considered to be masterpieces.

At the age of forty–two, Huang–fu Mi was struck with hemiplegia and confined to bed. It was during this period that he took up the study of medicine and began the great work of the *Jia Yi Jing*. Years later, another misfortune befell him. During the late Han Dynasty, many people fervently believed in the elixirs of the Daoists and became obsessed with distilling drugs of immortality from various minerals, including mercury. Such pursuits were especially popular among the upper classes and the intellectuals. Huang–fu Mi was one of the victims of this harmful epidemic of self–poisoning. He ingested a powder called Five Stone Powder (*Wu Shi San*) or Cold Stone Powder (*Han Shi San*) which nearly cost him his life. He subsequently remained so ill that he all but lost hope of recovery and almost committed suicide. This traumatic experience solidified his determination to pursue the study of medicine. Being a scholar of distinction, Huang–fu Mi had easy access to high positions within the government. However, Huang–fu Mi preferred a scholarly life, refusing all offers from the Emperor, and devoting the rest of his life to the study of medicine.

Huang–fu Mi was a prolific author and left behind him an extensive corpus of writing. Among these were *Wang Di Shi Ji* (*Biographies of Various Emperors and Kings*); *Gao Shi Zhuan* (*Biographies of the Lofty*); *Yi Shi Zhuan* (*Biographies of Hermits*); *Lie Nu Zhuan* (*Biographies of Women Martyrs*); and *Xuan Yan Chun Qiu* (*The Spring and Autumn of Yuan Yan*). But the most influential work of all was his medical magnum opus, the *Jia Yi Jing*, which took him twenty–six years to complete.

The Systematic Classic

Chinese medical classics often seem as if they are continually evolving, almost living entities. They are always being edited, annotated, and reinterpreted in the context of the time in which they are being read. This is particularly the case with *The Systematic Classic*. The *Jia Yi Jing* was first published in 282 CE, the year of Huang–fu Mi's death. But, thus far, the earliest version available is dated 1601 CE during the Ming dynasty. This leaves a gap of thirteen hundred and nineteen years during which we are unable to trace the manner in which the text was altered or edited. From the various versions now available, it is clear that it has been tampered with extensively during this time. Among the various extant editions, an enormous number of mistakes contradict each other in so many places that even editions supposedly based on the same prototype produce renditions that diametrically oppose one another and read like different books. There are three main versions of the *Jia Yi Jing* in circulation in China today, all of which were edited in or after the Ming dynasty. *Zhen Jiu Jia Yi Jing Jiao Shi (The Collated and Annotated Systematic Classic of Acupuncture and Moxibustion)*, hereafter referred to as the Shandong edition, by the Shandong College of Traditional Chinese Medicine, published by the People's Health & Hygiene Press in 1980 and the *Huang Di Zhen Jiu Jia Yi Jing ((The Newly Revised) Yellow Emperor's Systematic of Acupuncture and Moxibustion)* hereafter referred to as the Huang edition, by Huang Long–xiang, published by the China Medical Science & Technology Press in 1990, both claim to be based on the same prototype, the *Gu Jin Yi Tong Zheng Mai Quan Shu (The Comprehensive Collection of Ancient and Modern Medical Works Including Works on the Pulse)* version. In certain passages the two editions provide two very different readings. On page six of the Shandong edition there is the sentence, "If there is emptiness of lung qi, this results in difficult breathing..." The corresponding statement can be found on page thirty of the Huang edition which reads, "If there is emptiness of lung qi, breathing through the nose is smooth..." Here we have the same condition and the opposite conclusion. It is no wonder that many practitioners of Chinese medicine comment that no two persons will translate to a single paragraph of the *Jia Yi Jing* into modern Chinese in the same way, let alone into a foreign language.

About this translation

As translators, we have attempted to be as faithful to the author as possible. Our task has entailed not merely putting the Chinese into English, but the making editorial decisions as to the content of the material we would translate as well. Since there is no definitive version of the *Jia Yi Jing* we often compared the various versions to confirm the presence of a single word in the text. We feel this approach ensured a reliable English version of *The Systematic Classic* which reflects to the greatest extent possible what was contained in Huang–fu Mi's original *Jia Yi Jing*. We have based our English version of the *Jia Yi Jing* on the *Yi Tong Zheng Mai*, edited in the Ming dynasty and circulated in a photocopied form by the People's Health & Hygiene Press, Beijing. This version was supplemented by numerous references to *Huang Di Zhen Jiu Jia Yi Jing (The Yellow Emperor's Systematic Classic of Acupuncture and Moxibustion)* edited by Huang Xiang–long which is a most reliable edition. In addition, the many other versions of this classic which have become available over the past fifty years containing commentary or modern Chinese translation have contributed greatly to the completion of this English version. Among these are the *Zhen Jiu Jia Yi Jing Jiao Shi (Collated and Annotated Systematic Classic of Acupuncture and Moxibustion)* mentioned above; the *Zhong Guo Zhen Jiu Hui Cui (Collection of Outstanding Chinese Acupuncture and Moxibustion Works)* Wang Xue–tai published by the Hunan Science & Technology Press, 1988; *Huang Di Ming Tang Jing Ji Jiao (The Restored and Collated Yellow Emperor's Classic of the Enlightening Hall)* by Huang Xiang–long published by the China Medical Science & Technology Press; the *Zhen Jiu Jia Yi Jing Shu Xue Chong Ji (The Gathering of Channel Points in the Systematic Classic of Acupuncture and Moxibustion)* by Zhang Shan–zhen et al. published by the Shandong Science & Technology Press, 1979; the *Huang Di Nei Jing Su Wen Yi Shi (Collated and Illustrated Basic Questions of the Yellow Emperor's Inner Classic)* edited by the Office of Medical Classics, Nanjing College of TCM, published by the Shanghai Science & Technology Press, 1959; and the *Ling Shu Jing Jiao Shi (The Collated and Annotated Spiritual Pivot)* edited by the HBO College of TCM published by the People's Health & Hygiene Press, 1982. We are much indebted to the editors and authors of the above works.

On translation

It is always good to know just what it is one is reading. This is particularly true when reading a translation because the biases of the translator are inherent in any translation. With the increase in Chinese source materials now available in English, there is now a growing interest among translators and publishers of Chinese medical literature in making such biases clear to their readership. In May of 1993, a group of Chinese medical translators and publishers formed the Council of Oriental Medical Publishers (COMP). The intent of the council is to promote clarity in how writings pertaining to oriental medicine have been translated once they are presented to the public. At present few translators define just how they have gone about translating a given Chinese medical text, yet this is a pre–requisite for any critical evaluation of the translation itself or its contents. The council does not advocate any particular style of translation over another, only that the style of translation be clearly stated. As a means of assisting in this clarification, the council has outlined three styles of translation based on the writings of the American sinologist Edward H. Schafer. These are denotative, connotative, and functional translations.

A denotative translation provides as close to a word for word translation as possible. For instance, the words *xian sheng* (先生) might be translated denotatively as Elder Born or First Born, which are the most literal meanings of the Chinese words themselves. If the meaning of such a translation is not readily apparent to a contemporary reader then COMP proposes that the translator provide a footnote, gloss, or commentary, clarifying what he or she believes the term actually means in modern English. A connotative translation, on the other hand, directly reflects what the translator believes to be the intentional meaning of the Chinese words. Thus, translated connotatively, *xian sheng* might be rendered as teacher or Mister in modern English, depending on the context. Another example taken from the text at hand is the term *hou jie*. In our translation of *The Systematic Classic*, we have rendered this literally as throat knot in accordance with a denotative translation. However, in modern English the throat knot refers to the Adam's apple.

In a denotative translation there is a strict one for one relationship between the Chinese words and their English translation. The Council of Oriental Medical Publishers has proposed that denotative translations be based on an identifiable and freely available standard glossary. Such a glossary might be a particular Chinese English dictionary, a Chinese medical glossary such as Nigel Wiseman et al.'s *Glossary of Chinese Medical Terms and Acupuncture Points* or some privately compiled glossary which can be made available to scholars and other readers. The benefits of a denotative translation are that it should rely on a standard set of technical terms which can be cross referenced throughout the Chinese literature and that it has the potential to most closely preserve the original source text with its full range of implications. On the other hand, denotative translations can be very difficult to read. Furthermore, not all Chinese words can be rendered with a single English term which is applicable in all cases. Thus, it is often impossible or impractical to take a purely denotative approach to translation.

The intention of a connotative translation is to render the meaning of the text in a way most easily accessible the translator's audience. Thus Elder Born becomes Mister and throat knot becomes Adam's apple. A connotative translation need not translate a Chinese word the same way each time it is used. The translator is free to choose whatever English word he or she feels most accurately conveys the meaning of the original text. This approach to translation relies entirely upon the knowledge and skill of the individual translator and it may or may not be possible to cross reference the terms used in the translation back to the original text.

A functional translation is essentially a paraphrase of its source language original. While the information conveyed may be based on a non–English text, this information may be worded quite differently or may only, in fact, be a truncated abstract. In this case the translator is only interested in conveying to his or her audience certain information which happens be come from a Chinese source and there is only a very loose linguistic relationship between the original and the functional translation. COMP suggests that functional translations may or may not be based on a stated glossary.

In reality these categories are far from being rigid and most translations exist somewhere on the continuum between the two theoretical extremes of denotative and functional approaches. Obviously, a translation which comprises the best attributes of a denotative approach while precisely reflecting the intended meaning is the ideal. It is inherently impossible for a translator to achieve a perfect fit of word and meaning between two languages. There is a well known saying that "translators are traitors." Any departure from the source language is a form of linguistic treason. Thus, every translator attempting to produce an accurate denotative translation is sooner or later forced into making certain concessions. In particular, purely denotative translations of premodern Chinese tend to run into a number of problems and translating the same ideogram in the same manner while rigidly adhering to a standardized terminology quickly produces an unreadable and erroneous translation. The Chinese words *jia* and *yi* in the title of the *Jia Yi Jing* are a case in point. *Jia* and *yi* have no meaningful denotative English equivalent. In terms of translating the title of this book, one is left with the options of either leaving them untranslated or taking a more connotative approach and rendering the couplet as "systematic."

The goal of a standardized terminology is to ensure consistency in a translation and the capacity to cross reference information from text to text. When one uses any technical term in Chinese medicine the reader should be able to reference this term back to the original Chinese. This ensures that all parties are referring to the same thing or idea. We feel that Wiseman *et al.* have compiled the most philologically accurate glossary of Chinese medical terms to date. This list is not perfect. We have departed from it in a number of instances, and in no way do we advocate a blind adherence to its standard. Nevertheless, we feel that this glossary is by virtue of its comprehensiveness and scholarship, the ground upon which all terminological dialogue will be based.

The advent of a standardized terminology such as Wiseman's has produced a great deal of discussion among translators of Chinese Medicine. Some writers, including ourselves, have taken issue with some of the choices Wiseman has made in translating specific terms. This type of discourse is not only inevitable but is an essential part of evolving a truly consensual Chinese medical terminology. The glossary as it stands today is continually being revised by all who use it including Wiseman himself. Other writers have challenged the validity of the basic concept of a standardized terminology. They argue that meaningful word for word translations are essentially impossible since any word in Chinese may have any number of valid meanings and should be translated freely in accordance with the context in which it appears. They assert that simply plugging in English equivalents for Chinese terms is folly. Our approach to the question of denotative versus connotative translation has been to attempt to combine the best of both approaches. When Chinese words are used as medical terms they can and should be translated via a standardized terminology in accordance with a denotative translation style. Such an approach ensures the reader that a given English word denotes a specific Chinese medical term. The challenge for the translator is knowing when a word is used as a technical term and when it is employed simply as a part of the overall Chinese vocabulary. Chinese medicine does not posses a technical terminology that is fundamentally separate from the Chinese language as a whole. There are few words that are used solely in a narrow medical context. This is particularly the case as one moves back through time. The meaning that modern Chinese medical writings intend to convey is most often unambiguous. However, a multiplicity of meanings for any given word or phrase is a fundamental characteristic of pre–modern Chinese. Even within the context of a given sentence of a medical discussion, the same word may be used in both a technical and a non technical manner.

A case in point is the word *ni* (逆). *Ni* appears most commonly in Chinese medicine in the context of an abnormal flow of qi within the body, and in this context, it is most is often translated as counterflow or some approximate equivalent such as rebellion. Wiseman *et al.* also note that *ni* may mean abnormal or unfavorable, depending on the context. This is not the limit of its possible connotations as *ni* may in certain contexts imply frigid hands and feet resulting from counterflow. While some sort of "counterflow" is the causative factor, in this case it would nevertheless be erroneous to simply translate *ni* as counterflow. Furthermore, *ni* may in some contexts simply mean an upward flow and have no negative implications whatsoever.

Regardless of whether one prefers a denotative or connotative approach to translation, most translators would agree that when *ni* refers to a counterflow, it should always be translated in the same way, whatever word one actually selects. This is in the interest of maintaining a word for word equivalency of technical terms. In this work, we have translated *ni* as counterflow when the concept of counterflow is implied. When *ni* appears to connote one of its many other non technical meanings, then a more appropriate word has been selected.

There are times a given Chinese word such as *yin* (阴) may be used in a very specific context exclusive of its overall range of meaning. Yin has a such a well developed range of connotations for English readers that it is typically not translated. Nevertheless, it is sometimes necessary to translate yin in a specific manner to bring out the intent of the writer. For instance, yin may refer to "the two lower yin" meaning both the urethra and anus. It may also refer only to the genitals. When yin is used in the context of the genitals we have translated it as genitals. However, since there is no handy English word denoting the combination of the urethra and anus, when yin is used to imply these we have left it as "yin" and pointed out this meaning in a footnote.

Fa (发) is an example of very common Chinese word that most often occurs in a nontechnical context. It has a variety of meanings including to send out, deliver, to discharge, to shoot, to develop or expand, to open up or discover, and to feel, to name but a few. While *fa* most often appears in a non–technical context in Chinese medical writings, it may also convey a specific technical meaning of moving perspiration outward through the striations so that pathogens located in the exterior may escape. Wiseman suggests the verb "to effuse" when *fa* appears in this context, and so we have translated *fa* as "effuse" when we wish to denote its technical meaning.

Another example is *jing*. Wiseman translates *jing* (精) as essence, or semen. When it appears as a technical term in Chinese medicine, we have translated it as either essence or semen, depending on the context in accordance with Wiseman's standardized terminology. In the present work, *jing* appears in many non–technical contexts where it may mean refined, precise, skilled, clever, or proficient. In this context, we have translated it in whatever manner is appropriate. Clearly, inserting the word semen wherever *jing* appears in a text would yield a meaningless translation. At the same time, appropriate divergence from Wiseman's terminology in no way negates the value of a standardized terminology. Where the reader sees the technical term essence or semen in the text, she knows we are referring to the Chinese term *jing*.

Our approach to this text has been to provide a word for word denotative translation wherever this yielded a cogent and readable document. We have tried to maintain the integrity of the Chinese word order whenever possible as well. This, too, is a basic criteria of a denotative translation. Whenever a given word could not be correctly and meaningfully translated using Wiseman's standardized technical terminology, we have adopted a more connotative approach to ensure the meaning of the text is adequately conveyed. The are a few instances in which we have not used Wiseman's terminology but have adopted our own preference for a given technical term used in a technical context. For example, we have translated the acupoint name *Gong Sun* (Sp 4) as Offspring of Duke, rather than Wiseman's Yellow Emperor, because at the time the *Jia Yi Jing* was written, the term Yellow Emperor used in any context was reserved for the Emperor himself. We have footnoted such discrepancies the first time the word appears in the text. In this way, we feel that we have adopted the most appropriate methodology for any given situation and thus rendered the most effective translation.

About lexicological marks

Text appearing in brackets [] has been added by subsequent unknown pre–modern editors through the centuries and has come to be considered virtually a part of the original text. This material most often clarifies the original text, but at times is at odds with it, and we have pointed this out in the footnotes. Text appearing in parenthesis () represent the additions of the current translators. Text of this nature has been included for the purposes of clarifying the intent of the original text in English. The reader should be aware that such inclusions are editorial by their very nature. For instance, in Book 10, Chapter 2, the Chinese sentence reads,

> 虚邪。。与卫气相薄，阳胜则为热，阴胜则为寒，
> 寒则真气发，去则虚，虚则寒
>
> *"Xu xie...yu wei qi xiang bo, yang sheng ze wei re, yin sheng*
> *ze wei han, han ze zhen qi qu, qu ze xu, xu ze han."*

The English version is,

> Vacuity evil...wrestles together with the defensive qi. If yang triumphs, this leads to heat. If yin triumphs, this leads to cold. Cold makes the true qi depart, and in consequence, the true qi leaves behind it emptiness. In the end, emptiness leads to (more serious) cold.

In consideration of the fact that cold has already developed, we feel that it is quite logical to add the modifier, "more serious", to cold in the conclusion. However, there is another possible interpretation. The first cold means external cold, while the second cold may refer to internal or vacuity cold. If one interprets these lines in this way, then internal or empty should be added in parentheses instead of more serious. Where an alternative interpretation of the text is possible for whatever reason, we have included that reading or a paraphrase of it in an accompanying footnote.

Since the division of a classical Chinese passage into paragraphs is an arbitrary convention introduced into some Chinese versions of the *Jia Yi Jing*, we have rearranged the division of paragraphs in our English version to facilitate a more readable manuscript. The Arabic numerals appearing before a paragraph or group of paragraphs have been inserted by the translators to serve as an expedient mark that the entire following section comes from the same source, for instance from a chapter of the *Ling Shu* for which a cite can be found in the footnotes.

In this book, acupoints are identified first by the English translation of their name. This is then followed in parentheses by the *pinyin* spelling of their name, a comma, and a numerical identification based on the number of points located on each channel: *ergo* Life Gate, (*Ming Men*, GV 4). These numerical identifications are based on the World Health Organization's Proposed Standard International Acupuncture Nomenclature (WHO Geneva, 1991) except for the following discrepancies: For the lung channel, we use Lu instead of LU; for the stomach channel, we use St instead of ST; for the spleen we use Sp instead of SP; for the heart, we use Ht instead of HT; for the Bladder, we use Bl instead of BL; for the kidney we use Ki instead of KI; for the pericardium we use Per instead of PC; for the triple heater, we use TH instead of TE; and for the liver Liv instead of LR.

Book and chapter titles mentioned either in the text or the footnotes appear in English and *pinyin* the first time that they appear in a volume or book. For instance we refer to the *Spiritual Pivot (Ling Shu)* in Book One, Chapter One, but in subsequent chapters within Book One we have omitted the English, referring only to the *Ling Shu*. The reader can find an English translation for any book or chapter title by referring its first cite in the index.

Scholars of Chinese medicine have been writing commentaries on *The Systematic Classic* since it first appeared, but there are some passages which simply make no sense. In some instances, scholars through the ages have put forward wildly implausible interpretations of some of the more arcane passages in *The Systematic Classic*. In others, they have simply admitted defeat. While we have attempted to present the most cogent translation of *The Systematic Classic* possible, it must be acknowledged that there are some passages that no one seems to understand. While doing our best to present these passages in an accurate manner, we have pointed out their impenetrability in the footnotes to save the reader undue frustration.

The Systematic Classic was written in the form of a dialogue between the Yellow Emperor and his legendary physicians Qi Bo, Bo Gao, Lei Gong, and Shao Shi, all of whom were considered eminent scholars of medicine. Where Huang–fu Mi has not assigned a specific interlocutor, we have simply selected Qi Bo as the questioner since his name appears most frequently.

There has been a great deal of discussion within the sinological community as to whether the *Nei Jing* of Huang–fu Mi's time bears any resemblance to the *Nei Jing* as we know it today. Some scholars assert that it is inaccurate to say that a given passage in the *Jia Yi Jing* was taken from the *Nei Jing* because we have no real idea of what the *Nei Jing* looked like in Huang–fu's time. The *Nei Jing* has certainly undergone a great deal of supplementation, castration, editing and general tampering over the centuries. Nevertheless we are of the opinion that the *Nei Jing* Huang–fu read was essentially the book we recognise as the *Nei Jing* today. We base this opinion on the following facts. Huang–fu Mi was the first to describe the *Nei Jing* as being composed of the *Su Wen* and the *Ling Shu* (or *Jiu Juan, Ninefold Volume*), the format we recognise today. Prior to Huang–fu's time it was not referred to in this way. Since Huang–fu lived part of his life in the Han dynasty, which is the latest possible period in which the *Nei Jing* may first have appeared, it is reasonable to assume that he had more ready access to the original versions of the *Nei Jing* than his successors in later times. Even a cursory comparison of the *Jia Yi Jing* and the present editions of the *Ling Shu* are all but identical. This leads one to conclude that *Ling Shu* available to Huang–fu was basically the same that we have today except in those chapters which are recognised as being adulterations by Wang Bing. It is based on this line of reasoning that we cite the various chapters and passages in the *Jia Yi Jing* as being "derived from" the *Nei Jing*.

Acknowledgments

We would like to thank the senior physicians Han Bin, Zhang Tian–ren, and Wang Jun–tang at the No. 2 Teaching Hospital, Tianjin College of TCM for their encouragement and enlightening advice. In the US, the help of Dan Bensky, Miki Shima, and Bob Flaws has been invaluable. Without the help of these individuals this work would not have been possible. However, any errors and inaccuracies in this book are ours and ours alone.

Yang Shou-Zhong
Charles Chace
April 1994

FOREWORD BY GAO BAO-HENG

It is well known that any scholar with a profound knowledge of heaven, earth, and humanity is entitled to call himself a Confucian, and that such an understanding of heaven and earth, but not including humanity, is considered an art. Although the practice of medicine may seem to be little more than a skill, it is nonetheless, the concern of the Confucian. In his preface to *Yi Wen Zhi (The Records of Literature and Art,*[1] Ban Gu[2] asserts that a Confucian is a man equipped with the knowledge of how to assist the monarch in following the law of yin and yang and enlightening the people on civilized (behavior). Practically speaking, this is none other than the knowledge of heaven, earth, and man, although it is defined in another way. He also believed that a physician is qualified to shed light on an analysis of affairs of state by way of his studies in pathology and to provide a correct approach to government in the light of his clinical experience. How can a man be considered competent if he is not sufficiently competent in those affairs pertaining to heaven, earth, and humanity?

Huang-fu Mi of the Jin dynasty was a man of wide reading and was well learned in many disciplines. He was famous for his composed nature, his lofty aspirations, and his abstention from personal indulgence. He was struck with wind *bi* and undertook the study of medicine, studying the medical classics in an effort to achieve perfect mastery of them.

He compiled the twelve volume *Zhen Jiu Jing (Acupuncture and Moxibustion Classic),*[3] based on the three works *Huang Di Su Wen (Yellow Emperor's Basic Questions),*[4] *Zhen Jing (The Classic of Needles)* and the *Ming Tang (The Enlightening Hall).*[5] This has surpassed all other efforts that Confucian scholars have made in the domain of medicine thus far.

Some say that the above three classics were compiled during the Warring States period,[6] and therefore could not have been written by the Yellow Emperor. However, since man is a living creature with a variety of complicated organs hidden beneath the skin inside a body eight *chi*[7] in length, it is impossible to measure the firmness and fragility of the five viscera, or the largness and smallness of the six bowels, the amount of grain ingested, the length of the blood vessels, the freshness of the blood, and the approximate quantity of the qi and blood in the twelve primary channels. He who first learned all of these things must have been a consummate sage or an immortal, and was certainly not a man living in the Warring States period.

These great classics, the eighteen volume *Huang Di Nei Jing (Yellow Emperor's Inner Classic)* and the three volume *Ming Tang (Enlightening Hall)* are monumental works of remote antiquity. In view of the great many errors found in them, which have deterred many people from learning them such as misplacements, emasculations, omissions, and misspellings, all of which have confused the doctrines and distorted them monstrously, Huang–fu Shi–an[8] became determined to collate (these classics). This is the basis on which he compiled his book. Later, Zhen Quan[9] of the Tang dynasty executed the drawings of the *Ming Tang Tu (Ming Tang Atlas)* which was matched by the illuminating expositions of Sun Si-miao.[10] As for other works, they cannot all be enumerated here.

Upon the call of the sovereign, a number of Confucian scholars commenced reviewing previous significant medical works. They completed a revision of the *Zhen Jiu Jia Yi Jing* by referencing the immaculate editions of the *Su Wen Jiu Xu Ling Shu*, the *Tai Su*[11] the *Qian Jin Fang (Prescription Worth a Thousand Taels of Gold)* the *(Qian Jin) Yi (Fang)*,[12] *(The Supplement to the Prescriptions Worth a Thousand Taels of Gold)*, and the *Wai Tai Mi Yao (The Secret Essentials of a Provincial Governor)*.[13] They have made a fair copy to present to His Majesty for his personal examination. This is in the humble hope that His Enlightened Majesty, who is wisest of all, will shower his boundless grace, affection, and generosity over all of his subjects by having this work, originally of the Yellow Emperor and Qi Bo published to bring happiness, harmony, and peace to the entire land and thus benefit infinite generations to come. In so doing, these scholars are fulfilling their duty of assisting the Sovereign in following the law of yin and yang, and enlightening the people on civilized (behavior).

Gao Bao-heng
Chancellor of the Royal Academy

Sun Qi
Minister of Land Reclamation,
Governor of Bureau of General Palace Affairs

Lin Yi
Chief of the Imperial Secretariat

Endnotes

[1]The *Yi Wen Zhi* was part of the official history of the early Han dynasty, composed by Ban Gu.

[2]Ban Gu (32-92 CE), an eminent politician and scholar of the early Han Dynasty.

[3]The full name of this book is the *Huang Di San Bu Zhen Jiu Jia Yi Jing*.

[4]This is the first part of the *Nei Jing* and is often considered a separate volume. It is the foundation of Chinese medical theory.

[5]The *Ming Tang Zhen Jiu Zhi Yao (The Treatment Essentials of Acupuncture and Moxibustion from the Enlightening Hall)* was also allegedly written by the Yellow Emperor. This book has been lost for millennia. Many works of Chinese medicine are entitled *Ming Tang* and in this context it can be interpreted as referring specifically to acupuncture and moxibustion.

[6]A period in Chinese history 475 BCE–221 BCE characterized by continual warring between rival states.

[7]A Chinese unit of length. The present *chi* is equivalent to one third of a meter, however, in ancient times it was much shorter.

[8]This is the style name of Huang–fu Mi, his literary or scholastic name.

[9]Zhen Qian (541-643 CE) was an eminent scholar famous for his literary achievements. Later in his life he resigned his post of Secretary General to the Emperor and devoted himself to the study of medicine. He specialized in acupuncture and his primary contributions include the *Mai Jing (The Pulse Classic)*, *Zhen Fang (Acupuncture Prescriptions)*, and the *Ming Tang Tu Sheng Ren (The Ming Tang Atlas of Living Man.*

[10]Sun Si–miao (581-682 CE) was one of the most illustrious physician of ancient times. He was well known for his wide range of talents and on a number of occasions refused offers of high position from the Emperor himself.

[11]The *Huang Di Nei Jing Tai Su (The Yellow Emperor's Inner Classic on the Essentials)*, was edited by Yang Xiang–shan in the sixth and seventh centuries. It is one of the earlier versions of the *Huang Di Nei Jing* and contains annotations and commentaries by the author.

[12]The *Qian Jin Yi Fang* was written by Sun Si–miao.

[13]A medical work by Wang Tao (670-755) which has contributed greatly to the preservation of ancient medical classics.

HUANG–FU MI'S PREFACE

The way of medicine has had a long history. In remote antiquity, *Shen Nong*[1] acquired knowledge of medicines by tasting hundreds of plants. Later, the Yellow Emperor succeeded in tackling all of the relevant, abstruse and complicated problems and developed acupuncture based in theory, on the laws governing life. He did this by consulting with Qi Bo, Bo Gao, and Shao Yu,[2] by studying the five viscera and the six bowels deep in the interior of the body as well as the channels and their connecting vessels, the qi and blood, and the skin and complexion on the exterior aspect of the body. (In addition) he referred all of these things to heaven and earth to corroborate this lore regarding human physiology. As a result of all this the way of acupuncture came into being. These theories are magnificent. Afterwards, the Emperor received Lei Gong[3] as his disciple through whom these medical teachings were imparted to later generations. Yin Yi,[4] a great man who was almost a sage, wrote the *Tang Ye, (The Decoctions and Liquids)* [5] which was the result of his research into the *Shen Nong Ben Cao (Shen Nong's Pharmacopoeia).*[6]

Yu Fu, Yi Huan,[7] and Bian Que[8] of the middle and ancient times, Yi He of the Qin dynasty and Cang Gong[9] of the Han Dynasty are all renowned in history not only as brilliant physicians, but as outstanding scholars who possessed penetrating insight into the root and origin of things.

Hua Tuo[10] and Zhang Zhong–jing[11] lived during the Han dynasty. With a wealth of extraordinary formulas and treatments, and with rich experience in treating (unusual) cases, Hua Tuo worked wonders in curing countless difficult cases. No one has been able to give a comprehensive account of his achievements. (The following examples illustrate the skill of these two physicians.)

Once Hua Tuo was asked to treat a royal wine taster named Liu Ji–yan who was suffering from apprehension and malice (*wei e*)[12] and whom he treated and cured. (Hua Tuo) predicted: "In nine years Ji-yan will suffer a relapse and the root of this will be apprehension and malice. If this illness comes to pass he will die. In the end it was as (Hua Tuo) said.

One day upon meeting Wang Zhong–xuan who was just over twenty years of age, Zhang Zhong–jing observed: "Gentleman, you have (unknowingly) contracted an illness. At the age of forty your eyebrows will fall out, and one half a year after your eyebrows fall out you will die." He prescribed Five Stone Decoction (*Wu Shi Tang*) to avert this eventuality. However, Zhong–xuan found these remarks offensive so although he accepted the decoction he did not take it. Three days later Zhong–jing saw Zhong–xuan once again and said, "Didn't you take the decoction?" Zhong–xuan said, "But I have taken it." Zhong–jing replied, "Your complexion definitely indicates that you have not taken the decoction." Gentleman, how can you treat life so lightly?" Zhong–xuan however, did not heed the warning. After twenty years his eyebrows fell out, and after another one hundred and eighty seven days he died. In the end it was as (Zhong–jing) said. These two experiences cannot be surpassed by Bian Que and Cang Gong. Hua Tuo was haughty and conceited and in the end he died violently. Zhong–jing enriched and expanded the *Tang Ye* into a work of more than 10 volumes, (containing prescriptions) which are for the most part effective. In recent times the director of the Imperial Medical Bureau, Wang Shu–he[13] collated and expounded upon the works of Zhong–jing and this material is of great practical significance.

According to the *Qi Lue (The Outlines of the Seven Fields)*,[14] and the *Yi Wen Zhi (The Records of Literature and Art)*, the *Huang Di Nei Jing* (Yellow Emperor's Inner Classic) comprised 18 books. This is the total of the present nine book *Zhen Jing (Acupuncture Classic)* and the nine book *Su Wen (Basic Questions)* which comprise the current *Nei Jing*. Nonetheless, segments are missing from the original work and while it is true that (this classic) contains profound insights on a wide range of topics, it is characterized by expositions on general theories and inadequate discussion of practical applications. The biography of Cang Gong asserts that he learned his medicine from the *Su Wen*. The *Su Wen*'s discusses meticulous discussion of disease and the *Jiu Juan's (Ninefold Volume)* sections devoted specifically to the channels and vessels are so abstruse that they are not easily studied. The *Ming Tang Kong Xue Zhen Jiu Zhi Yao (The Acupuncture and Moxibustion Treatment Essentials of the Enlightening Hall)* is another legacy left by the Yellow Emperor and Qi Bo. All three works have the same origin and have much in common. They contain much of the same material and many of the same errors. During the reign of Gan Lu, I became ill with wind stroke and in addition I suffered from deafness for one hundred days. I began to study the primers of medicine and to compile this twelve volume work based upon the these three works. I reclassified the material according to its nature, deleted the superfluous materials, and commented on the essentials in a twelve volume (treatise). The *Yi Jing (The Change Classic)* says, "by observing the condensed form, one may perceive circumstances in heaven and earth." This epigram reveals a universal principle (in respect to the study). The classification of materials is just what is meant by condensation.

Although we receive the bodily form from our predecessors, with bodies which are eight *qi* in length, it can be said that we would be wandering ghosts but for a knowledge of medicine! For all our filial affection, loyalty and generosity which we cherish, if we are unfamiliar with medicine we shall have no means of rendering assistance when our sovereign or our parents are in distress or even when our naked babies are smeared with earth.[15] This is why the sages have beat their brains and contemplated deeply in order to perfect their medicine. From this it follows that (the study and practice of medicine) cannot be neglected.

While compiling this book, I rarely deleted even those materials which seemed to have little practical value. If the need arises for a more concise work, I will endeavor to collate these classic texts once again.

Huang-fu Mi

Endnotes

[1]A legendary emperor and the immediate predecessor to the Yellow Emperor. Shen Nong was the father of medicine and animal husbandry.

[2]Supposed contemporaries and subjects of the Yellow Emperor, all of whom were said to be authorities on medicine.

[3]This is a legendary figure who was a minister of the Yellow Emperor.

[4]Yin Yi (16-15th centuries BCE) was the alleged inventor of the technique of boiling medicinal herbs. He rose from an ordinary cook to the Premier entirely on the strength of his extraordinary wisdom.

[5]This was a medical work now lost, supposedly written by Yin Yi.

[6]This is the first pharmacopoeia, allegedly written by Shen Nong.

[7]Legendary physicians living in the Spring and Autumn Period (770-476 BCE)

[8]Bian Que (406-310 BCE) was among the most outstanding physicians in ancient times. His real name was Qin Yue–ren. However, he was called Bian Que because Bian Que was a legendary and divine physician.

[9]Cang Gong (205-140 BCE) was another eminent physician of ancient times. His real name was Chun Yu–yi, but he was called Cang Gong because he was once the manager (*gong*) of the imperial stable (*cang*). He was said to be capable of arriving at a diagnosis by merely glancing at the patient.

[10]Hua Tuo (141-208 CE) was believed to be the inventor of drug anesthesia and the founder of surgery in China. He was charged with attempted murder and sentenced to death when he attempted to perform a craniotomy on the supreme ruler at the time, Cao Meng–de.

[11]Zhang Zhong–jing (145-208 CE) is generally regarded as the founder of clinical therapeutics in Chinese medicine. His *Shang Han Lun (Treatise on Injury by Cold)* and *Jin Gui Yao Lue (Prescription From the Golden Cabinet)* are among the most important texts in the Chinese medical literature.

[12]A syndrome characterized by irritability and apprehension

[13]Wang Shu–he (170-255 CE) was an eminent physician whose major contribution was the *Mai Jing (Pulse Classic)*.

[14]The earliest Chinese work on literary systematics by Liu Sin (?-23 CE) of the Han dynasty.

[15]*i.e.*, when one's offspring are in grave danger

TABLE OF CONTENTS

BOOK THREE

BOOK FOUR

BOOK FIVE

BOOK SIX

BOOK SEVEN

BOOK EIGHT

BOOK ELEVEN

BOOK TWELVE

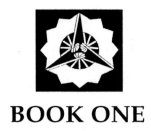

BOOK ONE

Chapter One

Treatise on Essence, Spirit, & the Five Viscera[1]

(1)

The Yellow Emperor asked:

All methods of needling must first have their basis in spirit. The blood, the vessels, the constructive *(qi)*, qi, essence, and spirit are all stored within the five viscera. Therefore, what are vitality *(de)*, qi, life *(sheng)*, essence, spirit, *hun, po*, the heart-mind *(xin)*, reflection *(yi)*, will *(zhi)*, thought *(si)*, wisdom *(zhi)*, and worry *(lu)*? Please tell me about these.

Qi Bo answered:

Heaven bestows vitality, while earth bestows qi. The coordinated flow of vitality and qi engenders life.[2] That which comes together with life is called essence. The interaction of the two essences is called the spirit. That which follows the spirit everywhere is called the *hun*. That which comes and goes with the essence is called the *po*. That which controls bodily substance is called the heart-mind. The heart's capacity for recollection is called reflection. The retention of a recollection is called the will. The retention and transformation of the will is called thought. Thought is engendered when consideration must be given to will. Worry develops when thought is infused

with expectation and anticipation. Worry results in wisdom when it is capable of coping with the affairs (of daily life). Therefore, in nurturing life the wise adapt (to the changes of) the four seasons, acclimatizing to cold and summer heat, leading a life of equanimity, free from either overjoy or anger, adjusting yin and yang, and regulating the unyielding and the pliant.[3] In so doing, evils will rarely arise, and a long life will be obtained.[4]

Apprehension, thought, and worry will damage the spirit. Damage to the spirit causes fright and incessant flux.[5] Since sadness and sorrow stir up the center, the spirit expires and eventually life is lost. Joy and delight dissipate the spirit and thus it cannot be stored. Worry and anxiety obstruct the qi which then cannot circulate. An exuberance of anger perplexes (the spirit which) will then run wild. Fright disturbs the spirit and leads it astray. [The *Tai Su (The Essentials)*[6] substitutes "loses control over" *(shi shou)* for "leads astray" *(bu shou)*.]

(2)

The *Su Wen (Basic Questions)* says: Anger causes the qi to counterflow and thus in the extreme, causes vomiting of blood and counterflow of qi while eating. Therefore the qi ascends. Joy keeps the qi in harmony and the emotions at peace. As a result, the constructive *(qi)* and the defensive *(qi)* are free and uninhibited. Therefore the qi is relaxed. Sorrow causes tension within the cardiac ligation[7] and elevates the lobes of the lung. The upper burner is inhibited and constructive and defensive cannot be dissipated. Thus, there is hot qi within (the upper burner) and therefore the (correct) qi becomes dispersed. Apprehension causes the spirit to retreat. This retreat leads to obstruction of the upper burner. Obstruction causes the qi to return (downward) and this return leads to distention in the lower burner. Therefore the qi fails to circulate. If there is cold, the interstices (cou li, 腠理) will become obstructed, the constructive and defensive cannot circulate and thus the qi is restricted. If there is heat, this causes the interstices to open, allowing the constructive and defensive to flow freely and promoting a massive discharge of sweat. Thus the qi is discharged as well. When there is fright, the heart has no place to rely upon, and the spirit has no place to gather, thus reflection has no place to concentrate and the qi therefore becomes chaotic. Exertion causes wheezing and sweating. The inside (due to the wheezing) and outside (due to the sweating) are both frittered away. Thus the qi is consumed. Thought engages the heart which arrests the spirit. The qi then becomes lodged and fails to circulate; therefore the qi becomes bound up. [The nine qi above differ little from one another and are largely the same.]

(3)

The liver stores the blood and it is the blood which houses the *hun*. The qi (of the liver) pertains to the speech, its fluid is the tears. A vacuity of liver qi leads to fright, and repletion fullness leads to anger. The *Su Wen* says: When a person lies down, blood returns to the liver, and when the liver receives blood, one is able to see. (The eye is associated with the liver.) When the feet receive blood, one is able to walk. When the hands receive blood, one is able to grasp, and when the fingers receive blood, one is able to clutch.

The heart stores the vessels and it is the vessels which house the spirit. The qi (of the heart) pertains to swallowing, and its fluid is sweat. A vacuity of heart qi leads to melancholy and sorrow, and repletion leads to incessant laughter.

The spleen stores the constructive and it is the constructive which houses reflection. The qi (of the spleen) pertains to swallowing and its fluid is saliva. A vacuity of spleen qi leads to loss of use of the four limbs and restlessness of the five viscera. A repletion leads to abdominal distention and inhibition of urination and defecation.

The lung stores the qi and the qi houses the *po*. The qi (of the lung) pertains to cough and the fluid of the lung is the nasal mucous. A vacuity of lung qi leads to nasal and respiratory inhibition and diminished qi. A repletion leads to asthma, fullness of the chest, and ease of respiration when lying down.

The kidney stores essence and it is the essence which houses the will [*Ling Shu Ben Shen Pian {Spiritual Pivot: On Spirit as Root}* substitutes "qi" for "will"]. The qi (of the kidney) pertains to yawning and its fluid is the spittle.[8] Kidney qi vacuity leads to inversion, and repletion leads to distention and restlessness of the five viscera.

Thus it is necessary to study the forms that disease takes within the five viscera in order to determine the state of vacuity and repletion within the qi and to therefore carefully restore balance.[9]

(4)

Sorrow or sadness stirring within the liver damages the *hun*. Damage to the *hun* leads to mania, frenzy, an insecurity of essence (a variant version gives "absence of or no essence" which is an abnormal state), retraction of the penis, contraction of the sinews, and inability to raise the ribs on both sides. Should the hair become brittle and the (facial) color faded or prematurely aged,[10] death will come in autumn.[11]

The *Su Wen* says: The sound of the liver is shouting, its manner of pathological change is gripping, and its emotion is anger. Anger injures the liver. The *Jiu Juan (Ninefold Volume)*[12] and the *Su Wen* both say: The merger of essence and qi in the liver leads to worry.

This can be explained as follows: liver vacuity

leads to fright, while repletion leads to anger. Anger if not appeased quickly also engenders worry and restriction. There are interrelationships between the liver and kidney, the liver and spleen, and the liver and lung. The spleen is earth and the other four viscera receive their nourishment from it. Therefore, fright develops within the liver but takes shape in the kidney, and worry develops within the spleen but takes shape in the liver. The liver is connected to the gallbladder and the gallbladder is the bowel of the central essence (zhong jing). The kidney treasures the essence and thus anger and fright are akin to one another. Once either of these has gone too far, this leads to injury of both viscera. The two classics seem to contradict each other, but in the final analysis, practically speaking, they are the same.

If the heart is affected by apprehension, thought, and worry, this injures the spirit. If the spirit is injured, this leads to fright and loss of control of oneself, cleaving of the major muscular masses, and shedding of the flesh. Should the hair become brittle and the (facial) color prematurely aged, death will come in winter.

The *Su Wen* says: The sound of the heart is laughing, its manner of pathological change is worry, and its emotion is joy. Joy injures the heart. The *Jiu Juan* and the *Su Wen* both say: The merger of essence and qi in the heart leads to joy.

Some people presume that these two classics are wrong in their discussion of joy affecting the heart and the lung and spleen. What can be said of this? This can be explained as follows: Heart vacuity leads to sorrow and sorrow leads to worry. Heart repletion leads to laughter and laughter to joy. The heart and lung and the spleen and heart are related to one another. Thus joy may start in the heart but takes shape in the lung, while thought starts in the spleen but takes shape in the heart. If either is in excess, this leads to injury to both viscera. Here the classics focus on articulating these interrelationships and there is no contradiction in their statements.[13]

If the spleen is afflicted by unresolved worry and anxiety, this leads to injury of reflection (*i.e.*, an impaired capacity for reflection). Injury of reflection leads to oppression and chaos, and this results in an inability to raise the four limbs. If the hair becomes brittle and the (facial) color prematurely aged, death will come in spring.

The *Su Wen* says: The sound of the spleen is singing and its manner of pathological change is belching. Its emotion is thinking and thinking injures the spleen. The *Jiu Juan* and *Su Wen* both say: The merger of essence and qi in the spleen leads to hunger.[14]

If the lung is afflicted by excessive joy and delight, this leads to injury of the *po*. Injury of the *po* leads to mania, while mania deprives one of the capability for reflection and the person's skin may also be parched. If the hair becomes brittle and the (facial) color prematurely aged, death will come in summer.

The *Su Wen* says: The sound of the lung is crying, their manner of pathological change is coughing, and their emotion is worry. Worry injures the lung. The *Jiu Juan* and the *Su Wen* both say: The merger of essence and qi in the lung leads to sorrow.

If the kidney is afflicted by a constant exuberance of anger, this leads to injury of the will. Injury of the will leads to an inability to remember what was previously said and an inability to bend forward and back. If the hair becomes brittle and the (facial) color prematurely aged, death will come during long summer.

The *Su Wen* says: The sound of the kidney is groaning, its manner of pathological change when affected is shivering, and their emotion is apprehension. Apprehension injures the kidney. The *Jiu Juan* and *Su Wen* both say: The merger of essence and qi in the kidney leads to apprehension. Constant and unresolved apprehension leads to injury of the essence. Injury of the essence leads to aching bones, atonic inversion, and frequent spontaneous seminal discharge.

Because the five viscera govern the storage of essence, they cannot be (allowed to become) injured. Such injury leads to loss (of essence) and yin vacuity. Yin vacuity results in a lack of qi, and a lack of qi leads to death.

Therefore, in employing needles, it is necessary to examine the bearing of the patient. Thus can one know whether essence or spirit, *hun* or *po* are obtained or lost, abundant or meager. If all five (viscera) have been injured, needles are not an acceptable form of treatment.

Chapter Two

The Five Viscera, Five Changes, & Five Transporting Points[15]

(1)

The Yellow Emperor asked:

Please tell me the details of the five viscera and the five transporting points.

Qi Bo answered:

People have five viscera. These viscera have five changes[16] and these changes have five transporting points. Hence there are five times five or twenty five transporting points which correspond to the five seasons.[17]

The liver is a masculine viscus, its color is green-blue, and its season is spring. Its days are *jia* and *yi*,[18] its sound is *jue*,[19] and its flavor is sour. [The *Su Wen* says: The flavor associated with the liver is acrid. The classic is inconsistent here.[20]]

The heart is a masculine viscus, its color is red, and its season is summer. Its days are *bing* and *ding*, its sound is *zhi*, and its flavor is bitter. [The *Su Wen* says: The flavor associated with the heart is salty. The classic is inconsistent here.]

The spleen is a feminine viscus, its color is yellow, and its season is long summer. Its days are *wu* and *ji*, its sound is *gong*, and its flavor is sweet.

The lung is a feminine viscus, its color is white, and its season is autumn. Their days are *geng* and *xin*, their sound is *shang*, and their flavor is acrid. [The *Su Wen* says: "The flavor of the lung is bitter." The classic is inconsistent here.]

The kidney is a feminine viscus, its color is black, and its season is winter. Its days are *ren* and *gui*, its sound is *yu*, and its flavor is salty. These are the so-called five changes.

The viscera rule winter. In winter, needle the well (*jing*) points. Color rules spring, and in the spring, needle the rapids (*ying*) points. The seasons rule summer. In summer, needle the brook (*shu*) points. Sound rules long summer. In long summer, needle the stream (*jing*) points. Flavor rules autumn. In autumn, needle the confluence (*he*) points. This is called the five changes which rule or govern the five transporting points.

The Yellow Emperor asked:

How are the source points united, thus resulting in the six transporting points?

Qi Bo answered:

The source (*yuan*) points do not correspond with any of the five seasons but are connected with the stream (*jing*) points and correspond with these. Thus six times six equals thirty-six transporting points (for the six bowels).[21]

The Yellow Emperor asked:

What does it mean that the viscera rule winter, the seasons rule summer, sound rules long summer, flavor rules autumn, and color rules spring?

Qi Bo answered:

When a disease is in the viscera, choose the well points. When a disease results in a change of color, choose the rapids points. When a disease is sometimes mild and sometimes severe, choose the brook points. When a disease results in changes in the voice or is due to repletion within a channel [a variant version says "network vessels"] and (stagnant) blood, choose the stream points. And when a disease is in the stomach [a variant version says "chest"] or is caused by irregularities in eating and drinking, choose the confluence points. Therefore this is spoken of as flavor ruling the confluence points. Together these are called the five changes (associated with the five transporting points).

(2)

If one runs counter to the qi of spring, *shao yang* will not grow and there will be internal changes within the liver.[22]

If one runs counter to the qi of summer, *tai yang* will not grow and the heart qi will be hollow within (*nei dong,* 內洞). If one runs counter to the qi of autumn, *tai yin* will not be hollow, and the lung qi will be scorched and stuffed full.[23]

If one runs counter to the qi of winter, *shao yin* will not store (the qi) and the kidney qi will become turbid and sink.[24]

As (the ebb and flow of) yin and yang in the four seasons is the root of all things, the sage acts in accordance with the root by nourishing the yang in spring and summer and nourishing the yin in fall and winter. To go against the root is to fell the stem.

Yin and yang act within all things from their beginning to their end. Following them leads to life and going against them leads to death. Habitual rebellion or disobedience results in internal separation.[25]

Thus the sage does not (wait to) treat until after the occurrence of disease but (treats) when there is as yet no disease.

According to the treatise (*i.e., Su Wen—Si Qi Tiao Shen Da Lun [Basic Questions—The Treatise on Regulating the Spirit in Accordance with the Four Seasonal Qi]*), (disease) spreads mutually between the five viscera via the control cycle.[26] (For instance,) if the heart becomes diseased, this may spread to the lung. Thus the lung should be treated before it becomes diseased.

Chapter Three

The Five Viscera & Six Bowels, Yin & Yang, Exterior & Interior[27]

(1)

The lung connects with the large intestine and the large intestine is the bowel of conveyance and conduction. The heart connects with the small intestine. The small intestine is the bowel of reception and retention. The liver connects with the gallbladder. The gallbladder is the bowel of central essence. The spleen connects with the stomach. The stomach is the bowel of the five grains. The kidney connects with the urinary bladder. The urinary bladder is the bowel of the fluids. Because *shao yin* pertains to the kidney, and the kidney links upwardly to the lung, it governs both viscera. Because the triple burner, the bowel of the central sluices providing the water passageways emerges into the urinary bladder, it is a solitary or unique bowel. These are the connections of the six bowels (with the five viscera).

(2)

The *Su Wen* says: As for the brain, marrow, bone, vessels, gallbladder, and the female's uterus, these six, are generated by earth qi and thus all store yin (essence). Like the earth, they store but do not discharge and, for that reason, are called the unusual bowels that persevere (remain unchanged) (*qi heng zhi fu,* 奇恒之腑).

As for the stomach, large intestine, small intestine, triple burner, and urinary bladder, these five are born of heavenly qi. Like the qi of heaven, they discharge but do not store. Because they receive turbid qi from the five viscera, they are named bowels of conveyance and transformation. They cannot retain (matter) for long because they are transporters and dischargers. The *po gate*[28] is also at the service of the five viscera and does not allow water and grains to be stored for long (within the body).

Because the five viscera store essence and spirit without discharging them, they are full but are not replete. Because the six bowels convey and transform matter without storing, they may be replete but are not (in actuality) full. When water and grains enter through the mouth, the stomach is first full, while the intestines are empty. As food moves downward, the intestines become full and the stomach becomes empty. Hence, (the six bowels are) replete but not full, while (the five viscera) are full but not replete.

Why does the *qi* mouth[29] alone rule all five viscera? The stomach is the sea of water and grains and the great source of the six bowels.[30]

Because the liver connects with the gallbladder, foot *jue yin* and foot *shao yang* have an interior/exterior relationship. Because the spleen connects with the stomach, foot *tai yin* and foot *yang ming* have an interior/exterior relationship. Because the kidney connects with the urinary bladder, foot *shao yin* and foot *tai yang* have an interior/exterior relationship. Because the heart connects with the small intestine, hand *shao yin* and hand *tai yang* have an interior/exterior relationship. And because the lung connects with the large intestine, hand *tai yin* and hand *yang ming* have an interior/exterior relationship.

As for the five viscera, the lung, which is their canopy, is revealed externally by the broadness of the shoulders and the sinking of the throat. The heart is the ruler, with the supraclavicular fossa as its pathway.[31] Its condition is indicated by the distance between the acromion processes of the shoulders and the size of the xiphoid process. The liver holds the office of general, and its strength is determined by the size of the eyes. The spleen holds the office of sentry and is in charge of receiving grains. (Its condition is) manifest in the preferences and aversions of the mouth and tongue. As the lookout, the kidney is in charge of hearing. Their condition can be known by the condition of the ears (including sensitivity to sound).

Of the six bowels, the stomach is the sea. If the skeleton is broad, the neck large, and the chest expansive, a large quantity of grains can be contained. The length of the nostrils reflects the condition of the large intestine. The thickness of the lips and the length of the philtrum reflect the condition of the small intestine. If the lower eyelids are large, then the gallbladder is staunch (i.e., firm). If the wings of the nose are out-turned, the urinary bladder leaks[32] and discharges. If the middle of the bridge of the nose is elevated, then the triple burner is closely fit (i.e., secure and concentrated). The six bowels are reflected in these places. If above and below are divided (equally) in three,[33] the viscera are calm and in good condition.

Chapter Four

The Five Viscera, Six Bowels, & the Sense Organs[34]

(1)

The nose is the sense organ of the lung. The eyes are the sense organs of the liver. The mouth is the sense organ of the spleen. The tongue is the sense organ of the heart. The ears are the sense organs of the kidney. These are the five sense organs and they reflect the condition of the five viscera.

If the lung is diseased, there is asthma, panting, and flaring of the nostrils. If the liver is diseased, the canthi of the eyes are blue-green. If the spleen is diseased, the lips are yellow. If the heart is diseased, the tongue retracts and the color of the cheeks are red. And if the kidney is diseased, the cheeks and forehead are black.

(2)

Because the lung qi opens into the nose, when the nose is harmonious, fragrance can be distinguished from fetor. Because the heart qi opens into the tongue, when the tongue is harmonious, the five flavors may be distinguished. The *Su Wen* says: The portal of the heart is the ears. [A variant version says "tongue".]

The heart is fire and the kidney is water. Water and fire promote each other. Heart qi should open through the tongue, but the tongue is not a portal.

Because it must open through a portal, it does so through the ears. [Wang Bing[35] states that the hand *shao yin* connecting vessel converges in the ears.]

(3)

Because liver qi opens through the eyes, when the eyes are in harmony (with the liver), the five colors can be seen. The *Su Wen* states: Most of the vessels home in the eyes. The *Jiu Juan* also states: The heart stores the vessels and the vessels house the spirit. Because spirit and brightness are intimately connected, they are said to home in the eyes.[36]

The spleen opens through the mouth. When the mouth is in harmony (with the spleen), it is able to distinguish the flavors of the five grains. The kidney opens through the ears. When the ears are harmonious, the five notes can be heard. The *Su Wen* says: The portals of the kidney are the ears. However, the kidney opens through the ears above, but opens through the lower *yin* below.[37]

Disharmony of the five viscera leads to blockage of the nine portals.[38] Disharmony of the six bowels leads to lingering and binding and thus to *yong*–abscesses.[39] Evils within the bowels lead to disharmony in the yang vessels. When there is a disharmony within the yang vessels, the qi becomes lodged. If the qi becomes lodged, this results in an exuberance of yang qi. Evils within the viscera lead to disharmony of the yin vessels. When there is a disharmony within the yin vessels, the blood becomes lodged. If the blood becomes lodged, this leads to an exuberance of yin qi. If there is too great an exuberance of yin qi, the yang qi cannot fulfill its functions. This is referred to as a (condition of) barricade (*guan*, 关). If there is too great an exuberance of yang qi, then the yin qi will be unable to flourish. This is called separation (*ge*, 格). If there is an exuberance of both yin and yang, neither may be able to fulfill its function. This is called barricade and separation. Barricade and separation is a mortal disease that results in premature death.[40]

Chapter Five

The Sizes of the Five Viscera & Reflections of the Six Bowels[41]

(1)

The Yellow Emperor asked:

All people receive the qi of heaven. Some live out their heavenly decreed life span while others fail to avert disease. Why is this?

Qi Bo answered:

The five viscera are innately large or small, positioned high or low, sturdy or fragile, and lie in an upright or inclined position. The six bowels may be large or small, long or short, thick or thin (walled), knotted or straight, slack or tense as well. Thus, there are twenty-five variations,[42] (relating to the size and shape of the viscera and bowels), each one differing from the next. Some are benign and some are malignant, some are propitious, and some are ominous.

A small heart is calm and cannot be injured by evil, [the *Tai Su*[43] says: "External evils are not able to injure"] yet it is easily injured by worry. A large heart cannot be injured by worry but is easily injured by evils. [The *Tai Su* again says: "external evil".]

An elevated heart leads to fullness within the lung, oppression, poor memory, and difficulty in speaking. A heart positioned low (in the chest) lies outside the viscera[44] and is easily damaged by cold and easily intimidated by the words of others. If the heart is sturdy then the viscera are calm, well guarded, and secure. If the heart is fragile there is a susceptibility to diseases of pure heat wasting thirst and heat in the center.[45] If the heart is upright it is harmonious, uninhibited, and so difficult to injure. If the heart is inclined it is irresolute and hesitant and thus insecure.[46]

If the lung is small, it is calm; one requires little to drink and does not become ill with by asthma. [A

7

variant version says: "asthma".] If the lung is large, one requires much to drink and is susceptible to illnesses of chest *bi*[47] and counterflow of qi. If the lung is elevated, the qi ascends. There is asthma, panting, and counterflow cough. If the lung is low (in the chest), it presses down on the liver and tends to cause pain in the hypochondrium. If the lung is sturdy, it does not become diseased by counterflow cough and rising qi. If the lung is fragile, it is susceptible to illnesses of pure heat wasting thirst and is easily injured by heat, (resulting in) asthma, panting, and epistaxis. If the lung is upright, it is in harmony; it is uninhibited and so is difficult to injure. If the lung is inclined to one side, illnesses characterized by pain at one side of the chest tend to develop.

If the liver is small, it is calm and the hypochondrium does not become diseased. If the liver is large, it oppresses the stomach and presses against the throat. Pressure on the throat obstructs the diaphragm [a variant version says: "affliction of the diaphragm" and "pain in the hypochondrium"]. If the liver is elevated (within the thorax), it pushes up against the heart above and presses and tenses the flanks below resulting in *xi ben*.[48] If the liver lies low (in the thorax) this leads to pressure on the stomach and a void in the hypochondrium, and a void here leaves one vulnerable to a contraction of evil. If the liver is sturdy, the viscera are calm and difficult to injure. If the liver is fragile, it may be easily damaged by diseases of pure heat wasting thirst. If the liver sits upright it is in harmony, uninhibited and difficult to injure. If the liver is inclined to one side, this causes one-sided pain in the hypochondrium.

If the spleen is small it is calm and it is difficult for evils to injure it. If the spleen is large, there is a tendency to contract pain in the sides of the abdomen and an inability to walk quickly. If the spleen is elevated, there is a dragging feeling in the sides of the abdomen and pain in the flanks. If the spleen is low, it pushes down on the large intestine. If the large intestine is depressed it lies outside the viscera (*i.e.* is displaced) and, therefore, may contract evils. If the spleen is sturdy, it is difficult to injure the viscera. If the spleen is fragile it may be easily damaged by diseases of

pure heat wasting thirst. If the spleen is upright it is in harmony, uninhibited, and difficult to injure. If the spleen is inclined to one side there is a tendency to fullness and distention.

If the kidney is small, it is calm and difficult to injure. If the kidney is large, there is a susceptibility to illnesses of low back pain [a variant version says: "deafness, ringing in the ears, and spontaneous sweating" {later editor}], inability to bend forward or back, and a susceptibility to injury by evils. If the kidney is elevated, there is a susceptibility to illnesses of the sinews on either side of the spine and an inability to bend forward and back. [A variant version says: "stiffness of the back and pus and polyps in the ears".] If the kidney is low, there is lumbosacral pain, inability to bend forward and back, and fox-like *shan*.[49] If the kidney is sturdy, illnesses such as pain of the lower and upper back will not occur. If the kidney is fragile, it may be easily damaged by pure heat wasting thirst. If the kidney stands upright, it is in harmony, uninhibited and difficult to injure. If the kidney is inclined to one side, there is a susceptibility to low back and sacral pain.

These are the twenty-five changes. They are responsible for the diseases commonly encountered in people.

The Yellow Emperor asked:

How can one recognize these conditions?

Qi Bo answered:

A red (facial) color with fine texture (*cou li*)[50] indicates a small heart, while (a red complexion with) coarse texture indicates a large heart. Absence of a xiphoid process indicates a high heart. While a short and (anteriorly) raised xiphoid process indicates a low heart. A long xiphoid process indicates a sturdy heart, while a small, weak, thin xiphoid process indicates a fragile heart. A straight xiphoid process that does not rise anteriorly indicates an upright heart, while a xiphoid process slanted to one side indicates an inclined heart.

A white (facial) color with fine texture indicates

small lungs, while (a white complexion with) coarse texture indicates large lungs. Broad shoulders with a sunken throat indicate high lungs, while an upper body narrowed at the axillae but widened at the level of the free ribs indicates low lungs. A thick upper back and shoulders indicate sturdy lungs, while thin shoulders and upper back indicate fragile lungs. Well proportioned shoulders and breast indicate upright lungs, whereas a breast raised to one side indicates inclined lungs.

A green-blue (facial) color and fine texture indicates a small liver, while (a green-blue complexion with) coarse texture indicates a large liver. A broad chest with bulging flanks indicates a high liver, while an upper body drawn inward at the flanks which are also lowered indicates a low liver. A well proportioned chest and flanks indicate a sturdy liver, while weak (floating) ribs indicate a fragile liver. A well proportioned chest, flanks, and abdomen indicate an upright liver. Whereas free ribs raised to one side indicate an inclined liver.

A yellow (facial) color with fine texture indicate a small spleen, while (a yellow complexion with) coarse texture indicates a large spleen. Out-turned lips indicate a high spleen. While slack, drooping lips indicate a low spleen. Firm lips indicate a sturdy spleen, while large lips which are not sturdy indicate a fragile spleen. Well proportioned upper and lower lips indicate an upright spleen. Whereas lips raised to one side indicate an inclined spleen.

A black (facial) color and fine texture indicate small kidneys, while (a black complexion with) coarse texture indicates large kidneys. High ears indicate high kidneys, while ears thrown backwards indicate low kidneys. Sturdy ears indicate sturdy kidneys. Thin ears indicate fragile kidneys. Well shaped ears thrown forward as far as the Jawbone (Jia Che)[51] indicate upright kidneys, whereas ears which are inclined and high indicate inclined kidneys.

Those with the above changes will be well if they take care of themselves. If they neglect themselves, however, this will result in disease.

The Yellow Emperor asked:

Tell me why it is that some people never become ill and live the full measure of their heavenly (decreed) span of life. Even deep worries, violent fright, and frustrations are not able to affect them nor can they be injured by great cold or heat. Others are never without disease even though they live their life indoors and are well-protected, free from worry and frustration.

Qi Bo answered:

The five viscera and six bowels may house evils. Those whose five viscera are small have less disease but are susceptible to anxiety and nervousness; those whose five viscera are large are habitually relaxed, and not easily worried. Those whose five viscera are high tend to be overambitious; those whose five viscera are low tend to be inferior people. Those whose five viscera are sturdy are free from disease; those whose five viscera are fragile are never separated from disease. Those whose five viscera are upright are harmonious, uninhibited, and are virtuous people at heart; those whose five viscera are inclined have evil hearts and are likely to be thieves. They are not level or honest people and their speech is capricious.[52]

The Yellow Emperor asked:

Tell me of the correspondences of the six bowels.

Qi Bo answered:

The lung connects with the large intestine and the skin corresponds to the large intestine. The *Su Wen* says: The lung is connected with the skin and the hair is their efflorescence. The heart is their ruler. [The explanation below that the fine hair corresponds to the kidney is wrong. {later editor}][53]

The heart connects with the small intestine. The vessels correspond to the small intestine. The *Su Wen* says: The heart is connected with the vessels and its efflorescence is the (facial) color. The kidney is its ruler. These statements are in accord with one another.

The liver connects with the gallbladder. The sinews correspond with the gallbladder. The *Su Wen* says: The liver is connected with the sinews and its efflorescence is the nails. The lung is its ruler. These statements agree with one another.

The spleen connects with the stomach. The flesh corresponds with the stomach. The *Su Wen* says: The spleen is connected with the flesh. Its efflorescence is the lips. Its ruler is the liver. These statements agree with one another.

The kidney connects with the triple burner and urinary bladder. The interstices and fine hair corresponds with the bladder. The *Jiu Juan* also says: The kidney connects with the bones. The *Su Wen* says: The kidney connects with the bones. Their efflorescence is the hair and they are ruled by the spleen. These statements are identical.

The Yellow Emperor asked:

What do these correspondences signify?

Qi Bo answered:

The lung corresponds with the skin. If the skin is thick, the large intestine is thick (walled); if the skin is thin, the large intestine is thin.[54] If the skin is slack and the belly is big, the large intestine is broad and long. If the skin is taut, the large intestine is taut and short. If the skin is moist the large intestine is upright. If the skin and flesh cannot be separated from one another, the large intestine is knotted.

The heart corresponds with the vessels. If the skin is thick, the vessels are thick. If the vessels are thick, the small intestine is thick. If the skin is thin, the vessels are thin. If the vessels are thin, the small intestine is thin. If the skin is slack, the vessels are relaxed. If the vessels are relaxed, the small intestine is broad and long. If the skin is thin and the vessels are flat and small, the small intestine is small and short. If the yang channels and vessels[55] are excessively twisted, the small intestine is knotted.

The spleen corresponds with the flesh. If the major muscular masses are strong and large, the stomach is sturdy. If the major muscular masses are slender, the stomach is not sturdy. If the major muscular masses are not proportionate to the body, the stomach is low. If the stomach lies low (in the abdomen), the lower venter is restricted and inhibited. [The *Tai Su* says: "The lower venter fails to restrict."] If the major muscular masses are not strong, the stomach is slack. If the major muscular masses are devoid of fine reticulations within them [a variant version does not have "within them" {later editor}], the stomach will be tense. If the major muscular masses are rich in fine reticulations, the stomach is knotted. If the stomach is knotted, the upper venter is restricted and inhibited.

The liver corresponds with the nails. If the nails are thick and their color is yellow, the gallbladder is thick. If the nails are thin and their color is red, the gallbladder is thin. If the nails are sturdy and their color is blue-green, the gallbladder is tense. If the nails are sodden and red, the gallbladder is slack. If the nails are straight and white, the gallbladder is straight. If the nails are grimy and colored black with excessive striations, the gallbladder is knotted.

The kidney corresponds with the bones. If the skin is thick with compact texture, the triple burner and urinary bladder are thick. If the skin is thin with coarse texture, the triple burner and urinary bladder are thin. If the interstices are sparse, the triple burner and urinary bladder are slack. If the skin is tense and without fine hairs, the triple burner and bladder are tense. If the fine hairs are beautiful and thick, the triple burner and urinary bladder are straight. If the fine hairs are sparse, the triple burner and urinary bladder are knotted.

The Yellow Emperor asked:

Thin or thick, beautiful or ugly, tell me how these variations in form indicate or reflect disease.

Qi Bo answered:

The (viscera) in the interior can be known by observing their external correspondences. Hence the (location of the) disease can be known.

Chapter Six

The Twelve Source Points[56]

The five viscera have the six bowels and the six bowels have the twelve source points. The twelve source points[57] are distal to the four passes (*i.e.*, the elbows and knees).[58] The four passes govern treatment of the five viscera. Therefore, when (any of) the five viscera are diseased, the most appropriate (point) among the twelve source points should be chosen. The twelve source points are the places by which the five viscera irrigate the three hundred sixty-five joints with the qi and flavors they have received. When the viscera become diseased, this will manifest at the twelve source points, each of which has its own manifestations. Awareness of (the functions of) the twelve source points and observation of their correspondences leads to knowledge of how the viscera may be harmed.

The lung, *shao yin* within yang,[59] has Great Abyss (*Tai Yuan*, Lu 9) bilaterally as their source point. The heart, *tai yang* within yang, has Great Mound (*Da Ling*, Per 7) bilaterally as its source point. The liver, *shao yang* within yin, has Supreme Surge (*Tai Chong*, Liv 3) bilaterally as its source point. The kidney, *tai yin* within yin, has Great Ravine (*Tai Xi*, Ki 3) bilaterally as its source point. The spleen, consummate yin within yin, has Supreme White (*Tai Bai*, Sp 3) bilaterally as its source point. The source point of the *gao*[60] is Turtledove Tail (*Jiu Wei*, CV 15), and the source point of the *huang*[60] is the navel (*bo yang*, 脖胦).[61] The above twelve source points govern the treatment of diseases involving either the five viscera or six bowels.

For distention, choose the three yang (channels). While for swill diarrhea,[62] choose the three yin. [A variant version says: "For stagnation, choose the three yin."]

Diseases occurring in the five viscera are likened to a thorn in the flesh, to a stain, to a knot, or to an obstruction. A thorn, though stuck for a long time, can be pulled out. A stain, though left for a long time, can be cleaned. A knot, though retained for long, can be untied. An obstruction, though bound up for long, can be broken. It is wrong to declare that there is no cure for long-standing disease. For one who is skilled in the use of needles, the cure of disease is like pulling out a thorn, cleaning a stain, untying a knot, or breaking an obstruction. However long it may have persisted, the disease will yield to treatment. To say something cannot be treated reflects a lack of attainment in this art.

Chapter Seven

The Twelve Channels & the Twelve Great Waters[63]

The Yellow Emperor asked:

There are twelve channels. In the external world they relate to the twelve great waters.[64] In the interior (of the body) they pertain to the five viscera and six bowels. Just as the twelve great waters receive and convey water, so the five viscera are associated with and store the spirit, qi, *hun*, and *po*. The six bowels receive and convey grain and receive and distribute qi. The vessels receive and manage blood. Please explain how these are combined in treatment and discuss the proper depths of needle insertion and the proper number of cones of moxa to be used.

Qi Bo answered:

The viscera may be sturdy or fragile; the bowels may be large or small; there may be greater or lesser amounts of grains; the vessels may be long or short; the blood may be pure or turbid; and there may be a greater or lesser amount of qi. Within the channels, there may be more blood and less qi, less blood and more qi, both more blood and qi, or both less blood and qi. These amounts are constant. Thus, when treating with acupuncture/moxibustion in order to regulate the qi of the channels, these constants should be kept in mind. These are the reflection of heaven and earth within humankind and resonate with yin and yang. Therefore, one must not fail to examine them carefully.

The foot *yang ming* relates to the River Hai in the external (world) and pertains to the stomach in the interior (of the body). The foot *tai yang* relates to the River Qing in the external (world) and pertains to the urinary bladder and ensures the free flow of the water passageways in the interior (of the body). The foot *shao yang* relates to the River Wei in the external (world) and pertains to the gallbladder in the interior (of the body). The foot *tai yin* relates to the River Hu in the external (world) and pertains to the spleen in the interior (of the body). The foot *jue yin* relates to the River Mian in the external (world) and pertains to the liver in the interior (of the body). The foot *shao yin* relates to the River Ru in the external (world) and pertains to the kidney in the interior of the (body). The hand *yang ming* relates to the River Jiang in the external (world) and pertains to the large intestine in the interior (of the body). The hand *tai yang* relates to the River Huai in the external (world) and pertains to the small intestine in the interior (of the body). The hand *shao yang* relates to the River Ta in the external (world) and pertains to triple burner and water passageways in the interior (of the body). The hand *tai yin* relates with the River He in the external (world) and pertains to the lung in the interior (of the body). The hand heart-governor *xin zhu*[65] relates to the River Zhang in the external (world) and pertains to the pericardium in the interior (of the body). The hand *shao yin* relates to the River Ji in the external (world) and pertains to the heart in the interior (of the body).

The twelve rivers, the five viscera, and six bowels have their external sources and their internal supplies. These external sources and internal supplies join to form endless ring-like flows. The channels of humans are like this as well. Heaven is yang and earth is yin. (The part of the body lying) above the lumbar region is heaven and (the part of the body lying) below the lumbar region is earth. North to the Hai is yin.[66] North to the Hu is yin within yin.[67] South to the Zhang is yang.[68] North to the He till the Zhang is yin within yang.[69] South of the Ta till the Jiang is yang with-in yang.[70] These are yin and yang in the districts of the country. This too refers to the mutual relationship of humankind to heaven and earth.

The Yellow Emperor asked:

Like the great rivers, the channels with which they resonate vary in the distances they cover, the depths to which they run, and the amount of water and blood they contain. Each (channel) differs from the other. How should these (individual characteristics) be integrated in needling?

Qi Bo answered:

The foot *yang ming* is the sea of the five viscera and the six bowels. Its vessel is large, abundant in blood, exuberant in qi, and extravagant in heat. If one does not needle deeply, one cannot scatter (the qi), and without retention (of the needle) drainage (of the qi) cannot occur.

The foot *yang ming* has more blood and more qi. Therefore, needle to a depth of six *fen* and retain (the needle) for a duration of ten exhalations.[71] The foot *shao yang* has less blood but more qi. Therefore, needle to a depth of four *fen* and retain (the needle) for a duration of five exhalations. The foot *tai yang* has more blood and more qi. Therefore, needle to a depth of five *fen* and retain the (needle) for a duration of seven exhalations. The foot *tai yin* has more blood and less qi. Therefore, needle to a depth of three *fen* and retain (the needle) for a duration of four exhalations. The foot *shao yin* has less blood but more qi. Therefore, needle to a depth of two *fen* and retain (the needle) for a duration of three exhalations. The foot *jue yin* has more blood but less qi. Therefore, needle one *fen* deep and retain (the needle) for a duration of two exhalations.

The yin and yang (channels) of the hands have ready access to the qi. Thus the qi arrives quickly (when needled) and the needle should be inserted to a depth not exceeding two *fen*, and it should be retained for a duration not exceeding one exhalation. These may vary depending whether one is young or mature, large or small, obese or emaciated. This approach is called compliance with natural law and applies to moxibustion as well. If excessive moxibustion produces malignant fire, this leads to a withering of the bones and an astringing of the vessels. If one is needled excessively, this gives rise to a desertion of the qi.

The Yellow Emperor asked:

Are there standard measures in regard to the largeness and smallness of the vessels, whether one has more or less blood, the thickness or thinness of the skin, the strength or fragility of the flesh, and the largeness or smallness of the muscular masses?

Qi Bo answered:

Those of medium size should be chosen as the norm. They should not be haggard or suffer from an exhaustion of blood and qi. How can those who are abnormally emaciated and haggard be considered the norm for needling! One should carefully press, palpate, touch and depress.[72] In pressing, one may perceive hot and cold, exuberance and exhaustion, and so regulate these. This is referred to as the "appropriate (examination) which leads to true knowledge."[73]

Chapter Eight

The Four Seas[74]

The human body has four seas. The twelve channels all pour into these seas. They are the sea of marrow, the sea of blood, the sea of qi, and the sea of water and grains. The stomach is the sea of water and grains. Its transporting points are Qi Thoroughfare (*Qi Jie*, St 30)[75] above and Three Li (*San Li*, St 36) below. The penetrating vessel is the sea of the twelve channels. Its transporting points are Great Shuttle (*Da Zhu*, BL 11) above and Upper and Lower Great Hollow (*Shang* and *Xia Ju Xu*, St 37 and St 39) below. The center of the chest is the sea of qi. Its transporting points are above and below (the end of) the neckbone[76] and at Man's Prognosis (*Ren Ying*, St 9) anteriorly. The brain is the sea of marrow. Its transporting points are at the top of the head (*Bai Hui*, GV 20) above and at Wind Pool (*Feng Fu*, GV 16) below. When the four seas proceed normally, this is life; when there is counterflow, this causes decay. Knowing how to regulate these is of benefit; not knowing is harmful.

The Yellow Emperor asked:

How can one tell if the four seas are normal or abnormal?

Qi Bo answered:

If there is a surplus within the sea of qi, there will be qi fullness and oppression within the chest, rapid breathing, and a red face; if there is an insufficiency of qi, there will not be enough (breath) for speech. If there is a surplus within the sea of blood, there will be the illusion of an enlarged body, depression and peevishness, and an inability to tell where one is diseased; if there is an insufficiency (of qi within the sea of blood) there is the illusion that ones body is small and cramped and an inability to tell where the disease is located. If there is a surplus within the sea of water and grains, there will be abdominal distention and stuffiness; if there is insufficiency (within the sea of water and grains), there will be constant hunger but an inability to ingest food. If there is a surplus within the sea of marrow, (the body will be) light, agile, possessed of great strength, and the ability to accomplish what is normally beyond one's self; if there is insufficiency (within the sea of marrow), the brain will spin, there will be ringing in the ears, aching pain in the lower legs, vertigo, loss of eyesight, fatigue, and somnolence.

The Yellow Emperor asked:

How can these be regulated?

Qi Bo answered:

Carefully observe their transporting points and regulate vacuity and repletion. Do nothing to violate (this principle) or this will be harmful. Acting in accord with these principles promotes recovery, and defiance of them causes failure.[77]

Chapter Nine

Breathing Vis-à-Vis the Fifty Circuits (of Qi) Around the Body, the Four Seasons, the Divisions of the Day, & Moments of Time of the Dripping (Clepsydra)[78]

(1)

The Yellow Emperor asked:

What are the fifty cycles of the constructive qi?

Qi Bo answered:

The heavenly circuit contains twenty-eight constellations. Each constellation has thirty-six minutes. One circuit of qi movement around the human (body equals) one thousand eight minutes (of the sun's movement through these constellations).[79] In the human body above and below, left and right, front and back, there are twenty-eight network vessels.[80] Their total length in the body is sixteen *zhang* and two *chi*.[81] These correspond to the twenty-eight constellations. One hundred moments of time measured in water dripping down (from the clepsydra) equals the divisions of one day and night.[82] Thus in humans, during one exhalation, the pulse beats twice and the qi moves three *cun*. During one inhalation, the pulse beats again two times and the qi moves three *cun*. During the interval of inhalation and expiration determining a breath, the qi moves six *cun*. During ten breaths, the qi moves six *chi* and the sun moves two minutes.[83] In two hundred seventy breaths, the qi moves sixteen *zhang* and two *chi*. The qi circulates and crosses through the center and this constitutes one cycle around the body. When the water drips two moments of time, the sun moves a little more than twenty minutes. In five hundred forty breaths, the qi moves two circuits around the body. When the water drips four moments, the sun moves a little more than forty minutes. In two thousand seven hundred breaths, the qi moves in ten cycles around the body. The water drips down twenty moments and the sun moves through five constellations and a little more than

twenty minutes. In thirteen thousand five hundred respirations, the qi moves in fifty cycles around the body. The water drips one hundred moments and the sun moves through (all) twenty-eight constellations. By the time the clepsydra is empty, the vessels reach their end. [Wang Bing[84] says: This is a rough estimation. Exactly speaking, the sun by now has travelled one thousand one minutes and six seconds.] What is referred to as reunion is the same movement of one circuit (through all twenty-eight channels and vessels). To mete out the full measure of the life span decreed by heaven and earth, the qi must travel fifty circuits covering eight hundred ten *zhang*. This is because, by travelling fifty circuits in one day and one night, the qi ensures that the five viscera are nurtured by their essence. If it fails to travel this many cycles, this is referred to as precarious existence (*kuang sheng*, 狂生). The reason that qi must travel fifty circuits is to guarantee that all five viscera receive (sufficient) qi. [This passage is found at the end of the *Jing Mai Gen Jie* {Chapter on the Channels & Vessels, Roots & Ends from the *Spiritual Pivot*}[85] but has been transferred to its present place in this text.]

(2)

The Yellow Emperor asked:

Where are the exits, entrances, and meeting places in the circulation of defensive qi?

Qi Bo answered:

There are twelve months in a year, and twelve watches in a day. *Zi* and *wu* are the warp, and *mao* and *you* are the weft.[86] There are seven constellations in each quarter of heaven. Therefore, there are seven times four or twenty-eight constellations in heaven. *Fang* and *mao* are the warp and *zhang* and *xu* are the weft. From *fang* to *bi* is yang. While from *mao* to *xin* is yin. Yang rules the day and yin rules the night. Since the movement of defensive qi completes fifty cycles around the body in one day and one night, it covers twenty-five cycles in the yang by day and another twenty-five in the yin by night, thus visiting all five viscera.

Therefore, at the calm dawn watch,[87] yin qi has reached the end and the yang qi issues from the eyes. When the eyes open, the qi circulates to the head, turns down the neck, proceeds further down along the foot *tai yang* and along the upper back to reach the tip of the small toe. One of the divergent (branches) deviates from the inner canthus and travels down along the hand *tai yang* to reach the lateral aspect of the little finger.[88] Another divergent (branch) also deviates from the inner canthus and travels down along the foot *shao yang*, finally pouring into the space between the small and fourth toe. Another branch follows the hand *shao yang* to arrive between the small finger (and the ring finger), its ramification ascends to the region anterior to the ear, joining the *han* vessel,[89] and pouring into the foot *yang ming*. Then this ramification travels downward to the dorsum and submerges between the five toes.[90] Another divergent (branch) starts from the ear and goes down along the hand *yang ming* to submerge between thumb and forefinger and into the palm.[91] The branch which goes down to the foot submerges into the heart of the foot and then emerges from below the medial malleolus, and, traveling along the yin aspect, returns to the eye[92] to complete one single cycle.

Thus, (during the time it takes) the sun to move one post,[93] human qi moves one circuit around the body plus eight tenths (of another circuit) around the body. When the sun moves two posts, human qi moves three circuits around the body plus six tenths (of another circuit) around the body. When the sun moves three posts, human qi moves five circuits around the body plus four tenths of (another circuit) around the body. When the sun moves four posts, human qi moves seven circuits around the body plus two tenths (of another circuit) around the body. When the sun moves five posts, human qi moves nine circuits around the body. When the sun moves six posts, human qi moves ten circuits around the body plus eight tenths (of another circuit) around the body. When the sun moves seven posts, human qi moves twelve circuits around the body plus six tenths (of another circuit) around the body. When the sun moves fourteen posts, human qi moves twenty-five circuits around the body plus two tenths (of

another circuit) around the body. (At this point,) yang ends in yin and yin receives the qi.

Beginning in the yin, (the defensive qi) first pours from the foot *shao yin* into the kidney. From the kidney it pours into the heart. From the heart it pours into the liver. From the liver it pours into the spleen. And finally, from the spleen it pours back into the kidney, thus completing a single circuit. When (the sun) moves one post in the night, human qi moves one viscus plus eight tenths in the yin. Also like its movement in the yang, (the qi) returns to the eyes after twenty-five complete circuits in the yin. One day and one night's movement in yin and yang does not equal a whole number of circuits, the fraction being two tenths of the body for the yang in the day and two tenths of a viscus in the yin during the night. Because of this, people get up and lie down (*i.e.*, go to bed) at varying hours.

The Yellow Emperor asked:

The defensive qi travels around the body, up and down, to and fro without a break. Then how should needling be timed in connection with the qi?

Qi Bo answered:

(During each season yin and yang) may be allotted into greater or lesser shares (in time). Days may be longer or shorter during the spring, summer, autumn, or winter, and each is divided according to (definite) principles.[94]

As a rule, the period of calm dawn when the night is at its end is taken as the starting point. However, because the water drips one hundred moments in one day and one night, twenty-five of these moments equal half a day. This counting can go on without limit. Sundown marks the stop (of yang). Irrespective of whether the day is long or short in each of the four seasons, the calm dawn and sundown should be made as the mark for the start and stop (of yang). Correct location of the qi and needling accordingly is said to be fortuitous. If the disease is in the yang division, the qi must first be located within the yang division and then it may be needled. If the disease is in the yin division, the qi must first be located within the yin division and then it may be needled. Careful timing guarantees a desirable effect on the disease. While if one loses the opportunity, none of the hundreds of diseases can be cured.

While the water drips one moment, human qi is in the *tai yang*.[95] When the water drips two moments, human qi is in the *shao yang*. When the water drips three moments, human qi is in the *yang ming*. When water drips four moments, human qi is in the yin division.[96] When the water drips five moments, human qi is in the *tai yang*. When the water drips six moments, human qi is in the *shao yang*. When the water drips seven moments, human qi is in the *yang ming*. When the water drips eight moments, human qi is in the yin division. When the water drips nine moments, human qi is in the *tai yang*. When the water drips ten moments, human qi is in the *shao yang*. When the water drips eleven moments, human qi is in the *yang ming*. When the water drips twelve moments, human qi is in the yin division. When the water drips thirteen moments, human qi is in the *tai yang*. When the water drips fourteen moments, human qi is in the *shao yang*. When the water drips fifteen moments, human qi is in the *yang ming*. When the water drips sixteen moments, human qi is in the yin division. When the water drips seventeen moments, human qi is in the *tai yang*. When the water drips eighteen moments, human qi is in the *shao yang*. When the water drips nineteen moments, human qi is in the *yang ming*. When the water drips twenty moments, human qi is in the yin division. When the water drips twenty-one moments, human qi is in the *tai yang*. When the water drips twenty-two moments, human qi is in the *shao yang*. When the water drips twenty-three moments, human qi is in the *yang ming*. When the water drips twenty-four moments, human qi is in the yin division. And when the water drips twenty-five moments, human qi is in the *tai yang*. This is how half a day is passed.

Fourteen posts from *fang* to *bi* or fifty moments of water dropping is the measure of half a day. Another fourteen posts from *mao* to *xin* or another fifty moments of water dropping is the measure of the rest of the day. The sun moves one post and water drips three moments plus four sevenths.

The *Da Yao (The Great Outlines)*[97] says that, just as the sun above stays in the first constellation, one also knows that the qi of the body is in the *tai yang*. Therefore, when the sun moves one post, human qi has been in three yang and one yin divisions. This is constant and without end. This circulation is carried out in accordance with heaven and earth, in a complicated but orderly fashion. Upon arriving at the end, it returns to the beginning. During the course of one day and one night, the water moves one hundred moments and (one round) is complete. It is said that, in needling fullness, one needles when (the qi) arrives. In needling a state of vacuity, one needles when (the qi) is in retreat. Here the instructions say that at the juncture of inflow and withdrawal of the qi, one should needle vacuity and repletion accordingly.

Chapter Ten

Constructive Qi[98]

The internal ingestion of grain is the treasure of the *dao* of the constructive qi. Grains enter the stomach and qi is transported to the lung. It flows in and pervades the center, spreading and dispersing over the exterior. The essence is refined and circulates within the channels, and the constructive qi moves constantly without cessation. It ends and returns to the beginning. This is called the law of heaven and earth.

Thus once the qi emerges from the hand *tai yin*, it goes along the inner aspect of the upper arm. It pours into the hand *yang ming* and then proceeds upward to the face. There it pours into the foot *yang ming*, circulating downward to the dorsum of the foot to pour into the big toe. There it joins the foot *tai yin*, where it moves upward to the spleen, and from the spleen it pours into the heart. It continues its journey along the hand *shao yin*, emerging from the axilla, moving down the arm, and pouring into the tip of the little finger. After joining the hand *tai yang*, it moves upward, passing the axilla, emerging from the suborbital region [the nape in a variant edition], and finally pours into the inner canthus. Then it moves up to the top of the head and turns down the nape to join the foot *tai yang* with which it goes downward along the spine to the sacrococcygeal region and further down to the tip of the small toe. Then it travels towards the center of the sole to pour into the foot *shao yin*. From there (the qi) circulates upward to pour into the kidney, subsequently pouring into the heart and spreading into the chest. Then it goes along the heart-governor,[99] emerging from the axilla, moving down the arm, submerging [emerging in a variant edition] between the two sinews (in the forearm), again submerging in the palm, emerging from the tip of the middle finger, and pouring into the ulnar aspect of the ring finger to join the hand *shao yang*. (The qi) then proceeds upward to pour into the center of the chest, spreading in the triple burner. From there it pours into the gallbladder and then emerges from the lateral costal region or flanks. After pouring into the foot *shao yang*, it moves downward to the dorsum and pours into the big toe. After joining the foot *jue yin*, (the qi) moves upward to the liver wherefrom it ascends and pours into the lung. Then it travels through the throat, submerging in the nasopharynx and terminating in the smelling portal[100] ["smelling bar" in a variant version]. A branch deviates from here, going upward to the forehead, along the top of the head, and then downward along the spine until it enters the sacrococcygeal region. This is the governing vessel. (The qi) continues, linking the genital organs, passing through the pubic hair region, and submerging into the umbilicus. From there it goes upward inside the abdomen, submerges in the supraclavicular fossa, pours down into the lung, and reemerges from the hand *tai yin*. This is the movement of the constructive *qi*, constantly flowing up and down, this way (*ni*, 逆) and that (*shun*, 順).[101]

Chapter Eleven

Constructive, Defensive, & the Triple Burner[102]

The Yellow Emperor asked:

How do humans receive qi? How do yin and yang meet? What qi is the constructive? What qi is the defensive? Where does the constructive arise? Where does the defensive meet (the constructive)? The aged and the young do not possess the same qi. Yin and yang differ in their routes. Please tell me of the meeting (of yin and yang, constructive and defensive).

Qi Bo answered:

Humans receive qi from grains. Grain enters the stomach and qi is transported to the lung. Thus all the five viscera and six bowels receive the qi. The clear part is constructive and the turbid is defensive. The constructive circulates within the vessels, and the defensive circulates outside the vessels. These two circulate endlessly and have a grand meeting[103] after fifty measures of movement around (the body). Thus yin and yang link together to form an endless ring. The defensive qi circulates twenty-five measures within the yin and twenty-five within the yang. This is divided by day and night. Therefore, people rise with yang and lie down with yin. At midday, yang is at high tide and this, therefore, is called double yang.[104] While at midnight, yin is at high tide and this, therefore, is called double yin.[105] The *tai yin* rules the interior and the *tai yang* rules the exterior.[106] Each moves twenty-five measures during a period of one day and one night respectively. At midnight, the yin is at high tide and after midnight it declines. At the time of the calm dawn the yin comes to an end and the yang begins to receive the qi. At midday, yang is at high tide. As the sun moves towards the west, yang declines. At sundown yang comes to an end and the yin receives the qi. At midnight there is a grand meeting when all people are asleep. This is called meeting of the yin.[107] At the calm dawn, yin comes to an end and the yang receives qi. This goes on without cessation in accordance with the laws of heaven and earth.

The Yellow Emperor asked:

The old cannot sleep at night while the young and strong never wake. What (condition of) the qi accounts for this?

Qi Bo answered:

The strong have an exuberance of qi and blood. They have slippery (*i.e.*, fatty) flesh and muscles, their pathways of qi are unimpeded, and their constructive and defensive are without irregularity. Thus they are energetic by day and sleep at night. As for the old, their qi and blood are diminished, their flesh and muscles are withered, their pathways of qi are astringed, the qi of the five viscera are in conflict with one another, constructive qi is decrepit and scant, and the defensive qi harasses the interior. Thus by day they are not energetic and by night they cannot sleep.

The Yellow Emperor asked:

Tell me about the circulation of the constructive and the defensive qi and from where these pathways originate.

Qi Bo answered:

The constructive issues from the middle burner. The defensive issues from the upper burner. The upper burner emerges from the upper opening of the stomach, ascending along the pharynx,[108] to penetrate the diaphragm and spread throughout the chest. It then travels towards the axilla, circulating along the route of the hand *tai yin*, and again pours into the hand *yang ming*. Ascending to the tongue, it then descends into the foot *yang ming*. Together with the constructive, it travels twenty-five measures as a single round within the yin and yang respectively. It travels fifty circuits over the course of one day and one night and then begins over again at its grand reunion in the hand *tai yin*.

The Yellow Emperor asked:

When a person takes hot food and drink it descends to the stomach. Before the qi is settled,[109] one may sweat from the face, the spine, or from the (upper) half of the body. [*Wai Tai San Jiao Mai Bing Lun {The Secret (Medical Essentials of) a Provincial Governor: "The Treatise on the Pulses & Diseases of the Triple Heater"}* says trunk and hands.] What causes the sweat to exit without following the route of the defensive qi?

Qi Bo answered:

If there is external injury due to wind, the interstices are opened from within. This steams the hair and the interstices discharge. This mobilizes the defensive qi and leads it astray. The defensive qi is quick and fierce, volatile and impetuous, and tends to escape at the first opening. As a result, it fails to follow its pathway. This is called leaking discharge (*lou xie*).[110]

The middle burner also originates near to the mouth of the stomach and it exits posterior to the upper burner.[111] After it has received the qi, it separates the waste, steams the fluids, transforms the fine essence, and pours (the essence from the fluid) upward into the lung vessel. There (this essence) is transformed into blood to nurture the body. As the most valuable substance, the blood has the singular privilege of travelling inside the channels. It is called the constructive qi.

The Yellow Emperor asked:

Why are blood and qi, having different names, considered to be of the same class?

Qi Bo answered:

The constructive and defensive are essence qi; the blood is the spirit qi. Therefore, blood and qi are named differently but considered to be in the same class. Thus, when deprived of blood, do not induce diaphoresis, and when deprived of sweat, do not bleed (acupoints). Hence humankind has two deaths but does not have two lives.[112]

The lower burner moves into the winding intestines (*hui chang*, 回肠)[113] and pours into the urinary bladder.[114] In the stomach, water and grains stay together and in due time are reduced to dregs. These are moved down into the large intestine in the precinct of the lower burner and percolated downward. After seeping and discharging, the sap seeps along the lower burner into the urinary bladder.

The Yellow Emperor asked:

A person may drink alcohol (over the course of a meal). The alcohol also enters the stomach, and yet one urinates before the grains have even ripened (in the stomach). Why is this?

Qi Bo answered:

Alcohol is a liquid from cooked grains. Its qi is fierce and slippery ["clear" in a variant version. {later editor}] Therefore, the liquid emerges prior to the grain even though it entered afterward.

Thus it is said the upper burner is like a mist. The middle burner is like a mash (*ou*).[115] The lower burner is like a sluice (*du*).[116]

Chapter Twelve

Yin & Yang, Clear & Turbid, Essence & Qi, Fluid & Humor, Blood & Vessels[117]

(1)

The Yellow Emperor asked:

Please tell me about the clear and turbid in the qi of humans. What are these?

Qi Bo answered:

That received from grains is turbid. That received from qi is clear.[118] The clear pours into the yin[119] and the turbid pours into the yang.[120] The clear of the turbid ascends to emerge at the pharynx; the turbid from the clear circulates downward to the stomach. The clear circulates upward and the turbid circulates downward. The interference of the clear and turbid with one another is called chaotic qi (*luan qi*).[121]

The Yellow Emperor asked:

Yin is clear and yang is turbid. Since there is clear within the turbid and turbid within the clear, how are these distinguished?

Qi Bo answered:

The major differentiation of the qi is that the clear ascends to pour into the lung and the turbid descends into the stomach. The clear qi from the stomach ascends and emerges from the mouth. The turbid qi from the lung descends, pouring into the channels, and accumulates in the sea of qi.[122]

The Yellow Emperor asked:

If all the yang are turbid, which alone of all the yang is the most turbid?

Qi Bo answered:

The hand *tai yang* alone receives (most) of the yang's turbid (qi).[123] The hand *tai yin* alone receives (most) of the yin's clear (qi).[124] What is clear ascends to the hollow orifices. What is turbid circulates downward into the channels. Thus all the yin are clear but the foot *tai yin* alone receives the turbid.[125]

The Yellow Emperor asked:

How are the different (kinds of qi) treated?

Qi Bo answered:

As a rule, the clear qi is slippery and the turbid qi is astringent. Therefore, when needling the yin, one must go deep and retain (the needle). When needling the yang, shallow insertion and rapid (needling) are indicated. When clear and turbid interfere with one another these must be regulated accordingly.[126]

(2)

The Yellow Emperor asked:

Humans have essence, qi, fluids, humor, blood, and vessels. What are these?

Qi Bo snswered:

Two spirits[127] communicate and combine to give

birth to form.[128] What existed prior to the birth of the body is called essence. What is diffused from the upper burner and distilled from the flavors of the five grains to fumigate the skin, replenish the body, and moisten the hair as a mist or dew moistens, is called the qi. What drains out in the form of sweat through the open interstices is called fluid. After grain has entered (the stomach), the qi (from it) fills (the body). That which lubricates and moistens, pours into the bones (and is discharged). It renders the joints flexible, supplementing and boosting the brain marrow, and moistening the skin. This is called the humor.[129] The sap received by the middle burner which had been turned red is called the blood. That which confines the constructive and causes it to flow along certain routes are called the vessels.

The Yellow Emperor asked:

There may be a surplus or insufficiency of the six qi.[130] (For instance,) there may be a greater or lesser amount of qi, the brain marrow may be replete or vacuous, and the blood vessels may be clear or turbid. How can these be recognized?

Qi Bo answered:

If there is desertion of essence, there is deafness. If there is desertion of qi, there is loss of brightness within the eyes. If there is a desertion of fluids, the interstices will open and there will be profuse sweating. If there is a desertion of humor, the bending and stretching of the joints is inhibited, the (facial) color is perished, the brain marrow is wasted, the lower legs ache, and the ears frequently ring. If there is desertion of blood, (the complexion is) white colored, withered and lusterless. If there is desertion of the vessels the pulses are empty and vacuous. These are the reflections (of the conditions of the six qi).

The Yellow Emperor asked:

What is the role and status of the six qi?

Qi Bo answered:

The six qi are each ruled by their respective regions. Although each of them has a (vital) role and status which is the same as that which rules it, the stomach with the five grains is the great sea.[131]

Chapter Thirteen

The Five Outlets (*Bie*, 別) of the Fluids & Humors[132]

The Yellow Emperor asked:

Water and grains enter the mouth, where they are transported to the intestines and stomach. The fluids from this process have five outlets. If one wears thin clothing in cold weather, (fluids) turn into urine and qi.[133] If one wears thick clothing during the heat of summer, they turn into sweat. If the qi is confined by sorrow, (these fluids) turn into tears. If heat in the center causes the stomach to be slack, they turn into drool. If there is an internal counterflow of evil qi, this causes the qi to become obstructed and to fail to circulate. This lack of circulation results in water distention or edema. I do not understand how these arise.

Qi Bo answered:

Water and grains enter through the mouth. These have five flavors which, when separated, pour into their own seas.[134] And the fluids and humors from them each go their (separate) ways as well. Hence the qi[135] exits from the upper burner ["triple burner" in a variant edition]. That which warms the flesh and muscles and which replenishes the skin are the fluids; that which becomes lodged and does not circulate (within the body) is humor. Thick clothing worn in the summer heat opens the interstices resulting in the discharge of sweat. If cold becomes lodged in the spaces between the flesh, fluid gathers as froth and causes pain. In cold weather, the interstices are shut. The flow of qi is astringed and does not circulate. As a result, water flows downward to the urinary bladder, turning into urine and qi.

Of the five viscera and six bowels, the heart is the ruler, with the ears as the scouts, the eyes are the lookouts, the lung is the minister, the liver is the general, the spleen is the sentry, and the kidney rules the exterior. Thus the fluids and humors of the five viscera and six bowels all percolate upward into the eyes. When the qi becomes confined because of sadness within the heart, the cardiac ligation becomes tense. This tenseness causes the lobes of the lung to become elevated, and when they are so elevated, the humors overflow in the upper (part of the body). If the cardiac ligation is tense, the lung cannot sustain this elevated position and so sometimes it rises and sometimes it falls. Hence there is coughing and tears emerge.

If there is heat in the center the grains within the stomach will be dispersed. If the grains are dispersed, worms will cavort up and down. The intestines and stomach become dilated and thus the stomach becomes slack. This slackness causes the qi to counterflow resulting in salivation.

The fluids and humor from the five grains mix to form a grease which percolates into the hollow cavities of the bones, supplements and boosts the brain marrow, and flows downward to the *yin*. When yin and yang are not in harmony, humor overflows and flows downward to the *yin*.[136] The marrow and humor may both be diminished and descend, and if (the marrow and humor) descends excessively vacuity ensues. This vacuity leads to low and upper back pain and aching in the lower legs.

If the passageways of yin and yang qi do not flow freely, the four seas will be blocked, the triple burner will fail to drain, and fluids and humor will not be transformed. In this case, water and grains are detained in the stomach. Although these depart into the winding intestine, (water) may become lodged in the lower burner. If it is unable to percolate into the urinary bladder, this may cause distention in the lower burner. Water spillage leads to water distention. This is the normal flow and counterflow of the five outlets of the fluid and humor.[137]

Chapter Fourteen

Peculiar Evils (*Qi Xie*, 奇邪) & the Blood network vessels[138]

The Yellow Emperor asked:

I have heard that peculiar evils do not lie within the channels. Where do they reside?

Qi Bo answered:

Within the blood network vessels.

The Yellow Emperor asked:

In needling the blood network vessels there may be collapse. Why is this? When blood emerges, it may shoot out. Why is this? When blood emerges, it may be black and turbid. Why is this? When blood emerges, it may be clear and half composed of sap (*i.e.*, serous fluid). Why is this? When a person is needled there may be swelling. Why is this? When blood emerges, whether more or less in amount, there may be a somber green-blue facial color. Why is this? When a person is needled, there may be no change in facial color and yet there is vexation and oppression. Why is this? A lot of blood may emerge and yet there is no vacillation (*i.e.*, detrimental effect from the treatment). Why is this? Let me hear about all of these.

Qi Bo answered:

When vessel qi is exuberant but there is a vacuity of blood, needling causes desertion of qi, and desertion of qi leads to collapse. If qi and blood are both exuberant and yang qi is excessive, the blood is slippery. Needling in this case causes (the blood) to shoot out. When yang qi (*i.e.*, heat) has accumulated and becomes lodged for a long time without being drained, the blood will be blackish and turbid and thus cannot shoot out. If freshly drunk liquids percolate as fluids into the network vessels without uniting with the blood, when blood emerges, there will be a discernable outflow of this sap (as well). Water existing within the body may accumulate and cause swelling in an individual who has not recently drunk. If yin qi (*i.e.*, water qi) accumulates for an extended period within the yang (*i.e.*, the surface), it will force its way into the network vessels. Therefore, in needling, before the blood has been allowed to emerge, the (yin qi) starts out. Then there is swelling. If one drains when yin and yang qi have just come together but have yet to join and harmonize, this will lead to a desertion of both yin and yang and the exterior and interior will separate from one another. Such desertion causes the (facial) color to be a somber blue-green. If, when needling, much blood emerges and, although the complexion does not change, there is vexation and oppression, needling the network vessels causes a vacuity within the channels. Channels which are now vacuous are categorized as yin. The yin qi deserts and thus there is vexation and oppression. If yin and yang are both affected and produce *bi*, (these evils) must have spilled into the channels internally and poured into the network vessels externally. Since this is characterized by a surplus of both yin and yang, even if much blood is discharged it is not able to cause vacuity.

The Yellow Emperor asked:

What are the signs (of the network vessels)?

Qi Bo answered:

The blood vessels are exuberant, sturdy, lie transversely, and are red. They lie up and down, in no constant place. They may be as small as a needle or as large as a chopstick. Needling with a draining technique (cures) all ten thousand (diseases). (However, this should be performed) without loss of measure (*i.e.*, with moderation), for if measure is lost there will be an adverse reaction, (the severity of which depends) upon the degree (of the error).

The Yellow Emperor asked:

The needle may enter the flesh and get stuck. Why is this?

Qi Bo answered:

Hot qi affects and heats the needle. When heated, the needle becomes stuck in the flesh and, therefore, difficult to extract.

Chapter Fifteen

The Five (Facial) Colors[139]

(1)

Lei Gong asked:

I have heard that hundreds of diseases are begun by wind and that counterflow inversion arises as a result of cold and dampness. How are these (various diseases) differentiated?

The Yellow Emperor answered:

It is necessary to investigate the region between the eyebrows. [The *Tai Su* says: "the middle gate tower".] (If the color here is) thin and lustrous, this is wind. If (the color here) is deep seated and turbid, this is *bi*. If in the earth (region),[140] this is inversion. These are constants. Thus one is able to identify the disease by color.

Lei Gong asked:

Some people die suddenly without disease. How can this be understood?

The Yellow Emperor answered:

When a major qi[141] has entered the viscera and bowels, sudden death will occur without disease (preceding it).

Lei Gong asked:

Sometimes the disease has improved somewhat when sudden death occurs. How can this be predicted?

The Yellow Emperor answered:

If a red color emerges at the cheeks the size of one's thumb, although the disease has improved slightly, sudden death may occur. If a black color emerges on the forehead large as a thumb, although there is no disease, there will also be sudden death.

Lei Gong asked:

Is the time of death predictable?

The Yellow Emperor answered:

Prediction is based on examination of the (facial) color. The forehead reflects the head and face; the region above the glabella, the throat [the *Tai Su* says: "upper gate tower"]; the region between the eyebrows [the *Tai Su* says: "middle gate tower"], the lung; and the region immediately below it,[142] the heart. The region further below[143] reflects the liver; the region to its left, the gallbladder; the lower tip,[144] the spleen; the region beside the tip of the nose, the stomach; the center of the face.[145] the large intestine; the region lateral to the large intestine region,[146] the kidney; the region straight under the kidney region, the umbilicus. The region above the king of the face[147] reflects the small intestine; the region below the king of the face[148] reflects the urinary bladder and uterus; the cheeks reflect the shoulder; the region lateral to the cheeks reflects the arms; the region below the arm region reflect the hands; the region above the inner canthi reflects the breasts; the region supralateral to the cheek reflects the spine; the region superior to the angle of the mandible[149] reflects the thighs; the center (of the cheeks) reflects the knees; the region below the knee region reflects the shins; the region further below reflects the feet; the nasolabial groove reflects the medial aspect of the thighs; the angle of the mandibles reflects the kneecaps. The above are the reflecting regions of the five viscera and six bowels and the limbs with their joints. The five colors of the five viscera should appear in their corresponding regions. The appearance (of a sickly color) deep to the bone reveals disease beyond a doubt. If a color appears in a location associated with its engendered phase (according to five phase) although a disease may be serious, it will not be fatal.[150]

Lei Gong asked:

What are the five officials (*guan*, 官) of the five colors?[151]

The Yellow Emperor answered:

Green-blue and black indicate pain. Yellow and red indicate heat. White indicates cold. These are the five officials.

Lei Gong asked:

By (examining) the colors the severity of diseases can be determined. How is this done?

The Yellow Emperor answered:

A coarse, bright color indicates a slight disease; a deep, dull color ["a withered color" in a variant edition], a serious disease. If the color moves upward, the disease is also serious; but if the color moves downward like scattered clouds, the disease is coming to an end. The five colors should appear in their (respective) visceral regions. There is an outer region and an inner region. If a color develops from the outer region to the inner region, disease develops from the outside to the inside. If a color develops from the inner region to the outer region, the disease progresses from the exterior to the interior. If a disease arises in the interior, the yin should be treated first and yang should be treated later. Reversal (of these treatment priorities) will exacerbate (the disease). If the disease arises in the exterior, yang should be treated first and yin should be treated later. [The *Tai Su* says: "If disease arises in the yang, the exterior should be treated first and the interior treated later." This statement corresponds with the above, only the wording is different.] Reversal will exacerbate the condition.

Use yang to harmonize yin. Use yin to harmonize yang.[152] If the regions are clearly discriminated, ten thousand cases will attain ten thousand cures. Ability to differentiate left from right,[153] this is called the great path. Men and women have different locations.[154] Thus they are classified as yin and yang. It is a good practitioner who carefully examines brilliance and dullness (in determining the severity of an illness).

A deep, turbid (color) indicates an internal (disease). While a superficial, clear (color) indicates an external (disease). Yellow and red indicate wind. Green-blue or black indicate pain. White indicates cold. A yellow, oily, lustrous (color) indicates pus. Extreme red indicates (heat in the) blood. Extreme pain is indicated by hypertonicity. Extreme cold is indicated by lack of sensitivity of the skin.

The five colors appear in their associated regions. By examining whether these are superficial or sinking, one can know whether (the disease) is shallow or deep. Careful examination of the lustre or dullness (of these colors) reveals whether (the disease) is amenable or recalcitrant (to treatment). By determining whether (the color) is scattered or concentrated one can know whether (the disease) is recent or old. By inspecting the color above and below one can know the position of the disease (in the body). Gathering spirit in the heart (*i.e.*, insightful examination of facial color) brings knowledge of past and present. Thus, unless these qi are minutely distinguished, one will not know what is wrong. Only by concentration without distraction can one determine whether the condition is recent or old. A bright color which is not coarse, but rather deep and dull, indicates a serious (disease. On the other hand,) if the color is neither bright nor lustrous, the disease is not extreme. If the color is dispersed, and is not firmly seated, there is no accumulation (within the body). The disease is dispersed and there is qi pain (*i.e.*, pain due to blockage of qi) because accumulation has not yet developed. If the kidney restrains the heart, the heart becomes diseased first and the kidney will correspondingly (become diseased secondarily). The other colors are (also) like this.[155]

In a male, if there is a (sickly) color in the king of the face,[156] there is lateral abdominal pain which radiates downward to the testicles. (If there is a sickly color) in the philtrum, there is pain in the penis. If in the upper part of the philtrum, there is pain in the root of the penis. If in the lower part of the philtrum, there is pain in the glans of the penis. These diseases are categorized as fox-like *shan*[157] and *yin tui*.[158]

In a female, if there is (a sickly color) in the king of the face,[159] there is disease in the urinary bladder and uterus. A scattered (color) means pain. A concentrated (color) means accumulation. The position (of the concentrated color), whether at the right or left, and its shape, round or square, is the same as the color. If (the color) tends to move downward, there is flux involving the lowest part (*i.e.*, the vagina).[160] If there is a moist, greasy (color), one has overeaten or eaten unclean food.

The left means the right ["the left" in a variant edition], and the right means the left ["the right" in a variant edition].[161] If the color is pathognomonic, either concentrated, accumulated, scattered, or not in its right position, (disease) is indicated by the position of the color on the face.

The colors green-blue, black, red, white, and yellow should be natural and full but (may appear) in another place (than their home region). (Take for instance), red in another place. A red color as large as an elm seed in a strange place, for example, in the king of the face, suggests lack of menses. If the color tapers at the top, there is emptiness in the upper part (of the body). If it tapers at the bottom, there is (disease) in the lower part (of the body). Color on either the right or left (can be read by utilizing the) same method.

In terms of the five colors named by the viscera, green-blue is the liver, red is the heart, white is the lung, yellow is the spleen, and black is the kidney. The liver is connected with the sinews and green-blue is matched with the sinews. The heart is connected with the vessels and red is matched with the vessels. The spleen is connected with the flesh and yellow is matched with the flesh. The lung is connected with the skin and white is matched with the skin. And the kidney is connected with the bones and black is matched with the bones.

(2)

The brightness of the five colors is the efflorescence of the qi. For red, the desirable (color) is like cinnabar screened by thin, transparent silk. The undesirable (color) is like burnt ocher. For white, the desirable is like brilliant white jade ["white goose plumage" in a variant edition], and the undesirable is like chalk ["salt" in a variant edition]. For green-blue, the desirable is like brilliant sky-blue jade, and the undesirable is like indigo. For yellow, the desirable is like realgar screened by thin silk gauze, and the undesirable is like yellow clay. For black, the desirable is like thick black lacquer, and the undesirable is like charcoal. [The *Su Wen* says: "the somber color of ground".] If the five colors manifest the finest essence (qi), longevity does not endure.[162]

(3)

Green-blue like faded grass, black like soot, yellow like citron,[163] red like coagulated blood, and white like dried bone, when these five colors appear, there is death. Green-blue like kingfisher feathers, black like crow feathers, red like the crest of a cock, yellow like the belly of a crab, and white like pig fat, these five colors appear and there is life. When (qi) is burgeoning in the heart, (the color) is like cinnabar screened by thin, white, silk gauze. When (qi) is burgeoning in the lung, (the color) is like red screened by thin, white, silk gauze. When (qi) is burgeoning in the liver, (the color) is like green-blue, bluish red screened by thin, white, silk gauze. When (qi) is burgeoning in the spleen, (the color) is like Trichosanthes seeds screened by thin, white, silk gauze. When (qi) is burgeoning in the kidney, (the color) is like purple screened by thin, white, silk gauze. These are the external efflorescences of the burgeoning (of qi) within the five viscera.

When examining the five colors, if the face is yellow and the eyes green-blue, the face is yellow and the eyes are red, the face is yellow and the eyes are white, or the face is yellow and the eyes are black, death will not occur. If the face is green-blue and the eyes are red ["green-blue" in a variant edition], the face is red and the eyes are white, the face is green-blue and the eyes are white, the face is black and the eyes are white, or the face is red and the eyes are cyan, all of these indicate death.

Chapter Sixteen

Twenty-Five Yin & Yang Types of Humans With Different Form & Disposition, Qi & Blood[164]

(1)

The Yellow Emperor asked:

Humans may be either yin or yang. What is a yin person? What is a yang person?

Shao Shi[165] answered:

Between heaven and earth, the number five is indispensable. Man also resonates with it. Therefore, humans cannot be merely divided into yin or yang (types). Roughly speaking, there is the *tai yin* person, the *shao yin* person, the *tai yang* person, the *shao yang* person, and the harmoniously balanced yin/yang person. These five types differ in terms of their bearing as well as in (the quality) of their sinews, bones, blood, or qi.

The *tai yin* person is avaricious, neither compassionate nor humane. He is good at pretending to be modest and generous while hiding his real intentions. He is grasping and not giving, susceptible to oppression without betraying it, and moves but only after (other) people. Such is the *tai yin* person.

The *shao yin* person is less avaricious but has a wicked heart, gloats over losses suffered by others as if he benefitted from them. He does not wince at injuring others, is jealous of others' success, envious, and lacks grace. Such is the *shao yin* person.

The *tai yang* person is easily complacent and self-satisfied, boastful, incompetent but never daunted from big words. He is overambitious and vain, impetuous and rash in handling affairs without regard to reason. He is obstinate and arbitrary in spite of his impotence, never mending his ways ["never knowing repentance" in a variant edition] even after failure. Such is the *tai yang* person.

The *shao yang* person is haughty and vain with apparent prudence and discretion, overweening and fond of self-publicity on acquiring a petty position. He is good at mixing externally but bad at administration. Such is the *shao yang* person.

The harmoniously balanced yin/yang person is calm and quiet in behavior, yet is fearless (in the face of trouble). He is without (excessive) joy or happiness, is tactful and correct but unhurried and easy, uninterested in contention and competition, punctual and orderly but also adaptable, respectful, and humble, polite but not obsequious. This is called consummate (self-)control or culture.

In ancient times, those who used acupuncture/moxibustion inspected the five physiques in people (and used them as the basis of) treatment. Thus in cases of abundance, they applied drainage techniques, and in cases of vacuity, they applied supplementation.

The *tai yin* person has lots of yin but is devoid of yang. His yin blood is turbid, his defensive qi astringent, his yin and yang are in disharmony, his sinews are slack, and his skin is thick. (In this type of situation,) unless rapid needling and draining (techniques are applied), no (illness) can be removed.

The *shao yin* person has lots of yin and scant yang. Their stomach is small but their intestines are large. Their six bowels are not balanced; their *yang ming* vessels are small but their *tai yang* vessels are large. Careful examination is necessary before regulating therapy is administered since the blood of such individuals is liable to desert and their qi is easily spoiled.

The *tai yang* person has lots of yang and no yin. Cautious regulation is necessary in order to drain yang without causing desertion of yin. Otherwise the yang may also desert, leading to mania. If there is a desertion of both yin and yang, there will be sudden death or loss of consciousness.

The *shao yang* person has lots of yang but scant yin. His channels are small and their network vessels are large. His blood is within and their qi is without. Their yin should be made replete and their yang evacuated. Excessive draining of the network vessels leads to sudden death. If qi deserts there will be illness and the central qi will also become insufficient. One cannot recover from such a disease.

In the harmoniously balanced yin/yang person, both the yin and yang qi are harmonious and the blood vessels are regulated. One must carefully study the yin and yang, examine both evil (factors) and the correct qi, calmly (deliberate) their facial expression and appearance, and then examine what is surplus and differentiate that from what is insufficient. Then that which is exuberant can be drained and that which is vacuous can be supplemented. If there is neither fullness or emptiness, choose (points) on the (affected) channel.

This is the regulation of yin and yang based on the differentiation of the five types of people.

The *tai yin* person is described as being sooty black in color, sulky but not reflective. They are tall and bulky and never bend.

The *shao yin* person is described as aloof but conniving and furtive. They conduct (their affairs) in secret. They rise up and are rash and impetuous in the face of danger and move as if in hiding.

The *tai yang* person is described as being haughty and complacent. Their body is straight and their chest protrudes.

The *shao yang* person is described as holding their head up when standing, flinging both arms when walking with both elbows held away from the upper back.

The harmoniously balanced yin/yang person is described as being stately and graceful, polite and courteous, genial, affable, and equanimitous. All of the multitudes call this person a gentleman.

(2)

The Yellow Emperor asked:

When I asked Shao Shi about the yin and yang (types) of people, Shao Shi said, "Between heaven and earth, the number five is indispensable." Thus humans may have five times five or twenty-five shapes or forms depending upon the growth of blood and qi. How are these differentiated and how can one know their interior (*i.e.*, internal organs) by inspection of their exterior?

Qi Bo answered:

One must first establish the five physiques, metal, wood, water, fire, and earth. Then these are subdivided in terms of the five colors and differentiated according to the five notes. This then makes up the twenty-five (types) of people.

The wood form person is analogous to the upper *jue*.[166] He has a green-blue (facial) color, a small head and a long face, broad shoulders with a flat upper back, small, nice hands and feet, and is talented. He is studious, lacks strength, and is fraught with worries. He is diligent, and endures spring and summer but does not endure autumn and winter. (During this time) he is (susceptible to) invasion and thus disease. (This form) is ruled by the foot *jue yin*. They are dignified and amiable.

The big *jue* ["left *jue*" in a variant edition {later editor}] person, analogous to the left foot *shao yang* and, (specifically,) the upper part of the *shao yang*, is obedient.

The right *jue* ["small *jue*" in a variant edition {later editor}] person, analogous to the right foot *shao yang* and, (specifically) the lower part of the *shao yang*, is meek.

The great *jue* ["right *jue*" in a variant edition {later editor}] person, analogous to the right foot *shao yang* and upper part of the *shao yang*, is quiet ["prefers to be in the background" in a variant edition].

The half *jue* person, analogous to the left foot *shao yang* and the lower part of the *shao yang*, is not contracted (*i.e.*, is upright).

The fire form person is analogous to the upper *zhi*,[168] has a red (facial) color, broad paravertebral muscles, a pointed face and small head, well proportioned shoulders, upper back, and thighs, small hands and feet, moves steadily on the earth, is quick witted, rocks when walking, is full fleshed in the shoulders and upper back, hot tempered, generous but neglectful of promises, thoughtful, observant and penetrating, good looking, impatient, is not long-lived but liable to sudden death, and endures spring and summer but does not endure autumn and winter. (During this time) he is susceptible to invasion and hence disease. He is ruled by the hand *shao yin* and has a knack for things ["honest" in a variant edition].

The supreme *zhi* person, analogous to the left hand *tai yang* and upper part of the *tai yang*, is shallow (in character).

The small *zhi* person, analogous to the right hand *tai yang* and the lower part of the *tai yang*, is full of doubt and suspicion.

The right *zhi* person, analogous to the right hand *tai yang* and upper part of the *shao yang*, is buoyant ["animated" in a variant edition].

The half *zhi* person, analogous to the left hand *tai yang* and lower part of the *tai yang*, is wavering, happy go lucky, and of mild disposition.

The earth form person is analogous to the upper *gong*,[168] has a yellow (facial) color, a big head and round face, beautiful shoulders and upper back, a big belly, well shaped legs, and small hands and feet. He has excessive flesh, his upper and lower limbs are mutually well proportioned, he walks calmly upon the earth, and he is reliable and has a calm heart. He is kindhearted and charitable, does not desire power, and endures autumn and winter but does not endure spring and summer. (During this time) they are susceptible to invasion and disease. They are ruled by the foot *tai yin* and have moral integrity.

The supreme *gong* person is analogous to the left foot *yang ming* and the upper part of the *yang ming* and is gentle.

The extra *gong* person is analogous to the left foot *yang ming* and the lower part of the *yang ming*, and is vigorous ["pleasant" in a variant edition].

The small *gong* person is analogous to the right foot *yang ming* and the upper part of the *yang ming* and is changeable.

The left *gong* person is analogous to the right foot *yang ming* and the lower part of the *yang ming* ["top of the *yang ming*" in a variant edition], is hard working ["a common man" in a variant edition].

The metal form person is analogous to the upper (*shang*),[168] has a white (facial) color, a small head and a round face, small shoulders and upper back, small abdomen, and small hands and feet, muscles of the outer ankles like bone, and nimbleness of the bones of the body ["swiftness of movement" in a variant edition]. He is honest and selfless, impatient, quiet yet fierce, and a good candidate for government office. He endures autumn and winter but does not endure spring and summer. (During this time) they are susceptible to invasion and disease. They are ruled by the hand *tai yin* and have moral integrity.

The supreme *shang* person is analogous to the left hand *yang ming* and the upper part of the *yang ming* and is truthful and righteous.

The right *shang* person is analogous to the left hand *yang ming* and the lower part of the *yang ming*, and is gallant.

The left *shang* person is analogous to the right hand *yang ming* and the upper part of the *yang ming* and is perceptive and judicious.

The small *shang* person is analogous to the right hand *yang ming* and the lower part of the *yang ming* and is awe-inspiring.

The water form person is analogous to the upper *yu*,[168] has a black (facial) color, a big head, an uneven face ["curved face" in a variant edition], a large chin, narrow shoulders, a big belly, small ["large" in a variant edition] hands and feet, and swings his body while walking. He has a lowered coccyx and long upper back, is disrespectful, deceitful, and treacherous. He is subject to violent death, endures autumn and winter but does not endure spring and summer. (During this time) he is susceptible to invasion and disease. He is ruled by the foot *shao yin* and is filthy and abject.

The big *yu* person is analogous to the right foot *tai yang* and the upper part of the *tai yang* and is happy and gay.

The small *yu* person is analogous to the left foot *tai yang* and the lower part of the *tai yang* and is constantly oppressed.

The common *yu* person is analogous to the right foot *tai yang* and the lower part of the *tai yang* and is tranquil.

The yoke *yu* person is analogous to the left foot *tai yang* and the upper part of the *tai yang* and is quiet and calm.

The Yellow Emperor asked:

If the form fits but the color does not, what then?

Qi Bo answered:

If either the form overwhelms the color or the color overwhelms the form,[167] one is liable to disease once impaired (by evil) in their starred year.[168] Neglect leads to sorrow (*i.e.*, to death). When form and color are in accord with one another, this ensures happiness and wealth.

The Yellow Emperor asked:

As to the years as they relate to the mutual overwhelming of the form and color, how can this be known?

Qi Bo answered:

A person's great fear recurs every nine years (beginning at) seven years, then sixteen, twenty-five, thirty-four, forty-three, fifty-two, sixty-one, (etc.) These (years) are fearful for all people. (During these times,) one must not fail to attempt to calm oneself. Invasion leads to disease and neglect leads to sorrow (i.e., death).

The Yellow Emperor asked:

As for the vessels above and below and the state of the blood and qi, how can one know these from the form qi?

Qi Bo answered:

(In terms of) the upper foot *yang ming*, exuberance of blood and qi results in a beautiful, long beard. An abundance of blood and little qi leads to a short beard. Abundant qi and scant blood leads to a sparse beard. Scantiness of both blood and qi results in no beard and many creases around both corners of the mouth.

(In terms of) the lower foot *yang ming*, exuberance of blood and qi results in long, beautiful hair in the lower (part of the body). An abundance of blood and scanty qi results in hair in the lower (part of the body) which is beautiful but short and limited to (regions below) the umbilicus and walking with the feet lifted high. There is scant flesh on the big toes and the feet are susceptible to cold. Scant blood and abundant qi result in flesh which is susceptible to chilblains. Scant blood and scant qi results in absence of (body) hair. If there is (hair), it is sparse, withered, and brittle and there is a susceptibility to atonic inversion and foot *bi* or obstruction.[169]

(In terms of) the upper foot *shao yang*, an exuberance of blood and qi leads to long, beautiful whiskers. An abundance of blood and scant qi results in short, beautiful whiskers. Scant blood and an abundance of qi leads to a scanty beard. Scanty blood and qi results in an absence of any beard and a (susceptibility to) invasion leading to *bi* obstruction, bone pain, and withered nails.

(In terms of) the lower foot *shao yang*, an exuberance of blood and qi results in long, beautiful hair on the shins and fat outer ankles. An abundance of blood and scant qi results in short, beautiful hair on the shins, and tough, thick skin on the outer ankle. Scant blood and an abundance of qi results in scant hair on the shins and thin, fragile skin on the outer ankles. Scanty blood and qi result in an absence of hair (on the shins) and skinny outer ankles with no flesh.

(In terms of) the upper foot *tai yang*, an exuberance of blood and qi results in beautiful eyebrow hairs. The eyebrows have long hairs. An abundance of blood and scanty qi results in bad eyebrows and many small creases in the face. Scant blood and an exuberance of qi results in a fleshy face. Harmony between the blood and qi results in beautiful (facial) color.

(In terms of) the lower foot *tai yang*, an exuberance of blood and qi results in fleshy, full heels and sturdy heels. Scant qi and an abundance of blood results in skinny, hollow heels. Scanty blood and qi results in a susceptibility to twisted sinews and pain under the heels (i.e., on the plantar surface).

(In terms of) the upper hand *yang ming*, an exuberance of blood and qi results in a beautiful moustache. Scant blood and an abundance of qi results in a poor moustache. Scanty blood and qi results in an absence of any moustache.

(In terms of) the lower hand *yang ming*, an exuberance of blood and qi results in beautiful hair in the axilla and a fleshy, warm thenar eminence. Scanty qi and blood results in cold and emaciated hands.

(In terms of) the upper hand *shao yang*, an exuberance of blood and qi results in long, beautiful eyebrows and beautiful, (well-)colored ears. Scant blood and qi results in burnt or withered ears with bad color.

(In terms of) the lower hand *shao yang*, an exuberance of blood and qi results in fleshy, warm hands. Scanty blood and qi results in emaciated, cold (hands). Scant qi and an abundance of blood results in emaciated hands with lots of vessels.

(In terms of) the upper hand *tai yang*, an exuberance of blood and qi results in abundant sideburns and a fleshy, smooth or even face. Scanty blood and qi both results in an emaciated, black colored face.

(In terms of) the lower hand *tai yang*, an abundance of blood and qi results in plump palms. Scanty blood and qi results in emaciated, skinny, cold palms.

Yellow and red (complexions) are indicative of an abundance of hot qi. Green-blue and white (complexions) are indicative of scanty hot qi. Black colored (complexions) are indicative of an abundance of blood but scanty qi. Beautiful eyebrows indicate an abundance of blood in the *tai yang*. Flourishing whiskers and beard indicate an abundance of blood in the *shao yang*. A beautiful beard indicates an abundance of blood in the *yang ming*. These are the correspondences. Ordinarily in people, the *tai yang* has more blood and less qi. Ordinarily the *shao yang* has more qi but less blood. Ordinarily the *yang ming* has an abundance of blood and scant qi. Ordinarily the *shao yin* has an abundance of qi and scant blood. Ordinarily the *jue yin* has an abundance of blood and scant qi. And ordinarily the *tai yin* has an abundance of qi and scant blood. These are the constant measures of heaven.

The Yellow Emperor asked:

Are there precepts for needling the twenty-five (types) of persons?

Qi Bo answered:

Those with beautiful eyebrows have an abundance of blood and qi in the *tai yang* vessel. Those with bad eyebrows have scant blood and qi. Those with a fat, lustrous (complexion) have a surplus of blood and qi. Those with a fat but lusterless complexion have a surplus of qi and an insufficiency of blood. Those with an emaciated and lusterless complexion have an insufficiency

of qi and blood. Regulating therapy must be administered based upon careful examination of the relative surplus or insufficiency of the form qi and conditions of normality or abnormality must be taken into account.

The Yellow Emperor asked:

How does one needle according to yin and yang?

Qi Bo answered:

One must palpate the *cun kou* and *ren ying*[170] before regulating yin and yang. One must also palpate along the channels and network vessels in search of congelation, binding, and lack of free flow. These cause pain and obstruction somewhere in the body and, in serious cases, lead to lack of movement and thus congelation. Congelation can be warmed by conducting qi to it[171] but will not be resolved until the blood is harmonized. In case of binding within the network vessels, the vessels are bound and the blood cannot circulate, and this circulation can be facilitated by dredging.[172] Thus it is said: If there is a surplus of qi above, conduct it downward.[173] If there is an insufficiency of qi, it should be pushed towards (where it is insufficient).[174] Where (qi) has lodged and become retarded, it should be met and ushered.[175] Therefore, one must be clear about the flow of channels and tunnels before one is able to oppose (the imbalance). In case of contention between cold and heat, conduct and circulate (the qi). In case of stale blood but without binding, immediately take aim at this.[176] If one is first clearly acquainted with the twenty-five (types) of persons, distinguishing where blood and qi are situated, left and right, above and below, needling will be simply accomplished.

(3)

The Yellow Emperor asked:

(In some cases) the spirit may be spry (*i.e.*, motile) and that, before needling the qi may arrive; (in some cases) the qi may come simultaneously with the needle; in some cases upon withdrawal of the needle, the qi may remain; in some cases the sensation may come only after repeated needling. Upon withdrawal of the needle, the qi may counterflow; or, (in some cases,) the disease may become more serious with repeated needling. Please tell me the reason for various manifestations of these six situations.

Qi Bo answered:

In those persons with double yang, their spirit is spry and their qi is easily activated. They are impressive and awe-inspiring, their speech is glib but they are susceptible to illness. When they walk they lift their feet high, and there is a surplus of the visceral qi of their heart and lung. Their yang qi is slippery, exuberant, and volatile. Thus their spirit is mobile and their qi circulates even before (it is stimulated directly). In those persons with double yang whose spirits do not move in advance, these people have no lack of yin. Those with an abundance of yang are mostly cheerful, while those with an abundance of yin are more irritable. When one is frequently angry but easily appeased, it is said that one has no lack of yin. Because yin and yang are difficult to separate, the spirit cannot move in advance. When yin and yang are harmonious and regulated, the blood and qi flourish, and thus, as soon as the needle is inserted, the qi exits as the needle is inserted. This occurs immediately as soon as the (needle and the qi) meet. In those with an abundance of yin and scant yang, yin qi sinks and the yang qi floats upward. Sinking here means that it is stored internally. Thus when the needle is withdrawn, the qi follows (the withdrawal) and remains behind. In those with abundant yin and scant yang, the qi sinks and moves towards (the needle) with difficulty, therefore one may needle repeatedly before there is sensation. In those whose qi counterflows (in the course of treatment) and whose disease worsens with repeated needling, this has nothing to do with yin or yang qi or the tendency (for the qi) to sink or float. It is lack of technique that should be held responsible. Their form qi has nothing to do with this.

Endnotes

[1] Part 1 is derived from Chap. 8, Vol. 2, *(Spiritual Pivot) Ling Shu*; Part 2 from Chap. 39, *(Basic Questions) Su Wen*; Part 3 from Chap. 8, Vol. 2, *Ling Shu*, the inserted quote being from Chap. 10, *Su Wen*; Part 4 from Chap. 8, *Ling Shu*, the inserted quote from Chap. 78, Vol. 2, *Ling Shu* and Chap. 5, *Su Wen*.

[2] This implies that it is intercourse between male and female which gives birth to a new life.

[3] Unyielding and pliant refers to various pairs of opposites and is an extension of yin and yang.

[4] The basis of life is essence. The interaction of the essences of female yin and male yang to produce new life is called spirit. The realm of sensory input and consciousness is the heart-mind. When recollection or intent becomes fixed and unchanging this is called will. When will and recollection become fixed and form the basis for consideration, this is called thought. When one thinks deeply and plans carefully, this is worry.

[5] Flux here means spermatorrhea in males and vaginal discharge in females.

[6] The *Huang Di Nei Jing Tai Su (The Yellow Emperor's Inner Classic: The Essentials)* in full, one of the earliest versions of the *Nei Jing*. It was collated by Yang Shang-shan in the early years of the 7th Century. See note 4, Foreword by Gao Bao-heng *et al*, for more explanation.

[7] The cardiac ligation is the major connecting vessel of the heart.

[8] Spittle (*tuo*) is the fluid which issues from under the tongue, which lies along the pathway of the foot *shao yin* vessel.

[9] "Qi in the context of the lung is strongly associated with the breath." What is being referred to here are essentially illnesses of the qi manifesting on the level of the breath. "It's qi pertains to . . . ": This is indicative of qi illnesses resulting from a loss of the regulation of the visceral qi. *Su Wen-Xuan Ming Wu Qi Pian (Simple Questions: On the Exposition of the Five Qi)* speaks of "illnesses of the five qi." The heart relates to swallowing, the lung relates to coughing, the liver relates to speech, the spleen relates to belching, and the kidney relates to yawning.

[10] The Chinese word *yao* means to die young or prematurely. However, in English, one cannot say that color or *se* is prematurely dead. One can say a color is faded, but then that does not convey the sense of premature decline leading to untimely death. If one translates the word *se* simply as complexion, then this word becomes meaningless in all its other contexts. Wiseman translates this as a perished complexion, which, while technically accurate, is not very evocative.

[11] Death occurs in the autumn as this is the season of metal which controls liver wood.

[12] This is another name for the *Spritual Pivot*. The titles of the *Basic Questions* and the *Spiritual Pivot* were not established at the time of Huang-fu Mi. See note #4 in the Foreword by Gao Bo-heng.

[13]Yang Shang-shan states that worry occurring in the heart is due to changes affecting the heart. While worry occurring in the lung is the emotion of the lung, since the lung rules autumn, worry is normal during that time. Since the heart rules summer, worry may also arise during that time.

[14]*Yi Xue Gang Mu (The Systematically Arranged Medical Work)* substitutes the word fearfulness for the word hunger in this passage.

[15]Part 1 is from Chap. 44, Vol. 7, *Ling Shu*; Part 2 from Chap. 2, *Su Wen*.

[16]The five changes referred to here are the five seasons, the five phases, the five notes or sounds, the five colors, and the five flavors.

[17]The five seasons are spring, summer, long summer, autumn, and winter.

[18]The ten heavenly stems are *jia* (S1), *yi* (S2), *bing* (S3), *ding* (S4), *wu* (S5), *ji* (S6), *geng* (S7), *xin* (S8), *ren* (S9), and *gui* (S10). They are used to denote the days within the sixty day Chinese cycle.

[19]In the ancient Chinese pentatonic scale, the five notes were *gong, shang, jue, zhi,* and *yu* corresponding to 3, 2, 1, 5, and 6 in numbered musical notation. According to five phase theory, *gong* corresponds to earth, *shang* to metal, *jue* to wood, *zhi* to fire, and *yu* to water. *Gong* is said to be characterized by richness and depth of sound, *shang* by briskness, *jue* by rotundity and fluency, *zhi* by modulation, and *yu* by obscurity and lowness. These tones of different properties are believed to reflect different states of mind and to cause different influences on the five viscera.

[20]In the current version of the *Su Wen*, no such statement is found.

[21]From this point on in the text, these points will be referred to only by their English names, *i.e.*, well, rapids, brook, stream, and confluence points.

[22]Internal changes within the liver refer to a failure in the production of qi and depressive restraint of the qi injuring the liver.

[23]The lung will be scorched and full. This implies that lung heat scorches the lobes of the lung and there is a fullness of qi within the chest.

[24]The *Lei Jing (The Classified Classic)* states: "Storage means storage within (the viscera), and deep means deep and descending. The kidney qi fails to store and accumulate, thus a pouring drainage of deep cold engenders illness."

[25]*Nei ge* refers to a pattern characterized by separation of yin and yang and loss of communication between the interior and the exterior.

[26]According to the control cycle, lung/metal restrains liver/wood. Liver/wood restrains spleen/earth. Spleen/earth restrains kidney/water. And kidney/water restrains heart/fire. According to this progression, disease in one viscus, the kidney for example, is most likely to spread to another viscus of the restrained or controlled phase, *i.e.*, the heart.

[27]Part 1 is from Chap. 2, Vol. 1, *Ling Shu*; Part 2 from Chap. 11, *Su Wen*; and Part 3 from Chap. 29, Vol. 6, *Ling Shu*.

[28]This is the anus.

[29]Also known as the *cun kou* or inch mouth or opening and *mai kou* or vessel opening. This refers to the pulse of the radial artery at the styloid processes.

[30]Speaking of the six bowels here makes little sense but makes for an elegant explanation.

[31]This is taken to mean that all the hand yang channels pass through the supraclavicular fossa.

[32]*Lou*, to leak, here does not imply a problem but is used in the same way one says colloquially in English to take a leak, or urinate.

[33]A well proportioned human face should have equal distances between the front hairline and the bridge of the nose, from the bridge of the nose to its tip, and from the philtrum to the tip of the chin. In a well shaped physique, the height of the head, the length of the feet, and the height of the waist should all be equal.

[34]Part 1 is from Chap. 73, Vol. 11, *Ling Shu*; Part 2 is a combination of parts of Chap. 8, Vol. 2 and Chap. 17, Vol. 4, *Ling Shu* and Chap. 5 & 10, *Su Wen*; and Part 3 is from Chap. 17, Vol. 4, *Ling Shu*.

[35]Wang Bing (710-804 CE) was a talented politician and scholar thanks to whom we have the *Huang Di Nei Jing* or *Su Wen* as it is. It took Wang approximately twelve years to finish collating his version of this preeminent classic.

[36]Spirit here pertains to the vessels and the heart. Brightness pertains to the eye.

[37]In Chinese Medicine, the *yin* (same yin as yin/yang) refer to the anus and urethra in a man and anus and urethra/vaginal meatus in a woman. Thus they are sometimes referred to as the front and rear yin or collectively as the two yin. In this context, yin can also mean secret, as in one's privates or genitalia.

[38]The nine portals is a collective term for the seven portals of the upper body (two eyes, two ears, two nostrils, and mouth) and the two of the lower body (the anus and urethra/vaginal meatus).

[39]*Yong* refers to acute, localized, suppurative, inflammatory lesions involving the skin, subcutaneous tissue, or internal organs.

[40]Barricade blockage is a condition whereby an exuberance of yin and yang results in a separation of yin and yang. The *Shang Han Lun (Treatise on Cold Damage)* written by Zhang Zhong-jing in the Han Dynasty described barricade as being associated with inhibited urination and blockage as being associated with counterflow vomiting. Vomiting and an inability to eat is also referred to as barricade blockage. The *Bing Yuan (An Exposition on External Pathogenic Factors as a Cause of Illness)* which was among the first prescription books), associated constipation with barricade and urinary blockage with blockage. In general, barricade blockage is associated with the physiological manifestation of obstruction.

[41]This entire chapter is a combination of parts of Chap. 47, Vol. 7, *Ling Shu* and Chap. 10, *Su Wen*.

[42]*Bian*, literally, changes

[43]See note 6 above for identification of this text.

[44]*I.e.*, out from under the protection of the lung

[45]Heat in the center, *re zhong*, can also be read as simply "heat within".

[46]Yang Shang-shan comments: "In discussing the heart, eight changes in spirit are listed. Afterwards, when discussing the other four viscera, only visceral changes are mentioned without referring to such changes in spirit. This is because the spirit rules the *hun, po,* reflection, and will. Therefore the discussion of spiritual changes above includes those of the four other viscera. Thus they are already implied and are therefore not discussed here." The so-called changes in spirit are worry, poor memory, irresoluteness, etc., appearing in the text.

[47]*Bi,* a condition mainly manifested by pain, swelling, and stiffness of the muscles and joints similar to rheumatoid and osteoarthritis. It is due to invasion and/or accumulation of cold, heat, wind, dampness, or other evils.

[48]*Xi ben,* homonymous with inverted cup surging in Chinese, refers to a syndrome of asthma and counterflow qi due to lung qi losing its function of depurative downbearing. This results from counterflow ascent of liver qi. See Chap. 3, Book 8.

[49]Similar to inguinal hernia and characterized by intermittent descent of a part of the small intestine into the scrotum. It is called fox-like *shan* since its appearance and disappearance suggests a fox running back and forth into its den.

[50]*Cou li* is commonly translated as "interstices" but here its meaning is different.

[51]There is no consensus about the location of *Jia Che*. Some believe it to be *Jia Che* (St 6), while others suppose it to mean the lower jaw.

[52]It is notable that what is being discussed here are the gross anatomical relationships of the viscera. Contrary to conventional belief, Chinese physicians were clearly concerned with the bowels and viscera as anatomical entities as well as spheres of energetic influence. The above passages also strike one as being particularly poignant in the light of such modern osteopathic techniques as visceral manipulation which both diagnose and treat disease states based upon the relative positioning of the viscera.

[53]In many versions, there are no brackets, but some scholars have produced convincing evidence that this remark was inserted by Lin Yi *et al.*, editors in the Song Dynasty.

[54]*Hou* means both thick and robust; *xi* means both thin and meager. Both connotations are implied here. The viscera in question is either thick walled and robust or thin walled and meager.

[55]Yang channels and vessels are those which are visible from the surface.

[56]This entire chapter is derived from Chap. 1, Vol. 1, *Ling Shu*.

[57]The viscera have no source points, but their *shu* rapids points are regarded and clinically used as source points. The twelve rapids points here include the *shu* transporting points of the five viscera plus *Jiu Wei* (Turtledove Tail, CV 15) and *Qi Hai* (Sea of Qi, CV 6), the source points of the *gao* and *huang*.

[58]Note that not all the twelve source points are located on the limbs as is described in the following paragraph.

[59]This refers to the fact that the lung is a feminine viscus but located in the upper or yang part of the body. The descriptions of the other viscera in this paragraph should be understood in the same way.

[60]Often collectively known as *gao huang,* this refers to the area below the heart but above the diaphragm. Seen separately, *gao* is the fatty membrane below the heart, while *huang* is the membrane just above the diaphragm.

[61]CV 6, more commonly known as *Qi Hai*, Sea of Qi.

[62]Swill diarrhea is diarrhea containing grains which are totally undigested.

[63]This entire chapter is derived from Chap. 12, Vol. 3, *Ling Shu*.

[64]These are the rivers Qing, Wei, Hai, Hu, Ru, Mian, Huai, Ta, Jiang, He, Ji, and Zhang. The identities of these rivers has been the subject of much controversy since there have been many rivers in China with the same name, and rivers in China have undergone tremendous changes over time. For instance, one river may have become two or more, while two may have joined into one.

[65]The author always calls the hand *jue yin* the hand *xin zhu* or heart-governor.

[66]"North to the Hai is yin" may be interpreted to mean that the stomach, the urinary bladder, and the gallbladder pertain to yin since all of them run mainly in the lower part of the body. As the stomach channel travels anterior to the urinary bladder and the gallbladder, the last two are north of the stomach channel (Hai) when the body faces south, the conventionally honored direction on formal occasions in Chinese culture.

[67]"North to the Hu is yin within yin" may be interpreted to mean that the three foot yin channels are yin within yin since all of them mainly travel on the inner or medial aspect of the lower limbs. Since the spleen channel (Huai) runs anterior to the liver and kidney channels, the last two are north of the spleen when the body faces south.

[68]"South to the Zhang is yang" may be interpreted to mean that the pericardium and lung channels belong to yang since both of them run mainly in the upper body and arms. Since the lung channel runs anterior to the pericardium (Zhang) in the arms, it lies south of the latter when the body faces south.

[69]"North to the He till the Zhang is yin within yang" may be interpreted to mean that the pericardium and the lung channels run in the inner aspect or yin of the arms which are yang.

[70]"South of the Ta till the Jiang is yang within yang" may be interpreted to mean that the triple burner and large intestine channels belong to yang since the large part of their journey occurs in the outer or yang aspect of the yang arm. Since the triple burner channel (Ta) is posterior to the large intestine channel (Jiang), it lies north of the latter when the body faces south.

[71]In Chinese medicine, "one exhalation" is often used as a unit of measurement of time. This refers to the time taken by the whole process of one inhalation and one exhalation and the brief interval between the two.

[72]*Qie xun men an*–in this context means taking the pulse; *xun*–palpating in this context means feeling the flesh to determine the size of the vessel and the thickness of the skin. This cannot be determined simply by touching and depressing, hence these four words are used.

[73]The *Lei Jing* states: "Based on the condition, appropriate (action) must emanate from the heart and be reflected in the hand. This reflects the true knack for treating diseases!"

[74]This entire chapter is taken from Chap. 33, Vol. 6, *Ling Shu.*

[75]This point is also named Qi Surge or *Qi Chong.*

[76]*Ya Men* (GV 15) and *Da Zhui* (GV 14) respectively

[77]This implies that the mistake of treating vacuity with drainage and repletion with supplementation should, by all means, be avoided.

[78]Part 1 is derived from Chap. 15, Vol. 4, *Ling Shu*; Part 2 from Chap. 76, Vol. 11, *Ling Shu.*

[79]The twenty-eight constellations were grouped into four clusters. The eastern green dragon area included the constellations *jue, gang, di, fang, xin, wei,* and *ji.* The northern *xuan wu,* a hybrid turtle and snake in Chinese mythology, included *dou, niu, nu, xu, wei, shi,* and *bi.* The western white tiger area included *kui, lou, wei, mao, bi, zi,* and *can.* And the southern red quail area included *jing, gui, liu, xing, zhang, yi,* and *zhen.* The ancients believed that the sun moved around the earth visiting each of the constellations one by one.

[80]These are the twelve regular channels bilaterally making twenty-four channels plus the conception and governing vessels and the yin motility and yang motility vessels for a total of twenty-eight.

[81]One *zhang* is ten *chi* or a hundred *cun.*

[82]The clepsydra was an ancient time keeping instrument which consisted of a kettle-like container with a hole at the bottom from which water was allowed to drip. A stick within the kettle was notched with one hundred divisions. When the water level dropped one notch, this equalled one division or moment in time. It equalled one quarter of an hour.

[83]According to the figures given in this text, the sun moves 0.07466 minutes.

[84]See note 35, Chap. 4, Book 1.

[85]This passage cannot be found in the place referred to by the author.

[86]Also refer to note 79 above. The matches between the heavenly stems, earthly branches, and constellations in relation to the directions, time, and the seasons are as follows:

Earthly branches/months: B1, 11th month; B2, 12th month; B3, 1st month; B4, 2nd month; B5, 3rd month; B6, 4th month; B7, 5th month; B8, 6th month; B9, 7th month; B10, 8th month; B11, 9th month; B12, 10th month

Earthly branches/hours: B1, 11 PM-1 AM; B2, 1-3 AM; B3, 3-5 AM; B4, 5-7 AM; B5, 7-9 AM; B6, 9-11 AM; B7, 11 AM-1 PM; B8, 1-3 PM; B9, 3-5 PM; B10, 5-7 PM; B11, 7-9 PM; B12, 9-11PM

Directions: South, *zhang*; east, *fang & xin*; north, *xu*; west, *bi & mao*

[87]B4 watch, 3-5 AM

[88]The points involved in the journey of the defensive qi include *Jing Ming* (Bl 1), *Shao Ze* (SI 1), *Zu Qiao Yin* (GB 44), *Guan Chong* (TH 1), and *Jia Che* (St 6) respectively.

[89]The artery in the region below the jaw

[90]The points involved in this leg of the defensive qi's journey include *Li Dui* (St 45) and *Shang Yang* (LI 11) respectively.

[91]Note that the hand *yang ming* does not enter the palm but the defensive qi does.

[92]The point involved in this leg of the defensive qi's journey is *Jing Ming* (Bl 1).

[93]From the ancients point of view, the way the sun travelled around in space visiting each of the twenty-eight constellations in turn was like that of a postman calling at various postal stations.

[94]This means that the duration of daylight and darkness is determined according to the season. For instance there is more daylight during the summer than during the winter.

[95]The human qi here is the defensive qi.

[96]The *shao yin* is implied in this context.

[97]A long lost ancient medical classic

[98]This chapter is derived from Chap. 16, Vol. 4, *Ling Shu*.

[99]The pericardium channel

[100]This is described as a passage leading to the brain.

[101]*Ni* may mean counterflow and *shun* may mean correct or suitable flow. However, here used in juxtaposition as a compound term, these words imply a flow which goes up and down, this way and that. *Ni* here does not imply a rebellious or improper flow as it usually does when describing the flow of qi.

[102]This chapter is derived from Chap. 18, Vol. 4, *Ling Shu*.

[103]This refers to the simultaneous meeting of yin and yang, *ying* and *wei*.

[104]Day is yang and the middle of the day is yang within yang.

[105]Night is yin and the middle of the night is yin within yin.

[106]The circulation of constructive qi begins and ends in the *tai yin*. Therefore, this channel is said to rule or govern the interior. The circulation of defensive qi begins and ends in the *tai yang*. Therefore, this channel is said to rule the exterior.

[107]The meeting of the yin differs from double yin, though both occur at midnight. The former implies that both the constructive and defensive are located in the yin phase at that moment.

[108]This refers to the alimentary tract.

[109]The phrase, "Before the qi is settled" implies that although the food has entered the stomach, it has not yet been distilled and refined.

[110]In this scenario, an attack of wind coerces the heat generated by food and drink, which steams open the interstices. This results in an abnormal circulation of defensive qi which in turn is unable to secure the exterior, allowing unbridled perspiration.

[111]The middle burner is understood by most to be located below the upper burner rather than behind it. This is an idiosyncratic perspective on the location of the middle warmer.

[112]Sweat belongs to yang or the defensive. While blood belongs to the constructive. These two, sweat and blood, stand in a interior/exterior relationship to protective and constructive respectively. Loss of either of them means loss of the other pair and life is consequently threatened. Therefore, humankind is said to face two deaths. However, even though one of these in either pair is normal, life is not necessarily secure. Thus, it is understandable to say that humankind does not have two lives.

[113]*I.e.*, the ileum

[114]This is understood to mean that the dregs from the stomach are moved into the large intestine and the water from it is poured into the urinary bladder.

[115]*Ou*, evoking macerated water and grain

[116]*Du*, evoking the free flow of fluids in the lower burner like water within a canal.

[117]Part 1 is derived from Chap. 40, Vol. 6, *Ling Shu*; Part 2 from Chap. 30, Vol. 6, *Ling Shu*.

[118]In this context qi implies air.

[119]In this context yin implies the five viscera.

[120]In this context yang implies the six bowels.

[121]*Luan qi*. Qi can be considered to be chaotic when the clear qi fails to ascend and the turbid qi fails to descend.

[122]See Chap. 8, Book 1.

[123]Because the small intestine, home of the hand *tai yang* channel, is the bowel of receiving bounty, it is the principal organ handling the chyme, *i.e.*, the turbid. Hence the hand *tai yang* is said to receive the turbid most of all.

[124]Because the lung, home of the hand *tai yin*, is the only viscus to let qi, *i.e.*, the clear, in and out, the hand *tai yin* is said to receive the clear more than the other yin viscera.

[125]Because the spleen, home of the foot *tai yin*, is the viscus in charge of conveyance of water and grains and the viscus

[125]to move fluids and humor for the sake of the stomach, the foot *tai yin* is said to be the only viscus to receive the turbid.

[126]This passage concerns the appropriate depth of needle insertion for the various channels.

[127]Here the two genders, male and female are implied.

[128]New life or offspring

[129]This phrase is puzzling and none of the commentaries of the past have given a plausible explanation. There is some speculation that there is a misprint here. It is notable here that fluid (*jin*) and humor (*ye*) are regarded as different things although in many contexts they are not.

[130]The six qi here refers to what is explained in the preceding paragraph, i.e., the essence, qi, fluids, humors, blood, and vessels.

[131]The regions of the six qi are the five viscera, namely the lung, the kidney, the spleen, the liver, and the heart, which each rule the qi, essence, fluids and humor, blood, and vessels respectively.

[132]This chapter is derived from Chap. 36, Vol. 6, *Ling Shu*.

[133]From the Chinese medical point of view, water, when steaming, turns into qi. While qi, when condensed turns into water. Therefore, water is just a form of qi and qi is just a form of water. Thus it follows that urine is water and qi or qi in the form of water.

[134]These are the sea of qi, sea of blood, sea of marrow, and sea of water and grains. Also see Chap. 8, Book. 1,

[135]In this context the qi is understood to be the fluids and humors.

[136]Yin in this context means the urethra and anus.

[137]Here it should be understood that the transformation of urine, sweat, tears, saliva, and marrow essence is normal, while water distention is abnormal.

[138]This chapter is derived from Chap. 39, Vol. 6, *Ling Shu*.

[139]Part 1 is derived from Chap. 49, Vol. 8, *Ling Shu*; Part 2 from Chap. 17, *Su Wen*; and Part 3 from Chap. 10, *Su Wen*.

[140]The chin is referred to as earth.

[141]This means an extraordinarily violent pathogen.

[142]The nasion or root of the nose

[143]The bridge of the nose

[144]The tip of the nose

[145]The area around Welcome Fragrance (*Ying Xiang*, LI 20)

[146]The cheek

[147]This should have been described as the region supralateral to the king of the face or between the nose and the cheekbone.

[148]The philtrum

[149]The region around the jawbone, (*Jia Che*, St 6)

[150]This means that if the colors appear in accordance with the engendering cycle of the five phases the condition is benign. For instance, a black color (water) appearing in the lung region (metal) or a red color (fire) appearing in the liver region (wood) are benign manifestations.

[151]The viscera are often referred to as *guan*, officials, and so the five officials are understood as the five viscera. *Guan* can also be interpreted as a derivative color sense.

[152]This concerns the surfeit of yin and yang. When, for example, yin is prevailing, yang is bound to be insufficient, and, therefore, only by supplementing yang can yin be restored to normalcy.

[153]This means familiarization with ascent and descent, turns and meetings, or the like of yin and yang on the left and right sides of the body.

[154]The statement that the male is associated with the left while the female with the right has a profound implication. Here only color is concerned. A color appearing on the left or developing towards the left in a male is a bad sign, while for a female it is a good sign.

[155]Black is the color of the kidney, and it occupies the area below the forehead, however the area above the nose is reflective of the heart.

[156]The location of the color should have been described as supralateral to the king of the face or tip of the nose.

[157]See note 49, Chap. 5, Book 1.

[158]*Tui* or *tui shan* may be subdivided into four types: 1) intestinal *tui*, 2) testicular *tui*, 3) qi *tui*, and 4) water *tui*. This is an extensive category including swelling in the testicles with hardening or numbness of the scrotum and a dragging pain in the lateral lower abdomen in men. In women it is characterized by heaviness, pain, and distention of the lower abdomen. See the appendix to view the characters for *tui shan*.

[159]This may be an erroneous reference since in females it is the philtrum which is associated with the urinary bladder and uterus rather than the king of the face.

[160]A collective term for conditions mainly characterized by abnormal vaginal discharge.

[161]This sentence implies that a color appearing on the left of the face reflects conditions on the right part of the body and *vice versa*.

[162]The fine or finest essence (qi) is understood to be the pith and quintessence of the viscera. If it is exposed, the color presents a bold shade without mellowness. It is also called the exposure of the true viscus.

[163]This is the small, dried fruit of citron or trifoliate orange which has dropped prematurely and is a common ingredient in many TCM formulas.

[164]Part 1 is derived from Chap. 72, Vol. 12, *Ling Shu*; Part 2 from Chap. 64, Vol. 9, and Chap. 65, Vol. 10, *Ling Shu*; and Part 3 from Chap. 67, Vol. 10, *Ling Shu*.

[165]A legendary figure, supposedly a subject of the Yellow Emperor

[166]The five notes: *jue, zhi, gong, shang,* and *yu,* corresponding to wood, fire, earth, metal, and water respectively. Each of the five notes, however, is divided into five subnotes which are said to share the qualities or properties of that note. *Jue* (wood), for example, is subclassified into *shang jue* or upper *jue,* which is said to cover the whole of *jue* in quality, and four other subnotes, namely, the right upper corner, the right lower corner, the left upper corner, and the left lower corner.

[167]According to five phase theory, a man of fire form may, for example, have a white (metal) complexion. This is called form overwhelming or victorious over color. If he has a black (water) complexion, this is called color victorious over or overwhelming form.

[168]A year which is bad for one's health and which is believed to repeat at regular intervals. See the later sections of the present chapter.

[169]See note 47, Chap. 5, Book 1.

[170]The *ren ying* is the carotid pulse lateral to the laryngeal prominence in the neck. See note 29, Chap. 3, Book 1.

[171]This implies retention of the needle.

[172]This implies the application of bleeding therapy.

[173]This implies the selection of points in the lower part of the body.

[174]This implies selecting points in the upper body and aiding in the ascension of qi by pushing the flesh upward along the channels once the needle is inserted.

[175]This is interpreted by some as meaning that the needling should be administered first where the qi is lodged.

[176]"Immediately take aim at" or attacking promptly may be interpreted as draining or pricking the vessel.

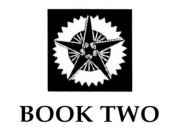

BOOK TWO

Chapter One

The Twelve Channels, Including Their Network Vessels & Branches (Part 1)[1]

Lei Gong[2] asked:

It is stated in the *Jin Mai*[3] that, with respect to needling, (a knowledge of) the channels and vessels is of foremost (importance). Please tell me why this is so.

The Yellow Emperor answered:

The (state of the) channels and vessels determines life or death. Hundreds of diseases are managed (according to their condition), and vacuity and repletion are regulated through them. Therefore one cannot be unfamiliar with them.

The vessel of the lung hand *tai yang* originates within the middle burner and descends to connect with the large intestine. It comes back up along the orifices of the stomach,[4] ascends through the diaphragm, and homes to the lung. From there it proceeds along the pulmonary ligation and moves transversely towards the axilla. It emerges from there, circulating downwards in front of the (hand) *shao yin* channel and the heart-governor channel in the anterior aspect of the upper arm to enter the elbow. It then continues along the anterior aspect of the forearm, passing by the medial border of the styloid process of the radius to submerge at the *cun kou*.[5] It ascends at the fish belly (*i.e.*, the thenar eminence) and, mov-ing along the fish belly, emerges from the tip of the thumb.

A branch diverges from the region distal to the wrist, moving along the radial border of the forefinger and emerging from its tip.

If there are (pathological) changes (within the channel), then there will be illnesses such as distention and fullness of the lung, inflation (*peng peng*, 膨膨),[6] pain in the supraclavicular fossa. In severe cases, the arms will fold (across the chest) and there will be visual distortion (*mao*, 瞀).[7] This is called arm inversion.

If the governing (viscus), the lung, becomes diseased, there will be cough, an ascent of qi, dyspneic rale, heart vexation, fullness in the chest, pain in the radial border of the anterior aspect of the upper arm and forearm, inversion, and heat in the palms. An exuberance of (lung) qi causing a surplus results in pain in the shoulder and the back, injury due to cold, spontaneous sweating in wind stroke, and frequent, scanty urination. A vacuity of (lung) qi results in pain and cold in the shoulder and back, insufficiency of qi causing shortness of breath, and a change in the color of the urine ["sudden violent diarrhea" in a variant version. {later editor}] All of these are illnesses (of the lung).

As for disorders involving any of the twelve channels, if there is an exuberance (of qi), then drain it; if there is a vacuity, then supplement it. If there is heat, (needle it) rapidly; if there is cold, retain (the needle). In the case of sinking (syndrome),[8] employ moxibustion. (In a case with) neither exuberance nor vacuity, select points on the related channel. Exuberance is determined by a *cun kou* pulse which is four times as large as the *ren ying*.[9] Vacuity, on the contrary, is determined by a *cun kou* pulse which is smaller than the *ren ying*.

The vessel of the large intestine hand *yang ming* originates at the tip of radial aspect of the index finger. It goes along the radial side of the finger to emerge between the two bones of the Valley Union (*He Gu*, LI 4) and then moves upwards to submerge between the two sinews. It continues up the radial border of the posterior surface of the forearm to enter the outer side of the elbow. (The large intestine channel) moves further up the radial side of the posterior surface of the upper arm to arrive at the shoulder (joint) where, ascending, it emerges from the anterior aspect of the *yu* bone[10] to rendezvous (with other channels) at the spinal column.[11] From there it proceeds downward, submerging at the supraclavicular fossa to connect with the lung, penetrating the diaphragm and homing to the large intestine.

A branch diverges from the supraclavicular fossa, ascending to the cheek via the neck and then descending to enter the teeth. It emerges again to encircle the mouth. Crossing at the philtrum, the left (channel crosses) to the right and the right to the left. It then ascends past the two nostrils.

If there are (pathological) changes within (the channel), then there will be illnesses such as toothache and swelling in the suborbital region. If the fluid governed (by the large intestine channel) becomes diseased, there will be yellowing of the eyes (along with) dryness of the mouth, runny snivel nosebleed, throat *bi*, pain in the anterior aspect of the shoulder and the anterior aspect of the upper arm, and pain and loss of use of the index finger.

An exuberance and surplus of qi (within the large intestine) is characterized by excessive heat and swelling along the route of the channel. If there is a vacuity of qi, there will be cold shuddering which is difficult to get over.

As for all of the above illnesses, exuberance is determined by a *ren ying* pulse which is four times as large as the *cun kou*; vacuity, on the contrary, is characterized by a *ren ying* pulse which is smaller than the *cun kou*.

The vessel of the stomach foot *yang ming* originates from the nose (and its right and left channels cross) at the root of the nose. It travels across and then beside the *tai yang* channel and runs by the side of the nose to enter the upper teeth. It emerges again to wrap the lips, with its right and left routes crossing at Sauce Receptacle (*Cheng Jiang*, CV 24). It travels below and behind the jowl and emerges at Great Reception (*Da Ying*, St 5). From there it proceeds along the mandibular border, up the region anterior to the ear, past Guest Host Person (*Ke Zhu Ren*, St 6), and then along the hairline to the corner of the forehead.

A branch diverges from in front of Great Reception (*Da Ying*) and goes down to the throat via Man's Prognosis (*Ren Ying*, St 9) to submerge at the supraclavicular fossa. From there it proceeds down through the diaphragm, homing to the stomach, and connecting with the spleen.

The straight branch[12] [a commentary in *Su Wen*, "*Wu Zang Sheng Cheng Pian*" (*Basic Questions: On the Generation & Development of the Five Viscera*) reads "A branch circulates"] deviates at the supraclavicular fossa, travelling down along the medial border of the breast and then alongside of the umbilicus, and finally entering into the qi thoroughfare [also known as *Qi Chong*, St 30, referring to the point of the same name].

Another branch originates at the lower opening of the stomach, travelling down the interior of the abdomen and arriving at the Qi Thoroughfare to join the preceding one. From there it continues downward, passing the anterosuperior portion of the thigh, arriving at the Crouching Rabbit[13] and then enters the knee cap. It continues down along the lateral aspect of the lower leg and, by way of the instep, arrives at the medial aspect of the second toe.

Another branch descends from a point three *cun*

below the knee[14] running downward to submerge at the lateral aspect of the middle toe.

Another branch (diverges) from the instep, enters the big toe and finally emerges at the tip of the toe.

If (there are pathological) changes (within the channel), then there will be illnesses such as quivering with cold, frequent stretching and yawning and a black complexion on the forehead. In a severe case there will be an aversion to the sight of people and fire, alarm and fright at hearing noise made by wood, palpitation, and a preference for privacy with doors and windows shut. If the disease is even more severe, there will be a desire to climb to heights while singing loudly and moving about naked and abdominal distention with thunderous rumbling in the intestines. This is lower leg inversion.

If the blood governed by (the stomach channel) becomes diseased, there will be mania, nue,[15] rampant thermic heat with spontaneous sweating, runny snivel nosebleeding, deviated mouth, labial papules, swelling of the neck, throat bi, enlarged abdomen with water swelling, pain and swelling in the knee cap, pain in the breast, at qi thoroughfare, the upper thigh, at Crouching Rabbit, and the lateral aspect of the lower leg down to the dorsum of the foot. There will also be loss of use of the middle toe.

If there is an exuberance of qi (within the stomach channel), there will be heat all over the front of the body; if there is a surplus of qi within the stomach (organ), grains will be digested swiftly, one will tend to be hungry and the urine will be a yellowish color. If there is an insufficiency of qi, there will be shuddering cold all over the front of the body. If there is cold in the stomach there will be distention and fullness.

As for all the above illnesses, exuberance is characterized by a ren ying pulse which is four times as great as the cun kou; vacuity, on the contrary, is characterized by a ren ying pulse which is smaller than the cun kou.

The vessel of the spleen foot tai yin originates at the tip of the great toe travelling upward along the white flesh of the medial aspect of the toe, past the posterior border of the kernal bone[16] to the front border of the medial malleolus. From there it proceeds upward, entering the calf, travelling along the posterior border of the tibia where it crosses in front of the (foot) jue yin. It ascends further along the anterior border of the medial aspect of the thigh. It enters the abdomen, homes to the spleen, and connects with the stomach. It then ascends through the diaphragm by the side of the throat to link with the root of the tongue, spreading over the underside of the tongue.

A branch diverges from the stomach and, ascending through the diaphragm, pouring into the heart.

If (there are pathological) changes (within the channel), there will be illnesses such as stiffness of the root of the tongue, retching upon intake of food, pain in the venter, abdominal distention, frequent belching and generalized heaviness which are temporarily relieved by defecation or passing flatus.

If the governing (viscus), the spleen, becomes diseased, then there will be pain in the root of the tongue, inability to turn over, failure of food to descend, heart vexation, urgency below the heart,[17] cold nue (虐), thin-stool diarrhea, conglomeration, swill diarrhea, water blockage,[18] jaundice, inability to eat, green-blue lips, pain and swelling in the thigh and knee (which occurs when attempting to) stand up, inversion and loss of use of the great toe.

As for all of the above illnesses, exuberance is characterized by a cun kou pulse which is four times as great as the ren ying; vacuity, on the contrary, is characterized by a cun kou which is smaller than the ren ying.

The vessel of the heart hand shao yin originates within the heart and emerges to home to the heart ligation. It then passes through the diaphragm and descends to connect the small intestine.

A branch follows the heart ligation and ascends

to the throat to link with the ocular ligation[19] [a variant version states "and then crosses the chest and comes out from the lateral costal region", as opposed to "follows the heart ligation"].

Its straight branch goes upward, also following the heart ligation to arrive in the lung, where it descends to emerge at the axilla. It then turns downward along the posterior border of the inner aspect of the upper arm, where it moves behind the (hand) *tai yin* and the heart-governor channels to enter the inner side of the elbow. Then it proceeds along the ulnar border of the anterior aspect of the forearm to the end of the styloid process of the ulna proximal to the palm. From there it enters the ulnar side of the palm, moving along the radial aspect of the small finger to emerge from its tip.

If there are (pathological) changes (within the heart channel), there will be illnesses such as dry throat, heart pain and thirst with desire to drink. This is arm inversion.

If the governing (viscus), the heart, becomes diseased, there will be yellowing of the eyes, fullness and pain in the lateral costal region, pain in the posterior border of the inner aspect of the upper arm and forearm, inversion, and heat and pain in the palm.

As for all the above illnesses, exuberance is determined by a *cun kou* pulse which is three times as large as the *ren ying*; vacuity, on the contrary, is characterized by a *cun kou* which is smaller than the *ren ying*.

The vessel of the small intestine hand *tai yang* originates from the tip of the small finger travelling along the outside of the hand up to the wrist to emerge at the styloid process of the ulna. It travels straight upward along the ulnar border of the forearm to emerge at the inside of the elbow between two bones. From there it proceeds further upward along the posterolateral aspect of the upper arm to emerge at the shoulder joint, wrapping the scapula. (Its right and left routes) cross above the shoulder and it submerges at the supraclavicular fossa, descending to connect with the heart. Following the esophagus it penetrates

the diaphragm to reach the stomach and homes to the small intestine.

A branch (deviates) at the supraclavicular fossa following the neck to the cheek, where it goes to the outer canthus and then enters the ear.

Another branch[20] deviates at the cheek, ascending to the suborbital region, then turning to the nose to reach the inner canthus, obliquely connecting with the zygoma.

If there are (pathological) changes (within the channel), this results in illnesses such as sore throat, swelling of the submandibular region, inability to turn the head, neck pain which feels as if it had ruptured, and upper arm pain which feels as if it had been broken.

If the humor governed (by the small intestine channel) becomes diseased, there will be deafness, yellowing of the eyes, swelling of the cheek, and pain in the neck, submandibular region, shoulder, upper arm, elbow, and the posterior aspect of the forearm.

As for all of the above illnesses, exuberance is determined by a *ren ying* pulse which is three times as great as the *cun kou*; vacuity, on the contrary, is characterized by a *ren ying* which is smaller than the *cun kou*.

The vessel of the urinary bladder foot *tai yang* originates in the inner canthus of the eye and ascends to the forehead where its right and left routes cross at the vertex. A branch diverges from the vertex toward the tip of the auricle.

Its straight branch diverges at the vertex, submerging to connect with the brain, and again emerging to descend to the nape. From there it proceeds along the medial side of the scapula, running parallel to the spinal column into the lumbar region. It then submerges, moving along the backbone, connecting with the kidney and homing to the urinary bladder.

Another branch diverges at the lumbar region, descending to join[21] at the posterior *yin* (i.e., the anus) and then entering the popliteal fossa via the gluteus.

Another branch diverges from around the medial aspect of the scapula, travelling downward along the linking sinews.[22] It passes through the thigh pivot,[23] travelling down the lateral-posterior border of the thigh to join into the hollow of the knee.[24] From there it descends through the calf, emerging out from behind the lateral malleolus along the base of the fifth metatarsal bone and arriving finally to the lateral aspect of the small toe.

If there are (pathological) changes (within the urinary bladder channel), then there will be illnesses such as (qi) surging headache, (pain in the) eyes as if they were about to burst (from their sockets), neck (pain) as if it were being pulled up, spinal pain, lumbar (pain) as if (the back) were broken, an inability to bend the thigh (i.e., hip joint, rigidity of the) popliteal fossa as if it were bound up, and (pain) in the calf as if it were split open. This is malleolus inversion.

If the sinew governed (by the channel) becomes diseased, there will be hemorrhoids, nue, mania, madness, pain in the fontanel, neck, and nape, yellowing of the eyes, lacrimation, runny snivel nosebleeding, pain all the way along the nape, spine, lumbus, sacrococcygeal region, popliteal fossa, calf, and foot, and loss of use of the small toe.

As for all of the above illnesses, exuberance is determined by a ren ying pulse which is three times as great as the cun kou; vacuity, on the contrary, is characterized by a ren ying pulse which is smaller than the cun kou.

The vessel of kidney foot shao yin originates at the underside of the small toe and travels transversely toward the center of the sole. It then emerges from under the navicular bone (Ran Gu, Ki 2) and passing behind to the medial malleolus, it enters the heel. From there it ascends through the calf, moving out from the medial side of the popliteal fossa and ascending along the posterior border of the medial aspect of the thigh. It then links up with the spine to home to the kidney and connect with the urinary bladder.

Its straight branch diverges from the kidney, ascending through the liver and diaphragm to enter the lung. It moves along the throat, bypassing the root of the tongue. [In a variant version it is described as "diverging at the pubic bone, travelling by the side of the umbilicus, up inside the abdomen to enter the lung"].

Another branch emerges from the lung to connect with the heart and pour into the chest.

If there are (pathological) changes (within the channel), there will be illnesses such as hunger with no desire to eat, a soot-black facial complexion, coughing and spitting of blood, dyspneic rale ["noise in the throat" in a variant version], hazy vision in rising from sitting position, and a sensation of the heart being suspended as in hunger. This is bone inversion.

If the governing viscus, the kidney, becomes diseased, there will be heat in the mouth, dry tongue, swelling of the pharynx, ascent of qi, dry and painful throat, heart vexation, heart pain, jaundice, intestinal pi, pain in the spine and posterior border of the medial aspect of the thigh, atonic inversion, somnolence, and heat and pain in the underside of the foot.

If moxibustion is applied, the patient is advised to force down raw meat, to loosen his belt and hair, to carry a large staff, and to walk in shoes with weights.[25]

As for all of the above illnesses, exuberance is determined by a cun kou pulse which is three times as great as the ren ying; on the contrary, vacuity is characterized by a cun kou which is smaller than the ren ying.

The vessel of the heart-governor hand jue yin, originates in the chest and homes to the pericardium. It then travels downward through the diaphragm, connecting sequentially with the three burners.

A branch follows the chest and emerges in the

costal region at a point three *cun* below the axilla. From there it ascends to the axilla and then travels along the anterior aspect of the arm, moving between the (hand) *tai yin* and *shao yin* to enter the elbow. Then it proceeds along the forearm circulating between the two sinews[26] to enter the palm. From there it moves along the middle finger and finally emerges from the tip of the finger.

Another branch diverges in the palm, travelling along the finger next to the small one to emerge from its tip.

If there are (pathological) changes (within the channel), there will be illnesses such as heat in the hand, hypertonicity of the elbow, and swelling of the axilla. In severe cases there will be fullness of the chest and the lateral costal region, a violent stirring of the heart with a rolling sensation, red facial complexion, yellowing of the eyes and incessant laughing.

If the vessel ["the pericardium" in a variant version] governed (by the channel), becomes diseased, there will be heart vexation, heart pain, and heat in the palm.

As for all of the above illnesses, exuberance is determined by a *cun kou* pulse which is twice as great as the *ren ying*. On the contrary, vacuity is characterized by a *cun kou* which is smaller than the *ren ying*.

The vessel of the triple burner hand *shao yang* originates from the tip of the finger next to the small finger. It emerges between the two fingers, travelling across the back of the wrist, between the two bones on the posterior aspect of the forearm, ascending to link with the elbow. It travels along the posterior aspect of the arm to arrive at the shoulder. From there it crosses and moves behind the foot *shao yang* channel, submerging at the supraclavicular fossa to spread over the center of the chest. It then disperses to connect with the pericardium, descending through the diaphragm and homing to the three burners consecutively.

A branch diverges from the center of the chest,

ascending to emerge at the supraclavicular fossa. It then ascends along the nape, curving behind the auricle, and moves straight upward to emerge from the upper aspect of the auricle. From there it turns down and then crosses the cheek to reach the suborbital region.

Another branch diverges from behind the auricle, entering the ear, and emerging anterior to the auricle. It then passes Guest Host Person (*Ke Zhu Ren*) to join the preceding branch at the cheek and ultimately reaches the outer canthus.

If there are (pathological) changes (within the heart-governor channel) there will be illnesses such as deafness, muddleheadedness, swelling of the throat, and throat *bi*.

If the qi governed (by the channel) becomes diseased, there will be spontaneous perspiration, pain in the outer canthus, swelling of the cheek, pain (radiating) along the back of the auricle and the posterior aspect of the shoulder, (down) the upper arm, elbow and forearm, and loss of use of the finger next to the small one.

As for all of the above illnesses, exuberance is determined by a *ren ying* pulse which is twice as large as the *cun kou*; vacuity, on the contrary, is characterized by a *ren ying* pulse which is smaller than the *cun kou*.

The vessel of the gallbladder channel of foot *shao yang* originates at the outer canthus and travels upward to the protrusion of the head.[27] It then descends behind the auricle, moving along the neck and passing in front of the hand *shao yang* to arrive at the shoulder. From there it crosses behind the hand *shao yang* to enter the supraclavicular fossa.

A branch diverges from behind the auricle, entering the ear and emerging in front of the ear to terminate in the region lateral to the outer canthus.

Another branch diverges from the outer canthus descending past Great Reception (*Da Ying*, St 5)[28] to unite with the hand *shao yang* in the suborbital region.[29] From there it descends through Jawbone

(*Jia Che*, St 6) and down the neck to join the preceding branch in the supraclavicular fossa. It then descends into the chest, penetrating the diaphragm, connecting with the liver, and homing to the gallbladder. From there it travels inside the lateral costal region, emerging at the Qi Thoroughfare, circling the region of the pubic hair to transversely enter the hip joint.

Its straight branch diverges at the supraclavicular fossa, travelling down to the axilla, penetrating the chest, and passing the region of the free ribs to join the preceding branch at the hip joint. From there it descends along the yang aspect of the thigh,[30] emerging at the lateral side of the knee, and descends anterior to the outer assisting bone,[31] travelling straight down to the tip of the severed bone.[32]

From there it passes in front of the lateral malleolus, travelling along the instep to emerge at the tip of the toe next to the small one.

Another branch diverges at the instep and enters the big toe. It passes between the first and second metatarsal bone to come out at the tip of the big toe in the aspect proximal to the second toe. From there it turns back into the nail to emerge at the three hairs region.

If there are (pathological) changes (within the gallbladder channel) there will be illnesses such as bitter taste in the mouth. The patient will frequently take great sighing breaths; there will be pain in the heart and lateral costal regions and inability to turn over. In severe cases there will be a slight dusty complexion, sheenless and lusterless skin, and heat in the lateral side of the foot. This is yang inversion.

If the bone governed (by the channel) becomes diseased, there will be headache, pain in the face and submandibular region, pain of the outer canthus, pain and swelling in the supraclavicular fossa, swelling of the axilla, and saber and pearl string lumps (*i.e.*, scrofula), shivering with cold after sweating, and *nue*. There will be pain all along the chest, including the lateral costal region, the lateral aspect of the thigh and knee,

the lower leg, the severed bone and region in front of the lateral malleolus, as well as all the joints on the way. There will also be loss of the use of the toe next to the small toe.

As for all of the above illnesses, exuberance is determined by a *ren ying* pulse which is twice as large as the *cun kou*; on the contrary, vacuity is characterized by a *ren ying* pulse which is smaller than the *cun kou*.

The vessel of the liver foot *jue yin* originates at the border of the three hairs region of the big toe and travels upward along the surface of the instep, through the point one *cun* anterior to the medial malleolus and up to a point eight *cun* above the medial malleolus. From there it crosses behind the (foot) *tai yin* channel, ascending along the medial side of the popliteal fossa and then along the yin [medial] aspect of the thigh, entering the region of the pubic hair and encircling the genitals. It then enters the lateral abdominal region,[33] by passing the stomach, and homes to the liver. It connects with the gallbladder, ascends to penetrate the diaphragm, and spreads over the lateral costal region. From there it passes behind the throat and, entering the nasopharynx, it links with the ocular ligation and ascends to emerge at the forehead and join the governing vessel at the vertex [a variant version reads "it meets the (foot) *tai yin* and *shao yang* in the ilium, and then goes along the spine to enter the third and fourth sacral perforation"].

A branch follows the ocular ligation, then descends inside the cheek, and encircles inside of the lips.

Another branch starts from the liver, penetrates the diaphragm, and ascends to pour into the lung.

If there are (pathological) changes (within the liver channel), then there will be illnesses such as lumbar pain, inability to bend either forward or backward, and *tui shan*[34] in males and lower abdominal swelling in females. [The *Lei Jing (The Classified Classic)* equates this condition with *shan* illness.] In severe cases there will be dry throat, dusty facial complexion, or ghostly complexion.

If its governing (viscus), the liver, becomes diseased, then there will be thoracic fullness, counterflow retching, throughflux diarrhea (*dong xie*, 洞泻),[35] fox-like *shan*, enuresis, and dribbling urinary block.

As for all of the above illnesses, exuberance is determined by a *cun kou* pulse which is twice as large as the *ren ying*; vacuity, on the contrary, is characterized by a *cun kou* which is smaller than the *ren ying*.

If the qi of foot *shao yin* expires, this causes withered bones. The (foot) *shao yin* is the winter vessel.[36] It runs deeply and nurtures the bone marrow. When the bone is not moistened ["softened" in a variant version], the flesh cannot adhere to the bone. Consequently there is a lack of affinity between the bone and the flesh. The flesh becomes sodden and declines (*i.e.*, becomes limp and flaccid). Flesh which is sodden and in decline results in lengthened teeth [*i.e.*, receding gum lines], tartar, and sheenless hair. Sheenless hair implies that the bone is already defunct. Deterioration happens on *wu* days and death on *ji* days, for earth is victorious over water.[37]

If the qi of hand *shao yin* expires, this causes stoppage of the vessels. Stoppage of the vessels impairs blood flow causing lusterless, sheenless hair. Therefore a soot-black complexion ["complexion like a dried faggot" in a variant version] implies that blood is already defunct. Deterioration occurs on *ren* days and death on *gui* days, for water is victorious over fire.[38]

The *Ling Shu*[39] states that the demise of the *shao yin* presents a picture of black facial complexion, lengthened teeth with tartar, abdominal distention and blockage, and stoppage between the upper and the lower (aspects of the body). All these are signs of death.

If the qi of foot *tai yin* expires, this causes a failure of the vessels to nurture the lips of the mouth. The lips of the mouth are the root of the flesh.

Once the vessels cease to nurture, the flesh becomes limp, causing fullness in the philtrum ["tongue atony" in a variant version]. Fullness in the philtrum causes the lips to be outturned. Outturned lips imply that the flesh is already defunct. Deterioration occurs on *jia* days and death on *yi* days, for wood is victorious over earth.[40]

If the qi of hand *tai yin* expires, this results in scorched skin and hair. It is the (hand) *tai yin* that circulates the qi to warm the skin and hair. If the qi fails to circulate, the skin and the hair become scorched. Scorched skin and hair causes an absence of fluid and humor. An absence of fluid and humor injures the skin and articulations. Once the skin and articulations have been injured, the skin withers and the hair becomes brittle. Brittle hair implies that the qi is already defunct. Deterioration occurs on *bing* days and death on *ding* days, for fire is victorious over metal.[41]

The *Jiu Juan (Ninefold Volume)* states: Abdominal distension and block and inability to get a breath (results in) a tendency toward eructation. Eructation brings about retching, retching gives rise to counterflow, and counterflow makes the face red. If counterflow does not occur, however, there must be an obstruction between the upper and the lower. An obstruction between the upper and lower leads to a black facial complexion and scorched skin and hair and means the end (*i.e.*, death).[42]

If the qi of foot *jue yin* expires, this causes the sinews to contract. The (foot) *jue yin* is the vessel of the liver. The liver is associated with the sinews. The sinews converge in the yin organ (*i.e.*, the genitals) and, moreover, its vessel connects the root of the tongue. Therefore, if the channel fails to nurture (the structures under its influence), then the sinews become contracted and tense, causing the retraction of the testicles and the tongue. Therefore, if the lips become green-blue, the tongue curls and the testicles retract. Then the sinews are already defunct. Deterioration occurs on *geng* days and death on *xin* days, for metal is victorious over wood.[43]

The *Jiu Juan* states that heat in the center, dry throat, frequent urination, heart vexation, and in serious cases, retracted testicles mean the end (*i.e.*, death).

When the qi of all five yin (viscera) expires, the ocular ligation rolls. This rolling causes visual dizziness, which implies that the spirit orientation is already defunct. As the spirit orientation is defunct, death comes in one and a half days at the latest.

If the *tai yang* vessel expires, that is the end. The death is preceded by upturned eyes, arched back rigidity, tugging and slackening,[44] a white complexion, and expiry sweating.[45] These all mean the end.

If the *shao yang* vessel expires, that is the end. The death is preceded by deafness, hundreds of articulations will go slack,[46] and the eyes will gape as in fright, reflecting the expiry of the (ocular) ligation. With the expiry of the ocular ligation, death follows in one and a half days. With death, the complexion turns green-blue and white.

If the *yang ming* vessel expires, that is the end. The death is preceded by twitching of the mouth and eyes, susceptibility to fright, raving, a yellow complexion, overexuberance within the channel above and below, and insensitivity (of the skin and muscle). All these mean the end.

If all of the six yang channels expire, yin and yang will separate from one another. If the yin and yang separate from one another causing the interstices to open and drain, this results in expiry sweating in drops big as pearls which seep out but do not roll. This implies that the qi is already defunct. If it happens in the morning, death comes in the evening; if it happens in the evening, death comes the next morning.

These are the manner in which the twelve channels collapse.

Chapter One

The Twelve Channels, Including Their Network Vessels & Branches (Part 2)[47]

(1)

The Yellow Emperor asked:

Of the twelve channels, the hand *tai yin* alone beats constantly. Why is this?

Qi Bo answered:

The foot *yang ming* is the vessel of the stomach. The stomach is the sea of the five viscera and the six bowels. The clear part of its qi ascends to pour into the lung, while the qi of the lung moves along the (hand) *tai yin*. The flow of the lung qi is closely related to breathing, therefore the pulse beats twice for one exhalation and twice for one inhalation as well. As long as the respiration does not cease, the pulse beats without end.[48]

(2)

The Yellow Emperor asked:

Why does the qi opening[49] alone reflect the five viscera?

Qi Bo answered:

The stomach is the sea of water and grain and the major source (of nourishment) for the six bowels. The five flavors enter the mouth and are stored in the stomach in order to nourish the qi of the five viscera. Although the qi opening also belongs to the (hand) *tai yin*,[50] all the qi and flavors of the five viscera and the six bowels come from the stomach. They are transmuted and are then reflected at the qi opening. Likewise, all five qi[51] enter through the nose, and are stored in the lung and the heart. Diseases involving the lung and the heart inhibit (the function of) the nose.[52] [The *Jiu Juan* emphasizes beating, while the *Su Wen* focuses on the qi, which is under the government of the five viscera. The two statements compliment one another.][53]

47

(3)

The Yellow Emperor asked:

The qi passes the *cun kou*. Where is its source in its upper reaches? Where does it submerge and run hidden? By which path does it return (to its beginning)? I do not thoroughly understand these things.

Qi Bo answered:

When qi leaves the viscera, it is as sudden as (an arrow) loosed from a bow or torrents rushing down against the banks of a river. However, when (the qi) arrives in the fish (margin, *i.e., Yu Ji*, Lu 10), it is on the decline. After that, the surplus of the qi diminishes further and becomes dispersed on its ascent upstream. It then circulates onward in a more subtle way.

The Yellow Emperor asked:

What causes the foot *yang ming* (vessel) to beat?

Qi Bo answered:

The stomach qi ascends to pour into the lung. The impetus of the qi[54] which surges into the head flows along the pharynx up to the hollow portals. It follows the ocular ligation to enter and connect with the brain and then emerges at *Han*.[55] From there it travels downward through Guest Host Person (*Ke Zhu Ren*, a.k.a. *Xia Guan*, St 7), along the tooth carriage (*i.e.*, the lower jaw bone). It meets the (foot) *yang ming*, finally descending to Man's Prognosis (*Ren Ying*, St 9). This is a special branch of the stomach qi attached to the (foot) *yang ming*. Therefore (it ensures) that the yin and yang, the upper and the lower[56] beat as one vessel.

Thus yang disease with small yang pulses reflect ominous (*ni*, 逆) conditions. (On the other hand,) yin diseases with a large yin pulse also reflect an ominous condition. The yin and yang should be both quiet and stirring (respectively) as if controlled by a (single) wire. Any incongruity (between them invariably) suggests disease.[57]

The Yellow Emperor asked:

What causes the foot *shao yin* to beat?[58]

Qi Bo answered:

The penetrating vessel is the sea of the twelve channels. Along with the connecting vessel of the (foot) *shao yin*, it originates below the kidney and emerges at the Qi Thoroughfare. It then travels along the medial aspect of the thigh, passing obliquely into the popliteal fossa, and travelling down the medial aspect of the lower leg bone. There it joins the channel of the (foot) *shao yin* and, moving behind the medial malleolus, it enters the sole.

A branch obliquely enters the (medial) malleolus and then emerges at the instep, entering the big toe in order to pour into all of the network vessels and warm the dorsum. This accounts for the constant beating of the vessel (of the foot *shao yin*).[59]

The Yellow Emperor asked:

The defensive qi circulates, linking above and below as if in an endless circuit. Suppose a man is caught unexpectedly by an evil qi or severe cold, such that he loses the use of his hands and feet. At the same time the yin and yang routes of his vessels as well as their meeting (points) and communication between them is in disarray. How can his qi still (manage to) circulate?

Qi Bo answered:

The four extremities are the places where the yin and yang (channels) meet and the sites where the major network vessels of qi travel. The four thoroughfares[60] are the roads along which the qi runs. When the network vessels are severed, these roads are open; and when the congestion in the four extremities is resolved, qi (automatically) resumes its flow there, circulating in a circular manner.

The Yellow Emperor exclaimed:

Very good! So that is what is called an endless circuit. It knows no termination, and upon reaching the end it returns to the beginning. Hence its name.

(4)

The twelve channels circulate deeply along the borders of the flesh. They lie deeply and cannot be seen. The one which can be seen, however, is the foot *tai yin* vessel, as it passes the region superior to the medial malleolus and is not (adequately) covered there. Therefore the vessels at the surface which can commonly be seen are all network vessels. Of the network vessels of the six (hand) channels, the hand *yang ming* and *shao yang* are the major vessels originating between the five fingers. They ascend to meet in the elbow.

When drinking alcohol, the defensive qi circulates first in the skin. It first replenishes the network vessels and these network vessels are the first to become exuberant. Once the defensive qi has leveled off, the constructive qi begins to fill up and then the channels become overexuberant.

An abrupt or violent beating within any of the vessels is indicative of an invasion of pathogenic qi. If the (evil qi) becomes lodged either in the root or in the end (of the channel) and is not moved out, this generates heat. The pulse must be hard, vacuous, or sunken, or otherwise abnormal. This is how one can tell which channel is affected.

Lei Gong asked:

How can the channels be distinguished from the network vessels?

The Yellow Emperor answered:

The channels typically cannot be seen. Vacuity and repletion can be evaluated via the qi opening (*i.e.*, the *cun kou* radial pulse). The vessels which can be seen are the network vessels. None of these network vessels pass through the major joints. They travel along paths which are inaccessible (to the channels), coming and going (to connect with the primary channels) and spreading throughout the skin. The places where these (network vessels) meet one another may be observed

on the exterior of the body.[61] Therefore whenever one needles the network vessels, it is essential to hit their binding places. If (static blood) is severe, although there is as yet no blood binding (*i.e.*, stasis), one must promptly treat (the connecting vessel) to drain (the pathogen) and remove the blood. (If the pathogen) is allowed to become lodged (within the network vessels), this gives rise to *bi*.

In diagnosing the network vessels, if the vessel is green-blue, this indicates cold and pain; if it is red, this indicates heat. When there is cold in the stomach, the vessels in the fish's margin of the hand are usually green-blue; when there is heat in the stomach, the network vessels in the fish's margin are red. Black network vessels in the fish's margin are indicative of enduring *bi*. Red, green-blue, and black motley network vessels are indicative of cold and heat. Short, green-blue network vessels indicate shortage of qi. Whenever needling cold and heat, one must treat the blood network vessels (by bleeding them), and this treatment must be performed once every other day until the static blood is removed completely. Vacuity and repletion must then be regulated. Small, shortened network vessels suggest shortage of qi. In severe cases draining therapy may give rise to oppression. Severe oppression may cause collapse with an inability to speak. Once oppression is felt, the patient should be helped to sit up instantly.

The (connecting) branch of the hand *tai yin* is called Broken Sequence (*Lie Que*, Lu 7).[62] It originates in the parting (of the muscles) in the wrist and, together with the *tai yin* channel, goes straight to enter the palm and disperse in the fish's margin. As for its illnesses, if there is repletion, there will be heat in the palm and the styloid process of the radius; if there is vacuity, there will be yawning, stretching, enuresis, or frequent urination. (To treat it,) select the point one and a half *cun* proximal to the wrist where the branch diverges into the (hand) *yang ming* (*i.e.*, Broken Sequence).

The (connecting) branch of the hand *shao yin* is called Connecting Li (*Tong Li*, Ht 5). At the point one *cun* proximal to the wrist, it diverges and circulates upward, following the channel (of the hand *shao yin*) into the heart. It links with the root of the tongue and homes to the ocular ligation. In the case of repletion the diaphragm will be propped up.[63] In the case of vacuity there will be loss of speech. (To treat it,) select the point one *cun* proximal to the wrist, where the branch diverges to the (hand) *tai yang* (*i.e.*, Connecting Li).

The connecting branch of the hand heart-governor is called Inner Pass (*Nei Guan*, Per 6). At a point two *cun* proximal to the wrist, it diverges at a point between the two sinews and then follows the channel (of the hand heart-governor) upward to link the pericardium and connect the heart ligation.[64] In the case of repletion there will be heart pain; in the case of vacuity there will be heart vexation. (To treat it,) select the point between two sinews (*i.e.*, Inner Pass).

The (connecting) branch of the hand *tai yang* is called Branch to the Correct (*Zhi Zheng*, SI 7). At a point five *cun* to the wrist, it passes internally to pour into the (hand) *shao yin*. A ramification travels upward through the elbow to connect with Shoulder Bone (*Jian Yu*, LI 15). In the case of repletion there will be slackened joints and loss of use of the elbow; in the case of vacuity there will be warts, which are as (numerous and) small as scabbed scabies. (To treat it,) select the branch (*i.e.*, Branch to the Correct).

The (connecting) branch of the hand *yang ming* is called Veering Passageway (*Pian Li*, LI 6). At a point three *cun* from the wrist (crease), it diverges toward the (hand) *tai yin*. One ramification travels upward along the forearm, into the shoulder joint, through the mandible, and finally to the lower teeth. Its other ramification enters the ear to meet the other gathering vessels. In the case of repletion there will be tooth decay and deafness; in the case of vacuity, the teeth will be cold and the diaphragm will be obstructed. (To treat it,) select the branch (*i.e.*, Veering Passageway).

The (connecting) branch of the hand *shao yang* is called Outer Pass (*Wai Guan*, TH 5). At a point

two *cun* to the wrist, it curves outward around the forearm to pour into the chest and unite with the heart-governor channel. In the case of repletion there will be hypertonicity of the elbow; in the case of vacuity there will be loss of use of the elbow. (To treat it,) select the branch (*i.e.*, Outer Pass).

The (connecting) branch of the foot *tai yang* is called Taking Flight (*Fei Yang*, Bl 58). At a point seven *cun* to the (lateral) malleolus it diverges toward the (foot) *shao yin*.

In the case of repletion there will be nasal congestion ["nosebleeding and nasal congestion" in a variant version], headache, and pain in the back; in the case of vacuity there will be runny snivel nosebleeding. (To treat it,) select the branch (*i.e.*, Taking Flight).

The (connecting) branch of the foot *shao yang* is called Bright Light (*Guang Ming*, GB 37). At a point five *cun* above the (lateral) malleolus, it diverges toward the (foot) *jue yin* and then follows the channel (of the foot *shao yang*) down to connect with the dorsum. In the case of repletion there will be inversion; in the case of vacuity there will be atonic limpness and inability to sit up. (To treat it,) select the branch (*i.e.*, Bright Light).

The (connecting) branch of the foot *yang ming* is called Bountiful Bulge (*Feng Long*, St 40). At a point eight *cun* to the (lateral) malleolus, it diverges toward the (foot) *tai yin*. A ramification travels upward along the lateral aspect of the tibia to connect the head and the nape where it unites with the qi of the other channels. It then connects with the throat below. If the illness is one of a counterflow of qi, there will be throat *bi* and sudden loss of voice. In the case of repletion there will be mania and withdrawal; in the case of vacuity there will be a loss of use of the foot and a withered lower leg. To treat it select the branch (*i.e.*, Bountiful Bulge).

The (connecting) branch of the foot *tai yin* is called Offspring of Duke (*Gong Sun*, Sp 4).[65] At one *cun* from the base joint (*i.e.*, the tubercle of the metatarsophalangeal articulation of the big toe), it diverges to the (foot) *yang ming*. A ramification enters the inside to connect with the stomach and the intestines. If there is a counterflow ascent of inversion qi, there will be choleraic disease. In the case of repletion there will be lancinating pain in the intestines; in the case of vacuity there will be drum distention. (To treat it) select the branch (*i.e.*, Offspring of Duke).

The (connecting) branch of the foot *shao yin* is called Large Goblet (*Da Zhong*, Ki 4). Starting from behind the (medial) malleolus, it diverges into the (foot) *tai yang*, wrapping the heel. A ramification follows the channel (of the foot *shao yin*) up to the pericardium and then descends penetrating the lumbar spine. If the illness is one of qi counterflow, there will be vexation and oppression. In the case of repletion there will be dribbling urinary block; in the case of vacuity there will be lumbago. To treat it, select the branch (*i.e.*, Large Goblet).

The (connecting) branch of the foot *jue yin* is called Woodworm Canal (*Li Gou*, Liv 5). At a point five *cun* above the medial malleolus, it diverges into the (foot) *shao yang*. Its ramification follows the channel (of the foot *jue yin*) up to the testicles, binding with the penis. If the illness is one of qi counterflow, there will be swelling of the testicles and sudden *shan*. In the case of repletion there will be a persistent erection and heat in (the penis); in the case of vacuity there will be fulminant itching (of the genitals). (To treat it) select the branch (*i.e.*, Woodworm Canal).

The (connecting) branch of the conception vessel is called Tail Screen (*Wei Yi*).[66] It descends to the turtledove tail (*i.e.,*. the xiphoid process) and disperses in the abdomen. In the case of repletion there will be pain in the skin of the abdomen; in the case of vacuity there will be itching. (To treat it) select the branch (*i.e.*, Tail Screen).

The (connecting) branch of the governing vessel is called Long Strong (*Chang Qiang*, GV 26). It travels parallel to the spine ascending to the nape, dispersing in the head. It then descends and, at the (medial border) of the scapula, it diverges into

the (foot) *tai yang*, penetrating the paravertebral muscles. In the case of repletion there will be stiffness of the spine; in the case of vacuity there will be heaviness and shaking of the head. These are disorders involving the paravertebral region[67] [the preceding seven words are absent from the *Jiu Juan*]. (To treat it) select the branch (*i.e.*, Long Strong).

The major connecting vessel of the spleen is called Great Envelope (*Da Bao*, Sp 20).[68] It emerges three *cun* below Armpit Abyss (*Yuan Ye*, GB 22) and spreads through the lateral costal region. In the case of repletion there will be pain all over the body; in the case of vacuity there will be slackness within the hundred articulations. If the blood vessel appears in a netlike pattern, it should be removed completely.

In regard to these fifteen network vessels, they will invariably be seen in conditions of repletion, while in cases of vacuity they will be submerged. When one looks for them but they are invisible (in their normal locations), one should search above and below (in areas adjacent to the point). The (locations) of the channels within each person varies, and so (the location of the) network vessels vary as well.

(5)

The Yellow Emperor asked:

The skin of the body is divided into (several cutaneous) regions, and the vessels (in each region) have the channels as their signposts. Please tell me the knowledge relevant (to this).

Qi Bo answered:

If one desires to understand the different cutaneous regions, (one must learn) the signs reflecting the distribution of the channels. All the channels function this way. The yang[69] of the *yang ming* is known as *hai fei* (害蜚).[70] This same examining (technique) may be applied to all twelve connecting (channels) both above and below.[71] The superficial network vessels observable in the (*yang ming*) regions constitute all of the network vessels of the *yang ming*. (As to the colors of the vessels,) if green-blue is the cardinal shade, this indicates pain; if black is the cardinal shade, this indicates *bi*; red or yellow indicates heat; if white is the cardinal shade, this indicates cold; if a combination of all five colors can be observed, this indicates chills and fever. When there is an exuberance (of pathogenic qi) within the connecting vessel, the (corresponding) channel will be the next to be visited. This is because yang governs the exterior while yin governs the interior.[72]

The yang of the *shao yang* is known as the gate pivot (*shu zhu*, 枢杼) ["pivot holder" in a variant version]. The superficial vessels observable in the (*shao yang*) regions constitute all of the network vessels of the *shao yang*. When there is an exuberance (of pathogenic qi) within the network vessels, next visited will be the (corresponding) channel. What is in the yang tends to (penetrate) to the interior; what is in the yin emerges and then percolates into the interior. This is the case with each of the channels.[73]

The yang of the *tai yang* is called shutting pivot (*guan shu*, 关枢).[74]

The superficial vessels observable in the (*tai yang*) regions constitute all of the network vessels of the *tai yang*. When there is an exuberance of (pathogenic qi) within the connecting vessel, the (corresponding) channel will be visited next.

The yin[75] of the *shao yin* is called window pivot (*shu ling*, 枢檽).[76]

The superficial vessels observable in the (*shao yin*) regions constitute all of the network vessels of the *shao yin*. When there is an exuberance (of pathogenic qi) within the connecting vessel, the (corresponding) channel will be visited next.

As to the entry of (pathogenic influences) into the channels, these (pathogenic influences) pour from the region of the yang connecting (vessels) into the channels. Upon emerging, these (pathogenic influences) pour from the region of the yin (network vessels) into the bones in the interior.

The yin of the heart-governor is called injured shoulder (*hai jian*).[77] The superficial vessels observable in the regions of the (heart-governor) constitute all of the network vessels of the heart-governor. When there is an exuberance of (pathogenic qi) within the network vessels, the (corresponding) channel will be visited next.

The yin of the *tai yin* is called *guan zhi*.[78] The superficial vessels observable in the (*tai yin*) regions constitute all of the network vessels of the *tai yin*. When there is an exuberance of (pathogenic qi) within the network vessels, the (corresponding) channel will be visited next.[79]

The network vessels of the twelve channels discussed above all belong to the cutaneous regions. Therefore hundreds of diseases will invariably begin here. (Pathogens) must first visit the skin and hair. When a pathogen strikes, it forces open the interstices. Once (the interstices) have been opened it will then visit the network vessels. If it becomes lodged and is not removed, (the pathogen) will be transferred into the channel. If it becomes lodged (within the channel) and is not removed, it will be transferred into the bowels, accumulating in the stomach and the intestines. At the onset of the pathogen just as it had entered the skin, there will be shivering causing the hair to stand on end and open interstices. Once (the pathogen) has invaded the connecting vessel, the vessel becomes exuberant and changes color. Once the pathogen has invaded the channel, the channel becomes exuberant. When the channel becomes vacuous, (the pathogen) has sunken deeper. If (the pathogen) becomes lodged in the sinew and bone and cold prevails, there will be hypertonicity of the sinew and pain in the bone. If heat prevails, the sinews will be slack and the bones wasted. There will be burning flesh, (*rou shuo*, 肉烁)[80] with a cleaving of the major muscle groups (*po jun*, 破䐃)[80] and brittle, dried hair.

The Yellow Emperor asked:

What kinds of disease develop within the twelve cutaneous regions?

Qi Bo answered:

The vessels of the (cutaneous) regions lie within the skin. When a pathogen visits the skin, the interstices are forced open. Once (the interstices) have been forced open, the pathogen may then enter more deeply, visiting the network vessels. Once (the pathogen) fills the connecting vessel, it then pours into the channel. Once (the pathogen) fills the channel, it will enter still deeper and become housed in the bowel or the viscus. Therefore if (the disease lies) in the cutaneous regions and is not cured (in a timely manner), a major disease may develop.

(6)

The Yellow Emperor asked:

In observing the network vessels, their respective colors vary. Why is this?

Qi Bo answered:

The channels have constant colors, while the network vessels do not.

The Yellow Emperor asked:

What are the constant colors for the channels?

Qi Bo answered:

The heart is red, the lung is white, the liver is green-blue, the spleen is yellow, and the kidney is black. These are the colors of their corresponding channels.

The Yellow Emperor asked:

Do the yin and yang[81] network vessels (have the same colors) as their corresponding channels as well?

Qi Bo answered:

The color of the yin network vessels (is the same color) as its corresponding channel. The color of the yang network vessels change and is not constant. It fluctuates in accordance with the four sea-

sons. When cold prevails, (the vessel) congeals, and, when it is so congealed, (the vessel will be) blue-green and black in color. When heat prevails (the vessel) is lubricated and brilliant, and, when it is so lubricated and brilliant, (the vessel will be) yellow or red in color. These colors are normal and do not suggest disease. If all of the five colors can be seen, there is said to be chills and fever.

(7)

The Yellow Emperor asked:

I have heard that humankind is in accord with the way of heaven. Thus (humans) have five viscera internally and these correspond to the five notes, five colors, five flavors, five seasons,[82] and five directions.[83] Humans also have six bowels externally which correspond with the six pitch-pipes.[84] These are analogous to the yin and yang channels[85] and in accordance with the twelve months, twelve *chen*,[86] twelve solar terms of the year,[87] twelve watches,[88] twelve great waters, and the twelve channels. Thus these five viscera and six bowels correspond to the way of heaven.

The twelve channels are responsible for life in humans and the development of illness. They concern the treatment of a person's (illness) and the origins of illness. They must be studied by the beginner and yet provide the skilled (practitioner) with limitations (they cannot exceed). The mediocre (practitioner) finds (the channels) easy (to understand), while the superior practitioner finds them difficult (to understand).[89]

The Yellow Emperor asked:

What are the separations and anastomoses, exits and entrances (of the channels)?

Qi Bo answered:

These (issues) are neglected by the mediocre, while the superior practitioner is familiar with them. Please allow me to inform you about them. The primary (*zheng*, 正) (channel) of the foot *tai yang* diverges (from the main channel) and enters the popliteal fossa. A branch (of the divergent pathway) ascends along its pathway to a point five *cun* below the coccyx and enters the anus. It homes to the urinary bladder and disperses in the kidney. (Another branch of the divergent pathway) continues along the paravertebral sinews and submerges at the region opposite to the heart, dispersing in the inside. A direct branch (of the divergent pathway) ascends along the paravertebral sinews to the nape where it homes to the (foot) *tai yang* channel.[90]

The primary (channel) of the foot *shao yin* reaches the popliteal fossa where it diverges toward and unites with the (foot) *tai yang*. It ascends to the kidney and, at the fourteenth vertebrae, emerges to home to the girdling vessel. A direct branch (of the divergent channel) links the root of the tongue and emerges again at the nape to unite with the (foot) *tai yang*. This is the first union.[91] [The *Jiu Xu {The Nine Hills}* states that the branches of all the yin channels are assumed by some to be the primary.][92]

The primary (channel) of the foot *shao yang* curves around the upper thigh and enters the pubic hair region to join the (foot) *jue yin*. A divergent (channel) enters between the free ribs and travels along the inside of the chest. (This divergent branch) then homes to the gallbladder, dispersing over the liver and penetrating the heart. It continues to ascend, passing by the pharynx where it emerges at the jowl and disperses in the face. It links the ocular ligation and finally joins the (foot) *shao yang* channel at the outer canthus.

The primary (channel) of the foot *jue yin* diverges from the dorsum of the foot. It ascends to the region of the pubic hair to unite with (foot) *shao yang* and continues its course with the (foot) *shao yang*. This is the second union.

The primary (channel) of the foot *yang ming* ascends to the upper thigh, then enters the abdomen. It homes to the stomach, dispersing in the spleen and communicating with the heart above. It proceeds upward, travelling along the pharynx,

emerging from the mouth and arriving at the root of the nose and the suborbital region to link the ocular ligation and join the (primary channel of foot) *yang ming*.

The primary (channel) of the hand *tai yang* points to the earth.[93] It diverges and enters the shoulder joint. It then enters the axilla, travelling toward the heart and finally linking the small intestine.

The primary (channel) of the foot *tai yin* diverges upward to the upper thigh and joins the (foot) *yang ming*, travelling together with its branch up to connect in the throat and penetrate the root of the tongue. This is the third union.

The primary (channel) of the hand *shao yin* diverges from the main channel. This branch travels inward and enters Armpit Abyss (*Yuan Ye*, GB 22) between two sinews, homing to the heart and following the throat up to emerge at the face and join (the hand) *tai yang* at the inner canthus. This is the fourth union.

The primary (channel) of the hand *shao yang* points to heaven.[94] It diverges at the vertex, entering the supraclavicular fossa, descending through the triple burner, and dispersing in the chest.

From the primary (channel) of the hand heart-governor, a channel diverges three *cun* below the axilla.[95] It enters the chest, homing to the triple burner and then coming out to follow the throat. After that, it emerges behind the auricle to join the (hand) *shao yang* below the mastoid bone. This is the fifth union.

The primary (channel) of the hand *yang ming* starts in the hand and travels to the breast. It diverges (from the main channel) at Shoulder Joint (*Jian Yu*, LI 15) to enter the neck bone. It descends to the large intestine, homing to the lung, then following the throat up to emerge at the supraclavicular fossa to join the *yang ming* (channel proper).

(Upon separation from the) primary (channel) of the hand *tai yin*, a divergent channel then enters

Armpit Abyss (*Yuan Ye*, GB 22), travelling in front of the (hand) *shao yin* to enter the lung, and disperses in the large intestine. It emerges at the supraclavicular fossa and then follows the throat to join the (hand) *yang ming*. This is the sixth union.

Chapter Two

Eight Extraordinary Vessels[96]

(1)

The Yellow Emperor asked:

What is the upflow and downflow (*ni shun*, 逆顺) of the vessels?

Qi Bo answered:

The three yin vessels of the hand travel from the viscera towards the hands; the three yang vessels of the hand from the hands towards the head; the three yang vessels of the foot from the head towards the feet; the three yin vessels of the foot from the feet towards the abdomen.

The Yellow Emperor asked:

Why is it that the foot *shao yin* alone circulates downward?[97]

Qi Bo answered:

The penetrating vessel is the sea of the five viscera and the six bowels. The five viscera and six bowels are dependent on it for nourishment. Its upward course emerges at the nasopharynx, percolating into all the yang (channels) and irrigating all the yin (channels). Its downward course pours into the major connecting vessel of the (foot) *shao yin*[98] and emerges at the Qi Thoroughfare. It continues along the posterior border of the medial aspect of the thigh and obliquely enters the popliteal fossa. It then runs hidden inside the tibia to the region posterior to the medial malleolus where it branches into two. The descending

branch joins the (foot) *shao yin* channel, percolating into the three (foot) yin channels; the anterior branch runs hidden to emerge at the joint of the tibia and the tarsus, travelling downward along the upper surface of the foot to enter the big toe, where it percolates into the network vessels and warms the flesh. Therefore, if the branched connecting vessel is bound up, the beating (of the vessel) on the dorsum stops. If there is no beating, then there will be inversion, and if there is inversion, then there will be cold.

The Yellow Emperor asked:

How may (inversion) be identified?

Qi Bo answered:

(Relax the patient) by way of (comforting) words and then palpate (the surface of the foot). If one ascertains whether or not (the vessel there) is beating, then one will know whether (the penetrating vessel) flows normally or abnormally.[99]

(2)

Both the penetrating vessel and the conception vessel originate in the uterus and travel upward inside the spine forming the seas of the channels and the network vessels. Their superficial and exterior courses travel upward along the abdomen ["separately" in a variant version] to meet each other at the throat. They then diverge and connect the lips of the mouth.

When there is an exuberance of both blood and qi, the skin may be replenished and the flesh warmed. If, however, the blood alone is exuberant, the skin is infiltrated and irrigated (with blood) and thus there is hair growth. Women have a surplus of qi and an insufficiency of blood and, as a result, during their menstrual flow they repeatedly experience a desertion of blood which impairs their conception and penetrating vessels. Since the conception vessel and penetrating vessel fail to nurture the lips of the mouth, neither beard nor moustaches grow (on women).

The conception vessel originates below Central

Pole (*Zhong Ji*, CV 3)[100] and ascends to the region of the pubic hair. From there it moves along the interior of the abdomen, through Origin Pass (*Guan Yuan*, CV 4) to the throat. It then ascends to the chin and, moving across the face, enters the eye.

The penetrating vessel originates in the Qi Thoroughfare and joins the channel of the (foot) *shao yin*.[101]

If the conception vessel is diseased, there is, in males, an internal binding resulting in the seven *shan*[102] and, in females, vaginal discharge and concretions and gatherings.

If the penetrating vessel is diseased, there will be qi counterflow and abdominal urgency.

If the governing vessel is diseased, there will be arched-back rigidity. [This explanation and that offered in the *Jiu Juan* complement one another.]

The Yellow Emperor asked:

When people suffer injury to the genitals, the qi of their genitals expires and will not return, causing the loss of the use of the organ. (In this case, a man's) moustache and beard will not leave him and yet in eunuchs alone it will. Why is this?

Qi Bo answered:

Because the eunuch has been deprived of his gathering sinew, his penetrating vessel has been damaged. In his case the lost blood cannot be restored, an internal binding within the skin has occurred, and the lips and mouth cannot be nurtured. As a result, he grows no moustache or beard.

Celestial eunuchs[103] whose conception and penetrating vessels are not exuberant and whose gathering sinews are not well developed have qi but do not have (enough) blood to nurture their lips and mouths, and so they do not grow moustaches or beards. [The description of the governing vessel is not found in the classics. A pertinent treatment which can be found in the "*Ying Qi* {On

Constructive Qi"} from the *Spiritual Pivot* is "What goes onto the forehead, up the vertex, down to the nape, along the spine to the coccyx is the governing vessel." {later editor}]

The *Su Wen* states that the governing vessel originates in the middle of the pubic bone below the lower abdomen. In women it links the court opening which is an orifice located at the upper end of the urethral meatus. From there its connecting vessel diverges, travelling in the genitals to join (the primary channel of the governing vessel) at the perineum and curving behind the perineum it then separately wraps the hip. There it joins (foot) *shao yin* together with the connecting vessel of the (foot) great yang.[104] United with (foot) *shao yin*, it ascends along the posterior border of the medial aspect of the thigh and then runs through the spine to home to the kidney. Together with the (foot) *tai yang*, (another branch) originates at the inner canthus, ascending to the forehead to join (the primary channel) at the vertex. It enters here to connect with the brain, and emerges again to descend separately to the nape. From there it (descends) along the medial border of the scapula, passing parallel to the spine and into the lumbar region. It then penetrates the paravertebral sinews to connect the kidney. In males (the governing vessel) follows the penis to the perineum, but the course of the rest of the vessel is the same as in females. The branch which travels straight upward from the lower abdomen runs through the center of the umbilicus, penetrates the heart, and enters the throat. From there it ascends to the chin, surrounding the lips, and ascends to link with the region just below the center of the eyes.[105]

If (the governing vessel) becomes diseased, there will be a surging ascension (of qi) from the lower abdomen into the heart and resultant (heart) pain and inability to defecate or urinate. This is surging *shan*. In females, there will be infertility, dribbling urinary block, hemorrhoids, enuresis and dry throat. If the governing vessel becomes diseased, it should be treated.

The *Nan Jing* states that the governing vessel originates at a point below Lower Extreme (*Xia Ji*, Ki

11)[106] and travels upward inside the spine to Wind Mansion (*Feng Fu*, GV 16) where it submerges to home to the brain. From there it ascends to the vertex and then moves down the forehead to the nose bridge. It is the sea of the yang vessels.[107]

(3)

The Yellow Emperor asked:

Where does the motility vessel[108] start and terminate, and what kind of qi manages it?

Qi Bo answered:

The motility vessel, a branch of the (foot) *shao yin*, originates in the region posterior to the navicular bone. It ascends to the region above the medial malleolus and then travels straight upwards along the medial aspect of the thigh to enter the genitals. From there it ascends along the inside of the abdomen to enter the supraclavicular fossa. It then proceeds upwards emerging in front of Man's Prognosis (*Ren Ying*, St 9), arriving in the suborbital region, and homing to the inner canthus. It unites with the (foot) *tai yang* and the yang motility vessel. (The two motility vessels) pool their qi and travel together to moisten ["deepen" in a variant version] the eyes; once the qi (of these two channels) fail to nourish one another, the eyes are unable to open.

The Yellow Emperor asked:

The qi (of the motility vessel) circulates solely to the five viscera and not to the six bowels. Why is this?

Qi Bo answered:

Qi never fails to circulate. It circulates forever like the flow of water or the sun and the moon. Therefore the yin vessel nurtures the viscera, while the yang vessel nurtures the bowels. Like an endless circuit, its period is unknown, for upon reaching the end it begins again. The flow of qi irrigates the viscera and the bowels in the interior and moistens the interstices in the exterior.[109]

The Yellow Emperor asked:

The motility vessel is classified into the yin and the yang (vessels) but which is counted?

Qi Bo answered:

For males it is the yang which is counted. For females it is the yin which is counted. The one which is counted in (should be regarded as) the channel, while the one which is not counted in, (should be regarded) as a connecting vessel.[110]

The *Nan Jing* states that the yang motility vessel originates within the heel and ascends along the lateral malleolus to Wind Pool (*Feng Chi*, GB 20).[111] The yin motility vessel also originates in the heel but ascends along the medial malleolus to enter the throat, meeting and joining the penetrating vessel. [These various expositions are cited for the purposes of cross-referencing. {later editor}]

It also says that the yang and yin linking vessels link (all the parts of) the body (into a whole). They collect and store but cannot circulate or irrigate. Therefore the yang linking vessel originates at the meeting place of the yang (channels) and the yin linking vessel originates at the joining place of all the yin (channels).

It also says that the girdling vessel originates in the free ribs, surrounding the body. [The vessels counting from the penetrating vessel on down {to the girdling vessel} are called the eight extraordinary vessels. {later editor}]

It also says that when the yin motility vessel becomes diseased, the yang[112] becomes slack and the yin becomes tense. (On the contrary,) when the yang motility vessel becomes diseased, the yin becomes slack and the yang becomes tense. The yang linking vessel links the yang and the yin linking vessel links the yin. When the yin and yang (linking vessels) can no longer link with one another, there will be melancholy, trance, slackening, and inability to contract and grasp things. When the girdling vessel becomes diseased, there will be abdominal fullness and lumbar dissolution as if one were sitting in water.

These are the diagnostics of the eight (extraordinary) vessels. [The linking vessels and girdling vessels are included. For details, refer to the "Wei Lun (Discourse on Atony)" in the *Su Wen*[113] and the *Jiu Juan*[114].]

Chapter Three

On the Measurements of the Vessels[115]

The Yellow Emperor asked:

Please tell me about the measurements of the channels and vessels.

Qi Bo answered:

The six yang (vessels) of the hand,[116] measured from the hand to the head, are (each) five *chi* in length. Their total length is five (*chi*) times six, which equals three *zhang*. The six yin (vessels) of the hand measured from the hand to the chest are three *chi* and five *cun* in length. Three (*zhang*) times six (channels) equals one *zhang*, eight *chi*, while five (*cun*) times six channels makes three *chi*, for a total of two *zhang* and one *chi*. The six yang (channels) of the foot measured from the head to the foot are eight *zhang* in length. Six times eight (*zhang*) unite to make four *zhang* and eight *chi*. The six yin (channels) of the foot measured from the foot to the chest are six *chi* and five *cun* in length. Six (*chi*) times six (channels) together make three *zhang* and six *chi*, while five (*cun*) times six (channels) together make three *chi* for a total of three *zhang* and nine *chi*. The motility vessels measured from the foot to the eye are each seven *chi* and five *cun* long. Two times seven (*chi*) equals one *zhang* and four *chi*, while two times five (*cun*) equals one *chi* for a total length of one *zhang* and five *chi*.[117] The governing vessel and the conception vessel each measure four *chi* and five *cun* in length. Four (*chi*) twice equals eight *chi*, while five (*cun*) twice equals one *chi* for a total of nine *chi*. (The sum of the lengths of) all the vessels together is sixteen *zhang* and two *chi*. These are the grand tunnels of the qi.[118]

The channels and vessels run through the interior. Their branches which run transversely are the network vessels. The ramifications (*bie*, 别) of the branches are the minute network vessels. If the minute network vessels are exuberant and contain (static) blood, it should be attacked without delay (*i.e.*, use rapid needling technique to eliminate blood stasis). Exuberance should be drained, while vacuity should be supplemented by drinking medicinals.

Chapter Four

Ends (*Biao*, 标) & Origins (*Ben*, 本)[119] of the Twelve Channels[120]

The Yellow Emperor said:

It is the five viscera which store essence, spirit, ethereal soul (*hun*), and corporeal soul (*po*), while it is the six bowels which receive water and grain and transform this material (into nutrients). The qi travels internally throughout the five viscera and externally connects the limbs and joints. The floating qi which does not travel inside the channels is the defensive qi, whereas the essential qi which circulates within the channels is the constructive qi. With yin and yang following one another, the interior and the exterior connect to form an endless ring-like circuit flowing forever.[121] Who (on earth) is familiar with the mysteries (of the circuit)? Aside from dividing (the channels) into yin and yang, they may be discriminated as to the locations of the roots and ends whether they are (in a state of) vacuity or repletion, and as to the locations of the separating (and meeting) places. In discriminating (the categories) of yin and yang within the twelve channels, one may understand the genesis of disease. In identifying where vacuity and repletion lies, the position of the disease may be ascertained. In knowing the qi thoroughfares[122] of the six bowels, one may understand how to resolve the entanglements at the right door. If one is able to determine vacuity and repletion based on the hardness and softness (of the affected area), one will know where to apply supplementation and drainage. If one knows the roots and the ends of the six channels (of yin and yang), there will be no perplexing (illnesses) under heaven.[123]

Qi Bo responded:

How profound is the discourse of the holy emperor! Please allow your subject to further detail (the origins and ends of the channels).

The origin of the foot *tai yang* lies at a point five *cun* above the heel, and its ends are in the Gate of Life, (*i.e.*, Bright Eyes [*Jing Ming*, Bl 1]). The Gate of Life is the eye.

The origin of the foot *shao yin* lies at a point three *cun* above the medial malleolus (Intersection Reach [*Jiao Xin*, Ki 8]) and it's ends are in its associated back point (Kidney Shu [*Shen Shu*, Bl 23]) and the two vessels beneath the tongue (Ridge Spring [*Lian Quan*, CV 23]).[124]

The origin of the foot *shao yang* lies within (the point) Yin Portal (*Qiao Yin*, GB 44) and its end is in front of the Window Panel (*Chuang Long*,[125] which is essentially) the ear. [The *Qian Jin* (*Essential Formulas Worth a Thousand Taels of Gold*) by Sun Si-miao says that the Window Panel is the vertical vessel anterior to the auricle, which may be felt pulsating when palpated with the hand. {later editor}]

The origin of the foot *yang ming* is (the point) Severe Mouth (*Li Dui*, St 45) and its end is Man's Prognosis (*Ren Ying*, St 9) by the side of the nasopharynx under the cheek. [The *Jiu Juan* places the end at Man's Prognosis (*Ren Ying*) on the cheek by the nasopharynx.[126] {later editor}][127]

The origin of the foot *jue yin* lies five *cun* above Moving Between (*Xing Jian*, Liv 2)[128] and its end is in its associated back point (*Gan Shu*, Bl 18).

The origin of the foot *tai yin* lies (at the point Three Yin Crossing [*San Yin Jiao*, Sp 6]) four *cun* anterior to Mound Center (*Zhong Feng*, Liv 4), and its ends are in its associated back point (*Pi Shu*, Bl 20) and the root of the tongue.

The origin of the hand *tai yang* lies on the dorsal surface of the styloid process of the ulna[129] and its end lies at the point one *cun* above the Life Gate (*i.e.*, Bright Eyes, *Jing Ming*). [The *Su Wen* places this point three *cun* above the life gate. The *Qian Jin* says that the Life Gate is one *cun* to the heart. {later editor}]

The origin of the hand *shao yang* lies two *cun* above the space between the little and ring fingers (at Humor Gate [*Ye Men*, TH 2]), and its ends lie in the point posterior to the upper tip of the auricle (at Angle Vertex [*Jiao Sun*, TH 20]) and the point below the outer canthus (Silk Bamboo Hole [*Si Zhu Kong*, TH 23]).

The origin of the hand *yang ming* lies in the point within the elbow bones (Pool at the Bend [*Qu Chi*, LI 11]) (below) and in Divergent Yang (*Bie Yang*)[130] above, while its end lies below the cheek at the collar iron (*qian*, 钳).[131]

The origin of the hand *tai yin* lies at the *cun kou*[132] and its end lies at a point below and in front of the axilla (at Celestial Storehouse [*Tian Fu*, Lu 3]) at a pulsing vessel.

The origin of the hand *shao yin* lies at the end of the styloid process of the ulna (at Spirit Gate [*Shen Men*, Ht 7]) and its end lies in its associated back point, (Heart Transport [*Xin Shu*, Bl 15]).

The origin of the hand heart-governor lies in the point proximal to the wrist between the two sinews, (Inner Pass [*Nei Guan*, Per 6]) and its end is at the point three *cun* below the axilla, (Celestial Pool [*Tian Chi*, Per 1]).

In examining these (origins and ends) they are as follows: If there is vacuity below there is inversion, while if there is exuberance below there is heat. If there is vacuity above there is dizziness, while if there is exuberance above there is heat and pain. Therefore, in the case of repletion, (treat it via) exhaustion and arrest,[133] while in the case of vacuity, (treat it via) conduction and promotion.[134, 135]

Please allow me to speak (further) on the qi thoroughfares.[136]

The stomach qi has its thoroughfare; the abdominal qi has its thoroughfare; the qi of the head has its thoroughfare; and the qi of the lower leg has its thoroughfare. When qi (becomes lodged) in the head, a cure is found in the brain.[137] When qi (becomes lodged) in the chest, a cure is found in the breast and the back points;[138] when qi lodges in the abdomen, a cure is found in the back points,[139] the penetrating vessel, and the pulsing vessels left and right of umbilicus.[140] When the qi (becomes lodged) in the lower leg, a cure is found at Qi Thoroughfare (*Qi Jie*, a.k.a. *Qi Chong*, St 30) and Mountain Support (*Cheng Shan*, Bl 57) as well as above and below the malleoli.

In needling (the qi thoroughfares), the filiform needle is used. Before (inserting the needle), it is necessary to press the points and maintain the pressure for a long time until a response is felt in the hand (of the practitioner). Those (illnesses) which may be needled are headache, dizziness and collapse, abdominal pain, fullness in the center, and fulminant distention. Recent accumulations with pain, if movable, are easy to treat, but accumulation without pain is difficult to treat.[141]

Chapter Five

Roots (*Gen*, 根) & Terminations (*Jie*, 结) of the Twelve Channels[142]

The Yellow Emperor said:

Heaven and earth act upon one another, and cold and heat supersede one another. As to the amount of yin and yang, which is smaller and which is greater? Yin's share consists of odd (numbers), while yang's share consists of even (numbers). Suppose (an illness) develops during the spring and summer, when there is less yin qi and more yang qi. Given that there is a lack of regulation between yin and yang, what (conditions) should be supplemented and what (conditions) should be drained? Suppose (an illness) arises during the autumn and winter when there is less yang qi and more yin qi and when the yin qi is exuberant while the yang qi is in decline. At that time the stems and leaves of the plants are withered and the rainwater seeps downward and saturates (the soil). Given that (the illness) is one of a separation of yin and yang, what (conditions) should be supplemented and what (conditions) should be drained? Extraordinary pathogens assail the channels in countless ways. Ignorance of the roots and terminations (and their physiological relationships with the) five viscera and the six bowels (during treatment) wrecks the passes, damages the pivots, and causes failures in opening and closure. Once there has been a substantial loss of yin and yang, they cannot be restored.[143]

The most important aspects of the nine needles (treatment modality) lie in the endpoints and origins. If one has knowledge of the endpoints and origins, then with one word one may have mastery (of needling). Without the knowledge of endpoints and origins, mastery in the way of needling is out of the question.

The (foot) *tai yang* is rooted at Reaching Yin (*Zhi Yin*, Bl 67) and it terminates at life gate[144] which is the eye.

The (foot) *yang ming* is rooted at Severe Mouth (*Li Dui*, St 45) and it terminates at the nasopharynx. The nasopharynx (is called) the great vices, and the great vices are the ears.[145]

The (foot) *shao yang* is rooted at Portal of Yin (*Qiao Yin*, GB 44) and it terminates at the window panel. The window panel is the ear.

Tai yang is the opening, *yang ming* is the closure, and *shao yang* is the pivot. When the opening has been wrecked, the soft tissue and articulations are corrupted and, as a result, sudden disease breaks out.[146] Therefore, in the case of sudden disease, the *tai yang* should be chosen (and treated) based on whether the condition is one of surplus or insufficiency. By corruption, it is meant that the skin and flesh become slack, dried, emaciated, and weak.

When the closure has been wrecked, qi cannot be checked and so cannot be reproduced (*qi wu suo zhi xi*, 气无所止息),[147] and this gives rise to atonic disease. In the case of atonic disease, the *yang ming* should be chosen (and treated) based on whether the condition is one of surplus or insufficiency.

Failure to check and reproduce itself means that the true qi is hindered, while the evil has taken up residence.

When the pivot has been wrecked, bone shaking occurs and one is unable to stand calmly on the earth. In the case of bone shaking, the *shao yang* should be chosen (and treated) based on whether the condition is one of either surplus or insufficiency. Bone shaking means that the joints are slack and fail to contract.[148]

(Regarding the above syndromes,) the problem should be traced back to its root.

The (foot) *tai yin* has its root in Hidden White (*Yin Bai*, Sp 1) and it terminates at Supreme Granary (*Tai Cang*, CV 12).

The (foot) *jue yin* is rooted at Large Pile (*Da Dun*, Liv 1), and it terminates at Jade Hall (*Yu Tang*, CV 18) and connects with Central Altar (*Dan Zhong*, CV 17). [The *Su Wen* substitutes the character *zhong* for *luo*. Thus the line reads ". . . and terminates at *Dan Zhong*"].

The (foot) *shao yin* is rooted at Gushing Spring (*Yong Quan*, KI 1) and it terminates at Ridge Spring (*Lian Quan*, CV 23).

Tai yin is the opening, *jue yin* is the closure, and *shao yin* is the pivot. Therefore, when the opening has been wrecked, the granaries fail to transport and diaphragmatic throughflux diarrhea (*ge dong*, 膈洞)[149] results. In the case of diaphragmatic throughflux diarrhea, choose the *tai yin* (for treatment) based on whether the condition is one of surplus or insufficiency. Once the opening has been wrecked, the qi becomes insufficient and disease is generated.

When the closure has been wrecked the qi runs loose and one is apt to be sentimental. In the case of such sentimentality, choose the *jue yin* (and

treat it) based on whether the condition is one of surplus or insufficiency.

When the pivot has been wrecked, the vessels bind up and cease to flow freely. In the case of such a lack of free flow, choose *shao yin* (and treat it) based on whether the condition is one of surplus or insufficiency. If any bind is found it should be removed completely.

The foot *tai yang* is rooted at Reaching Yin (*Zhi Yin*, Bl 67) and flows to Capital Bone (*Jing Gu*, BL 64), pouring into Kun Lun Mountain (*Kun Lun*, Bl 60) and emerging at Celestial Pillar (*Tian Zhu*, Bl 10) and Taking Flight (*Fei Yang*, Bl 58).

The foot *shao yang* is rooted at Portal Yin (*Qiao Yin*, GB 44) and flows to Hill Ruins (*Qiu Xu*, GB 40), pouring into Yang Assistance (*Yang Fu*, GB 38) and emerging at Celestial Surge (*Tian Chong*, GB 9) and Bright Light (*Guang Ming*, GB 37).

The foot *yang ming* is rooted at Severe Mouth (*Li Dui*, St 45) and flows to Thoroughfare Yang (*Chong Yang*, St 42), pouring into Lower Mound (*Xia Ling*, St 36) and emerging at Man's Prognosis (*Ren Ying*, St 9) and Bountiful Bulge (*Feng Long*, St 40).

The hand *tai yin* is rooted at Lesser Marsh (*Shao Ze*, SI 1) and flows to Yang Valley (*Yang Gu*, SI 5), pouring into Lesser Sea (*Shao Hai*)[150] and emerging at Celestial Window (*Tian Chuang*, SI 16) [this is possibly mistaken, {later editor}[151]] and Branch to the Correct (*Zhi Zheng*, SI 7).

The hand *shao yang* is rooted at Passage Hub (*Guan Chong*, TH 1) and flows to Yang Pool (*Yang Chi*, TH 4), pouring into Branch Ditch (*Zhi Gou*, TH 6) and emerging at Celestial Window (*Tian You*, TH 16) and Outer Pass (*Wai Guan*, TH 5).

The hand *yang ming* is rooted at Shang Yang (*Shang Yang*, LI 1) and flows to Uniting Valley (*He Gu*, LI 4), pouring into Yang Ravine (*Yang Xi*, LI 5) and emerging at Protuberance Assistant (*Fu Tu*, LI 18) and Veering Passageway (*Pian Li*, LI 6).

The above are the so called roots (*ben*) of the

twelve channels. They should be treated when the network vessels are exuberant.[152]

Chapter Six

Channel Sinews[153]

The sinew of the foot *tai yang* originates at the small toe. It ascends to bind at the (lateral) malleolus and then moves obliquely further up to bind in the knee. Its lower aspect travels along the lateral aspect of the foot to bind at the heel and ascends past the heel to bind at the popliteal fossa. Its divergent branch binds at the lateral aspect of the calf and then travels towards the medial border of the popliteal fossa. In the popliteal fossa it joins the sinew proper and from there it ascends to bind at the hip. It then ascends running parallel to the spine to arrive in the nape. One of its ramifications (*zhi*, 支) diverges inward to bind at the root of the tongue. The straight ramification binds at the occipital bone, ascending to the head and then down along the forehead to bind at the nose. Another ramification forms the upper ocular ligation[154] which descends to bind at the suborbital region. Yet another ramification starts from the region posterior and lateral to the axilla to bind at the shoulder bone. Another ramification enters the axilla, and, upon emerging from the supraclavicular fossa, it ascends upward to bind at the completion bone (*i.e.*, the mastoid process) of the temporal bone. Another ramification leaves the supraclavicular fossa and then ascends obliquely to enter the suborbital region.

Illnesses (involving this sinew include) dragging pain between the small toe and the heel, hypertonicity of the popliteal fossa, arched back rigidity, tension of the nape sinew, inability to raise the shoulder, and propping of the axilla initiating a contracting pain in the supraclavicular fossa with inability to move (the axilla and the supraclavicular fossa) left or right. In treatment, surprise manipulation with the red-hot needle[155] is effective and should be performed repeatedly at the points of pain until recovery. (The syndrome) is called mid spring *bi*.

The sinew of the foot *shao yang* originates from the toe next to the small one and ascends, converging in the lateral malleolus. It then ascends running along the lateral aspect of the lower leg to bind at the lateral border of the knee. One of its branches diverges from the outer assisting bone, ascending along the thigh. Its anterior (branch) binds at the crouching rabbit, (*i.e.*, the thigh) and its posterior (ramification binds at) the sacrum. A straight branch ascends across the lateral abdomen and the region of the free ribs and then travels along the anterior aspect of the axilla going up to link with the breast and bind at the supraclavicular fossa. A (ramification) of this straight branch emerges from the axilla to penetrate the supraclavicular fossa and emerges in front of the *tai yang* (sinew). It then runs behind the ear and ascends to the corner of the forehead where (the ramifications on either side of the body) join at the vertex. From there it turns downward into the submandibular region and at the same time it passes upward to bind at the suborbital region. Its branch binds at the outer canthus, forming the outer connecting system.

Illnesses (involving this sinew) include cramps of the toe next to the small toe triggering cramps in the outer aspect of the knee, inability to stretch or bend the knee, tension of the popliteal sinew affecting the anterior aspect of the thigh and the sacrum at the back, provoking pain along the lateral abdomen and the lateral costal region and triggering tension of the sinew up through the supraclavicular fossa, to the breast, nipple, and neck. (If the illness) runs from the left toward the right, the right eye cannot open[156] since the sinew passes through the right corner of the head. And after joining the motility vessel, the left route connects with the right one and, subsequently, injury to the left corner of the head can disable the right foot. This is called crossing the linking sinew. In treating (the above), surprise manipulation with the red-hot needle is effective. It should be performed at the painful places such as the points and repeated until recovery. The syndrome is termed as early spring *bi*.

The sinew of the foot *yang ming* originates at the

third (middle) toe and ascends to bind at the instep. It ascends obliquely and laterally to the (outer) assisting bone, ascending further to bind at the lateral aspect of the knee. It then continues straight upward to bind at the hip joint, and from there it runs up to the lateral costal region and homes to the spine. A straight (branch) ascends along the tibia to bind at the knee. A ramification of this straight branch binds at the outer assisting bone and unites with the (sinew of) the *shao yang*. The straight branch continues to ascend along the crouching rabbit, converging in the upper thigh and, gathering in the the genitals, it then ascends and spreads over the abdomen. It reaches the supraclavicular fossa and binds there, then ascends along the neck and, surrounding the mouth, it unites with (other sinews) at the suborbital region. From there it descends to bind with the nose and then turns up to unite with (the sinew of) the (foot) *tai yang*. The *tai yang* (sinew) forms the rim of the upper eyelid, while the *yang ming* (sinew) forms the rim of lower eyelid. A branch from the cheek binds in front of the auricle.

Illnesses (involving this sinew) include spasms of the sinew of the middle toe provoking spasms in the lower leg, twitching and rigidity of the foot, spasm of the crouching rabbit, swelling of the anterior part of the thigh, *tui shan*, tension of the abdominal sinew radiating up to the supraclavicular fossa and cheek, and sudden deviated mouth. In the acute case there will be an inability to shut the eyes and, if there is heat, there will be slackness and dyskinesia of the sinew and inability to open the eyes. If the sinew of the cheek is cold it will become tense, pulling the cheek and dislocating the mouth, whereas heat (in the cheek) will cause the sinew to become slack and disabled resulting in deviation (of the cheek and mouth. The deviation) can be treated with horse's lard. (Apply the) lard to the tense cheek and apply a tincture of alcohol with cinnamon to the slack one, all the while pulling with the mulberry hook. (Have the patient) sit opposite to a pot containing a live mulberry charcoal fire which is placed level (with his cheek). The fire heats up his tense cheek (which is covered with the lard), and all the while (the patient is instructed to) drink

wine and eat cooked meat. If one is a teetotaler, they should, nevertheless, be enjoined to force the wine down. Throughout the course of their therapy, massage should be applied. (If treated in) this manner the disorder is sure to yield.[157]

In treating (sinew illnesses of this channel in general), surprise manipulation with the red-hot needle is effective. It should be performed at the points of pain and repeated until recovery. This syndrome is called late spring *bi*.

The sinew of the foot *tai yin* originates at the tip of the medial aspect of the big toe and ascends to bind at the medial malleolus. A straight (branch) ascends to bind at the inner assisting bone, then ascends along the medial aspect of the thigh to bind at the upper thigh and gather at the genitals. From there it ascends to the abdomen, converging in the umbilicus, and, running along the inside of the abdomen, it then binds in the lateral costal region and disperses in the chest. An interior branch runs all along the spine.

Illnesses (involving this sinew) include contracture of the big toe with pain in the medial malleolus and spasms of the sinew. There may be pain in the inner assisting bone at the medial side of the knee, pain in the medial aspect of the thigh which radiates to the hip, wrenching pain in the genitals which radiates upward to the umbilical region, pain in the lateral costal regions, and pain in the breast and the spine. In treatment, surprise manipulation with the red-hot needle is effective and should be performed repeatedly at the places of pain until recovery. This syndrome is termed as middle autumn *bi*. [The *Tai Su (Primary Origination)* calls this early spring *bi*.]

The sinew of the foot *shao yin* originates at the inferior aspect of the small toe and then enters the center of the sole. It joins with the sinew of the foot *tai yin*, traveling obliquely towards the region inferior to the medial malleolus to bind at the heel. There it joins and follows the sinew of the (foot) *tai yang* upward to bind below the inner assisting bone.[158] Joining the sinew of the (foot) *tai yin*, it ascends along the medial aspect of the thigh to converge at the genitals. It then runs from the medial border of the paravertebral muscles to the nape converging at the occipital bone and joining the sinew of the foot *tai yang*.

Illnesses involving (this sinew channel) include spasms of the plantar part of the foot, and pain and spasms of the sinews along the entire course of the channel and all of its bindings. If the sinew proper is diseased, epilepsy, tugging, and tetany mainly result. If the illness is in the outer aspect of the body, one cannot bend forward; if the illness is in the inner aspect of the body, one cannot bend backward. That is to say, when the yang is diseased, there is arched back rigidity and an inability to bend forward, while if the yin is diseased the body cannot bend backward.[159] To treat (the above), surprise manipulation with the red-hot needle is effective, and should be performed repeatedly at the places of pain until recovery. For problems found in the interior, ironing, cultivation of qi,[160] and drinking medication is indicated. If the sinew turns and twists[161] too frequently, the case is fatal and cannot be cured. This syndrome is called early autumn *bi*. [The *Su Wen* calls this pattern midautumn *bi*.]

The sinew of the foot *jue yin* originates at the big toe and ascends to bind at the region in front of the medial malleolus. It continues upward along the tibia to bind at the region below the inner assisting bone. From there it ascends along the medial aspect of the thigh to bind at the genitals and connect all the sinews there.

Illnesses involving (this sinew) includes spasms of the big toe triggering pain in the region anterior to the medial malleolus, pain in the inner assisting bone, pain in the medial aspect of the thigh with spasms of the sinew, and loss of use of the yin organ. If there is damage to the interior, the penis cannot effect an erection. If there is damage due to cold, the testicles retract. If there is damage due to heat, (the penis) remains erect and does not contract. Treatment efforts should be directed at circulating water and clearing the yin qi.[162] In the case of illnesses characterized by spasms of the sinew, surprise manipulation with the red-hot needle is effective and should be performed repeatedly at the places of pain until

recovery. This syndrome is called late autumn *bi*.

The sinew of the hand *tai yang* originates at the small finger, converging at the wrist, and ascends along the inner aspect of the forearm up to bind at the inside of the elbow behind the olecranon, a place which, when flicked [*tan*, as in testing for a reflex], will elicit a response in the small finger. Finally it enters and binds at the axilla. A branch travels along the posterior border of the axilla, onto the scapula, and then along the neck where it goes in front of the sinew of the foot *tai yang* to bind at the completion bone (the mastoid process) behind the ear. Another branch enters the ear. Its straight (branch) emerges above the ear, descending to bind at the submandibular region below and then turning upward to home to the outer canthus.

Illnesses (involving this sinew) include spasms of the small finger triggering pain on the inner side of the elbow in the region proximal to the olecranon which travels along the anterior aspect of the arm and into the axilla. Thus there will be axillary pain, pain in the region posterior to the axilla, pain around the scapula, dragging pain in the neck and ringing in the ear, dragging pain in the submandibular region, and the eyes will be closed for a long time before one is able to see.[163]

If the neck sinew is tense, there is atony of the sinew, while if there is swelling in the neck, there is cold and heat in the neck.[164]

In treating (the above illnesses) surprise manipulation with a red-hot needle is effective and should be performed repeatedly at the points of pain until recovery. If the swelling persists, the sharp needle should be employed.

Another branch (of the channel sinew) travels upward to the teeth opposite the cheek wherefrom it passes the region anterior to the auricle to home to the outer canthus and then through *Han* to bind at the corner of the head. Syndromes involving the branch include spasms along the length of the branch. In treatment, surprise manipulation with the red-hot needle is effective and should be performed repeatedly at the points of pain until recovery. The illness is called mid-summer *bi*.

The sinew of the hand *shao yang* originates from the tip of the finger next to the small one. It binds at the wrist and then travels up the forearm to bind at the elbow. From there it proceeds upward, curving around the posterior aspect of the upper arm, travelling up the shoulder and moving past the neck to unite with (the sinew of) the hand *tai yang*. A branch ascends to the curve of the cheek (*qu jia*, i.e., the coracious process of the mandible) and enters the root of the tongue. Another branch ascends past the curve of the teeth (*qu ya*, i.e., the teeth opposite the cheek, the front molars) where it passes in front of the ear and homes to the outer canthus. It then ascends past *Han* to bind at the corner of the head.

Illnesses (involving this sinew) include spasms of the sinew along the length (of the channel) and retracted tongue. In treatment, surprise manipulation with a red-hot needle is effective and should be performed repeatedly at the points of pain until recovery. The illness is called late summer *bi*.

The sinew of the hand *yang ming* originates at the tip of the finger next to the thumb and binds at the wrist. It then ascends along the forearm to bind at the outer aspect of the elbow. From there it ascends, wrapping the upper arm, to bind at the shoulder bone. A branch wraps the scapula and then travels parallel to the spine. A straight branch leaves the shoulder bone and ascends to the neck. Another branch ascends to the cheek to bind at the suborbital region. From there a straight branch emerges in front of (the sinew of) the hand *tai yang*, rising to the left corner of the head to connect the head and then descending to the right submandibular region.[165]

Illnesses (involving this sinew) include a dragging pain and spasms of the sinew along the length of the channel, inability to raise the shoulder, and inability to turn the neck to the left or right to see. In treatment surprise manipulation with a red-hot needle is effective and should be performed repeatedly at the points of pain until recovery. The illness is called early summer *bi*.

The sinew of the hand *tai yin* originates at the thumb, and ascends along the finger to bind proximal to the fish's margin. It then travels past the outer border of the *cun kou* and ascends along the forearm to bind at the anterior side of the elbow. From there it ascends along the inner aspect of the upper arm where it enters the axilla and emerges at the supraclavicular fossa to bind in front of the shoulder bone. Above, it binds at the supraclavicular fossa and below it binds at the inside of the chest where it disperses over and penetrates the cardia.[166] It then unites with (the sinew of the hand *jue yin*) at the lateral costal region and terminates in the region of the free ribs.

Illnesses (involving this sinew) include spasms of the sinew and pain along the length of the channel and, in the case of the inverted cup syndrome,[167] lateral costal tension, and ejection of blood. In treating the above, surprise manipulation with a red-hot needle is effective and should be performed repeatedly at the points of pain until recovery. The syndrome is called midwinter *bi*.

The sinew of the hand heart-governor originates at the middle finger and travels together with the sinew of the (hand) *tai yin* to bind at the inner side of the elbow. It then travels up the anterior border of the upper arm to bind at the axilla where it disperses downward, passing both in front of and behind lateral costal region. Its branch enters the axilla to disperse in the chest and bind at the cardia.

Illnesses (involving this sinew) include spasms and pain along the length of the channel, chest pain, and inverted cup syndrome. In treatment, surprise manipulation with a red-hot needle is effective and should be performed repeatedly at the points of pain until recovery. The syndrome is called early winter *bi*.

The sinew of the hand *shao yin* originates from the inside (radial aspect) of the small finger and ascends to bind at the styloid process of the ulna. Further up it binds at the inner side of the elbow and then ascends to enter the axilla. After crossing the (sinew of the hand) *tai yin*, it runs inside the breast, converging in the chest and penetrating the cardia to link with the umbilicus.

Illnesses (involving the sinew) include a sense of urgent restraint in the interior (of the thoracic cavity) and deep-lying beam below the heart causing a binding of the elbow. Illnesses may include spasms and pain along the length of the channel. In treatment, surprise manipulation with a red-hot needle is effective and should be preformed repeatedly at the places of pain until recovery. If deep-lying beam has developed with ejection of blood and pus, the condition is fatal and cannot be cured. The illness is called late winter bi.[168]

As for diseases of the channel sinews (in general), if there is cold there will be arched back rigidity and sinew tension. If there is heat there will be slackness and dyskinesia of the sinew and inability of the penis to produce an erection. Yang tension leads to arched back rigidity, while yin tension to a posture which is bent forward where one cannot stretch out. Red-hot needling is for tension due to cold. Heat results in slackness and debility of the sinew, so surprise manipulation with the red-hot needle is not indicated.

As for the foot yang ming and the hand tai yang, sinew tension leads to deviation of the mouth and eye, tense canthi, and inability to see promptly. To treat this apply the above treatment modalities.

Chapter Seven

Measurements of the Bones & Intestines and Capacities of the Stomach & Intestines[169]

(1)

The Yellow Emperor asked:

The "Mai Du (Vessel Measures)"[170] deal with the lengths of the channels and the vessels. How are these (measurements) established?

Bo Gao answered:

The size, breadth, and length of the bones and

articulations is measured first. The measurements of the channels and vessels are then determined.

The Yellow Emperor asked:

Take for instance a man seven chi and five cun in height. What are the size and length of his bones?

Bo Gao answered:

The great bone of the head [neck in a variant version, {later editor}] measures two chi and six cun in circumference.[171] The circumference of the chest is four chi and five cun. The circumference of the waist is four chi and two cun.

The part (of the head) that is covered by hair is one chi and two cun from the forehead to the nape. It is one chi from the hair to (the tip of) the chin and this divided (into three equal parts) in a gentleman.[172]

From the throat knot[173] to the point between the supraclavicular fossa is four cun in length.[174] From the supraclavicular fossa to (the lower end of) the xiphoid process is nine cun in length. The greater this distance, the larger the lung, and the smaller this distance is, the smaller the lung. From the xiphoid process to Celestial Pivot (Tian Shu, St 25) is eight cun in length. The greater this distance, the larger the stomach; the smaller this distance, the smaller the stomach. From the Celestial Pivot to the pubic bone is six and a half cun in length. The greater this distance, the longer and broader the large intestine. The shorter this distance the shorter and narrower it is.

The pubic bone is six and a half cun in length. From the upper margin of the pubic bone to the inner assisting bone is one chi and eight cun in length. From the upper margin of the inner assisting bone down to it's lower margin is three and a half cun in length. From the lower margin of the inner assisting bone to the medial malleolus is one chi and three cun in length. From the medial malleolus to the ground is one chi and three cun. From the popliteal fossa to the instep is one chi and six cun in length. From the instep to the ground is three cun. The larger the circumference of a bone, the larger the bone is. The smaller (the circumference) the smaller it is.

It is one *chi* from the corner of the head to the pillar bone,[175] and it is four *cun* from there to the hidden place in the axilla.[176] From the axilla to (the lower border of) the region of the free ribs[177] is one *chi* and two *cun* in length. From the free ribs to the hip joint is six *cun* in length. From the hip joint to the midpoint (of the lateral side) of the knee it is one *chi* and nine *cun*. From the knee to the lateral malleolus it is one *chi* and six *cun*. From the lateral malleolus to the capital bone [the base of the fifth metatarsal] is three *cun* and from there to the ground is one *cun*.

(The space between) the two completion bones posterior to the auricles is nine *cun* in width. (The space between) the two ear gates[178] in front of the ears is one *chi* and two *cun* in width [three *cun* in a variant version. {later editor}] (The space between) the two cheeks is nine and a half *cun*[179] in width [seven *cun* in the *Jiu Xu (Nine Hills)*. {later editor}] The (space between the) two nipples is nine and a half *cun* in width. The (space between) the two thighs is six and a half *cun* in width.[180] The length of the foot is one *chi* and two *cun*, and the width of the foot is four and a half *cun*.

From the shoulder to the elbow is one *chi* and seven *cun* in length. From the elbow to the wrist is one *chi* and two point five *cun* in length. From the wrist to the base joint of the middle finger is four *cun* in length. From the base joint to the tip (of the finger) is four and a half *cun* in length.

From the nuchal hairline to the spinal bone[181] is three and a half *cun* [two *cun* in a variant version. {later editor}] From the spinal bone to the coccyx with the twenty-one vertebrae (in between) it is three *chi* in length. The first vertebra is one *cun* four and one tenth *fen* in length, and the length of the first seven veterbrae is nine *cun* eight and seven eighths of *fen*. The residue after the division of the total spinal length is shared by the inferior vertebrae.[182]

These are the measurements of the bones in an ordinary human, which may be employed to establish the length of the channels and vessels. In examining the channels and vessels in the body, the (vessels) which are superficial and tight or are bright and large ones are indicative of an abundance of blood. Those (vessels) which are fine and deep ones are indicative of an abundance of qi. These are the lengths of the channels.[183]

(2)

The Yellow Emperor asked:

Please tell me about the conveyance of grains within the six bowels. What is the size and length of the intestines and stomach, and what is their capacity for receiving grains?

Bo Gao answered:

The depth, distance, and length covered by the grain from entrance to exit (in various organs) are as follows: The distance from the lips to the teeth is nine *fen* and the width of the mouth is two and a half *cun*. The depth from the teeth to the epiglottis is three and a half *cun*, and (this cavity) has a capacity of five *he*.[184] The tongue weighs ten taels, is seven *cun* in length, and two and a half *cun* in width. The pharynx[185] weighs ten taels and is two and a half *cun* in width. From (the pharynx) to the stomach it is one *chi* and six *cun* in length. The stomach is curved and bent and, when stretched (to its full length), it measures two *chi* and six *cun* in length, one *chi* and five *cun* in circumference, and five *cun* in diameter with a capacity of three [two in a variant version {later editor}] *dou* and five *sheng*.

The small intestine is attached to the spine and begins by turning left, its coils overlapping one another, then pouring downward to join the large intestine and attach itself to the umbilicus in the front (of the body). It has sixteen coils which twist and bend. It is two and a half *cun* in circumference, eight *fen* and a little less than one half a *fen* in diameter, and three *zhang* and two *chi* [three *chi* in a variant version {later editor}] in length. The large intestine begins by turning left at the umbilicus, its coils turning round and round and then descends. There are sixteen coils which are four *cun* in circumference, one and a little less than a half *cun* in diameter, and two *zhang* and one *chi* in length. The broad intestine is attached to the spine to receive the large intestine where it coils left moving from above downward. It is eight *cun* in circumference at its broadest point, two and a little more than a half a *cun* in diameter, and two *chi* eight *cun* in length. From entrance to exit (including) the intestines and stomach measure six *zhang*, four *cun*, and four *fen* and have thirty-two coils.[186]

(3)

The Yellow Emperor asked:

If a person does not eat for seven days they will die. Why is this?

Bo Gao answers:

The stomach is one *chi* and five *cun* in perimeter, five *cun* in diameter, two *chi* and six *cun* in length, and has a capacity of three *dou* and five *sheng* of grain and water. Ordinarily it can contain two *dou* of grain, and one *dou* and five *sheng* of water before it becomes full. The upper burner dissipates the qi from which the finest essence is buoyant and swift, volatile and impetuous, and disturbed. The lower burner irrigates, discharging (what is left) into the small intestine. The small intestine is two and a half *cun* in circumference, eight and a little less than one half a *fen* in diameter, and three *zhang* and two *chi* in length. It has a capacity to receive two *dou* and four *sheng* of grain and six *sheng* and a little more than three and a half *he* of water. The large intestine is four *cun* in circumference, one and a little less than a half *cun* in diameter, and two *zhang* and one *chi* in length. It has a capacity to receive one *dou* of grain and seven and a half *sheng* of water. The broad intestine is eight *cun* in circumference, two and a little more than a half *cun* in diameter, and two *chi* and eight *cun* in length. It has a capacity to receive nine *sheng* and three and one eighth *he* of grain. The total length of the intestines and stomach is five *zhang* eight *chi* and four *cun*, and

they have a capacity to receive nine *dou* two *sheng*, one and a little more than a half *he* of water and grain. This is the amount of water and grain that the intestines and stomach can hold.

In ordinary people, however, this is not the case. (Generally) when the stomach is filled up, the intestines are empty (*xu*), while when the intestines are filled up, the stomach is empty. Under such conditions, the qi moves up and down (freely), the five viscera are quiet and calm, the blood vessels are in harmony and disinhibited, and (as a result) the essence spirit is in equilibrium. This is because spirit is the essential qi from grain and water. Ordinarily the intestines and stomach contain two *dou* and four *sheng* of grain and one *dou* and five *sheng* of water. People defecate twice daily and each elimination is two and a half *sheng*, totaling five *sheng* in a day. Five (*sheng* times) seven (days) is equal to three *dou* and five *sheng* and this denotes the exhaustion of grain and water (within the body). Therefore if a person does not drink or eat for seven (consecutive) days, they will die. The water, grain, essence, qi, fluid, and humor have all become exhausted and on the seventh day one naturally dies.

Endnotes

[1] The whole chapter is a combination of parts of Chap. 10, Vol. 3 and Chap. 9, Vol. 2, *Ling Shu (Spiritual Pivot).*

[2] See note 3, author's preface.

[3] See Chap. 48, Vol. 8, *Ling Shu.* The *Jin Mai* is the title of Chapter 48 of the *Ling Shu* but in the most current edition of the *Ling Shu* it is titled *Jin Fu (Prohibition of Importation [of Medicine]).*

[4] This is understood to be the upper and the lower openings of the stomach.

[5] This phrase can be interpreted in two ways. The symptoms which follow may be understood as the result of an external pathogen or as the result of pathological changes of an internal nature. The passage as it appears within the text is meant to convey both ideas.

[6] *Peng peng* implies a failure of qi diffusion and distended enlargement of the lung.

[7]Wiseman defines *mao* as visual distortion, however a textual annotation adds that *mao* may also mean cardiac vexation.

[8]Falling or sinking here is referred to as a syndrome of insufficiency of the yang qi in which the vessel or pulse is sunken or deep lying.

[9]The *cun kou* refers to the *cun kou* on the hand *tai yin* channel which governs the yin. The *ren ying* refers to the point Man's Prognosis (St 9) on the foot *yang ming* channel which governs the yang.

[10]A.k.a. Shoulder Bone (*Jian Yu*, LI 15)

[11]Point Great Vertebra (*Da Zhui*, GV 14) in the back of the neck is implied. Note that the term "meeting" or "rendezvous" throughout the book never fails to imply that a number of channels, vessels or some other entities join in a place, and that Great Vertebra is the rendezvous for six yang channels.

[12]A straight branch implies a channel which travels in essentially a straight line and does not curve or run transversely along its course.

[13]The Crouching Rabbit is the flesh above the knee.

[14]*I.e.*, at Leg Three Li (*Zu San Li*, St 36)

[15]Strictly speaking, the rendering of "malaria" for "*nue*" in Chinese medicine is misleading, for *nue*, in a wide sense, covers any syndrome characterized by alternating fever and chills, and, therefore, it has a wider application than malaria in modern Western medicine. Hence we have chosen not to translate this term.

[16]*Yi Xue Gang Mu* (*Systematically Arranged Medical Work*) defines this bone as being two *cun* posterior to the joint of the great toe and three *cun* anterior to the medial malleolus. It is as big around as a date seed and lies at the border of the red and white flesh. It is the head of the first metatarsal.

[17]*Ling Shu* and *Mai Jing* (*Pulse Classic*) specify pain below the heart.

[18]Since the spleen is diseased, it cannot nourish the urinary bladder and thus urination is inhibited.

[19]The ocular ligation is a structure which includes blood vessels and nerves to link the eyes and the brain. It is essentially the optic nerve.

[20]Some versions say "a straight branch".

[21]Like the word "meet" or "meeting", the term "join" or "joining" often suggests that some channels or vessels meet at a given location unless it is explained otherwise.

[22]*I.e.*, the paravertebral muscles

[23]*I.e.*, the hip joint

[24]*I.e.*, the popliteal fossa

[25]Book 8 of the *Tai Su* specifies that raw food (*sheng shi*) should be consumed. Book 6 of the *Mai Jing* says (the patient will) become sick (*sheng hai*). Another annotation says (*yi zuo rou*) eat meat. This passage is rather vague and open to interpretation. Loosening of the belt allows free flow within the kidney and lumbar region. Loosening of the hair allows for the free ascent of the yang qi and the diffusion of fire qi. The *tai yang* channel runs down the shoulder and arm. In the case of kidney disease, carrying a large staff permits the free flow of fire qi in the shoulder and arm. The weights referred to here are magnets, the weight of which is gradually increased to benefit the flow of fire qi.

[26]The tendons of the muscular palmaris longus and muscular flexor carpi radialis.

[27]This is the frontal eminence.

[28]Here the region of the cheekbone is implied.

[29]This branch is described in a variant version as "diverging from the outer canthus, directly ascending to meet the hand *shao yang* in the suborbital region."

[30]*I.e.*, the lateral aspect of the thigh

[31]*I.e.* the fibula

[32]The *Lei Jing Shi Er Jing Mai* (*The The Classified Classic: On the Twelve Channels & Vessels*) commentary states: The bony region above the lateral malleolus is called the severed bone, and the tip of the severed bone is the point Yang Assistance, (*Yang Fu*, GB 38). The severed bone in this context refers to the lower portion of the tibia.

[33]Nigel Wiseman translates *shao fu* as lower abdomen.

[34]See Book I, Chap. 15, note 159.

[35]Throughflux diarrhea is characterized by incessant diarrhea with generalized heaviness, chest dis-

tress, absence of thirst, little or no abdominal pain, and scanty dark urine.

36According to the five phases, the *shao yin* kidney corresponds to water, north, and the winter season.

37Since the *wu* and *ji* days are associated with earth and the kidney is analogous to water, it may be easily understood that from the point of view of the five phases restraining cycle that disease involving the kidney is dangerous on these days. Long summer, for example, pertains to earth, and therefore it is also a precarious and dangerous period for the kidney.

38The *ren* and *gui* days are associated with water and the hand *shao yin*, *i.e.* the heart, pertains to fire.

39The mention of the *Ling Shu* is quite incompatible with the author's habit of calling this medical classic the *Jiu Juan (Ninefold Volume)*. Therefore, it may well be the blunder of some unknown careless editor.

40The *jia* and *yi* days are associated with wood while the foot *tai yin*, *i.e.* the spleen, pertains to earth.

41The *bing* and *ding* days are associated with fire while the lung pertains to metal.

42According to the *Lei Jing*, a lack of counterflow means that there is an obstruction in the middle impeding the free flow of qi. If the spleen qi is impaired, it cannot control water, and this results in a black facial color. If the lung qi is impaired, the articulations do not allow circulation and this leads to scorched skin and hair.

43The *geng* and *xin* days are associated with metal while the liver pertains to wood.

44Tugging and slackening, *qi zong*. Tension within the sinews is qi, and, when the sinews become slack, this is *zong*. When the hands and feet alternate between contracture and relaxation, this is tugging and slackening.

45 Sweat breaking out in big drops which strangely do not run.

46The reference here is to the three hundred and sixty five articulations cited in the *Nei Jing*.

47Part 1 is derived from Chap. 62, Vol. 9, *Ling Shu*; Part 2 from Chap. 11, *Su Wen*; Part 3 from Chap. 62, Vol. 9, *Ling Shu*; Part 4 from Chap. 10, Vol. 3, *Ling Shu*;

Part 5 from Chap. 56, *Su Wen*; Part 6 from Chap. 57, *Su Wen*; and Part 7 from Chap. 11, Vol. 3, *Ling Shu*.

48This passage points out the intimate relationship between the hand *tai yin* and foot *yang ming* channels. The stomach is the sea of water and grains and transforms their finest essence. This clear qi ascends to the lung where it is mixed with air to produce ancestral qi. The circulation of qi therefore begins in the lung and, from there, circulates throughout the entire body, returning to the lung to repeat the circuit. This continual production and circulation of qi is the reason the hand *tai yin* beats constantly. It pumps qi in much the same way that the heart pumps blood.

49The term qi opening has many implications. First, it suggests a window which shows the rise and fall, the exuberance and insufficiency of qi, since the hand *tai yin*, *i.e.*, the lung, governs all kinds of qi. Secondly, the lung faces hundreds of vessels and the qi opening is just the converging place of all these vessels.

50It is implied that qi from grain and water has to be first transported to the lung, the governing viscus of the hand *tai yin*, which takes the responsibility of further moving it to other places.

51The five qi, here, means wind, cold, heat, dampness, and dryness. They are the qi of heaven.

52This section is inconsistent with the rest of the text. Many researchers suspect that something may be missing here. The commentary remarks in the brackets are vague in meaning as well.

53The editor's point is that the first paragraph in this section is from the *Jiu Juan* and emphasizes the conditions necessary for the ongoing " beating" of the qi. The second paragraph is excerpted from the *Su Wen* and focuses on the qi as it relates to the five viscera.

54The impetus of the qi is the clear qi or the yang qi.

55Another name for the point *Han Yan* (GB 4).

56The *cun kou* pulse is located in the lower part, while the *ren ying* in the upper part; accordingly the former is yin and the latter is yang. From another angle, the *cun kou* is yin because it is the vessel of the hand *tai yin*, while the *ren ying* is yang because it is ascribed to the foot *yang ming*.

57A yang illness here implies an exuberance of pathogenic qi and the pulse at *Ren Ying* should be large. If, however, this pulse is small, this implies a counterflow condition. By the same token, a yin disease here implies a condition of internal depletion which should be reflected in a small *cun kou* pulse. A large *cun kou* pulse implies a condition of counterflow as well. The size and activity of the yin and yang pulses should be in a state of balance with respect to one another. If there is a tendency towards abnormal activity or quietude, or a significant variation in size or strength, this reflects illness.

58The answer below apparently concerns the penetrating vessel rather than the foot *shao yin* vessel, but observant readers will not fail to notice that an account for the beating of the foot *shao yin* is implicit here.

59There are three places within the twelve channels where a vessel beats constantly. One is at the qi mouth at the radial aspect of the wrist on the hand *tai yin* channel. Another is at Man's Prognosis (*Ren Ying*, St 9) on the neck on the hand *yang ming* channel. The last is at Great Stream (*Tai Xi*, Ki 3) behind the medial malleolus on the foot *shao yin* channel. The movement of the first two pulses is a result of their relationship to the lung and stomach qi, while the movement of the last is a result of its relationship to the penetrating vessel. The lung rules the qi, the stomach is the sea of grains, and the penetrating vessel is the sea of blood. The viscera and bowels rely upon these three for nourishment and they form an integrated whole. Therefore pathological developments within the viscera and bowels will manifest at these three pulses.

60The head, abdomen, chest, and leg.

61The binding places of the network vessels are those places where they are the widest and most elevated. These are determined by the observation of changes in the color of the skin and by prominences in the surface of the skin which may be palpated.

62A (connecting) branch is a connecting vessel which links one channel with another and is usually named after the point from which it branches.

63Propped up implies a state of fullness to the point of bursting.

64The branch deviates to the hand *shao yang*, but the text does not state it explicitly.

65At the time this text was written acupoints and the like were not named after the emperor, as this is a relatively modern practice. We have therefore not employed Wiseman's translation of Yellow Emperor, and have used a more appropriate translation for the time.

66There has been controversy over the identity of the point *Wei Yi*. A majority of scholars hold that it should be Turtledove Tail (*Jiu Wei*, CV 15), but many maintain that it may be Meeting of Yin (*Hui Yin*, CV 1).

67This sentence appears incomplete and there is a general consensus that something is missing from it.

68There are actually two network vessels of the spleen. One is Offspring of Duke (*Gong Sun*, Sp 4) which links the spleen to the stomach and Great Envelope (*Da Bao*, Sp 20), which irrigates the areas neighboring the spleen.

69Here yang means the network vessels of a yang channel.

70There is more than one understanding of the term, since the characters *hai* and *fei* both have more than one meaning. *Hai* can be interpreted as "doing harm to", "impeding" or "shutting", while *fei* may mean, "door", "window", "soaring", "floating" or "propagating". They combine to give 1) yang at its summit and about to decline; 2) inhibition of yang; 3) closing the entrance, etc. At this point there is no consensus about the interpretation of the term in Chinese circles.

71The hand channels are the upper channels, and the foot channels, the lower ones.

72In this context, the yang refers to the connecting vessel in the exterior, while yin refers to the primary channel in the interior.

73The term "gate pivot" (*shu zhu*) is used to articulate the function the connecting vessel serves as a valve between the exterior and the interior, and between the *tai yang* and the *yang ming*. An exuberance within the *shao yang* connecting channels will spill into the main channels, thus "penetrating the interior". An exuberance within the primary channels spills outward "emerging" from the channels only to return and percolate into the interior.

74The use of the term "shutting pivot" (*guan shu*) points out that the vessel serves in a defensive capacity against invading pathogenic factors.

[75]The connecting vessel of a yin channel.

[76]The use of the term "window pivot" (*shu ling*) points out the location of the connecting vessel between the *tai yin* and *jue yin* and hence its capacity of facilitating communication between yin and yang.

[77]The character of *hai* is the same as in *hai fei* (see note 70 above), while *jian* may have the meaning of the shoulder or to the shoulder. The term may be interpreted in the following different ways: 1) the yin of the *jue yin* being at the summit and about to decline; 2) the yin of the *jue yin* being harmful; 3) shutting the window; 4) the yin of the *jue yin* is shutting, etc.

[78]The term *guan zhi* is untranslatable. It can be understood to be 1) confining the insect (as in hibernation), meaning that the *tai yin* is responsible for sealing in the yin qi which lies in the interior of the body; 2) the latch on the sill of the gate, etc.

[79]These passages point out the pathological and physiological functions of the superficial network vessels of the twelve channels by the use of their figurative nominations. Changes in each of these vessels suggests disease in its corresponding channel or organ and such diseases can be treated via treatment of the superficial network vessels. These passages are credited with the establishment of the relationships between changes in skin color and a specific physical condition. They also provide the basis for clarifying the terse statements which often appear in other texts such as "prick the connecting vessel when there is repletion in the viscus". Plum blossom needling and hair needling are expressions of the development of this theory.

[80]*Rou shuo* is an exuberant heat in the flesh causing emaciation. *Po jun* pertains to the skin and flesh of the shoulder, elbow, and thigh region. For example, in cases of high fever the skin in these areas will crack.

[81]A *yang luo* (connecting vessel) is a shallow connecting vessel, while a *yin luo* is a deep one.

[82]Spring, summer, long summer, autumn, and winter. Also see Chap. 2, Book 1, of this work.

[83]East, south, west, north, and center.

[84]These are twelve bamboo pipes of varied lengths, giving twelve standardized pitches of half tones, each having a specific name, from the lowest to the highest being *Huang Zhong, Da Lu, Tai Cu, Jia Zhong, Gu Xi, Zhong Lu, Rui Bin, Lin Zhong, Yi Ze,* *Nan Lu, Wu She,* and *Ying Zhong.* They are evenly divided into two groups, those numbered odd as the yang, those numbered even as yin.

[85]The channels are grouped in terms of yin and yang in order to match the six pitch-pipes. There are actually twelve pipes, but they are divided into yin and yang groups of six pipes each.

[86]These are the twelve earthly branches. They were widely employed to denote the order of things.

[87]They are the Beginning of Spring, Waking of Insects, Clear Brightness, Beginning of Summer, Grain in Ear, Slight Heat, Beginning of Autumn, White Dew, Cold Dew, Beginning of Winter, Great Snow, and Slight Cold.

[88]They are Midnight (B1), Cockcrow (B2), Calm Dawn (B3), Sunrise (B4), Breakfast (B5), Outlying Region (B6), Midday (B7), Sun Descent (B8), Late Afternoon (B9), Sundown (B10), Dusk (B11), and Serenity (B12). Note that after the Han dynasty, the twelve watches began to be called after the twelve earthly branches. See Book 1, note 87.

[89]The inference here is that the channels provide the essentials for study by beginning students of acupuncture and yet offer even the most erudite fertile ground for research.

[90]The primary channel (*zheng*) in this context is in actuality a branch which is a part of the channel proper but is not the channel proper itself.

[91]This refers to the meeting between a yin channel with its associated yang channel. These six unions serve as main links between the yin channels and their respective associated yang channels. It is notable that the yin channels alone travel toward the associated yang channel to form the unions, while the yang channels do not.

[92]*The Nine Hills* is a shortened form of *The Nine Hills of the Spiritual Pivot,* the ancient title of the *Spiritual Pivot.*

[93]There are several different plausible interpretations of the term "point to the earth", but there is currently no consensus among Chinese medical researchers.

[94]There are several plausible interpretations of the term "points to heaven", but there is currently no consensus among Chinese medical researchers.

[95]*I.e.,* Celestial Pool (*Tian Chi, Per 1*)

[96]Part 1 is derived from Chap. 38, Vol. 6, *Ling Shu*; Part 2 from a combination of Chap. 65. Vol. 10, *Ling Shu*, Chap. 60, *Su Wen*, and the 28th Difficult Issue of the *Nan Jing (Classic of Difficult Issues)*; and Part 3, a combination of Chap. 17, *Ling Shu* and the 28th and 29th Difficult Issue of the *Nan Jing*.

[97]The subsequent answer to the emperor's question pertains to the penetrating vessel rather than the foot *shao yin*. In the corresponding part of the *Ling Shu*, the answer is preceded by a negative response to the question.

[98]*I.e.*, Large Goblet (*Da Zhong*, Ki 4)

[99]If the vessel on the dorsum of the foot is not palpable, there is inversion.

[100]Note that the description of the routes of the vessel is different from that above. This is also seen concerning its consort vessel below.

[101]The *Su Wen* states that the penetrating vessel joins with the channel of foot *shao yin*. The *Nan Jing*, however, states that it joins with the *yang ming* channel. In addition it joins with the *shao yin* channel running up 5 *fen* lateral to the umbilicus. It also runs up the *yang ming* channel 2 *cun* lateral to the umbilicus. Thus the penetrating vessel originates within the Qi Thoroughfare and ascends along both the *yang ming* and *shao yin* channels. It ascends by the umbilicus to the chest, where it disperses. This description of the penetrating vessel is different from that in the *Jiu Juan (Ninefold Volume)*.

[102]Prior to the Sui and Tang dynasties, the seven *shan* were classified as inversion *shan*, concretion *shan*, cold *shan*, qi *shan*, dish *shan*, infraumbilical *shan*, and wolf *shan*. After the Yuan dynasty they were called cold *shan*, sinew *shan*, water *shan*, qi *shan*, blood *shan*, fox *shan*, and *tui shan*. All of the different types of *shan* are manifestations of qi stasis of one sort or another and of abnormal vaginal discharge and conglomerations and gatherings in females.

[103]Celestial eunuchs are also known as celestial castrati (*tian yan*). The genitalia of these individuals are undeveloped; they are incapable of achieving an erection or reproducing.

[104]Another name for the *tai yang* channel

[105]The route of the governing vessel is described as identical to that of the conception vessel. The two vessels are considered by some to be in fact a single vessel carrying different names over different aspects of their course.

[106]A.k.a. Pubic Bone (*Heng Gu*, Ki 11)

[107]The *Jiu Juan* is referring to the circulation of the constructive qi within the governing vessel which is, therefore, from above to below. The *Nan Jing* is dealing with the origination of the vessel itself which is from below to above. The two statements compliment one another. The *Su Wen* states that the governing vessel runs together with the penetrating vessel.

[108]The term motility vessel always means the yin motility vessel throughout this book unless defined otherwise.

[109]The answer to this question essentially refutes the contention that the qi of the yin and yang motility vessels travels only to the five viscera. The qi of the yin motility vessel travels to the viscera and then spills over into the bowels. The qi of the yang motility vessel first travels to the bowels and then spills over into the viscera. In reality, it is unproductive to differentiate the viscera and bowels in this context as both motility vessels ultimately irrigate both the viscera and the bowels. See Chap. 4, Book 2 for a more detailed discussion of the measurements of the channels.

[110]The total length of a man's channels and vessels is estimated to be sixteen *zhang* and two *chi*. Besides the twelve channels, some vessels are counted in this tally and some are not. The vessels counted in are the governing, the conception, and the yang motility in males or the yin motility in females.

[111]The yang motility is believed to be a branch of the foot *tai yang* channel.

[112]Yin is referred to as the yin or medial aspect; yang as the yang or lateral aspect of the body.

[113]Chap. 44, but there is little in this section on the vessels.

[114]Chap. 17, Book 4, *Ling Shu*.

[115]This entire chapter is derived from Chap. 17, Vol. 4, *Ling Shu*.

[116]All the channels are counted bilaterally thoughout this book.

[117]Although the motility vessel is comprised of two channels, *i.e.*, the yin and yang motility vessels, it is only counted as a single vessel.

[118]1 *chi* = 0.33m
   0.1 *zhang* = 10 *cun*
   1 *cun* = 3.33cm = 1.3123 in.
   1 *chi* = 0.333m = 1.0936 ft.
   1 *zhang* = 10 *chi*}

[119]*Biao* is most commonly translated as "branch"; however, in this context, it means the end, as in the end or tip of a branch as juxtaposed with the root.

[120]This whole chapter is derived from Chap. 52, Vol. 8, *Ling Shu*.

[121]The allusion here is that the constructive (yin) and defensive (yang) qi move like water.

[122]This does not merely refer to point *Qi Chong* (St 30), the Qi Thoroughfare of the stomach, but infers the main passageways of qi within the body as a whole.

[123]Pathogenic factors most often attack the body along the pathways of the correct qi. In understanding the pathways of the six channels, an understanding can be gained of where entanglements of pathogenic qi lie. The doors referred to here, *hu men*, are the thoroughfares through which the qi and blood circulate.

[124]CV 23 is the meeting point of the yin linking and the conception vessels.

[125]Also called Auditory Palace (*Ting Gong*, SI 19)

[126]This description is ambiguous.

[127]Some scholars feel that two points are actually being referred to here. One is Man's Prognosis (*Ren Ying*, St 9), and the other is located somewhere next to the nasopharynx on the cheeks, probably Earth Granary (*Di Cang*, St 4).

[128]Five *cun* above Moving Between suggests Mound Center (*Zhong Feng*, Liv 4).

[129]Possibly Nursing the Aged (*Yang Lao*, SI 6).

[130]The same as Upper Arm (*Bi Nao*, LI 14)

[131]*Qian Shang* refers to the point in the neck one *cun* under the mandibular border posterior to Man's Prognosis (*Ren Ying*, St 9) and above Protuberance Assistant (*Fu Tu*, LI 18). It is named after a contrivance worn around the neck by convicts as a punishment in ancient China.

[132]At the point Great Abyss (*Tai Yuan*, Lu 9)

[133]Draining therapy is implied.

[134]Supplementing therapy is implied.

[135]Vacuity here implies a depletion of yang below resulting in inversion. Exuberance here implies the presence of evil heat. The *Su Wen* substitutes the word *tong*, pain, for heat. Vacuity above resulting in dizziness implies a failure of the clear yang to ascend. Exuberance above implies an upward flaring of evil heat.

The origins and ends cannot be literally interpreted as the beginning and terminations of the channels and some of them are not even on the route of their corresponding channels. Origins and ends are best understood as influential spheres of the channels. Origins lie low on the body and so are termed "below". Ends, because they lie in the upper part of the body, are termed "above".

[136]Qi thoroughfares here refer to the main passage through which the various channels flow. There are altogether four: the abdomen, the heart, the chest (and back), and the legs.

[137] The point Hundred Convergences (*Bai Hui*, GV 20) is implied.

[138]This refers to the points of the foot *tai yang* above the eleventh vertebra.

[139]I.e., the points of the foot *tai yang* below the eleventh vertebra.

[140]This refers to part of the penetrating vessel in the abdomen and the points of the foot *shao yin* in the area.

[141]Accumulation without pain implies that the evil qi has consolidated its presence within the body and has become deeply lodged. Hence it is difficult to treat.

[142]This entire chapter is derived from Chap. 5, Vol. 2, *Ling Shu*.

[143]The roots (*gen*) and terminations (*jie*) are indicative of the beginnings and ends of the circulation of the yin and yang, qi and blood, and the channels and vessels. Pathogenic qi may invade the body in a myriad of ways. Ignorance of the origins and terminations of the channels and the physiological relationships of the organs and viscera will therefore negatively influence therapy. This allows the pathogenic qi to become even more chaotic. The pivots of three yin and the three yang become damaged, there is a separation of yin and yang, and injury to the essence resulting in an untreatable situation.

[144]The earliest reference to Life Gate (*Ming Men*) occurs in the *Ling Shu* where it refers to the eye and not the moving qi between the kidneys.

[145]There is probably a textual error here, since nasophar-

ynx (*han sang*) cannot be at the ear, nor is it certain whether naming it the window panel is correct.

[146]The *Su Wen* contains the character *nei* (internal) rather than *rou*, thus making the line read...."the internal articulations become corrupted."

[147]*Qi wu suo zhi xi.* The *Tai Su* speaks of "the capacity of the qi for quiescence which prevents it from being drained off and the capacity for circulation which promotes respiration.

[148]Since the *shao yang* governs the sinew, when the *shao yang* pivot becomes diseased the sinew and bones are not nourished, the articulations lose their strength, then shake, and become agitated.

[149]*Ge dong* is a syndrome caused by the enfeebled qi of the diaphragm which leaves the lower burner wide open.

[150]*Shao Hai* (Ht 3) is mistaken for *Xiao Hai* (SI 8), but the mistake was made by the author, Huang-fu Mi himself.

[151]There is no mistake. The commentary remark might have been inserted by some careless editor of later times.

[152]The endpoints and origins (*biao ben*) and the roots and terminations (*gen jie*) are identical in some channels. This is true of the foot *shao yang*, and *yang ming*. In some channels they are located near to each other and in some channels the root and the origin are the same but the termination and endpoints vary.

The endpoints (*biao*) and terminations (*jie*) are all located relatively high in the body on the head, face, and chest, while the origin (*ben*) and the roots (*gen*) have a relatively lower position in the body below the knee and the elbow. In the sense that these two pairs both provide the theoretical framework for the practice of treating the upper part of the body to treat a problem below and *vice versa*, they possess the same function.

The endpoints and origins, and the roots and terminations are not always identical. All roots are well points but all origins are not. The ramification of this is that all the points below the knee and elbow are significant in treating the body as a whole and one is not limited to the use of the five *shu* points.

The roots and terminations underscore the connection between the two extremes of the channel qi. The root is always the starting point of the channel qi. The endpoints and origins, however, stress the spread and diffusion of channel qi which is evident in the discussion of the qi thoroughfare. This functions when the qi spreads and flows.

With a few exceptions, roots (*gen*) are well (*jing*) points, flowing (*liu*) are source (*yuan*) points, and entering (*ru*) are connecting (*luo*) points. Only the roots and terminations are illustrated in the yin channels.

A few entering points (*ru*) specifically, Protuberance Assistant (*Fu Tu*, LI 18) and Celestial Window (*Tian You*, TH 16), are located above the four passes (*i.e.*, the knees and elbows), while all of the five *shu* points are located below this point.

The descriptive terms of the five *shu* points are designed to show the depth, width, and direction of the channel of a given point. The endpoints and origins, and the roots and terminations primarily describe the spread, concentrations, and influences of a given point. The same point may be given different names which represent different aspects of its function. For instance, Surging Yang (*Chong Yang*, St 42) is a pouring point but it is also a source point.

[153]This entire chapter is derived from Chap. 13, Vol. 4, *Ling Shu*.

[154]This is the upper eyelid.

[155]Surprise needling is a method of quick insertion and withdrawal of the needle.

[156]A contralateral disorder is implied here, that is, when the disorder travels from the right towards the left, the left eye is unable to open. The discussion following should be understood in the same way.

[157]The *Ben Cao Gang Mu* (*Detailed Outline of Materia Medica*) explains;"Horse lard is sweet, neutral, and emolliating. Applied to the tense side, it moistens *bi* and unblocks the blood vessels. Cinnamon wine is pungent, warm, and invigorating. Applied to the flaccid side, it harmonizes the constructive and defensive, and unblocks the channels and collaterals. Mulberry twig is used to treat wind *bi* and unblock the articulations. (In the treatment) of the above illness, the wine helps to promote circulation, and the sweet tastes serve as assistants. Therefore one also drinks wine and eats cooked meat."

[158]The inner assisting bone referred to here is the prominence at the medial aspect of the knee, which is part of the joint formed by the lower end of the femur and upper end of the tibia.

[159]The inner or the yin is referred to as the anterior aspect of the body while the outer or the yang means the posterior aspect of the body.

[160]It is the early name of modern *gigong*, an exercise characterized by deep breathing and tranquil

movements or postures, designed to keep fit and cure disease.

[161]Descriptive definition of spasms.

[162]Note that all therapies are included in medication.

[163]During an attack of this disorder one cannot see until one has left one's eyes closed for some time.

[164]This may also be read "If the neck sinew is tense, there is atony of the sinew and swollen neck which is due to cold and heat."

[165]Although the description is confined to one route, another route is implied since the sinew of each channel has the left and right pathways.

[166]Here the word cardia implies the diaphragm. While the word cardia is an accurate analog to the Chinese in this context, the cardia implies the diaphragm in this case.

[167]The *Tai Su* explains, "The inverted cup is the diaphragm and although the sinew (channel) does not penetrate the viscera and bowels, it is dispersed throughout the diaphragm". Thus disorders within the sinew channel may result in symptoms of diaphragmatic dysfunction.

[168]The *Tai Su* states, "Accumulations of the heart are called deep-lying beam which rise up from the umbilicus like an arm, ascending to just below the heart. The sinew (channel) descends from the diaphragm to the umbilicus. If there is subcardiac pain this is called *cheng*. If ones elbow binds up upon flexion and extension this is called *gang*."

[169]Part 1 is derived from Chap. 14, Vol. 4, *Ling Shu*; Part 2 from Chap. 31, Vol. 6, *Ling Shu*; Part 3 from Chap. 32, Vol. 6, *Ling Shu*.

[170]This is Chap. 17, Vol. 4, *Ling Shu*. It is the title of a chapter in an ancient edition of the *Ling Shu* which corresponds with Chap. 14 of the current edition.

[171]The *Tai Su* defines the great bone of the head (*tou da gu*) as consisting of the cranial bones between the neck and forehead.

[172]Of the face, the three parts are that from the front hairline to the line of the eyebrows, that from the line of the eyebrows to the tip of the nose, and that from the tip of the nose to the end of the chin.

[173]This is commonly translated today as the Adam's apple. However, in Huang-fu Mi's time there would have been no such term as Adam's apple.

[174]The distance is measured from the Adam's apple to the point Celestial Chimney (*Tian Tu*, CV 22).

[175]This is understood to be the root of the neck, *i.e.*, the joining place between the shoulder and the neck at the side, where the neck becomes abruptly thick.

[176]The center of the axilla.

[177]It is referred to in fact as the edge of the eleventh rib, or more exactly, Camphorwood Gate (*Zhang Men*, LV 13).

[178]*I.e.*, the tragus or, more exactly, Auditory Palace (*Ting Gong*, SI 19).

[179]Considering that the distance between the two breasts is said to be also nine and a half *cun* in the immediately later place in the text, the measurement must be wrong.

[180]Note that the distance happens to be equal to the length of the pubic bone. It is no coincidence, since this is, practically speaking, just the measure of the pubic bone between the groins.

[181]The upper border of the first thoracic vertebra or Great Vertebrae (*Da Zhui*, GV 14).

[182]The length of each individual vertebra below is not the result of the total length divided by twenty-one. It is conventionally estimated that the first seven vertebrae each is 1.41 *cun*; the second seven vertebrae each is 1.61 *cun*; the third seven vertebrae each is 1.26 *cun*. Counting in this way, the total length of the twenty-one vertebrae is not exactly 3 *chi*. The residue, according to the author, should be shared by the vertebrae below the first seven. Clinically, however, the practitioner measures the lengths by counting the vertebrae rather than employing the standards.

[183]The narration in this paragraph lacks consistency and is not logically connected with the preceding one.

[184]These are all units of volume and capacity. 1 *dou* = 10 *sheng* = 100 *he*. 1 *sheng* = liter.

[185]It is referred to as the upper opening of the epiglottis.

[186]This measurement covers the distance from the lips to the end of the large intestine including the stomach and intestines.

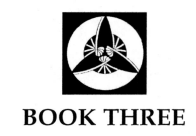

BOOK THREE

Chapter One

Seven Points[1] Located on the Head Directly Above the Nose at the Front Hairline & Located Laterally to Head Corner (*Tou Wei*, St 8)[2]

(1)

The Yellow Emperor asked:

There are three hundred and sixty-five qi points that correspond to a single year. Please tell me whether the minute network vessels (*sun luo*,)[3] and ravines and valleys have similar correspondences as well.

Qi Bo answered:

The minute network vessels and the ravines and valleys have three hundred and sixty-five meeting points[4] which correspond to a single year. They provide outlets through which extraordinary evils[5] (may pass) and passageways for the free flow of constructive and defensive (qi). The grand meetings of the flesh constitute the valleys and the minor meetings of the flesh constitute the ravines. The partings of the flesh and the meetings of the ravines and valleys constitute the passageways for the circulation of the constructive and defensive, as well as the dwelling place ["the

meeting places" in the *Su Wen*] of the great qi.[6]

(2)[7]

Spirit Court (*Shen Ting*, GV 24) is located in the hairline, directly above the nose and is a meeting point of the governing vessel, the foot *tai yang*, and *yang ming*.[8] It is prohibited to needling as it may cause madness and loss of the essence in the eye, but it may be moxaed with three cones.

Deviating Turn (*Qu Cha*, Bl 4)), also known as Nose Flush (*Bi Chong*), is located in the hairline one *cun* and five *fen* lateral to Spirit Court and belongs to the qi of foot *tai yang* vessel. It is located with the (patient's) head upright. It is needled to a depth of three *fen* and is moxaed with five cones.

Root Spirit (*Ben Shen*, GB 13) is located in the hairline, one *cun* and five *fen* lateral to Deviating Turn (a variant version places it four *fen* from the hairline straight above the auricle) and is a meeting point of the foot *shao yang* and the yang linking vessel. It is needled to a depth of five *fen* and moxaed with three cones.

Head Corner (*Tou Wei*, St 8)) is located in the hairline at the corner of the head one *cun* and five *fen* lateral to Root Spirit and is a meeting point of the foot *shao yang* and *yang ming*. It is needled to a depth of five *fen* and is prohibited to moxibustion.

Chapter Two

Eight Points on the Head Directly Above the Nose Located Along the Governing Vessel from One *Cun* Posterior to the Hairline to Wind Mansion (*Feng Fu*, GV 16)[9]

Upper Star (*Shang Xing*, GV 23) is located on the scalp, directly above the nose and one *cun* posterior to the hairline in a depression the size of a pea, and belongs to the qi of the governing vessel. It is needled to a depth of three *fen*, (the needle) is retained for a duration of six exhalations, and it is moxaed with five cones.

Fontanel Meeting (*Xin Hui*, GV 22) is located one *cun* posterior to Upper Star in a depression between the bones and belongs to the qi of the governing vessel. It is needled to a depth of four *fen* and moxaed with five cones.

Before the Vertex (*Qian Ding*, GV 21) is located one *cun* and five *fen* posterior to Fontanel Meeting in a depression between the bones and belongs to the qi of the governing vessel. It is needled to a depth of four *fen* and moxaed with five cones.

Hundred Convergences (*Bai Hui*, GV 20) is also known as the Quinary Meeting of Three Yang (*San Yang Wu Hui*). It is located one *cun* five *fen* behind Before the Vertex at the crown at the epicenter of hair (growth) in a depression as large as the tip of a finger. It is a meeting point of the governing vessel and the foot *tai yang*. It is needled to a depth of three *fen* and moxaed with five cones.

Behind the Vertex (*Hou Ding*, GV 19) is also known as Cross Surging (*Jiao Chong*). It is located one *cun* and five *fen* posterior to Hundred Convergences on the occipital bone and belongs to the qi of the governing vessel. It is needled to a depth of four *fen* and is moxaed with five cones.

Unyielding Space (*Qiang Jian*, GV 18) is also known as Big Plume (*Da Yu*). It is located one *cun* and five *fen* posterior to Behind the Vertex and belongs to the qi of the governing vessel. It is nee-dled to a depth of three *fen* and is moxaed with five cones.

Brain's Door (*Nao Hu*, GV 17) is also known as Whirling Wind (*Za Feng*) and Scalp Meeting (*Hui Lu*). It is located in the occipital bone one *cun* and five *fen* posterior to Unyielding Space and is the meeting point of the governing vessel and the foot *tai yang*. It is needled to a depth of three *fen* and (the needle) is retained for a duration of two exhalations. Moxibustion is prohibited as it may cause loss of voice. [The "*Ci Jin Lun* {The Treatise on Needling Commandments}" in the *Su Wen*[10] says that inadvertent penetration of the brain when needling Brain's Door on the head causes immediate death. In his notes, Wang Bing[11] holds that it may be moxaed with five cones. The *Gu Kong Lun*,[12] however, warns against moxibustion. The *Tong Ren Jing (The Classic of the Bronze [Acupuncture] Statue)*[13] says that moxibustion is prohibited, as it may cause dumbness.]

Wind Mansion (*Feng Fu*, GV 16) is also known as Root of the Tongue (*She Ben*). It is located on the nape one *cun* above the hairline in a depression in the major sinew where the muscle protrudes during rapid speech but falls flat when speech ceases. It is a meeting point of the governing vessel and the yang linking vessel. Moxibustion is prohibited as it may cause loss of voice. It is needled to a depth of four *fen*, and (the needle) is retained for a duration of three exhalations.

Chapter Three

Ten Points on the Head Along the Governing Vessel & One *Cun* & Five *Fen* Lateral to It as Far Back as Jade Pillow (*Yu Zhen*, Bl 9)[14]

Fifth Place (*Wu Chu*, Bl 5) is located one *cun* and five *fen* lateral to Upper Star (*Shang Xing*, GV 23) of the governing vessel and belongs to the qi of the foot *tai yang*. It is needled to a depth of three *fen*, (the needle) is retained for a duration of seven exhalations, and it is moxaed with three cones.

Light Guard (*Cheng Guang*, Bl 6) is located two *cun* posterior to Fifth Place and belongs to the qi of the foot *tai yang* vessel. It is needled to a depth of three *fen* and is prohibited to moxibustion.[15]

Celestial Connection (*Tong Tian*, Bl 7) is also known as Celestial Mortar (*Tian Jiu*) and is located one *cun* and five *fen* posterior to Light Guard. It belongs to the qi of the foot *tai yang* vessel. It is needled to a depth of three *fen*, (the needle) is retained for a duration of seven exhalations, and it is moxaed with three cones.

Declining Connection (*Luo Que*, Bl 8) is also known as Strong Yang (*Qiang Yang*) and Brain Cover (*Nao Gai*) and is located one *cun* and five *fen* posterior to Celestial Connection. It belongs to the qi of the foot *tai yang* vessel. It is needled to a depth of three *fen*, (the needle) is retained for a duration of five exhalations, and it is moxaed with three cones.[16]

Jade Pillow (*Yu Zhen*, Bl 9) is located seven *fen* behind Declining Connection (*Luo Que*), one *cun* three *fen* lateral to Brain's Door (*Nao Hu*, GV 17) at the rise of the pillow bone (*i.e.*, the occipital bone) and three *cun* from the hairline. It belongs to the qi of the foot *tai yang* vessel. It is needled to a depth of two *fen*, (the needle) is retained for a duration of three exhalations, and it is moxaed with three cones.

Chapter Four

Ten Points on the Head Directly Above the Eye Located Five *Fen* from the Hairline Back to Brain Hollow (*Nao Kong*, GB 19)[17]

On the Verge of Tears (*Lin Qi*, GB 15)[18] is located above the canthus of the eye in a depression five *fen* behind the hairline. It is a meeting point of the foot *tai yang*, the (foot) *shao yang* and the yang linking vessels. It is needled to a depth of three *fen*, (the needle) is retained for a duration of seven exhalations, and it is moxaed with three cones.[19]

Eye Window (*Mu Chuang*, GB 16) is also known as Reaching Camp (*Zhi Ying*) and is located one *cun* posterior to On the Verge of Tears. It is a meeting point of the foot *shao yang* and the yang linking vessel. It is needled to a depth of three *fen* deep and moxaed with five cones.

Upright Nutrition (*Zheng Ying*, GB 17) is located one *cun* posterior to Eye Window and is a meeting point of the foot *shao yang* and the yang linking vessel. It is needled to a depth of three *fen* and moxaed with five cones.

Intelligence Support (*Cheng Ling*, GB 18)[20] is located one *cun* and five *fen* posterior to Upright Nutrition and is a meeting point of the foot *shao yang* and the yang linking vessels. It is needled to a depth of three *fen* and moxaed with five cones.

Brain Hollow (*Nao Kong*, GB 19) is also known as Temple Region (*Nie Nao*) and is located one *cun* and five *fen* posterior to Intelligence Support in a depression below the occipital bone. It is a meeting point of the foot *shao yang* and the yang linking vessels. It is needled to a depth of four *fen* and moxaed with five cones. [A note in the "*Qi Fu Lun*"[21] locates this point on the lateral border of the occipital bone.]

Chapter Five

Twelve Points on the Head & Around the Auricle Extending Back to Completion Bone (*Wan Gu*, GB 12)[22]

Celestial Thoroughfare (*Tian Chong*, GB 9)[23] is located three *cun* anterior and superior to the auricle. It is needled to a depth of three *fen* and moxaed with nine cones. [A note in the "*Qi Fu Lun*"[24] states that it is a meeting point of the foot *tai yang* and *shao yang*. {later editor}]

Winding Valley (*Shuai Gu*, GB 8) is located above the auricle one *cun* and five *fen* from the hairline. It is a meeting point of the foot *tai yang* and *shao yang*. Chewing locates the point.[25] It is needled to a depth of four *fen* and moxaed with three cones.

Temporal Hairline Curve (*Qu Bin*, GB 7) is located above the auricle in a depression on the temporal hairline where a hollow appears when drumming the chin.[26] It is a meeting point of the foot *tai yang* and *shao yang*. It is needled to a depth of three *fen* and moxaed with three cones.

Floating White (*Fu Bai*, GB 10)[27] is located posterior to the auricle one *cun* from the hairline and is a meeting point of the foot *tai yang* and *shao yang*. It is needled to a depth of three *fen*, and moxaed with two cones. [A note in the "*Qi Xue Lun*"[28] prescribes moxibustion with three cones and an insertion depth of three *fen*.]

Portal Yin (*Qiao Yin*, GB 15) is located on the completion bone below the occipital bone where a twitch may be felt (when shaking the head). It is the meeting point of the foot *tai yang* and *shao yang*. It is needled to a depth of four *fen*, and moxaed with five cones. [A note in the "*Qi Xue Lun*" prescribes moxibustion with three cones and an insertion of three *fen*. {later editor}]

Completion Bone (*Wan Gu*, GB 12) is located posterior to the auricle four *fen* from the hairline and is a meeting point of the foot *tai yang* and *shao yang*. It is needled to a depth of two *fen*, (the needle) is retained for a duration of seven exhalations, and it is moxaed with seven cones. [A note in the "*Qi Xue Lun*" prescribes an insertion of three *fen* and moxibustion with three cones. {later editor}]

Chapter Six

Five Points on the Head Along the Hairline Running Laterally from the Midline[29]

Loss of Voice Gate (*Yin Men*)[30] is also known as Tongue's Horizontal (*She Heng*) and Tongue Repression (*She Yan*) and is located on the nape of the neck in a depression in the hairline. It enters to connect with the root of the tongue[31] and is a meeting point of the governing vessel and the yang linking vessel. Have (the patient) bend his head backward to locate the point. It is needled to depth of four *fen* and moxibustion is prohibited as it may cause loss of voice. [A note in the "*Qi Fu Lun*"[32] locates this point one *cun* from Wind Mansion {*Feng Fu*, GV 16}.]

Celestial Pillar (*Tian Zhu*, Bl 10) is located on the nape of the neck on the hairline in a depression by the lateral border of the major sinew and belongs to the qi of the foot *tai yang* vessel. It is needled to a depth of two *fen*, (the needle) is retained for a duration of six exhalations, and it is moxaed with three cones.

Wind Pool (*Feng Chi*, GB 20) is located posterior to the temple in a depression on the hairline and is a meeting point of the foot *shao yang* and the yang linking vessel. It is needled to a depth of three *fen*, (the needle) is retained for a duration of three exhalations, and it is moxaed with three cones. [A note in the "*Qi Fu Lun*" locates this point in a depression behind the auricle where the application of pressure provokes a trigger response in the ear, and it claims that it is the meeting point of the *shao yang* vessels of the hand and foot. It prescribes an insertion of four *fen*. {later editor}]

Chapter Seven

Eleven Points on the Back Along the Governing Vessel from the First Vertebra Down to the End of the Coccyx[33]

A note in the "*Qi Fu Lun*"[34] locates Spirit Tower (*Ling Tai*, GV 10) below the sixth vertebra, Central Pivot (*Zhong Shu*, GV 7) below the tenth vertebra, and Lumbar Yang Pass (*Yang Guan*, GV 3) below the sixteenth vertebra.

Great Vertebra (*Da Zhui*, GV 14) is located above the first vertebra in a depression and is a meeting point of the three yang (vessels) and the governing vessel. It is needled to a depth of five *fen* and is moxaed with nine cones.[35]

Kiln Path (*Tao Dao*, GV 13) is located at the joint space below the great vertebra[36] (*Da Zhui*, GV 14) and is a meeting point of the governing vessel and the foot *tai yang*. Bend (the patient's head forward) to locate it. It is needled to a depth of five *fen*, (the needle) is retained for a duration of five exhalations, and it is moxaed with five cones.

Body Pillar (*Shen Zhu*, GV 12) is located in the joint space below the third vertebra and belongs to the qi of the governing vessel. Bend (the patient's head forward) to locate it. It is needled to a depth of five *fen* deep, (the needle) is retained for a duration of five exhalations, and it is moxaed with five cones.

Spirit Path (*Shen Dao*, GV 11) is located in the joint space below the fifth vertebra. It belongs to the qi of the governing vessel. Bend (the patient's head forward) to locate it. It is needled to a depth of five *fen*, (the needle) is retained for a duration of five exhalations, and it is moxaed with five cones.

Consummate Yang (*Zhi Yang*, GV 9) is located in the joint space below the seventh vertebra and belongs to the qi of the governing vessel. Bend (the patient's head forward) to locate it. It is needled to a depth of five *fen* and moxaed with three cones.[37]

Sinew Contraction (*Jin Suo*, GV 8) is located in the joint space below the ninth vertebra and belongs to the qi of the governing vessel. Bend (the patient's head forward) to locate it. It is needled to a depth of five *fen* and moxaed with three cones. [A note in the "*Qi Fu Lun*" prescribes moxibustion with five cones. {later editor}]

Spinal Center (*Ji Zhong*, GV 6) is located in the joint space below the eleventh vertebra and belongs to the qi of the governing vessel. Bend (the patient's body forward) to locate it. It is needled to a depth of five *fen* and moxa is prohibited. Moxibustion may cause atony. [The source texts do not say this. The *Su Wen* states that moxibustion may cause rickets. *Tong Ren, Sheng Ji Zong*

Lu (Complete Records of Life Securing [Classics Complied Under the Decree] of His Majesty) and *Zi Sheng Jing (The Classic of Nourishing Life)* all state that if moxibustion is applied then the lumbar spine will become bent.]

Suspended Pivot (*Xuan Shu*, GV 5) is located in the joint space below the thirteenth vertebra and belongs to the qi of the governing vessel. Lie (the patient's body) prostrate to locate it. It is needled to a depth of three *fen* and it is moxaed with three cones.

Life Gate (*Ming Men*, GV 4) is also called Multiple Connection (*Shu Lei*) and is located in the joint space below the fourteenth vertebra. It belongs to the qi of the governing vessel. Lie (the patient's body) prostrate to locate it. It is needled to a depth of five *fen* and moxaed with three cones.

Lumbar Shu (*Yao Shu*, GV 2) is also called Back's Resolution (*Bei Jie*), Marrow Hole (*Sui Kong*), or Lumbar Door (*Yao Hu*). [*Wai Tai Mi Yao {Secret (Medical) Essentials of a Provincial Governor}* includes Lumbar Pivot (*Yao Shu*) in this list.] It is located in the joint space below the twenty-first vertebra and belongs to the qi of the governing vessel. It is needled to a depth of three *fen*, (the needle) is retained for a duration of seven exhalations, and it is moxaed with five cones.

Long Strong (*Chang Qiang*, GV 1) is also known as Yin Cleft of Qi (*Qi Zhi Yin Xi*), and, (from this point,) the connecting vessel of the governing vessel diverges (into the paravertebrals). It is located at the end of the coccyx and the *shao yin* binds here. It is needled to a depth of three *fen*. [Notes in both the "*Qi Xue Lun {Treatise on Points of Qi}*" and "*Shui Xue Lun {Treatise on Water Points}*" give two *fen* deep insertion. {later editor}] (The needle) is retained for a duration of seven exhalations, and it is moxaed with three cones.[38]

Chapter Eight

Forty-Two Points on the Back Located One *Cun*, Five *Fen* Lateral to Either Side of the Spine from the First Vertebrae Down to the Last Vertebra[39]

(1)

The associated points of the five viscera in the back should elicit a painful response when pressed and this identifies them as associated points. They may be moxaed but cannot be needled.[40] If there is an exuberance of qi, they should be drained; while if there is a vacuity of qi, they should be supplemented. In supplementing with fire (*i.e.*, moxibustion), do not blow on the fire, as it must be left to die on its own. When draining with (moxa), blow vigorously on the fire while holding (the moxa) steady until it burns out.[41]

(2)

Great Shuttle (*Da Zhu*, Bl 11) is located in the nape below the first vertebra in depressions one *cun* and five *fen* bilateral to the midline and is a meeting point of the foot *tai yang* and hand *shao yang*. It is needled to a depth of three *fen*, (the needle) is retained for a duration of seven exhalations, and it is moxaed with seven cones. [A note in the "*Qi Xue Lun*"[42] states that this point is a divergent connecting vessel of the governing vessel and the meeting point of the governing vessel and the hand and foot *tai yang*. {later editor}][43]

Wind Gate (*Feng Men*, Bl 12), also known as Heat Mansion (*Re Fu*), is located below the second vertebra one *cun* and five *fen* bilateral to the midline. It is a meeting point of the governing vessel and the foot *tai yang*. It is needled to a depth of five *fen*, (the needle) is retained for a duration of five exhalations, and it is moxaed with five cones.

Lung Shu (*Fei Shu*, Bl 13) is located below the third vertebra one *cun* and five *fen* bilateral to the midline. It is needled to a depth of three *fen*, (the needle) is retained for a duration of seven exhalations, and it is moxaed with three cones. [A note

in the "*Qi Fu Lun*"[44] states that is it an associated point of the five viscera and meeting point in the foot *tai yang*. {later editor}][45]

Heart Shu (*Xin Shu*, Bl 15) is located below the fifth vertebra one *cun* and five *fen* bilateral to the midline. It is needled to a depth of three *fen*, (the needle) is retained for a duration of seven exhalations, and it is prohibited to moxibustion.[46]

Diaphragm Shu (*Ge Shu*, Bl 17) is located below the seventh vertebra one *cun* and five *fen* bilateral to the midline. It is needled to a depth of three *fen*, (the needle) is retained for a duration of seven exhalations and it is moxaed with three cones.

Liver Shu (*Gan Shu*, Bl 18) is located below the ninth vertebra one *cun* and five *fen* bilateral to the midline. It is needled to a depth of three *fen*, (the needle) is retained for a duration of six exhalations, and it is moxaed with three cones.

Gallbladder Shu (*Dan Shu*, Bl 19) is located below the tenth vertebra one *cun* and five *fen* bilateral to the midline of the body and belongs to the qi of the foot *tai yang*. Locate it with the (patient's) body seated upright. It is needled to a depth of five *fen* and moxaed with three cones. [A note in the "*Qi Fu Lun*" prescribes needle retention for a duration of seven exhalations. In the "*Bi Lun* [Treatise on *Bi*]",[47] it is said to be the associated point of the gallbladder, the stomach, the triple burner, the large intestine, the small intestine, and the urinary bladder, and is supplied by the qi of the foot *tai yang* vessel. {later editor}][48]

Spleen Shu (*Pi Shu*, Bl 20) is located below the eleventh vertebra one *cun* and five *fen* bilateral to the midline. It is needled to a depth of three *fen*, (the needle) is retained for a duration of seven exhalations, and it is moxaed with three cones.

Stomach Shu (*Wei Shu*, Bl 21) is located below the twelfth vertebra one *cun* and five *fen* bilateral to the midline. It is needled to a depth of three *fen*, (the needle) is retained for a duration of seven exhalations, and it is moxaed with three cones.

Triple Burner Shu (*San Jiao Shu*, Bl 22) is located

below the thirteenth vertebra one *cun* and five *fen* bilateral to the midline, and belongs to the qi of the foot *tai yang* channel. It is needled to a depth of five *fen* and moxaed with three cones.[49]

Kidney *Shu* (*Shen Shu*, Bl 23) is located below the fourteenth vertebra one *cun* and five *fen* bilateral to the midline. It is needled to a depth of three *fen*, (the needle) is retained for a duration of seven exhalations, and it is moxaed with three cones.

Large Intestine Shu (*Da Chang Shu*, Bl 25) is located below the sixteenth vertebra one *cun* and five *fen* bilateral to the midline. It is needled to a depth of three *fen*, (the needle) is retained for a duration of six exhalations, and it is moxaed with three cones.

Small Intestine Shu (*Xiao Chang Shu*, Bl 27) is located below the eighteenth vertebra one *cun* and five *fen* bilateral to the midline. It is needled to a depth of three *fen*, (the needle) is retained for a duration of six exhalations, and it is moxaed with three cones.

Urinary Bladder Shu (*Pang Guang Shu*, Bl 28) is located below the nineteenth vertebra one *cun* and five *fen* bilateral to the midline. It is needled to a depth of three *fen*, (the needle) is retained for a duration of six exhalations, and it is moxaed with three cones.

Central Backbone Shu (*Zhong Lu Shu*, Bl 29) is located below the twentieth vertebra one *cun* and five *fen* bilateral to the midline. It is located on the prominent muscle running parallel to the spine. It is needled to a depth of three *fen*, (the needle) is retained for a duration of ten exhalations, and it is moxaed with three cones.[50]

White Ring Shu (*Bai Huan Shu*, Bl 30) is located below the twenty-first vertebra one *cun* and five *fen* bilateral to the midline and belongs to the qi of the foot *tai yang*. Locate it with the (patient's) body prostrate. It is needled to a depth of eight *fen*, and moxibustion is prohibited. [A note in the "*Shui Xue Lun*" (Treatise on Points for Heat & Water) says: "It is allowed to be needled five *fen* deep and moxaed with three cones." From the

Large Intestine *Shu* to this point are all said to belong to the qi of the foot *tai yang* channel. {later editor}][51]

Upper Bone Hole (*Shang Liao*, Bl 31) is located in the first hole (*i.e.*, sacral foramina) one *cun* below the iliac crest in the depressions lateral to the spine and is a connecting vessel of the foot *tai yang* and *shao yang*. It is needled to a depth of two *cun*, (the needle) is retained for a duration of seven exhalations and moxaed with three cones.

Second Bone Hole (*Ci Liao*, Bl 32) is located in the second hole (*i.e.*, sacral foramina) in the depressions bilateral to the spine. It is needled to a depth of three *cun*, (the needle) is retained for a duration of seven exhalations, and is moxaed with three cones. [The *Tong Ren Jing* prescribes needling to a depth of three *fen* and moxibustion with seven cones. {later editor}][52]

Middle Bone Hole (*Zhong Liao*, Bl 33) is located in the third hole (*i.e.*, sacral foramina) in the depressions bilateral to the spine. It is needled to a depth of two *cun*, (the needle) is retained for a duration of ten exhalations, and it is moxaed with three cones. [The *Tong Ren Jing* prescribes needling this point to a depth of two *fen*. {later editor}]

Lower Bone Hole (*Xia Liao*, Bl 34) is located in the fourth hole (*i.e.*, sacral foramina) in the depressions bilateral to the spine. It is needled to a depth of two *cun*, (the needle) is retained for a duration of ten exhalations, and it is moxaed with three cones. [The *Tong Ren Jing* prescribes needling this point to a depth of two *fen*. In the "*Mao Ci Lun* (Treatise on Cross Needling)" in the *Su Wen*,[53] it is said to be the converging point of the foot *tai yang*, the foot *jue yin* and the foot *shao yang*. {later editor}]

Meeting of the Yang (*Hui Yang*, Bl 35) is also known as Crux Disinhibitor (*Li Ji*) and is located bilateral to the tail bone. It belongs to the qi of the governing vessel. It is needled to a depth of eight *fen* and moxaed with five cones. [A note in the "*Qi Fu Lun*" prescribes moxibustion with three cones. {later editor}]

Chapter Nine

Twenty-Six Points on the Back Located Bilaterally from Three *Cun* Lateral to the Spine from the Second to the Twenty-First Vertebra[54]

Attached Branch (*Fu Fen*, Bl 41) is located bilaterally below the level of the second vertebra at the medial border of the scapula three *cun* (from the midline) and is a meeting point of the hand and foot *tai yang* channels. It is needled to a depth of eight *fen* and moxaed with five cones.

Po Door (*Po Hu*, Bl 42) is located bilaterally below the level of the third vertebra three *cun* from the midline of the body and belongs to the qi of the foot *tai yang* channel. It is needled to a depth of three *fen* and moxaed with five cones.

Spirit Hall (*Shen Tang*, Bl 44) is located bilaterally below the level of the fifth vertebra in depressions three *cun* (from the midline). It belongs to the qi of the foot *tai yang* channel. It is needled to a depth of three *fen* and moxaed with five cones.

Yi Xi (*Yi Xi*, Bl 45) is located at the medial border of the scapula below the level of the sixth vertebra three *cun* bilateral to the midline. When one exerts pressure (at this point), the patient will let out a groan. This is the point. It belongs to the qi of the foot *tai yang* vessel. It is needled to a depth of six *fen* and moxaed with five cones. [A note in the "*Gu Kong Lun*"[55] states that a vibration can be palpated here if one presses one's hand on the point and the patient is instructed to say *yi xi*. {later editor}]

Diaphragm Pass (*Ge Guan*, Bl 46) is located bilaterally below the level of the seventh vertebra in depressions three *cun* from the midline and belongs to the qi of the foot *tai yang* vessel. Locate it with the (patient) seated upright, shoulders extended. It is needled to a depth of five *fen* and moxaed with three cones. [A note in the "*Qi Fu Lun*" gives five cones for moxibustion. {later editor}]

Hun Gate (*Hun Men*, Bl 47) is located bilaterally below the level of the ninth vertebra in depressions three *cun* from the midline and it belongs to the qi of the foot *tai yang* vessel. Locate it with the (patient) seated upright. It is needled to a depth of five *fen* and moxaed with five cones.

Yang Headrope (*Yang Gang*, Bl 48) is located bilaterally below the level of the tenth vertebra in depressions three *cun* from the midline and belongs to the qi of the foot *tai yang* vessel. Locate it with the (patient) seated upright. It is needled to a depth of five *fen* and moxaed with three cones.

Reflection Abode (*Yi She*, Bl 49) is located bilaterally below the level of the eleventh vertebra in depressions three *cun* bilateral to the midline of the body and belongs to the qi of the foot *tai yang* vessel. Locate it with the (patient) seated upright. It is needled to a depth of five *fen* and moxaed with three cones.

Stomach Granary (*Wei Cang*, Bl 50) is located bilaterally below the level of the twelfth vertebra in depressions three *cun* from the midline and belongs to the qi of the foot *tai yang* vessel. It is needled to a depth of five *fen* and moxaed with three cones.

Huang Gate (*Huang Men*, Bl 51) is located bilaterally below the level of the thirteenth vertebra, three *cun* from the midline in the forked free rib region.[56] It belongs to the qi of the foot *tai yang* vessel. It is needled to a depth of five *fen* and moxaed with three cones. [The classic[57] says that "it is located on the same level as Turtledove Tail (*Jiu Wei*, CV 15)." {later editor}]

Will Chamber (*Zhi Shi*, Bl 52) is located bilaterally below the level of the fourteenth vertebra in depressions three *cun* from the midline and belongs to the qi of the foot *tai yang* vessel. Locate it with (the patient) seated upright. It is needled to a depth of five *fen* and moxaed with three cones. [A note in the "*Qi Fu Lun*" prescribes five cones. {later editor}]

Bladder Huang (*Bao Huang*, Bl 53) is located bilaterally below the level of the nineteenth vertebra in depressions three *cun* from the midline and belongs to the qi of the foot *tai yang* vessel. Locate it with (the patient) prostrate. It is needled to a depth of five *fen* and moxaed with three cones.

Sequential Limit (*Zhi Bian*, Bl 54) is located bilaterally below the level of the twenty-first vertebra in depressions three *cun* from the midline and belongs to the qi of the foot *tai yang* vessel. Locate it with (the patient) prostrate. It is needled to a depth of five *fen* and moxaed with three cones.

Chapter Ten

Thirty-Nine Points on the Face[58]

Suspended Skull (*Xuan Lu*, GB 5) is located in the temporal hairline and belongs to the qi of the foot *shao yang* vessel. It is needled to a depth of three *fen*, (the needle) is retained for a duration of seven exhalations, and it is moxaed with three cones. [A note in the *"Qi Fu Lun"*[59] locates this point in the temples in the hairline. {later editor}][60]

Mandibular Movement (*Han Yan*, GB 4) is located in the hairline on the upper border of the temples and is the meeting point of the foot *shao yang* and the foot *yang ming*. It is needled to a depth of seven *fen*, (the needle) is retained for a duration of seven exhalations, and it is moxaed with three cones. [A note in the *"Qi Fu Lun"* locates this point in the hairline superior to the temples and deep insertion is said to cause loss of hearing acuity. {later editor}][61]

Suspended Tuft (*Xuan Li*, GB 6) is located in the hairline on the lower border of the temples and is the meeting point of the *shao yang* and *yang ming* of the hand and foot. It is needled to a depth of three *fen*, (the needle) is retained for a duration of seven exhalations, and it is moxaed with three cones. [A note in the *"Qi Fu Lun"* locates this point in the hairline superior to the temples, and deep insertion is said to cause loss of hearing acuity. {later editor}]

Yang White (*Yang Bai*, GB 14) is located one *cun*

directly above the pupils of the eyes and is the meeting point of the foot *shao yang* and the yang linking vessel. It is needled to a depth of three *fen* and moxaed with three cones. [A note in the *"Qi Fu Lun"* states that it is the meeting point of the foot *yang ming* and the yin linking vessel. Since the foot *yang ming* is found to have no access here and, additionally, the foot *yang ming* and the yin linking vessel have no chance to meet, this note lacks credibility. {later editor}]

Bamboo Gathering (*Zan Zhu*, Bl 2), also known as Pillar Border (*Yuan Zhu*), Beginning of Light (*Shi Guang*), Night Light (*Ye Guang*), and Bright Light (*Ming Guang*), is located in a depression at the (medial) ends of the eyebrows and belongs to the qi of the foot *tai yang* channel. It is needled to a depth of three *fen*, (the needle) is retained for a duration of six exhalations, and it is moxaed with three cones.

Silk Bamboo Hole (*Si Zhu Kong*, TH 23), also known as Eye Bone-Hole (*Mu Liao*), is located in depressions at the lateral ends of the eyebrows and belongs to the qi of the foot *shao yang* channel. It is needled to a depth of three *fen* deep, (and the needle) is retained for a duration of three exhalations. Moxibustion is prohibited as it may cause unfortunate narrowing of the eyes and blindness. [A note in the *"Qi Fu Lun"* states that it belongs to the hand *shao yang* and prescribes needle retention for a duration of six exhalations. {later editor}]

Bright Eyes (*Jing Ming*, Bl 1), also known as Tear Hole (*Lei Kong*), located at the inner canthi, is the meeting point of the hand and foot *tai yang* and the foot *yang ming*. It is needled to a depth of six *fen*, (the needle) is retained for a duration of six exhalations, and it is moxaed with three cones. [A note in the *"Qi Fu Lun"* states that it is the meeting point of five vessels, the hand and foot *tai yang*, the foot *yang ming*, and the yin and yang motility vessels. {later editor}]

Pupil Bone Hole (*Tong Zi Liao*, GB 1) is located five *fen* lateral to the outer canthi and is the meeting point of the hand *tai yang*, and the hand and foot *shao yang*. It is needled to a depth of three *fen* and moxaed with three cones.

Tear Container (*Cheng Qi*, St 1) is also known as Mouse Hole (*Xi Xue*) and Face Bone Hole (*Mian Liao*) and is located seven *fen* inferior to the eyes directly below the pupils. It is the meeting point of the yang motility vessel, the conception vessel, and the foot *yang ming*. It is needled to a depth of three *fen*, and moxibustion is prohibited.

Four Whites (*Si Bai*, St 2) is located one *cun* inferior to the eyes in the suborbital foramina and belongs to the qi of the foot *yang ming* vessel. It is needled to a depth of three *fen* and moxaed with seven cones. [A note in the "*Qi Fu Lun*" prescribes an insertion of four *fen* but prohibits moxibustion. {later editor}]

Cheek Bone Hole (*Quan Liao*, SI 18), also known as Sharp Bone (*Rui Gu*), is located in the depressions at the lower borders of the zygomatic bones and is the meeting point of the hand *shao yang* and *tai yang*. It is needled to a depth of three *fen*.

White Bone Hole (*Su Liao*, GV 25), also known as King of Face (*Mian Wang*), is located at the tip of the nose bridge and belongs to the qi of the governing vessel. It is needled to a depth of three *fen*.

Welcome Fragrance (*Ying Xiang*, LI 20), also known as Surging Yang (*Chong Yang*), is located above Harmony Bone Hole by the side of the nostrils. It is the meeting point of the *yang ming* of the hand and foot and is needled to a depth of three *fen*.

Great Bone Hole (*Ju Liao*, St 3) is located eight *fen* lateral to the nostrils directly below the pupils of the eyes and is the meeting point of the motility vessel and the foot *yang ming*. It is needled to a depth of three *fen*.

Harmony Bone Hole (*He Liao*, LI 19), also known as Suborbital (*Zhou*), is located directly below the nostrils, five *fen* bilateral to the philtrum, and belongs to the qi of the hand *yang ming* channel. It is needled to a depth of three *fen*.

Water Trough (*Shui Gou*, GV 26) is located in the philtrum under the nose bridge and is the meeting point of the governing vessel and the hand *yang ming*. Locate it with the (patient's) lip straightened. It is needled to a depth of three *fen*, (the needle) is retained for a duration of six exhalations, and it is moxaed with three cones.

Extremity of the Mouth (*Dui Duan*, GV 27) is located at the tip of the (upper) lip and belongs to the qi of the hand *yang ming*. It is needled to a depth of two *fen*, (the needle) is retained for a duration of six exhalation, and it is moxaed with three cones.

Gum Seam (*Yin Jiao*, GV 28)[62] is located inside the (upper) lip above the teeth at the center of the gum seam. It is needled to a depth of three *fen* and moxaed with three cones. [A note in the "*Qi Fu Lun*" states that it is the meeting point of the conception and governing vessels. {later editor}]

Earth Granary (*Di Cang*, St 4) is also known as Stomach Link (*Wei Wei*). It is located four *fen* lateral to the corners of the mouth, a little above a palpable beating vessel, and is the meeting point of the motility vessel and the hand and foot *yang ming*. It is needled to a depth of three *fen*.

Nectar Receptacle (*Cheng Jiang*, CV 24),[63] also known as Celestial Pool (*Tian Chi*), is located in the middle of the chin under the lower lip and is the meeting point of the foot *yang ming* and the conception vessel. Locate it with the (patient's) mouth shut.[64] It is needled to a depth of two *fen*, (the needle) is retained for a duration of six exhalations, and it is moxaed with three cones. [A note in the "*Qi Xue Lun*"[65] prescribes needle retention for a duration of five exhalations. {later editor}]

Jawbone Carriage (*Jia Che*, St 6) is located in the depressions at the angles of the lower jaw where a hole appears when the mouth opens and belongs to the qi of the foot *yang ming*. It is needled to a depth of three *fen* and moxaed with three cones.

Great Reception (*Da Ying*, St 5), also known as Marrow Hole (*Sui Kong*), is located in depressions one *cun* and two *fen* to (the lower border of) the mandible where vessels beat and belongs to the qi of the foot *yang ming*. It is needled to a depth of three *fen*, (the needle) is retained for a duration of seven exhalations, and it is moxaed with three cones.

Chapter Eleven

Twenty Points Anterior & Posterior to the Auricles[66]

Upper Pass (*Shang Guan*, GB 3), also known as Guest Host Person (*Ke Zhu Ren*), is located at the upper border of the rising bone (*i.e.*, the zygomatic arch) anterior to the auricle where a hole appears when the mouth opens and is the meeting point of three vessels, the hand and foot *shao yang*, and the foot *yang ming*. It is needled to a depth of three *fen*, (the needle) is retained for a duration of seven exhalations, and it is moxaed with three cones. [A note in the "*Qi Fu Lun*"[67] describes this point as the meeting point of the hand and the foot *tai yang* and the foot *yang ming*. The note in the "*Qi Xue Lun*",[68] however, agrees with the *Jia Yi Jing*. {later editor}][69]

Lower Pass (*Xia Guan*, St 7)[70] is located below Guest Host Person (*Ke Zhu Ren*), at the lower border of the zygomatic arch anterior to the auricle and near the pulsating vessel where a hole appears when the mouth is shut but disappears when it opens. It is the meeting point of the foot *yang ming* and the foot *shao yang*. It is needled to a depth of three *fen*, (the needle) is retained for a duration of seven exhalations, and it is moxaed with three cones. Moxibustion is prohibited when there is earwax in the ear. [A variant version also prohibits moxibustion. However, it prescribes prolonged needle retention in the case with dry earwax. {later editor}]

Ear Gate (*Er Men*, TH 21) is located on the ear in the dent above the fleshy protuberance [*i.e.*, the tragus]. It is needled to a depth of three *fen*, (the needle) is retained for a duration of three exhalations, and it is moxaed with three cones. Moxibustion is forbidden when there is pus and earwax in the ear.

Harmony Bone Hole (*He Liao*, TH 22) is located

near the transverse pulsating vessel under the lock (of hair) anterior to the auricle and is the meeting point of the hand and the foot *shao yang* and the hand *tai yang*. It is needled to a depth of three *fen* and is moxaed with three cones. [A note in the "*Qi Fu Lun*" states that it is the meeting point of the hand and foot *shao yang*. {later editor}]

Auditory Convergence (*Ting Hui*, GB 2) is located anterior to the auricle in a depression which appears on opening of the mouth and where a pulsating vessel is palpable. It belongs to the qi of the (hand) *shao yang*. It is needled to a depth of four *fen* and moxaed with three cones. [A note in the "*Miu Ci Lun*"[71] states that it is located at the parting of the hand yang channels. {later editor}]

Auditory Palace (*Ting Gong*, SI 19) is located in the tragus of the ear, which is as large as a red bean, and it is the meeting point of the hand and foot *shao yang* and the hand *tai yang*. It is needled to a depth of three *fen* and is moxaed with three cones. [A note in the "*Qi Xue Lun*" prescribes needling to a depth of one *fen*. {later editor}]

Angle Vertex (*Jiao Sun*, TH 20) is located (on the scalp) above the tip of the auricle where a hole appears upon opening the mouth and is the meeting point of the hand and the foot *shao yang* and the hand *yang ming*. It is needled to a depth of three *fen* and is moxaed with three cones. [A note in the "*Qi Fu Lun*" locates this point below the hairline in the crevice between the auricle and the scalp and describes it as the meeting point of three vessels, the hand *tai yang*, and foot and hand *shao yang*. {later editor}]

Spasm Vessel (*Chi Mai*, TH 18), also known as Supporting Vessel (*Zi Mai*), is located among the chicken-foot like green-blue vessels (on the scalp) posterior to the root of the auricle. Blood issues out in bean-like drops when the point is pricked. It is needled to a depth of one *fen* and is moxaed with three cones.

Skull Rest (*Lu Xi*, TH 19) is located among the green-blue vessels behind the auricle and belongs to the qi of the foot *shao yang*. It is needled to a depth of one *fen* and is moxaed with three cones.

Excessive bleeding at this point is fatal.

Wind Screen (*Yi Feng*, TH 17) is located in a depression behind the auricle where pressure radiates into the ear and is the meeting point of the hand and the foot *shao yang*. It is needled to a depth of four *fen* and is moxaed with three cones.[72]

Chapter Twelve

Seventeen Points on the Neck[73]

Ridge Spring (*Lian Quan*, CV 23), also known as Root Pool (*Ben Chi*), is located in the submandibular region above the throat knot (*i.e.*, Adam's apple) and is the meeting point of the root of the tongue,[74] the yin linking and conception vessels. It is needled to a depth of two *fen*, (the needle) is retained for a duration of three exhalations, and it is moxaed with three cones. [A note in the "*Qi Fu Lun*"[75] prescribes needle insertion to a depth of three *fen*. {later editor}]

Man's Prognosis (*Ren Ying*, St 9), also known as Celestial Fivefold Confluence (*Tian Wu Hui*), is located at the major pulsating vessel in the neck which may be palpated on either side of the throat knot. It reflects the qi of the five viscera and belongs to the qi of the foot *yang ming*. Moxibustion is prohibited although it is needled to a depth of four *fen*. Needling too deeply may unfortunately be fatal. [A note in the "*Yin Yang Lei Lun* (Treatise on Analogizing with Yin & Yang)" in the *Su Wen*[76] locates *Ren Ying* one *cun* and five *fen* bilateral to the throat knot, where the pulsating vessel is palpable. {later editor}]

Celestial Window (*Tian Chuang*, SI 16), also known as Window Basket (*Chuang Long*), is located below the angle of the mandible posterior to Protuberance Assistant in a depression where a pulsating vessel is palpable. It belongs to the qi of the hand *tai yang*. It is needled to a depth of six *fen* and is moxaed with three cones.

Celestial Casement (*Tian You*, TH 16) is located between two sinews above the supraclavicular fossa posterior to Celestial Countenance and anterior to Celestial Pillar (*Tian Zhu*, Bl 10) below the completion bone within the hairline. It belongs to the qi of the hand *shao yang*. It is needled to a depth of one *fen* and is moxaed with three cones.

Celestial Countenance (*Tian Rong*, SI 17) is located below the auricle posterior to the angle of the mandible and belongs to the qi of the hand *tai yang*. It is needled to a depth of one *cun* deep and is moxaed with three cones.

Water Prominence (*Shui Tu*, St 10), also known as Water Gate (*Shui Men*), is located on the neck anterior to the grand sinew[77] directly below Man's Prognosis (*Ren Ying*, St 9) and above Qi Abode and belongs to the qi of the foot *yang ming*. It is needled to a depth of one *cun* and is moxaed with three cones.

Qi Abode (*Qi She*, St 11) is located in the neck directly under Man's Prognosis in a depression lateral to Celestial Chimney (*Tian Tu*, CV 22) and belongs to the qi of the foot *yang ming*. It is needled to a depth of three *fen* and moxaed with five cones.

Protuberance Assistant (*Fu Tu*, LI 18), also known as Water Point (*Shui Xue*), is located one *cun* and five *fen* lateral to Man's Prognosis and belongs to the qi of the hand *yang ming*. Locate it with (the patient) prostrate. It is needled to a depth of four *fen* and is moxaed with three cones. [The *Zhen Jing*[78] locates this point one *cun* and five *fen* posterior to Qi Abode. {later editor}]

Celestial Tripod (*Tian Ding*, LI 17) is located (in the neck) above the supraclavicular fossa directly below Protuberance Assistant and one *cun* and five *fen* posterior to Qi Abode and belongs to the qi of the hand *yang ming*. It is needled to a depth of four *fen* and is moxaed with three cones. [A note in the "*Qi Fu Lun*" locates this point half a *cun* posterior to Qi Abode. {later editor}]

Chapter Thirteen

Twenty-Eight Points on the Shoulders[79]

Shoulder Well (*Jian Jing*, GB 21) is located in a depression on the shoulder above the supraclavicular fossa and anterior to the grand bone[80] and is the meeting point of the hand and foot *shao yang* and the yang linking vessel. It is needled to a depth of five *fen* and is moxaed with five cones. [A note in the *"Qi Fu Lun"*[81] prescribes three cones. {later editor}]

Shoulder True (*Jian Zhen*, SI 9) is located inferior to the (lateral) curve of the scapula between two bones in a depression behind the shoulder bone and belongs to the qi of the hand *tai yang*. It is needled to a depth of eight *fen* and moxaed with three cones.

Great Bone (*Ju Gu*, LI 16) is located in a depression in the clavicular acromion between two bones[82] and is the meeting point of the hand *yang ming* and the motility vessel. It is needled to a depth of one *cun* and five *fen* and is moxaed with five cones. [A note in the *"Qi Fu Lun"* prescribes three cones. {later editor}]

Celestial Bone Hole (*Tian Liao*, TH 19) is located in a depression at the spina scapulae in line with the middle of, but superior to the supraclavicular fossa and is the meeting point of the hand *shao yang* and the yang linking vessel. It is needled to a depth of eight *fen* and moxaed with three cones.

Shoulder Bone (*Jian Yu*, LI 15) is located between two bones[83] at the end of the shoulder and is the meeting point of the hand *yang ming* and the motility vessel. It is needled to a depth of six *fen*, (the needle) is retained for a duration of six exhalations, and it is moxaed with three cones.

Shoulder Bone Hole (*Jian Liao*, TH 14) is located on the upper arm at the end of the shoulder. Locate it with the (patient's) arm raised obliquely. It is needled to a depth of seven *fen* and moxaed with three cones. [A note in the *"Qi Fu Lun"*

describes this point as belonging to the channel qi of the hand *shao yang*. {later editor}]

Upper Arm Shu (*Nao Shu*, TH 13) is located medial to Shoulder Bone Hole in a depression at the upper border of the scapula under the grand bone,[84] and is the meeting point of the hand and the foot *tai yang*, the yang linking vessel, and the motility vessel. Locate it with the (patient's) arm raised. It is needled to a depth of eight *fen* and it is moxaed with three cones.

Grasping the Wind (*Bing Feng*, SI 12) is located lateral to Celestial Bone Hole (*Tian Liao*, TH 15) behind the prominence of the shoulder where a hole appears when the arm is raised and is the meeting point of the hand *yang ming*, the hand *tai yang*, and the hand and foot *shao yang*. Locate it with the (patient's) arm raised. It is needled to a depth of five *fen*, and is moxaed with five cones. [A note in the *"Qi Fu Lun"* prescribes three cones. {later editor}]

Celestial Gathering (*Tian Zong*, SI 11) is located in a depression behind Grasping the Wind inferior to the great bone and belongs to the qi of the hand *tai yang*. It is needled to a depth of five *fen*, (the needle) is retained for a duration of six exhalations, and it is moxaed with three cones.

Outer Shoulder Shu (*Jian Wai Shu*, SI 14) is located at the upper border of the scapula in a depression three *cun* bilateral to the spine. It is needled to a depth of six *fen* and it is moxaed with three cones.

Central Shoulder Shu (*Jian Zhong Shu*, SI 15) is located at the medial border of the scapula in a depression two *cun* bilateral to the spine. It is needled to a depth of three *fen*, (the needle) is retained for a duration of seven exhalations, and it is moxaed with three cones.

Crooked Wall (*Qu Yuan*, SI 13) is located in the middle of the shoulder in a depression at the spina scapulae where a pulsing vessel is felt when pressure is applied. It is needled to a depth of nine *fen* and moxaed with ten cones.

Empty Basin (*Que Pen*, ST 12), also known as

Celestial Cover (*Tian Gai*), is located in the curve of the clavicle on the shoulder. It is needled to a depth of two *fen*, (the needle) is retained for a duration of seven exhalations, and it is moxaed with three cones. Unduly deep insertion causes counterflow breathing. [A note in the *"Gu Kong Lun"*,[85] states that it belongs to the qi of the hand *yang ming*, while a note in the *"Qi Fu Lun"* states that it belongs to the qi of the foot *yang ming*. {later editor}][86]

Upper Arm Convergence (*Nao Hui*, TH 13), also known as Upper Arm Bone Hole (*Nao Liao*), is located on the anterior aspect of the upper arm three *cun* from the shoulder and is the connecting vessel of the hand *yang ming*.[87] It is needled to a depth of five *fen* and moxaed with five cones. [A note in the *"Qi Fu Lun"* states that it is the meeting point of the hand *yang ming* and the hand *shao yang*. {later editor}]

Chapter Fourteen

Seven Points on the Chest Located from Celestial Chimney (*Tian Tu*) Downward Along the Conception Vessel to Center Palace (*Zhong Ting*)[88]

Celestial Chimney (*Tian Tu*, CV 22), also known as Jade Door (*Yu Hu*), is located in the center of a depression two *cun* inferior to the throat knot and is the meeting point of the yin linking vessel and the conception vessel. [A note in the *"Qi Fu Lun"* states that it is five *cun*. {later editor}] Locate it with the (patient's) head bent down. It is needled to a depth of one *cun*, (the needle) is retained for a duration of seven exhalations, and it is moxaed with three cones. [A note in the *"Qi Fu Lun"*[89] prescribes five cones. {later editor}]

Jade Pivot (*Xuan Ji*, CV 21) is located in the center of a depression one *cun* below Celestial Chimney and belongs to the qi of the conception vessel. Locate it with the (patient's) head bent back. It is needled to a depth of three *fen* and moxaed with five cones.

Florid Canopy (*Hua Gai*, CV 20) is located in a depression one *cun* under Jade Pivot and belongs to the qi of the conception vessel. Locate it with the (patient's) head bent back. It is needled to a depth of three *fen* and moxaed with five cones.

Purple Palace (*Zi Gong*, CV 19) is located in a depression one *cun* and six *fen* below Florid Canopy and belongs to the qi of the conception vessel. Locate it with the (patient's) head bent back. It is needled to depth of three *fen* and moxaed with five cones.

Jade Hall (*Yu Tang*, CV 18), also known as Jade Beauty (*Yu Ying*), is located in a depression one *cun* and six *fen* below Purple Palace and belongs to the qi of the conception vessel. Locate it with the (patient's) head bent back. It is needled to a depth of three *fen* and moxaed with five cones.

Chest Center (*Dan Zhong*, CV 17), also known as Original Child (*Yuan Er*), is located in a depression one *cun* and six *fen* below Jade Hall at the midpoint between the two breasts and belongs to the qi of the conception vessel. Locate it with the (patient) lying supine. It is needled to a depth of three *fen* and is moxaed with five cones.

Center Palace (*Zhong Ting*, CV 16) is located in a depression one *cun* and six *fen* below Chest Center and belongs to the qi of the conception vessel. Locate it with (the patient) lying supine. It is needled to a depth of three *fen* and moxaed with five cones.

Chapter Fifteen

Twelve Points on the Chest Located Two *Cun* Bilateral to the Conception Vessel from Shu Mansion (*Shu Fu*) Down to Corridor Walk (*Bu Lang*)[90]

Transport Mansion (*Shu Fu*, Ki 27) is located in a depression under the clavicle two *cun* bilateral to Turning Pivot (*Xuan Ji*, CV 21) and belongs to the qi of the foot *shao yin*. Locate it with (the patient) lying supine. It is needled to a depth of four *fen* and is moxaed with five cones.

Thriving Center (*Yu Zhong*, Ki 26)[91] is located in a depression one *cun* and six *fen* below Shu Mansion and belongs to the qi of the foot *shao yin*. Locate it with (the patient) lying supine. It is needled to a depth of four *fen* and moxaed with five cones.

Spirit Storehouse (*Shen Cang*, Ki 25) is located in a depression one *cun* and six *fen* below Thriving Center and belongs to the qi of the foot *shao yin*. Locate it with (the patient) lying supine. It is needled to a depth of four *fen* and is moxaed with five cones.

Spirit Homeland (*Ling Xu*, Ki 24)[91] is located in a depression one *cun* and six *fen* below Spirit Storehouse and belongs to the qi of the foot *shao yin*. Locate it with (the patient) lying supine. It is needled to a depth of four *fen* and is moxaed with five cones.

Spirit Seal (*Shen Feng*, Ki 23) is located in a depression one *cun* and six *fen* under Spirit Homeland and belongs to the qi of the foot *shao yin*. Locate it with (the patient) lying supine. It is needled to a depth of four *fen* and moxaed with five cones.

Corridor Walk (*Bu Lang*, Ki 22) is located in a depression one *cun* and six *fen* under Spirit Seal and belongs to the qi of the foot *shao yin*. Locate it with (the patient) lying supine. It is needled to a depth of four *fen* and is moxaed with five cones.

Chapter Sixteen

Twelve Points on the Chest from Qi Door (*Qi Hu*) Two *Cun* Lateral to Transport Mansion (*Shu Fu*) Down to Breast Root (*Ru Gen*)[92]

Qi Door (*Qi Hu*, St 13) is located in a depression under the clavicle two *cun* lateral to Transport Mansion (*Shu Fu*, Ki 27) and belongs to the qi of

the foot *yang ming*. Locate it with (the patient) lying supine. It is needled to a depth of four *fen* and is moxaed with five cones. [A note in the "*Qi Fu Lun*"[93] states that this point is four *cun* and eight *fen* above Breast Window and prescribes moxibustion with three cones. {later editor}]

Storeroom (*Ku Fang*, St 14) is located in a depression one *cun* and six *fen* below Qi Door and belongs to the qi of the foot *yang ming*. Locate it with (the patient) lying supine. It is needled to a depth of four *fen* and is moxaed with five cones. [A note in the "*Qi Fu Lun*" prescribes moxibustion with three cones. {later editor}]

Eave (*Wu Yi*, St 15)[94] is located one *cun* and six *fen* below Storeroom and belongs to the qi of the foot *yang ming*. Locate it with (the patient) lying supine. It is needled to a depth of four *fen* and moxaed with five cones. [A note in the "*Qi Fu Lun*" locates this point three *cun* and two *fen* below Qi Door and prescribes moxibustion with three cones. {later editor}]

Breast Window (*Ying Chuang*, St 16) is located one *cun* and six *fen* below Eave. It is needled to a depth of four *fen* and moxaed with five cones. [A note in the "*Qi Fu Lun*" states that it is located four *cun* bilateral to the midline of the body in a depression four *cun* and eight *fen* below the clavicles, that it belongs to the qi of the foot *yang ming*, and that it should be located with the body lying supine. {later editor}]

Breast Center (*Ru Zhong*, St 17) is contraindicated to needling or moxibustion. If (this point is) moxaed or needled, there will be the unfortunate development of corroding sores. Breast sores with pus, blood, and serum are curable. Breast sores with polyps looking like the corroding sore are fatal.

Breast Root (*Ru Gen*, St 18) is located in a depression one *cun* and six *fen* below the breast and belongs to the qi of the foot *yang ming*. Locate it with (the patient) lying supine. It is needled to a depth of four *fen* and is moxaed with five cones. [A note in the "*Qi Fu Lun*" prescribes three cones. {later editor}]

Chapter Seventeen

Twelve Points on the Chest Located from Cloud Gate (*Yun Men*) Two *Cun* Lateral to Qi Door (*Qi Hu*) Down to Food Duct (*Shi Dou*)[95]

Cloud Gate (*Yun Men*, Lu 2) is located under the clavicle in a depression two *cun* lateral to Qi Door (*Qi Hu*, St 13) where a pulsating vessel is palpable. It belongs to the qi of the foot *tai yin*. Locate it with the (patient's) arm raised. It is needled to a depth of seven *fen* and moxaed with five cones. Unduly deep insertion causes counterflow breathing. [A note in the "*Qi Fu Lun*"[96] locates it under the clavicle six *cun* bilateral to the conception vessel. In a note in the "*Ci Re Xue Lun*",[97] it is said to belong to the channel qi of the hand *tai yang*. {later editor}]

Central Treasury (*Zhong Fu*, Lu 1) is the alarm point of the lung and is also known as Breast Center Shu (*Ying Zhong Shu*). It is located one *cun* below Cloud Gate in a depression in the breast above the third rib where a pulsating vessel is palpable. Locate it with (the patient) lying supine. It is the meeting point of the hand and foot *tai yin*. It is needled to a depth of three *fen*, (the needle) is retained for a duration of five exhalations, and it is moxaed with five cones.

All Around Flourishing (*Zhou Rong*, Sp 20) is located in a depression one *cun* and six *fen* under Central Treasury and belongs to the qi of the foot *tai yin*. Locate it with (the patient) lying supine. It is needled to a depth of four *fen* and it is moxaed with five cones.

Chest Home (*Xiong Xiang*, Sp 19)[98] is located in a depression one *cun* and six *fen* below All Around Flourishing and belongs to the qi of the foot *tai yin*. Locate it with (the patient) lying supine. It is needled to a depth of four *fen* and moxaed with five cones.

Celestial Ravine (*Tian Xi*, Sp 18) is located in a depression one *cun* and six *fen* below Chest Home and belongs to the qi of the foot *tai yin*. Locate it with (the patient) lying supine. It is needled to a depth of four *fen* and is moxaed with five cones.

Food Duct (*Shi Dou*, Sp 17)[99] is located in a depression one *cun* and six *fen* below Celestial Ravine and belongs to the qi of the foot *tai yin*. Locate it with the (patient's) arm raised. It is needled to a depth of four *fen* and moxaed with five cones. [A note in the "*Qi Fu Lun*" states that it belongs to the qi of the hand *tai yin*. {later editor}]

Chapter Eighteen

Eight Points Below the Axilla in the Lateral Costal Region[100]

Armpit Abyss (*Yuan Ye*, GB 22) is located in a depression three *cun* below the axilla. Locate it with the (patient's) arm raised. It is needled to a depth of three *fen*, but moxibustion is contraindicated as moxibustion may unfortunately cause swelling corrosion and saber lumps.[101] Saber lumps which fester inward are fatal, but those due to cold and heat are curable. [A note in the "*Qi Xue Lun*",[102] states that this point belongs to the qi of the foot *shao yang*. {later editor}]

Great Embracement (*Da Bao*, Sp 21) is located three *cun* below Armpit Abyss and is the major connecting vessel of the spleen. It spreads in the chest and the lateral costal region, emerging below the ninth rib and at the ends of the free ribs,[103] and links all the yin (channels) there. It is needled to a depth of three *fen* and is moxaed with three cones.

Sinew Rut (*Zhe Jin*, GB 23)[104] is located three *cun* below and one *cun* anterior to the axilla bordering on the rib at the side, and belongs to the qi of the foot *shao yang* vessel. It is needled to a depth of six *fen* and is moxaed with three cones.

Celestial Pool (*Tian Chi*, Per 1), also known as Celestial Convergence (*Tian Hui*), is located one *cun* lateral to the breast ["two *cun*" in a note in the "*Qi Fu Lun*"[105] {later editor}] three *cun* below the axilla. It borders on the rib in the lateral costal region between the free ribs straight under the axilla[106] and is the meeting point of the hand *jue yin* and foot *shao yang* ["the meeting point of the hand heart-governor and the foot *shao yang*" in a variant version. {later editor}] It is needled to a depth of seven *fen*, and moxaed with three cones. [A note in the *"Qi Fu Lun"* prescribes a needle insertion of three *fen*. {later editor}]

Chapter Nineteen

Fifteen Points on the Abdomen Located from Turtledove Tail (*Jiu Wei*) Downward Along the Conception Vessel to Meeting of Yin (*Hui Yin*)[107]

Turtledove Tail (*Jiu Wei*, CV 15), also known as Tail Screen (*Wei Yi*) and Breast Bone (*He Yu*), is located five *fen* under the xiphoid process on the chest. It is a branch of the conception vessel and both needling and moxibustion are prohibited.[108] [Turtledove Tail is approximately opposite to the heart and can be located one *cun* and a half under the seventh sternocostal juncture in the case of the absence of the xiphoid process. A note in the *"Qi Fu Lun"*[109] locates it one *cun* under or at the midpoint between the juncture and Great Tower Gate (*Ju Que*, CV 14). If the xiphoid process is shorter than normal as is the case with some people, the point can be determined a little less than one *cun* under the process.]

Great Tower Gate (*Ju Que*, CV 14) is the alarm point of the heart and is located one *cun* below Turtledove Tail. It belongs to the qi of the conception vessel. It is needled to a depth of six *fen*, (and the needle is) retained for a duration of seven exhalations. It is moxaed with five cones. [A note in the *"Qi Fu Lun"* indicates it is to be needled to a depth of one *cun* and two *fen*.]

Upper Venter (*Shang Wan*, CV 13) is located one *cun* and five *fen* below Great Tower Gate or three *cun* below the xiphoid process. It is the meeting point of the conception vessel, the foot *yang ming*,

and the hand *tai yang*. It is needled to a depth of eight *fen* and moxaed with five cones.

Central Venter (*Zhong Wan*, CV 12) is also known as Supreme Granary (*Tai Cang*). It is the alarm point of the stomach and is located one *cun* below Upper Venter or at the midpoint between the xiphoid process and the umbilicus. It is engendered by the hand *tai yang* and *shao yang* and the foot *yang ming*. (These channels) meet with the conception vessel here. It is needled to a depth of one *cun*, two *fen* and moxaed with seven cones. [The *Jiu Juan (Ninefold Volume)* states that Supreme Granary lies in the center of the eight *cun* space between the xiphoid process and the umbilicus or four *cun* above the umbilicus. Its location in the *Mu Xue Jing (Classic of Alarm Points)* by Lu Guang[110] of three *cun* above the umbilicus is mistaken.]

Interior Strengthening (*Jian Li*, CV 11) is located one *cun* below Central Venter. It is needled to a depth of five *fen* and (the needle is) retained for a duration of ten exhalations. It is moxaed with five cones. [A note in the *"Qi Fu Lun"* prescribes needling to a depth of six *fen* with needles retained for seven exhalations.]

Lower Venter (*Xia Wan*, CV 10) is located one *cun* below Interior Strengthening and is a meeting point of the foot *tai yin* and the conception vessel. It is needled to a depth of one *cun* and moxaed with five cones.

Center of the Navel (*Qi Zhong*, CV 8) is also known as Spirit Gate (*Shen Que*) and Qi Abode (*Qi She*). It may be moxaed with three cones, but needling is contraindicated. Needling may cause malignant sores and ulcerations with fecal incontinence, an incurable and fatal syndrome.

Water Divide (*Shui Fen*, CV 9) is located one *cun* below Lower Venter and one *cun* above the umbilicus and is supplied by the qi of the conception vessel. It is needled to a depth of one *cun* and moxaed with five cones.

Yin Intersection (*Yin Jiao*, CV 7) is also known as Scarce Pass (*Shao Guan*) and Horizontal Door

(*Heng Hu*). It is located one *cun* below the umbilicus and is the meeting point of the conception vessel and the yin penetrating vessel.[111] It is needled to a depth of eight *fen* and moxaed with five cones.

Sea of Qi (*Qi Hai*, CV 6) is also known as Navel (*Bo Yang*) and Lower Huang (*Xia Huang*). It is located one *cun* and five *fen* below the umbilicus and belongs to the qi of the conception vessel. It is needled to a depth of one *cun* and two *fen* and moxaed with five cones.

Stone Door (*Shi Men*, CV 5) is the alarm point of the triple burner and is also known as Crux Disinhibitor (*Li Ji*), Essential Dew (*Jing Lu*), Cinnabar Field (*Dan Tian*), and Life Gate (*Ming Men*). It is located two *cun* below the umbilicus and belongs to the qi of the conception vessel. It is needled to a depth of five *fen*, (the needle is) retained for a duration of ten exhalations and it is moxaed with three cones. Needling and moxibustion are prohibited in females as it may cause infertility. [A note in the "*Qi Fu Lun*" prescribes a needle insertion of six *fen*, which is retained for seven exhalations, and moxibustion with three cones.]

Origin Pass (*Guan Yuan*, CV 4) is the alarm point of the small intestine and is also known as Second Gate (*Ci Men*). It is located three *cun* below the umbilicus and is the meeting point of the foot and the conception vessel. It is needled to a depth of two *cun*, (the needle) is retained for a duration of seven exhalations, and it is moxaed with seven cones. [A note in the "*Qi Fu Lun*" prescribes a needle insertion on one *cun* and two *fen*.]

Central Pole (*Zhong Ji*, CV 3) is the alarm point of the urinary bladder and is also known as Qi Source (*Qi Yuan*) and Jade Spring (*Yu Quan*). It is located four *cun* below the umbilicus and is the meeting point of the three yin channels of the foot and the conception vessel. It is needled to a depth of two *cun*, (the needle is) retained for a duration of seven exhalations, and it is moxaed with three cones. [A note in the "*Qi Fu Lun*" prescribes a needle insertion of one *cun* and two *fen*.]

Curved Bone (*Qu Gu*, CV 2) is located at the pubic bone one *cun* below *Zhong Ji* in a depression in the hairline where a pulsating vessel can be palpated. It is a meeting point of the conception vessel and the foot *jue yin*. It is needled to a depth of one *cun* and five *fen*, (the needle is) retained for a duration of seven exhalations, and it is moxaed with three cones. [A note in the "*Qi Fu Lun*" states that there are altogether fourteen points from the xiphoid process to the pubic bone, and all of them belong to the qi of the conception vessel.]

Meeting of Yin (*Hui Yin*, CV 1) is also known as Screen (*Ping Yi*) and is located anterior to the anus but posterior to the urethral meatus, *i.e.*, between the two yin (organs. From here) a branch connecting vessel of the conception vessel runs along the governing vessel. It is the meeting point of the governing and penetrating vessels (and the conception vessel). It is needled to a depth of two *cun*, (the needle is) retained for a duration of seven exhalations, and it is moxaed with three cones.

Chapter Twenty

Twenty-Two Points on the Abdomen Located from Dark Gate (*You Men*) Half a *Cun* Bilateral to Great Tower Gate (*Ju Que*) Down Along the Penetrating Vessel to Pubic Bone (*Heng Gu*)[112]

Dark Gate (*You Men*, Ki 21) is also known as Upper Gate (*Shang Men*). It is located in a depression five *fen* bilateral to Great Tower Gate, and is a point at which the penetrating vessel and the foot *shao yin* meet. It is needled to a depth of five *fen* and moxaed with five cones. [A note in the "*Qi Fu Lun*"[113] prescribes needling to a depth of one *cun*.]

Open Valley (*Tong Gu*, Ki 20) is located in a depression one *cun* below Dark Gate. It is a meeting point of the penetrating vessel and the foot *shao yin*. It is needled to a depth of five *fen* and moxaed with five cones. [A note in the "*Qi Fu*

Lun" prescribes needling to a depth of one *cun*.]

Yin Metropolis (*Yin Du*, Ki 19), also known as Food Palace (*Shi Gong*), is located one *cun* below Open Valley and is a meeting point of the penetrating vessel and the foot *shao yin*. It is needled to a depth of one *cun* and moxaed with five cones.

Stone Pass (*Shi Guan*, Ki 18) is located one *cun* below Yin Metropolis. It is a meeting point of the penetrating vessel and the foot *shao yin*. It is needled to a depth of one *cun* and moxaed with five cones.

Shang Bend (*Shang Qu*, Ki 17) is located one *cun* below Stone Pass and is a meeting point of the penetrating vessel and the foot *shao yin*. It is needled to a depth of one *cun* and moxaed with five cones.

Huang Shu (*Huang Shu*, Ki 16) is located one *cun* below Shang Bend and five *fen* bilateral to the umbilicus. It is a meeting point of the penetrating vessel and the foot *shao yin*. It is needled to a depth of one *cun* and moxaed with five cones.

Central Islet (*Zhong Zhu*, Ki 15) is located five *fen* below Huang Shu, and is a meeting point of the penetrating vessel and the foot *shao yin*. It is needled to a depth of one *cun* and moxaed with five cones. [A note in the *"Shui Re Xue Lun"* {Treatise on Points for Water & Heat Disorders} in the *Su Wen*[114] states that this point is located five *fen* below the umbilicus and five *fen* bilateral to the conception vessel.]

Fourfold Fullness (*Si Man*, Ki 14) is also known as Marrow Mansion (*Sui Fu*) and is located one *cun* below Central Islet. It is a meeting point of the penetrating vessel and the foot *shao yin*. It is needled to a depth of one *cun* and is moxaed with five cones.

Qi Point (*Qi Xue*, Ki 13) is also known as Wrapper Gate (*i.e.*, Uterine Gate, *Bao Men*) and Infant's Door (*Zi Hu*) and is located one *cun* below Fourfold Fullness. It is a meeting point of the penetrating vessel and the foot *shao yin*. It is needled to a depth of one *cun* and moxaed with five cones.

Great Manifestation (*Da He*, Ki 12) is also known as Yin Link (*Yin Wei*) and Yin Gate (*Yin Men*) and is located one *cun* below Qi Point. It is a meeting point of the penetrating vessel and the foot *shao yin*. It is needled to a depth of one *cun* and moxaed with five cones.

Horizontal Bone[115] (*Heng Gu*, Ki 11) is also known as Lower Extreme (*Xia Ji*) and is located one *cun* below Great Manifestation. It is a meeting point of the penetrating vessel and the foot *shao yin*. It is needled to a depth of one *cun* and moxaed with five cones.

Chapter Twenty-One

Twenty-Four Points on the Abdomen from Not Contained (*Bu Rong*) One *Cun* & Five *Fen* Lateral to Dark Gate (*You Men*) Down to Surging Qi (*Qi Chong*)[116]

Not Contained (*Bu Rong*, St 19) is located one *cun* and five *fen* lateral to Dark Gate, two *cun* bilateral to the conception vessel, or four *cun* from the tip of the fourth rib. It belongs to the qi of the foot *yang ming* vessel. It is needled to a depth of five *fen* and moxaed with five cones. [A note in the *"Qi Fu Lun"*[117] prescribes an insertion of eight *fen* and additionally states that, from Not Contained on down to Supreme Unity, each point lies one *cun* from the point adjacent to it.]

Assuming Fullness (*Cheng Man*, St 20) is located one *cun* below Not Contained and belongs to the qi of the foot *yang ming* vessel. It is needled to a depth of eight *fen* and moxaed with five cones.

Beam Gate (*Liang Men*, St 21) is located one *cun* below Assuming Fullness and belongs to the qi of the foot *yang ming*. It is needled to a depth of eight *fen* and moxaed with five cones.

Pass Gate (*Guan Men*, St 22) is located below Beam Gate and above Supreme Unity and belongs to the qi of the foot *yang ming* vessel.[118] It is needled to a depth of eight *fen* and moxaed with five cones.

Supreme Unity (*Tai Yi*, St 23) is located one *cun* below Pass Gate and belongs to the qi of the foot *yang ming*. It is needled to a depth of eight *fen* and moxaed with five cones.

Slippery Flesh Gate (*Hua Rou Men*, St 24) is located one *cun* below Supreme Unity and belongs to the qi of the foot *yang ming* vessel. It is needled to a depth of eight *fen* and moxaed with five cones.

Celestial Pivot (*Tian Shu*, St 25) is the alarm point of the large intestine and is also known as Long Stream (*Chang Xi*) and Valley Gate (*Gu Men*). It is located in a depression one *cun* and five *fen* lateral to Huang Shu and two *cun* bilateral to the umbilicus and belongs to the qi of the foot *yang ming* vessel. It is needled to a depth of five *fen*, (the needle) is retained for a duration of seven exhalations, and it is moxaed with three cones. [A note in the "*Qi Fu Lun*" states that it is one *cun* below Slippery Flesh Gate, just lateral to the umbilicus.]

Outer Mound (*Wai Ling*, St 26) is located below Celestial Pivot but above Great Gigantic and belongs to qi of the foot *yang ming* vessel. It is needled to a depth of eight *fen* and moxaed with five cones. [A note in the "*Qi Fu Lun*" states that it is located one *cun* below Celestial Pivot, while, in a note in the "*Shui Re Xue Lun*"[119] it is located one *cun* below the umbilicus one *cun* and five *fen* lateral to the penetrating vessel.]

Great Gigantic (*Da Ju*, St 27), also known as Armpit Gate (*Ye Men*), is located two *cun* below Long Stream and belongs to the qi of the foot *yang ming*. It is needled to a depth of eight *fen* and is moxaed with five cones. [A note in the "*Qi Fu Lun*" states that it is located one *cun* below Outer Mound.]

Water Way (*Shui Dao*, St 28) is located three *cun* below Great Gigantic and belongs to the qi of the foot *yang ming* channel. It is needled to a depth of two *cun* and five *fen* and moxaed with five cones.

Return (*Gui Lai*, St 29) is also known as Stream Hole (*Xi Xue*), and is located two *cun* below Water Way. It is needled to a depth of eight *fen* and moxaed with five cones. [A note in the "*Shui Xue Lun*" states that it belongs to the qi of the foot *yang ming*.]

Surging Qi (*Qi Chong*, St 30) is located below Return, one *cun* above the groin, where a pulsating vessel is palpable, and belongs to the qi of the foot *yang ming* vessel. It is needled to a depth of three *fen*, (the needle) is retained for a duration of seven exhalations, and it is moxaed with three cones. Moxibustion may unfortunately cause difficult breathing. [A note in the "*Qi Fu Lun*" states it is at the ends of the pubic bone, one *cun* above the groin. A note in the "*Ci Jin Lun*" [120]states that it is four *cun* below and bilateral to the umbilicus and one *cun* above the groin, where a pulsating vessel is palpable. A note in the "*Gu Kong Lun*"[121] states that it is bilateral to the pubic hair region one *cun* above the groin.]

Chapter Twenty-Two

Fourteen Points on the Abdomen from Cycle Gate (*Qi Men*) Directly Below the Breast One *Cun* & Five *Fen* Lateral to Not Contained (*Bu Rong*) Down to Surging Gate (*Chong Men*)[122]

Cycle Gate (*Qi Men*, Liv 14) is the alarm point of the liver. It is located at the tip of the angle of the second rib, one *cun* and five *fen* lateral to Not Contained directly inferior to the breast and is a meeting point of the foot *tai yin*, *jue yin*, and the yin linking vessel. It is located with the (patient's) arm raised, needled to a depth of four *fen*, and moxaed with five cones.

Sun and Moon (*Ri Yue*, GB 24) is the alarm point of the gallbladder. It is located five *fen* below Cycle Gate and is a meeting point of the foot *tai yin* and *shao yang*. It is needled to a depth of seven *fen* and moxaed with five cones. [A note in the "*Qi Fu Lun*"[123] states that it is located at the tip of the angle of the third rib, two *cun* and five *fen* just bilateral to the xiphoid process directly below the breast.]

Abdominal Lament (*Fu Ai*, Sp 16) is located one *cun* and five *fen* below Sun and Moon and is a meeting point of the foot *tai yin* and the yin linking vessel. It is needled to a depth of seven *fen* and moxaed with five cones.

Great Horizontal (*Da Heng*, Sp 15) is located three *cun* below Abdominal Lament lateral to the umbilicus and is a meeting point of the foot *tai yin* and the yin linking vessel. It is needled to a depth of seven *fen* and moxaed with five cones.

Abdominal Bend (*Fu Qu*, Sp 14) is also known as Abdominal Bind (*Fu Jie*) and is located one *cun* and three *fen* below Great Horizontal. It is needled to a depth of seven *fen* and moxaed with five cones.

Bowel Abode (*Fu She*, Sp 13) is located three *cun* below Abdominal Bend and is a meeting point of the foot *tai yin* and the yin linking vessel. The vessel[124] enters the abdomen to connect with the chest and bind at the heart and the lung. It then ascends via the lateral costal region to the shoulder. It is the cleft point of the (foot) *tai yin* and the branch of the three (foot) yin and the (foot) *yang ming* channels. It is needled to a depth of seven *fen* and moxaed with five cones.

Surging Gate (*Chong Men*, Sp 12) is also known as Palace of Charity (*Ci Gong*) and is located at the pulsating vessel in the groin, five *cun* below Great Horizontal, at the ends of the pubic bone below Bowel Abode. It is needled to a depth of seven *fen* and moxaed with five cones.

Chapter Twenty-Three

Twelve Points on the Abdomen from Camphorwood Gate (*Zhang Men*) Down to Squatting Bone Hole (*Ju Liao*)[125]

Camphorwood Gate (*Zhang Men*, Liv 13) is the alarm point of the spleen and is also known as Long Level (*Chang Ping*) and Lateral Costal Bone Hole (*Xie Liao*). It is located lateral to Great Horizontal, directly (level) with the umbilicus at the end of a free rib, and is the meeting point of the foot *jue yin* and *shao yang*. To locate Camphorwood Gate, the patient should lie on his side with the upper leg bent, the lower extended, and the arm raised. It is needled to a depth of eight *fen*, and (the needle) is retained for a duration of six exhalations. It is moxaed with three cones.

Girdling Vessel (*Dai Mai*, GB 26) is located one *cun* and eight *fen* below the region of the free rib. It is needled to a depth of six *fen* and moxaed with five cones. [A note in the *"Qi Fu Lun"*[126] states that it is the meeting point of the foot *shao yang* and the girdling vessel.]

Fifth Pivot (*Wu Shu*, GB 27) is located three *cun* below Girdling Vessel. It is also said to be one *cun* and five *fen* lateral to Water Way (*Shui Dao*, St 28). It is needled to a depth of one *cun* and moxaed with five cones. [A note in the *"Qi Fu Lun"* states that it is the meeting point of the foot *shao yin* and the girdling vessel.]

Capital Gate (*Jing Men*, GB 25) is the alarm point of the kidney and is also known as Qi Mansion (*Qi Fu*) and Qi Transport. It is located below the hip bone in the lumbar region lateral to the spine, one *cun* and eight *fen* below the region of the free ribs.[127] It is needled to a depth of three *fen* and (the needle) is retained for a duration of seven exhalations. It is moxaed with three cones.

Linking Pivot (*Wei Dao*, GB 28) is also known as Outer Pivot (*Wai Shu*) and is located five *cun* and three *fen* below Camphorwood Gate. It is a meeting point of the foot *shao yang* and the girdling vessel. It is needled to a depth of eight *fen* and moxaed with three cones.

Squatting Bone Hole (*Ju Liao*, GB 29) is located eight *cun* and three *fen* below Camphorwood Gate in a depression on the hipbone and is a meeting point of the yang motility vessel and the foot *shao yang*. It is needled to a depth of eight *fen* and moxaed with three cones. [A note in the *"Qi Fu Lun"* states that the hipbone is the ilium.]

Chapter Twenty-Four

Eighteen Points of the Hand
Tai Yin on the Arm[128]

The Yellow Emperor asked:

Tell me about the places where the five viscera and the six bowels[129] exit.

Qi Bo answered:

(Each of) the five viscera has five transporting points and, therefore, there are five times five, *i.e.*, twenty-five transporting points in all. Each of the six bowels has six transporting points and, subsequently, there are six times six, *i.e.*, thirty-six transporting points in all. There are twelve channels and fifteen network vessels, producing a total of twenty-seven (vessels of) qi running up and down in the body. The place where (the qi) emerges is the well (*jing*). The place where (the qi) gushes forth is the brook (*ying*). The place where (the qi) pours forth (*zhu*) is the rapids (*shu*). The place of effluence is the source (*yuan*). The place where (the qi) flows mightily is the stream (*jing*). The place where (the qi) submerges is the confluence (*he*). In a narrow sense, only the confluence can be called the transporting point. Generally speaking, however, the well, brook, source, stream, and confluence points of the hand *tai yin*, for example, are all called transporting points. Points other than these six (but located between them on a channel) are called intermediate points.

The points are as follows:

The vessel of hand *tai yin* emerges at the tip of the (palmar) surface of the thumb, travelling along the border of the white flesh to Great Abyss (*Tai Yuan*, Lu 9) proximal to the base joint of the phalanx of the thumb where it ripples, beating (palpably). It then proceeds, turning outward and ascending to the region distal to the base joint [a variant version reads "ascending from the base joint"], where it turns inward to meet there with the yin network vessels and to meet the other yin

channels at the fish's margin where several channels[130] have their confluences. [A later editor notes that it is likely that something is missing here.]

At this point the qi of the channel is smooth and swift, running deeply through the metacarpal bone. It then turns outward to emerge at the *cun kou* where it flows mightily. It continues to ascend, arriving in the inner aspect of the elbow where it submerges below the major sinew,[131] and then turns inward to ascend along the yin (in this case anterior) aspect of the upper arm. After entering the armpit, it turns inward toward the lung. This illustrates the turns and bends in the flow (of the hand *tai yin*).

The lung issues at Lesser Shang (*Shao Shang*, Lu 11) and Lesser Shang is associated with wood. It is located at the tip of the inner (radial) aspect of the thumb, the distance of a leek leaf from the corner of the nail. It is the place where the hand *tai yin* vessel issues and is, therefore, its well point. (Lesser Shang) is needled to a depth of one *fen* and (the needle) is retained for a duration of one exhalation. It is moxaed with one cone. [The "*Qi Xue Lun*"[132] prescribes three cones.]

Fish Border (*Yu Ji*, Lu 10) is associated with fire. It is located at the radial border of the thumb proximal to the base joint of the phalanx among the dispersing vessels. [This means that the vessels disperse and circulate from here.] It is the point where the hand *tai yin* channel gushes forth and is, therefore, the spring point. (Fish Border) is needled to a depth of two *fen*, and (the needle) is retained for a duration of three exhalations. It is moxaed with three cones.

Great Abyss (*Tai Yuan*, Lu 9) is associated with earth. It is located in a depression proximal to the wrist and is the point where the hand *tai yin* channel pours forth. Therefore, it is the rapids point. (Great Abyss) is needled to a depth of two *fen* and (the needle) is retained for a duration of two exhalations. It is moxaed with three cones.

Channel Ditch (*Jing Qu*, Lu 8) is associated with metal. It is located in a depression at the *cun kou* and is the point where the hand *tai yin* channel flows mightily. Therefore, it is the stream point. Channel Ditch is needled to a depth of three *fen* and (the needle) is retained for a duration of three exhalations. Moxibustion is prohibited because it may damage spirit-brightness.[133]

Broken Sequence (*Lie Que*, Lu 7) is the connecting vessel of the hand *tai yin* and is located one *cun* and five *fen* proximal to the wrist. It is the (meeting point of a branch) which diverges to the (hand) *yang ming*. Broken Sequence is needled to a depth of three *fen* and (the needle) is retained for a duration of three exhalations. It is moxaed with five cones.

Collection Hole (*Kong Zui*, Lu 6) is the cleft point of the hand *tai yin* and is located seven *cun* proximal to the wrist. Specially [a later editor notes that there is a lacunae here] metal twenty-seven are the parents of water.[134] (Collection Hole) is needled to a depth of three *fen* deep and (the needle) is retained for a duration of three exhalations. It is moxaed with five cones.

Cubit Marsh (*Chi Ze*, Lu 5) is a point associated with water. It is located at the pulsating vessel at the elbow crease and is the point where the hand *tai yin* vessel submerges. Therefore, it is the confluence point. (Cubit Marsh) is needled to a depth of three *fen* and moxaed with three cones. [A note in the "*Qi Xue Lun*" of the *Su Wen* states that the needle should be retained for the duration of three exhalations.]

Guarding White (*Xia Bai*, Lu 4) is located below Celestial Storehouse (*Tian Fu*) at a pulsating vessel five *cun* proximal to the elbow. It is a divergent branch of the hand *tai yin*. (Guarding White) is needled to a depth of four *fen* and (the needle) is retained for a duration of three exhalations. It is moxaed with five cones.

Celestial Storehouse (*Tian Fu*, Lu 3) is located three *cun* below the axilla at a pulsating vessel in the anterior aspect of the upper arm and belongs to the qi of the hand *tai yin* vessel. Moxibustion is prohibited since it may cause a counterflow of qi. It is needled to a depth of four *fen* and (the nee-

dle) is retained for a duration of three exhalations.

Chapter Twenty-Five

Sixteen Points of the Hand *Jue Yin* Heart-Governor on the Arm[135]

The vessel of the hand heart-governor emerges at the tip of the middle finger and then curves inward to run along the (palmar) aspect of the middle finger. It ascends, flowing into the palm, and passes deeply between two metacarpal bones. Upon emerging, it curves outward flowing between two sinews[136] at the border of the bone and the flesh where its qi is smooth and uninhibited. From there, it ascends for two *cun* before it turns outward [a variant version adds the word "emerging"] and flows between two sinews to the inner side of the elbow. There it submerges beneath a minor sinew [a variant version inserts the word "flowing"] at the juncture of two bones. It then ascends into the chest, internally connecting with the pericardium.

The heart-governor emerges at Central Hub (*Zhong Chong*, Per 9). Central Hub is associated with wood. It is located at the tip of the middle finger in a depression the distance of a leek leaf from the corner of the nail. It is the point where the hand heart-governor vessel emerges and is, therefore, the well point. (Central Hub) is needled to a depth of one *fen*, and (the needle) is retained for a duration of three exhalations. It is moxaed with one cone.

Palace of Toil (*Lao Gong*, Per 8) is associated with fire. It is also known as Five Li (*Wu Li*) and is located at the pulsating vessel in the middle of the palm. It is the point where the hand heart-governor channel gushes and is, therefore, the brook point. (Palace of Toil) is needled to a depth of three *fen*, and (the needle) is retained for a duration of six exhalations. It is moxaed with three cones.

Great Mound (*Da Ling*, Per 7) is associated with

99

earth. It is located in a depression between two sinews proximal to the wrist. It is the point where the hand heart-governor vessel pours forth and is, therefore, the rapids point. (Great Mound) is needled to a depth of six *fen*, and (the needle) is retained for a duration of seven exhalations. It is moxaed with three cones.

Inner Pass (*Nei Guan*, Per 6) is the connecting (point) of the hand heart-governor and is located two *cun* proximal to the wrist. It is (a point at which a branch) diverges to the (hand) *shao yang*. It is needled to a depth of two *fen* and moxaed with three cones.

Intermediary Courier (*Jian Shi*, Per 5) is associated with metal. It is located three *cun* proximal to the wrist in a depression between two sinews. Here the hand heart-governor flows mightily and it is, therefore, the stream point. It is needled to a depth of six *fen*, (the needle) is retained for a duration of seven exhalations, and it is moxaed with three cones.

Cleft Gate (*Xi Men*, Per 4) is the cleft point of the hand heart-governor and is located five *cun* proximal to the wrist. It is needled to a depth of three *fen* and moxaed with three cones. [The *Wai Tai* says five cones.]

Marsh at the Bend (*Qu Ze*, Per 3) is associated with water. It is located in a depression on the inner side of the elbow. Locate it with the (patient's) elbow bent. It is the point where the hand heart-governor vessel submerges and is, therefore, the confluence point. (Marsh at the Bend) is needled to a depth of three *fen*, and (the needle) is retained for a duration of seven exhalations. It is moxaed with three cones.

Celestial Spring (*Tian Quan*, Per 2) is also known as Celestial Warmth (*Tian Wen*) and is located below (the end of) the fold of the axilla, two *cun* (down) the upper arm. Locate it with the (patient's) arm raised. It is needled to a depth of six *fen* and moxaed with three cones.

Chapter Twenty-Six

Sixteen Points of the Hand *Shao Yin* on the Arm[137]

The Yellow Emperor asked:

The vessel of the hand *shao yin* has no transporting points.[138] Why is this?

Qi Bo answered:

The (hand) *shao yin* is the vessel of the heart. The heart is the supreme sovereign of the five viscera and the six bowels, the emperor where the essence-spirit is housed. Its viscus is strong and cannot be visited by pathogens [some sources say "cannot contain pathogens"]. Should it ever be visited (by pathogens), the heart becomes damaged. Whenever the heart becomes damaged, the spirit departs. When the spirit departs, death is inevitable. Therefore, whenever (one speaks of) any pathogen settling within the heart, it is always (within the context of) the enveloping connecting vessel of the heart (*i.e.*, the pericardium, *bao luo*, 包络). This enveloping connecting vessel is the vessel of the (hand) heart-governor. Therefore, the heart alone has no transporting points.

The Yellow Emperor asked:

Because the *shao yin* vessel alone has no transporting points, does the heart never become diseased?

Qi Bo answered:

Its external channel is subject to disease, but the viscus itself is not. Therefore, in order to treat the channel, it is effective to merely select the point at the end of the ulnar styloid process proximal to the wrist.[139] As for the vessel's exiting and submerging, its turns and bends, the channel is similar to the hand *shao yin*, [A later editor states that the *shao* of *shao yin* should be replaced by *tai*. The *Tong Ren Jing* substitutes *shao* for *jue*.] and the hand heart-governor vessel in these respects. The points of the (hand *shao yin* vessel) should be treated in accordance with vacuity and repletion, and the swiftness and sluggishness of the (qi within the channel). It is said that, in the case of surgance,[140] then drainage should be executed, and, in the case of debilitation, then supplementation is to be carried out. In this way, pathogenic qi is removed and the true qi is fortified. That is called compliance with universal order (*tian xu*).

The heart emerges at Lesser Surge (*Shao Chong*, Ht 9). Lesser Surge is associated with wood and is also known as Channel Beginning (*Jing Shi*). It is located at the tip of the radial aspect of the small finger, the distance of a leek leaf from the corner of the nail. It is the point where the hand *shao yin* emerges and is, therefore, the well point. (Lesser Surge) is needled to a depth of one *fen*, (the needle) is retained for a duration of one exhalation, and it is moxaed with one cone. There are eight points on the (hand) *shao yin*, seven of which have curative properties while one does not. Because pathogens cannot visit it, the heart is said to have no transporting points.

Lesser Mansion (*Shao Fu*, Ht 8) is associated with fire. It is located in a depression proximal to the base joint of the phalanx of the small finger at the same level with Palace of Toil (*Lao Gong*, Per 8). It is the point where the hand *shao yin* vessel gushes, and is therefore the brook point. It is needled to a depth of three *fen*, and moxaed with three cones.

Spirit Gate (*Shen Men*, Ht 7) is associated with earth. It is also known as Protuberant Hub (*Rei Chong*) and Central Metropolis (*Zhong Du*) and is located in a depression at the end of the styloid process of the ulna proximal to the palm. It is the point where the hand *shao yin* vessel pours forth and is, therefore, the rapids point. (Spirit Gate) is needled to a depth of three *fen*, (the needle) is retained for a duration of seven exhalations, and it is moxaed with three cones. [A note in the *"Yin Yang Lei Lun* (Treatise on Analogizing with Yin & Yang)" in the *Su Wen*[141] states that it is located five *fen* proximal to the wrist in line with the small finger.]

The hand *shao yin* cleft point (*Yin Xi*, Ht 6) is located at the vessel proximal to the palm, five *fen* to

the wrist. It is needled to a depth of three *fen* and moxaed with three cones. [A note in the *"Yin Yang Lei Lun"* states that it is located proximal to the small finger.]

Connecting Li (*Tong Li*, Ht 5) is the connecting vessel of the hand *shao yin* and is located one *cun* proximal to the wrist. It is the connecting point to the (hand) *tai yang*. (Connecting Li) is needled to a depth of three *fen* and moxaed with three cones.

Spirit Pathway (*Ling Dao*, Ht 4) is associated with metal. It is located one *cun* and five *fen* proximal to the palm; some say one *cun*. It is the point where the hand *shao yin* channel flows mightily and is, therefore, the stream point. (Spirit Pathway) is needled to a depth of three *fen* and moxaed with three cones.

Lesser Sea (*Shao Hai*, Ht 3) is associated with water. It is also known as Bending Joint (*Qu Jie*) and is located in a depression proximal to the joint on the ulnar side of the elbow where a pulsating vessel is palpable. It is the point where the hand *shao yin* vessel submerges and is, therefore, the confluence point. (Lesser Sea) is needled to a depth of five *fen* and moxaed with three cones.

Highest Spring (*Ji Quan*, Ht 1) is located in the axilla between two sinews[142] where a pulsating vessel enters the chest. It belongs to the qi of the hand *shao yin* vessel. (Highest Spring) is needled to a depth of three *fen* and moxaed with five cones.

Green-blue Spirit (*Qing Ling*, Ht 2) is located three *cun* above the elbow. Locate it with the (patient's) elbow straightened and arm raised. It is moxaed with seven cones.

Chapter Twenty-Seven

Twenty-Eight Points of the Hand *Yang Ming* on the Arm[143]

The large intestine in the upper part of the body is united with the hand *yang ming* which emerges at Shang Yang (*Shang Yang*, LI 1). Shang Yang is associated with metal. It is also known as Yang Extremity (*Jue Yang*) and is located on the radial aspect of the finger next to the thumb, the distance of a leek leaf from the corner of the nail. It is the point where the hand *yang ming* channel emerges, and is, therefore, the well point. It is needled to a depth of one *cun*, (the needle) is retained for a duration of one exhalation, and it is moxaed with three cones.

Second Space (*Er Jian*, LI 2) is associated with water. It is also known as Space Valley (*Jian Gu*) and is located in a depression on the finger next to the thumb and distal to the phalanx on the inside (*i.e.*, radial side). It is the point where the hand *yang ming* vessel gushes and is, therefore, the brook point. It is needled to a depth of three *fen*, (the needle) is retained for a duration of six exhalations, and it is moxaed with three cones.

Third Space (*San Jian*, LI 3) is associated with wood. It is also known as Lesser Valley (*Shao Gu*) and is located in a depression on the finger next to the thumb proximal to the base of the phalanx on the inside (*i.e.*, radial side). It is the point where the hand *yang ming* vessel pours forth and is, therefore, the rapids point. It is needled to a depth of three *fen*, (the needle) is retained for a duration of three exhalations, and it is moxaed with three cones.

Union Valley (*He Gu*, LI 4) is also known as Tiger's Mouth (*Hu Kou*) and is located at the articulation of the forking (metacarpal) bones of the thumb and index fingers. It is the point of efflux of the hand *yang ming* vessel and is, therefore, the source point. It is needled to a depth of three *fen*, (the needle) is retained for a duration of three exhalations, and it is moxaed with three cones.

Yang Ravine (*Yang Xi*, LI 5) is associated with fire. It is also known as Central Eminence (*Zhong Kui*) and is located in a depression between two sinews[144] on the upper side of the wrist. It is the point where the hand *yang ming* vessel flows mightily and is, therefore, the stream point. It is needled to a depth of three *fen*, (the needle) is retained for a duration of seven exhalations, and it is moxaed with three cones.

Veering Passageway (*Pian Li*, LI 6) is the connecting vessel of the hand *yang ming* and is located three *cun* proximal to the wrist. Here (a branch) diverges into the (hand) *tai yin*. It is needled to a depth of three *fen*, (the needle) is retained for a duration of seven exhalations, and it is moxaed with three cones.

Warm Dwelling (*Wen Liu*, LI 7) is also known as Counterflow Pouring (*Ni Zhu*) and Snake Head (*She Tou*). It is the cleft point of the hand *yang ming* and is located five *cun* proximal to the wrist in those of small build and six *cun* in those of large build. It is needled to a depth of three *fen* and moxaed with three cones. [A later editor notes that a large build implies adults and small build, children. In the *Zhen Jiu Jing Xue Tu Kao* [*Atlas and Collation of the Channels and Acupuncture Points*], Lu Shi states "A large build {means an individual is possessed of} a long body, while a small build means a short body." Most texts cite it's location as either five or six *cun* above the wrist.]

Lower Ridge (*Xia Lian*, LI 8) is located at the radius one *cun* distal to Upper Ridge, presumably [a later editor suggests that this may be mistaken] in a fissure within the external irregular (*i.e.*, external oblique) and muscles. It is needled to a depth of five *fen*, (the needle) is retained for a duration of five exhalations, and it is moxaed with three cones.

Upper Ridge (*Shang Lian*, LI 9) is located one *cun* distal to Three Li at the place where the external oblique (muscle) (*wai xie*) meets the yang (*ming* vessel).[145] It is needled to a depth of five *fen* and moxaed with three cones.

Hand Three Li (*Shou San Li*, LI 10) is located one *cun* distal to Pool at the Bend at a place where pressure causes the end of a tapering muscle[146] to be raised up. It is needled to a depth of three *fen* and moxaed with three cones.

Pool at the Bend (*Qu Chi*, LI 11) is associated with earth and is located between the elbow bones at the outer side of the elbow. It is the point where the hand *yang ming* channel submerges and is, therefore, the confluence point. It is needled to a depth of five *fen*, (the needle) is retained for a duration of seven exhalations, and it is moxaed with three cones.

Elbow Bone Hole (*Zhou Liao*, LI 12) is located at the elbow in a depression on the outer aspect of the large bone (*i.e.*, the humerus). It is needled to a depth of four *fen* and moxaed with three cones.

Five Li (*Wu Li* or *Shou Wu Li*, LI 13) is located three *cun* above the elbow, interior (*i.e.*, anterior) (to the preceding point) in the middle of a major vessel. [*Zhen Jiu Jing Xue Tu Kao {The Atlas and Collation of Channel Points for Acupuncture & Moxibustion}* states that the word sinew should be substituted for vessel so that the line reads "in the middle of a major sinew".] Needling is prohibited, but it may be moxaed with three cones. [The *Wai Tai* prescribes moxibustion with ten cones on this point.]

Upper Arm (*Bi Nao*, LI 14) is located seven *cun* above the elbow at the end of a muscular mass.[147] It is the meeting point of the network vessels of the hand *yang ming*. It is needled to a depth of three *fen* and moxaed with three cones.

Chapter Twenty-Eight

Twenty-Four Points of the Hand *Shao Yang* on the Arm[148]

The triple burner in the upper part of the body is united with the hand *shao yang* and emerges at Passage Hub (*Guan Chong*, TH 1). Passage Hub is associated with metal and is located at the tip of the finger next to the small one (*i.e.*, the ring finger), the distance of a leek leaf from the corner of the nail. It is the point where the hand *shao yang* vessel emerges, and is, therefore, the well point. It is needled to a depth of one *fen*, (the needle) is retained for a duration of three exhalations, and it is moxaed with three cones.

Armpit Gate (*Ye Men*, TH 2) is associated with water. It is located in a depression in the web between the small finger and the one next to it. It is the point where the hand *shao yang* vessel gushes, and is, therefore, the brook point. (Armpit Gate) is needled to a depth of two *fen* and moxaed with three cones.

Central Islet (*Zhong Zhu*, TH 3) is associated with wood. It is located in a depression proximal to the base joint of the phalanx of the finger next to the small one. It is the point where the hand *shao yang* pours forth, and is, therefore, the rapids point. It is needled to a depth of two *fen*, (the needle) is retained for a duration of three exhalations, and it is moxaed with three cones.

Yang Pool (*Yang Chi*, TH 4) is also known as Divergent Yang (*Bie Yang*) and is located on the outside of the hand in a depression at the back of the wrist. It is the point of efflux of the hand *shao yang* vessel, and is, therefore, the source point. It is needled to a depth of two *fen*, (the needle) is retained for a duration of six exhalations, and it is moxaed with three cones. [The *Tong Ren Jing* prohibits moxibustion.]

Outer Pass (*Wai Guan*, TH 5) is (the point of) the connecting vessel of the hand *shao yang*. It is located in a depression two *cun* proximal to the wrist and, (at this point, a branch) diverges to the heart-governor. It is needled to a depth of three *fen*, (the needle) is retained for a duration of seven exhalations, and it is moxaed with three cones.

Branch Ditch (*Zhi Gou*, TH 6) is associated with fire. It is located in a depression three *cun* above the wrist between two bones. It is the point where the hand *shao yang* vessel flows mightily, and is, therefore, the stream point. It is needled to a depth of two *fen*, (the needle) is retained for a duration of seven exhalations, and it is moxaed with three cones.

Convergence and Gathering (*Hui Zong*, TH 7) is the cleft point of the hand *shao yang* and is located in a fissure three *cun* proximal to the wrist. It is needled to a depth of three *fen* and moxaed with three cones.

Three Yang Connecting (*San Yang Luo*, TH 8) is

located on the arm at a major crossing vessel,[149] one *cun* above Branch Ditch. Needling is prohibited. However, it is moxaed with nine cones.

Four Rivers (*Si Du*, TH 9) is located in a depression on the posterior aspect of the arm five *cun* distal to the elbow. It is needled to a depth of six *fen*, (the needle) is retained for a duration of seven exhalations, and it is moxaed with three cones.

Celestial Well (*Tian Jing*, TH 10) is associated with earth. It is located on the outer aspect of the elbow posterior to the large bone (*i.e.*, the humerus) [*Sheng Ji Zong Lu (Complete Records of Life-Securing Classics)* and *Tong Ren* simply state that it is "one *cun* above the posterior aspect of the elbow"], in a depression between two sinews. Locate it with the (patient's) elbow bent. It is the point where the hand *shao yang* vessel submerges, and is, therefore, the confluence point. It is needled to a depth of one *fen*, (the needle) is retained for a duration of seven exhalations, and it is moxaed with three cones.

Clear Cold Abyss (*Qing Leng Yuan*, TH 11) is located one *cun* above the elbow. [The twenty-ninth volume of *Qian Jin Yao Fang (Essential Formulas Worth a Tousand Taels of Gold)* states it is three *cun* above the elbow, *Wai Tai*, *Tong Ren*, *Sheng Ji Zong Lu*, and *Zi Sheng Jing* claim it is two *cun* above the elbow.] Locate it with the (patient's) arm raised and elbow stretched. It is needled to a depth of three *fen*, and it is moxaed with three cones.

Dispersing Riverbed (*Xiao Luo*, TH 12) is located below the shoulder on the lateral aspect of the upper arm when the armpit is opened and the elbow is rotated obliquely. It is needled to a depth of six *fen* and is moxaed with three cones. [A later editor cites a note in the "*Qi Fu Lun*"[150] that it is the meeting point of the hand *shao yang* channel.]

Chapter Twenty-Nine

Sixteen Points of the Hand *Tai Yang* on the Arm[151]

The small intestine in the upper body unites with the hand *tai yang* and emerges at Lesser Marsh (*Shao Ze*, SI 1). Lesser Marsh is associated with metal. It is also known as Small Propitiousness and is located at the tip of the small finger in a depression one *fen* from the nail. It is the point where the hand *tai yang* channel emerges, and is, therefore, the well point. It is needled to a depth of one *fen*, (the needle) is retained for a duration of two exhalations, and it is moxaed with one cone.

Front Valley (*Qian Gu*, SI 2) is associated with water. It is located on the outside (*i.e.*, the ulnar aspect) of the small finger in a depression distal to the base joint of the phalanx. It is the point where the hand *tai yang* vessel gushes, and is, therefore, the brook point. It is needled to a depth of one *fen*, (the needle) is retained for a duration of three exhalations, and it is moxaed with three cones.

Back Ravine (*Hou Xi*, SI 3) is associated with wood. It is located on the outside of the small finger in a depression proximal to the base joint of the phalanx. It is the point where the hand *tai yang* vessel pours forth, and is, therefore, the rapids point. It is needled to a depth of two *fen*, (the needle) is retained for a duration of two exhalations, and it is moxaed with one cone.

Wrist Bone (*Wan Gu*, SI 4) is located on the outside (*i.e.*, the ulnar aspect) of the hand in a depression inferior to the carpal bone. It is the point where the hand *tai yang* vessel has its efflux, and is, therefore, the source point. It is needled to a depth of two *fen*, (the needle) is retained for a duration of three exhalations, and it is moxaed with three cones.

Yang Valley (*Yang Gu*, SI 5) is associated with fire. It is located on the outside of the hand on the wrist in a depression inferior to the styloid process of the ulna. It is the point where the hand *tai yang* vessel flows mightily, and is, therefore, the stream point. It is needled to a depth of two *fen*, (the needle) is retained for a duration of two exhalations, and it is moxaed with three cones. [A note in the "*Qi Xue Lun*"[152] prescribes three exhalations long.]

Nursing the Aged (*Yang Lao*, SI 6) is the cleft point of the hand *tai yang*. It is located in a hole on the styloid process of the ulna or, (to put it another way,) in a depression one *cun* proximal to the wrist. It is needled to a depth of three *fen*, and it is moxaed with three cones.

Branch to the Correct (*Zhi Zheng*, SI 7) is (the point) of the connecting vessel of the hand *tai yang*. It is located five *cun* proximal to the wrist. (At this point, a branch) diverges to the (hand) *shao yin*. It is needled to a depth of three *fen*, (the needle) is retained for a duration of seven exhalations, and it is moxaed with three cones.

Small Sea (*Xiao Hai*, SI 8) is associated with earth. It is located on the inner side of the elbow, lateral to the large bone (*i.e.*, the humerus),[153] in a depression five *fen* from the tip of the elbow. Locate it with the (patient's) elbow bent. It is the point where the hand *tai yang* vessel submerges and is, therefore, the confluence point. It is needled to a depth of two *fen*, (the needle) is retained for a duration of seven exhalations, and it is moxaed with seven cones. [A note in the "*Qi Xue Lun*" calls it *Shao Hai*.]

Chapter Thirty

Twenty-Two Points of the Foot *Tai Yin* (from the Foot) Through the Thigh[154]

The spleen emerges at Hidden White (*Yin Bai*, Sp 1) and is associated with wood. Hidden White is located at the tip of the medial aspect of the big toe, the distance of a leek leaf from the corner of the nail. It is the point where the foot *tai yin* vessel emerges, and is, therefore, the well point. It is needled to a depth of one *fen*, (the needle) is retained for a duration of three exhalations, and it is moxaed with three cones.

Great Metropolis (*Da Du*, Sp 2) is associated with fire. It is located in a depression proximal to the base joint of the phalanx of the big toe. It is the point where the foot *tai yin* vessel gushes, and is, therefore, the brook point. It is needled to a depth of three *fen*, (the needle) is retained for a duration of seven exhalations, and it is moxaed with three cones.

Supreme White (*Tai Bai*, Sp 3) is associated with earth. It is located in a depression inferior to the kernal bone on the medial aspect of the foot. It is the point where the foot *tai yin* vessel pours forth, and is, therefore, the rapids point. It is needled to a depth of three *fen*, (the needle) is retained for a duration of seven exhalations, and it is moxaed with three cones.

Offspring of Duke (*Gong Sun*, Sp 4) is located on the foot one *cun* proximal to the base joint of the phalanx of the big toe. (At this point, a branch) diverges to the (foot) *yang ming* and this is a (starting point of a) connecting vessel of the (foot) *tai yin*. It is needled to a depth of four *fen*, (the needle) is retained for a duration of twenty exhalations, and it is moxaed with three cones.

Shang Hill (*Shang Qiu*, Sp 5) is associated with metal. It is located on the foot in a depression inferior and a little anterior to the medial malleolus. It is the point where the foot *tai yin* vessel flows mightily, and is, therefore, the stream point. It is needled to a depth of three *fen*, (the needle) is retained for a duration of seven exhalations, and it is moxaed with three cones. [A note in the "*Qi Xue Lun*"[155] prescribes an insertion of three *fen*.]

Three Yin Intersection (*San Yin Jiao*, Sp 6) is located in a depression on the border of the lower bone (*i.e.*, the tibia, *gu xia*) three *cun* above the medial malleolus. It is the meeting point of the foot *tai yin*, *jue yin*, and *shao yin*. It is needled to a depth of three *fen*, (the needle) is retained for a duration of seven exhalations, and it is moxaed with three cones.

Leaking Valley (*Lou Gu*, Sp 7) is located in a depression on the border of the tibia six *cun* above the medial malleolus and is the point of the connecting vessel of the foot *tai yin*. It is needled to a depth of three *fen*, (the needle) is retained for a duration of seven exhalations, and it is moxaed with three cones.

Earth's Crux (*Di Ji*, Sp 8) is also known as Spleen Abode (*Pi She*) and is the cleft point of the foot *tai yin*. It is found at a place one more *cun* up[156] or in a hole five *cun* below the knee. It is needled to a depth of three *fen* and moxaed with five cones.

Yin Mound Spring (*Yin Ling Quan*, Sp 9) is associated with water. It is located below the knee on the medial aspect of the leg in a depression below the assisting bone. Locate it with the (patient's) leg stretched. It is the point where the foot *tai yin* channel submerges, and is, therefore, the confluence point. It is needled to a depth of five *fen*, (the needle) is retained for a duration of seven exhalations, and it is moxaed with three cones.

Sea of Blood (*Xue Hai*, Sp 10) is located in the white flesh on the medial aspect of the leg two *cun* above the knee cap and belongs to the qi of the foot *tai yin* vessel. It is needled to a depth of five *fen* and is moxaed with five cones.

Winnower Gate (*Ji Men*, Sp 11) is located on the fish belly[157] between two sinews[158] where a pulsating vessel is palpable level with Yin Market (*Yin Shi*, St 33). It belongs to the qi of the foot *tai yin* vessel. It is needled to a depth of three *fen*, (the needle) is retained for a duration of six exhalations, and it is moxaed with three cones. [A note in the "San Bu Jiu Hou Lun" in the *Su Wen*[159] locates this point straight below Five Li {*Wu Li*}[160] where a pulsating vessel may be palpated if pressed hard when the (patient), dressed in thin clothes, is instructed to arch his foot.]

Chapter Thirty-One

Twenty-Two Points of the Foot *Jue Yin* (from the Foot) Up Through the Thigh[161]

The liver emerges at Large Pile (*Da Dun*, Liv 1) and Large Pile is associated with wood. It is located at the tip of the big toe, the distance of a leek leaf from the corner of the nail in the three hair region. It is the point where the foot *jue yin* vessel emerges, and is, therefore, the well point. It is needled to a depth of three *fen*, (the needle) is retained for a duration of ten exhalations, and it is moxaed with three cones.

Moving Between (*Xing Jian*, Liv 2) is associated with fire. It is located on the foot in a depression in the web of the big toe, where a pulsating vessel is palpable. It is the point where the foot *jue yin* vessel gushes, and is, therefore, the brook point. It is needled to a depth of six *fen*, (the needle) is retained for a duration of ten exhalations, and it is moxaed with three cones.

Supreme Surge (*Tai Chong*, Liv 3) is associated with earth. It is located in a depression either two *cun* or one *cun* and five *fen* proximal to the base joint of the phalanx of the big toe. It is the point where the foot *jue yin* vessel pours forth, and is, therefore, the rapids point. It is needled to a depth of three *fen*, (the needle) is retained for a duration of ten exhalations, and it is moxaed with three cones. [A note in the "Ci Yao Tong Lun"[161] locates this point in a depression on the lateral border of the big toe two *cun* proximal to the base joint of the phalanx of the toe where a pulsating vessel is palpable.]

Mound Center (*Zhong Feng*, Liv 4) is associated with metal. It is located one *cun* anterior to the medial malleolus. Locate it in a depression when the (patient's) foot is bent upward or (between two sinews) when the (patient's) foot is straightened. It is the point where the foot *jue yin* vessel flows mightily, and is, therefore, the stream point. It is needled to a depth of four *fen*, (the needle) is retained for seven exhalations, and it is moxaed with three cones. [A note in the "Qi Xue Lun"[162] locates this point one *cun* and five *fen* anterior to the medial malleolus.]

Woodworm Canal (*Li Gou*, Liv 5) is (the point of) the connecting vessel of the foot *jue yin* and is located on the foot five *cun* above the medial malleolus. (At this point, a branch) diverges to the (foot) *shao yang*. It is needled to a depth of two *fen*, (the needle) is retained for a duration of three exhalations, and it is moxaed with three cones.

Central Metropolis (*Zhong Du*, Liv 6) is the cleft point of the foot *jue yin* and is located seven *cun* above the medial malleolus on the tibia. It lies directly across from the *shao yin*.[164] It is needled to a depth of three *fen*, (the needle) is retained for a duration of six exhalations, and it is moxaed with five cones.

Knee Joint (*Xi Guan*, Liv 7) is located in a depression two *cun* below the calf's nose and belongs to the qi of the foot *jue yin* vessel. It is needled to a depth of four *fen* and moxaed with five cones.

Spring at the Bend (*Qu Quan*, Liv 8) is associated with water. It is located on the inside of the knee below the inner assisting bone in a depression above the major sinew and beneath the lesser one.[165] Locate it with the (patient's) leg bent. It is the point where the foot *jue yin* vessel submerges, and is, therefore, the confluence point. It is needled to a depth of six *fen*, (the needle) is retained for a duration of ten exhalations, and it is moxaed with three cones.

Yin Bladder (*Yin Bao*, Liv 9) is located four *cun* above the knee on medial aspect of the thigh between two sinews. (At this point, a branch) of the foot *jue yin* diverges to the (foot) *tai yin*. It is needled to a depth of six *fen* and moxaed with three cones.

Five Li (*Wu Li*, Liv 10) is located below Yin Corner three *cun* distal to Qi Surge (*Qi Chong*, St 30) at a pulsating vessel on the yin (medial) aspect of the thigh. It is needled to a depth of six *fen* and moxaed with five cones.[166] [The *Wai Tai Mi Yao* [167] locates this point three *cun* distal to Surging Qi (*Chong Qi*, St 30) and two *cun* from the outer border of the thigh. It prescribes an insertion of eight *fen* and three cones for moxibustion.]

Yin Corner (*Yin Lian*, Liv 11) is located below Goat Arrow (*Yang Shi*, Liv 12), two *cun* distal to Surging Qi where there is a pulsating vessel. It is needled to a depth of three *fen*, and it is moxaed with three cones.

Chapter Thirty-Two

Twenty Points of the Foot *Shao Yang* Through the Thigh Including the Yin Motility & Yin Linking Vessels[168]

The kidney emerges at Gushing Spring (*Yong Quan*, Ki 1) and Gushing Spring is associated with wood. It is also known as Earth Surge (*Di Chong*) and is located in a depression in the center of the sole where a hole appears when the foot is arched and the toes bent downward. It is the point where the foot *shao yin* channel emerges, and is, therefore, the well point. It is needled to a depth of three *fen*, (the needle) is retained for a duration of three exhalations, and it is moxaed with three cones.

Burning Valley (*Ran Gu*, Ki 2) is associated with fire. It is also known as Dragon Abyss (*Long Yuan*) and is located anterior to the medial malleolus on the foot in a depression inferior to the rise of the large bone (*i.e.*, the tuberosity of the navicular bone). It is the point where the foot *shao yin* gushes, and is, therefore, the brook point. It is needled to a depth of three *fen*, (the needle) is retained for a duration of three exhalations, and it is moxaed with three cones. Pricking the point often produces blood and results in instant hunger and a good appetite.

Great Ravine (*Tai Xi*, Ki 3) is associated with earth. It is located in a depression at a pulsating vessel on the calcaneus posterior to the medial malleolus. It is the point where the foot *shao yin* vessel pours forth, and is, therefore, the rapids point. It is needled to a depth of three *fen*, (the needle) is retained for a duration of seven exhalations, and it is moxaed with three cones.

Large Goblet (*Da Zhong*, Ki 4) is located in the hollow behind the heel. (Here, a branch) diverges to the (foot) *tai yang*, and this is the point of the connecting vessel of the foot *shao yin*. It is needled to a depth of two *fen*, (the needle) is retained for a duration of seven exhalations, and it is moxaed with three cones. [A note in the "*Shui Re Xue Lun*" in the *Su Wen*[169] locates this point behind the medial malleolus, while in a note in the "*Ci Yao*

Tong Lun"[170] locates it in the hollow place on the posterior part of the heel where a pulsating vessel is palpable.]

Shining Sea (*Zhao Hai*, Ki 6) is engendered by the yin motility vessel and is located one *cun* below the medial malleolus. It is needled to a depth of four *fen*, (the needle) is retained for a duration of six exhalations, and it is moxaed with three cones.

Water Spring (*Shui Quan*, Ki 5) is the cleft point of the foot *shao yin* and is located below the medial malleolus one *cun* below Great Ravine (*Tai Xi*, Ki 3). It is needled to a depth of four *fen* and moxaed with five cones.

Recover Flow (*Fu Liu*, Ki 7) is associated with metal. It is also known as Deep-lying White (*Fu Bai*) or Glorious Yang (*Chang Yang*) and is located in a depression two *cun* above the medial malleolus. It is the point where the foot *shao yin* vessel flows mightily, and is, therefore, the stream point. It is needled to a depth of three *fen*, (the needle) is retained for a duration of three exhalations, and it is moxaed with five cones. [A note in the "*Ci Yao Tong Lun*" locates this point at the pulsating vessel two *cun* above the medial malleolus.]

Intersection Reach (*Jiao Xin*, Ki 8) is located two *cun* above the medial malleolus in front of the *shao yin*[171] and behind the *tai yin*[171] between the sinew and the bone.[172] It is the cleft point of the yin motility vessel. It is needled to a depth of four *fen*, (the needle) is retained for a duration of five exhalations, and it is moxaed with three cones.

Guest House (*Zhu Bin*, Ki 9) is the cleft point of the yin linking vessel and is located on the calf above the medial malleolus. It is needled to a depth of three *fen* and moxaed with five cones. [A note in the "*Ci Yao Tong Lun*" locates this point behind the medial malleolus.]

Yin Valley (*Yin Gu*, Ki 10) is associated with water. It is located posterior to the inner assisting bone at the knee, below the major sinew and above the lesser one[173] where (a pulsating vessel) is palpable. Locate it with the (patient's) knee bent. It is the point where the foot *shao yin* vessel submerges,

and is, therefore, the confluence point. It is needled to a depth of four *fen* and moxaed with three cones.

Chapter Thirty-Three

Thirty Points of the Foot *Yang Ming* (from the Foot) Through the Thigh[174]

The stomach emerges at Severe Mouth (*Li Dui*, St 45). Severe Mouth is associated with metal and is located at the tip of the toe next to the big one, the distance of a leek leaf from the corner of the nail. It is the point where the foot *yang ming* channel issues, and is, therefore, the well point. It is needled to a depth of one *fen*, (the needle) is retained for a duration of one exhalation, and it is moxaed with one cone.

Inner Court (*Nei Ting*, St 44) is associated with water and is located in a depression on the lateral border of the toe next to the big one. It is the point where the foot *yang ming* channel gushes, and is, therefore, the brook point. It is needled to a depth of three *fen*, (the needle) is retained for a duration of twenty exhalations, and it is moxaed with three cones. [A note in the "*Qi Xue Lun*"[175] prescribes needle retention for a duration of ten exhalations and moxibustion with three cones. {later editor}]

Sunken Valley (*Xian Gu*, St 43) is associated with wood and is located on the lateral border of the toe next to the big one, in a depression proximal to the base joint of the phalanx two *cun* proximal to Inner Court. It is the point where the foot *yang ming* channel pours forth, and is, therefore, the rapids point. It is needled to a depth of five *fen*, (the needle) is retained for a duration of seven exhalations, and it is moxaed with three cones.

Surging Yang (*Chong Yang*, St 42) is also known as Meeting Source (*Hui Yuan*) and is located on the instep five *cun* (to the second toe) at a pulsating vessel three *cun* proximal to Sunken Valley (*Xian Gu*). It is the point where the foot *yang ming* has its efflux, and is, therefore, the source point. It is needled to a depth of three *fen*, (the needle) is retained for a duration of ten exhalations, and it is moxaed with three cones.

Ravine Divide (*Jie Xi*, St 41) is associated with fire and is located one *cun* and five *fen* proximal to Surging Yang, in a depression at the ankle. It is the point where the foot *yang ming* flows mightily, and is, therefore, the stream point. It is needled to a depth of five *fen*, (the needle) is retained for a duration of five exhalations, and it is moxaed with three cones. [A note in the "*Qi Xue Lun*" locates this point two *cun* and five *fen* proximal to Surging Yang, while in a note in the "*Ci Nue Lun*" {Treatise on Needling for Nue} locates it three *cun* and five *fen*. {later editor}]

Bountiful Bulge (*Feng Long*, St 40) is the connecting vessel of the foot *yang ming* and is located eight *cun* above the lateral malleolus at the level of the Lower Ridge,[176] in a depression at the lateral border of the tibia. It is the point diverging to the (foot) *tai yin*. It is needled to a depth of three *fen* and moxaed with three cones.

Lower Ridge of the Great Hollow (*Ju Xi Xia Lian*, St 39)[177] is the uniting point of the foot *yang ming* and the small intestine. It is located three *cun* below Upper Ridge and belongs to the channel qi of the foot *yang ming*. It is needled to a depth of three *fen* and is moxaed with three cones.

Ribbon Opening (*Tiao Kou*, St 38), is located one *cun* above the Lower Ridge and belongs to the qi of the foot *yang ming* vessel. It is needled to a depth of eight *fen* (one text states that "the needle is retained for a duration of three breaths"), and it is moxaed with three cones.

Upper Ridge of the Great Hollow (*Shang Ju Xu*, St 37) is a uniting point of the foot *yang ming* and the large intestine. It is located three *cun* below Three Li and belongs to the qi of the foot *yang ming* vessel. It is needled to a depth of eight *fen* and is moxaed with three cones.

Three Li (*San Li*, St 36) is associated with earth and is located three *cun* below the knee on the lateral border of the tibia. It is the point where the qi of the foot *yang ming* vessel submerges, and is, therefore, the confluence point. It is needled to a depth

of one *cun* and five *fen*,[178] (the needle) is retained for a duration of seven exhalations, and it is moxaed with three cones. [The *Su Wen* locates this point three *cun* below the knee at the lateral border of the tibia between two sinews. {later editor}]

Calf's Nose (*Du Bi*, St 35) is located in the hole below the knee cap and above the tibia in the major sinew and belongs to the qi of the foot *yang ming* vessel. It is needled to a depth of six *fen*, and it is moxaed with three cones.

Beam Hill (*Liang Qiu*, St 34) is the cleft point of the foot *yang ming* and is located two *cun* proximal to the knee between two sinews. It is needled to a depth of three *fen* and moxaed with three cones.

Yin Market (*Yin Shi*, St 33) is also known as Yin Tripod (*Yin Ding*) and is located three *cun* above the knee below Crouching Rabbit (*Fu Tu*, St 32). Locate it with (the patient) in a kneeling posture. It belongs to the qi of the foot *yang ming* vessel. It is needled to a depth of three *fen*, (the needle) is retained for a duration of seven exhalations, and moxibustion is prohibited. [A note in the "*Ci Yao Tong Lun*"[179] locates this point in a depression below Crouching Rabbit, and prescribes moxibustion with three cones. {later editor}]

Crouching Rabbit (*Fu Tu*, St 32) is six *cun* above the knee on a prominence of the flesh and belongs to the qi of the foot *yang ming* vessel. It is needled to a depth of five *fen*, and moxibustion is prohibited.

Thigh Joint (*Bi Guan*, St 31) is located above the knee proximal to Crouching Rabbit in the parting (of the flesh). It is needled to a depth of six *fen* and moxaed with three cones.

Chapter Thirty-Four

Twenty-Eight Points of the Foot *Shao Yang* (from the Foot) Through the Thigh Inclusive of Four Points of the Yang Linking Channel[180]

The gallbladder emerges at Portal Yin (*Qiao Yin*,

GB 44). Portal Yin is associated with metal. It is located at the tip of the toe next to the small one, the distance of a leek leaf from the corner of the nail. It is the point where the foot *shao yang* vessel emerges, and is, therefore, the well point. It is needled to a depth of one *fen*,[181] (the needle) is retained for a duration of three exhalations, and it is moxaed with three cones. [A note in the "*Qi Xue Lun*"[182] prescribes needle retention for a duration of one exhalation. {later editor}]

Pinched Ravine (*Xia Xi*, GB 43) is associated with water. It is located between the small and the fourth toe in a depression distal to the base joint of the phalanx. It is the point where the foot *shao yang* vessel gushes, and is, therefore, the brook point. It is needled to a depth of three *fen*, (the needle) is retained for a duration of three exhalations, and it is moxaed with three cones.

Earth Fivefold Convergence (*Di Wu Hui*, GB 42) is located in a depression proximal to the base joint of the phalanx between the small and the fourth toe. It is needled to a depth of three *fen*, and moxibustion is prohibited since it may cause a person to become emaciated and to eventually die in no more than three years.

On the Verge of Tears (*Lin Qi*, GB 41) is associated with wood. It is located proximal to the base joint of the phalanx in a depression one *cun* and five *fen* from Pinched Ravine. It is the point where the foot *shao yang* channel pours forth, and is, therefore, the rapids point. It is needled to a depth of two *fen*, (the needle) is retained for a duration of five exhalations, and it is moxaed with three cones.

Hill Ruins (*Qiu Xu*, GB 40) is located inferior and a little anterior to the lateral malleolus in a depression three *cun* proximal to Overlooking Tears (*Lin Qi*). It is the point where the foot *shao yang* channel has its efflux, and is, therefore, the source point. It is needled to a depth of five *fen*, (the needle) is retained for a duration of seven exhalations, and it is moxaed with three cones.

Suspended Bell (*Xuan Zhong*, GB 39) is located at a pulsating vessel three *cun* above the lateral malleolus and is the connecting vessel of the three foot yang. Locate it by occluding the foot *yang ming* vessel.[183] It is needled to a depth of six *fen*, (the needle) is retained for a duration of seven exhalations, and it is moxaed with five cones.

Yang Assistance (*Yang Fu*, GB 38) is associated with fire. It is located four *cun* above the lateral malleolus [the two words "four *cun*" are absent from a note in the "*Qi Xue Lun*" {later editor}] at the end of the severed bone, three *fen* anterior to the assisting bone, seven *cun* proximal to Hill Ruins. It is the point where the foot *shao yang* channel flows mightily, and is, therefore, the stream point. It is needled to a depth of five *fen*, (the needle) is retained for a duration of seven exhalations, and it is moxaed with three cones.

Bright Light (*Guang Ming*, GB 37) is the connecting vessel of the foot *shao yang* and is located five *cun* above the lateral malleolus wherefrom the vessel diverges to the (foot) *jue yin*. It is needled to a depth of six *fen*, (the needle) is retained for a duration of seven exhalations, and it is moxaed with five cones. [A note in the "*Gu Kong Lun*"[184] prescribes a needle insertion of seven *fen* with retention for ten exhalations. {later editor}]

Outer Hill (*Wai Qiu*, GB 36) is the cleft point of the foot *shao yang* and is engendered by the (foot) *shao yang*. It is located seven *cun* above the lateral malleolus. It is needled to a depth of three *fen* and moxaed with three cones.

Yang Intersection (*Yang Jiao*, GB 35) is also known as Divergent Yang (*Bie Yang*) or Leg Bone Hole (*Zu Liao*) and is the cleft point of the yang linking vessel. It is located seven *cun* above the lateral malleolus. It points obliquely to the parting of flesh of the three yang.[185] It is needled to a depth of six *fen*, (the needle) is retained for a duration of seven exhalations, and it is moxaed with three cones.

Yang Mound Spring (*Yang Ling Quan*, GB 34) is associated with earth. It is located one *cun* below the knee in a depression at the lateral aspect (of the leg). It is the point where the foot *shao yang* channel submerges, and is, therefore, the confluence point. It is needled to a depth of six *fen*, (the needle) is retained for a duration of ten exhalations, and it is moxaed with three cones.

Yang Joint (*Yang Guan*, GB 33) is located three *cun* above Yang Mound Spring in a depression lateral to the Calf's Nose. It is needled to a depth of five *fen*, and moxibustion is prohibited.

Central River (*Zhong Du*, GB 32) is located at the lateral aspect of the thigh in a depression of the flesh five *cun* above the knee and belongs to the qi of the foot *shao yang* vessel. It is needled to a depth of five *fen*, (the needle) is retained for a duration of seven exhalations, and it is moxaed with five cones.

Jumping Round (*Huan Tiao*, GB 30) is located in the hip joint and belongs to the qi of the foot *shao yang* vessel. Locate it with the (patient) lying on their side, the lower leg stretched while the upper one is bent. It is needled to a depth of one *cun*, (the needle) is retained for a duration of twenty exhalations, and it is moxaed with five cones.

Chapter Thirty-Five

Thirty-Four Points of the Foot *Tai Yang* (from the Foot) Through the Thigh Including The Six Points of the Yang Motility[186]

The urinary bladder emerges at Reaching Yin (*Zhi Yin*, Bl 67), and Reaching Yin is associated with metal. It is located at the lateral aspect of the small toe, the distance of a leek leaf from the corner of the nail. It is the point where the foot *tai yang* emerges, and is, therefore, the well point. It is needled to a depth of one *fen*, (the needle) is retained for a duration of five exhalations, and it is moxaed with three cones.

Valley Passage (*Tong Gu*, Bl 66) is associated with water. It is located at the lateral aspect of the small toe in a depression distal to the base joint of the phalanx. It is the point where the foot *tai yang*

channel gushes, and is, therefore, the brook point. It is needled to a depth of two *fen*, (the needle) is retained for a duration of five exhalations, and it is moxaed with three cones.

Bundle Bone (*Shu Gu*, Bl 65) is associated with wood. It is located on the lateral aspect of the small toe in a depression proximal to the base joint of the phalanx. It is the point where the foot *tai yang* channel pours forth, and is, therefore, the rapids point. It is needled to a depth of three *fen*, (the needle) is retained for a duration of three exhalations, and it is moxaed with three cones. [A note in the "*Qi Xue Lun*"[187] locates this point on the border of the red and white flesh proximal to the base joint of the phalanx. {later editor}]

Capital Bone (*Jing Gu*, Bl 64)[188] is located on the lateral aspect of the foot below the major bone in a depression on the border of the red and white flesh which can be located by palpation. It is the point where the foot *tai yang* has its efflux, and is, therefore, the source point. It is needled to a depth of three *fen*, (the needle) is retained for a duration of seven exhalations, and it is moxaed with three cones.

Extending Vessel (*Shen Mai*, Bl 62) is engendered by the yang motility vessel, and is located below the lateral malleolus in a depression as large as the edge of the fingernail. It is needled to a depth of three *fen*, (the needle) is retained for a duration of six exhalations, and it is moxaed with three cones. [A note in the "*Ci Yao Tong Lun*"[189] locates this point five *fen* below the lateral malleolus. {later editor}]

Metal Gate (*Jin Men*, Bl 63) is the cleft point of the foot *tai yang* and is located in a hole below the lateral malleolus. Also known as Gate Beam (*Guan Liang*), it is shared by the yang linking vessel.[190] It is needled to a depth of three *fen* and moxaed with three cones.

Kneeling Servant (*Pu Can*, Bl 61) is also known as Quieting of Evil (*An Xie*) and is located below the heel bone in a depression which can be found with the foot arched. It is the point where the foot *tai yang* channel flows mightily, and is, therefore, the stream point. It is needled to a depth of five *fen*, (the needle) is retained for a duration of ten exhalations, and it is moxaed with three cones. [A note in the *"Ci Yao Tong Lun"* states that "a fine pulsating vessel is palpable in the depression". {later editor}]

Kun Lun Mountain (*Kun Lun*, Bl 60) is associated with fire and is located behind the lateral malleolus in a depression in the heel, where a fine pulsating vessel is palpable. It is the point where the foot *tai yang* channel flows mightily, and is, therefore, the stream point (*sic*). It is needled to a depth of five *fen*, (the needle) is retained for a duration of ten exhalations, and it is moxaed with three cones.

Instep Yang (*Fu Yang*, Bl 59), the cleft point of the yang linking vessel, is located three *cun* above the lateral malleolus between the bone and the sinew[191] in front of the *tai yang* and behind the *shao yang*.[192] It is needled to a depth of six *fen*, (the needle) is retained for a duration of seven exhalations, and it is moxaed with three cones.

Taking Flight (*Fei Yang*, Bl 58) is also known as Jue Yang (*Jue Yang*) and is located seven *cun* above the lateral malleolus. It is the connecting vessel of the foot *tai yang* which diverges to the (foot) *shao yin*. It is needled to a depth of three *fen* and moxaed with three cones.

Mountain Support (*Cheng Shan*, Bl 57) is also known as Fish Belly (*Yu Fu*), Intestine Mount (*Chang Shan,*) and Flesh Column (*Rou Zhu*) and is located in a depression at the parting of the flesh at the lower end of the calf. It is needled to a depth of seven *fen*, and moxaed with three cones.

Sinew Support (*Cheng Jin*, Bl 56) is also known as Calf Intestine (*Chuai Chang*) and Straight Intestine (*i.e.*, Rectum, *Zhi Chang*) and is located in a depression in the center of the calf. It belongs to the qi of the foot *tai yang* vessel. Needling is prohibited, but it may be moxaed with three cones. [A note in the *"Ci Yao Tong Lun"* locates this point in the center of *nao*.[193] {later editor} The *Zi Sheng Jing* advises needling to a depth of three *fen*.]

Yang Union (*He Yang*, Bl 55) is located two *cun* below the midpoint of the fold of the popliteal

fossa. It is needled to a depth of six *fen* and moxaed with five cones.

Bend Middle (*Wei Zhong*, Bl 54) is associated with earth and is located in the center of the popliteal fossa at the pulsating vessel in the crease. It is the point where the foot *tai yang* submerges, and is, therefore, the confluence point. It is needled to a depth of five *fen*, (the needle) is retained for a duration of seven exhalations, and it is moxaed with three cones. [A note in the *"Gu Kong Lun"*[194] locates this point at the back of the knee joint with the (patient's) foot bent upward, while a note in the *"Ci Yao Tong Lun"*[195] locates it at the posterior flexor side of the knee. {later editor}]

Bend Yang (*Wei Yang*, Bl 53) is the lower assisting point of the triple heater.[196] It is located in front of the foot *tai yang* and behind foot *shao yang*,[197] between two sinews at the lateral side of the popliteal fossa, and six *cun* below Support (*Fu Cheng*).[198] It is the point at which the connecting vessel of the foot *tai yang* diverges. It is needled to a depth of seven *fen*, (the needle) is retained for a duration of five exhalations, and it is moxaed with three cones. Locate it with the (patient's) body[199] bent forward.

Superficial Cleft (*Fu Xi*, Bl 52) is located one *cun* above Bend Yang (*Wei Yang*). Locate it with the (patient's) knee stretched. It is needled to a depth of five *fen* and moxaed with three cones.

Gate of Abundance (*Yin Men*, Bl 51) is located six *cun* below Flesh Cleft (*Rou Xi*).[200] It is needled to a depth of five *fen*, (the needle) is retained for a duration of seven exhalations, and it is moxaed with three cones.

Support (*Fu Cheng*, Bl 50) is also known as Flesh Cleft (*Rou Xi*), Yin Joint (*Yin Guan*), or Skin Region (*Pi Bu*). It is located at the fold in the medial aspect of the thigh below the hip. It is needled to a depth of two *cun*, (the needle) is retained for a duration of seven exhalations, and it is moxaed with three cones.

To induce a moxa (sore), old shoes are heated to iron (the part that has been moxaed), and a sore arises in three days.[201]

Endnotes

[1]In actuality there are only four points described in this chapter. The first is a single point and the other three are bilateral. A similar system of counting is used throughout the volume.

[2]Part 1 is derived from Chap. 58, *Su Wen (Basic Questions)*; Part 2 from *Ming (Zhen Jiu Ming Tang Zhi Yao [Acupuncture & Moxibustion Treatment Essentials of the Enlightening Hall])*.

[3]*Sun luo*, i.e., the branch divergences of the connecting channels

[4]This sentence can be rendered in another way, *i.e.*, "The minute... meet with the three hundred and sixty-five points..."

[5]Extraordinary evil (*qi xie*) are pathogens which may spontaneously enter the skin and hair and spill over into the network vessels. They may be on the left and pour into the right, or vice versa. They have no fixed location and do not enter the channels. These are referred to as extraordinary evils.

[6]The great qi here refers to the channel qi. The great qi may also mean evil qi in other contexts.

[7]In the passages that follow a specific number of moxa cones has been prescribed for many of the acupoints. It should be kept in mind that the number of moxa cones primarily infers the duration of time the point should be stimulated.

[8]A meeting point is an acupoint on a channel intersected by one or more other channels. These points are capable of treating disorders not only related to the channel on which they lie but also disorders related to the channels which intersect it as well. These points therefore treat a wide range of problems which are often quite distal to the point itself.

[9]This entire chapter is derived from the *Zhen Jiu Ming Tang Zhi Yao*.

[10]Chap. 52, *Su Wen*

[11]Refer to Note 35, Chap. 4, Book. 1.

[12]"Treatise on Bone Cavities", Chap. 60, *Su Wen*.

[13]This is a work by Wang Wei-yi (cir 987B1067), who contributed much to acupuncture by compiling the work and designing the bronze acupuncture statues.

[14]This chapter is derived from the *Zhen Jiu Ming Tang Zhi Yao*.

[15]The name Light Guard is derived from the habit people have of closing their eyes to concentrate. Thus, in a sense, thought is assisted by the eyes (*i.e.*, light). *Cheng Guang*, therefore, means "benefitting from light".

[16]*Luo Que* is, in fact, a common mispronunciation of *Luo Xi*, the proper translation of which is Connection Cleft.

[17]This chapter is derived from the *Zhen Jiu Ming Tang Zhi Yao*.

[18]A.k.a. *Tou Lin Qi*, i.e., Head On the Verge of Tears.

[19]The *Su Wen* and the *Tong Ren Jing* locate this point "directly above the eye", while *Wai Tai Mi Yao (The Secret [Medical] Essentials of a Provincial Governor)* and *Qian Jin Yao Fang (Essential Formulas Worth a Thousand Taels of Gold)* place the point above the canthus of the eye (*mu zi*). Wiseman translates this point as Overlooking Tears.

[20]Wiseman renders this point as Spirit Support.

[21]"Treatise on the Qi Abodes" Chap. 59, *Su Wen*.

[22]This chapter is derived from the *Zhen Jiu Ming Tang Zhi Yao*.

[23]Wiseman translates this point as Celestial Surge.

[24]Chap. 59, *Su Wen*.

[25]The motion of clenching the teeth causes movement at this point. See Chap. 7. Wiseman translates this point as Valley Lead.

[26]Drumming the chin (*gu han*) means to clench the teeth rapidly as if they were chattering from the cold.

[27]*Fu Bai* means "bottoms up" in the sense of a toast. The point acquired the name due to its use in treating patterns resembling intoxication. Wiseman translates this as Floating White.

[28]"Treatise on the Points of Qi", Chap. 58, *Su Wen*.

[29]This chapter is derived from the *Zhen Jiu Ming Tang Zhi Yao*.

[30]Now commonly known as *Ya Men* (GV 15).

[31]This implies that the governing vessel starts from this point to connect the root of the tongue.

[32]Chap. 59, *Su Wen*.

[33]This whole chapter is derived from the *Zhen Jiu Ming Tang Zhi Yao*.

[34]Chap. 59, *Su Wen*

[35]Wiseman translates this point as Great Hammer.

[36]The seventh cervical vertebra is called the great vertebra.

[37]Wiseman translates this point as Extremity of Yang.

[38]The *Su Wen* states: "The two vessels of the *shao yin* bind here." *Sheng Ji Zong Lu (Complete Records of the Life Securing [Classics])* states, "The foot *shao yin* and *shao yang* bind and unite here." It is basically a meeting point of the *shao yin* and *shao yang* vessels.

[39]Part 1 is from Chap. 51, Vol. 8, *Ling Shu*; Part 2 from the *Zhen Jiu Ming Tang Zhi Yao*.

[40]In many versions, needling is not prohibited, and there are needle prescriptions for many of these points even in this text.

[41]On the issue of needling the associated points on the back, a modern commentary suggests that, while the associated points may be needled, caution should be exercised and that they should not be needled excessively deeply. When supplementing with moxa, the ember must be allowed to burn slowly and be extinguished of its own accord. This allows for the accumulation of correct qi at the point. When draining with moxa, the ember should be blown and also allowed to go out on its own. Blowing on the moxa causes the heat to penetrate, thus purging the illness and is therefore draining.

[42]Chap. 58, *Su Wen*

[43]Many other classics including the *Wai Tai, Tong Ren,* and the *Zhen Jiu Da Cheng (The Great Compilation of Acupuncture & Moxibustion)* include this point as a meeting point of the *shao yang* as well.

[44]Chap. 59, *Su Wen*

[45]An associated point of the five viscera is simply a back *shu* or transport point.

[46]The *Wai Tai Mi Yao (Secret [Medical] Essentials of a Provincial Governor),* and *Zi Sheng Jing (Classic of Nourishing Life)* prescribe moxa with three and five cones respectively.

[47]Chap. 43, *Su Wen.*

[48]At the time of Huang-fu Mi's writing, although the 14 channels were described, the ascription of acupoints to specific channels was not as firmly established as it is today. Huang-fu Mi himself in this book contributed to the standard ascription of points to the channels we have today.

[49]No retention time is given.

[50]The *Su Wen* and *Wai Tai* refer to this point as Inner Central Backbone *Shu (Zhong Lu Nei Shu).*

[51]A number of variant editions contain the additional characters: *de qi zi xie, xie qi duo bu zhi* (得气

之泻，泻多之补治), thus making the final line read: "It is needled to a depth of eight *fen*. Getting the qi causes drainage, and, once having drained the point, then supplement it further." In *Tong Ren, Zi Sheng Jing,* and *Sheng Ji Zong Lu* the passage reads: "Get the qi and drain (the point) first. Having drained the point, then supplement it further. (*De qi qi xian xie, xian qi duo bu zhi*)", Both of these sentences, however, are absolutely inconsistent with Huang-fu Mi's treatment of all the other points, and the text may have been corrupted.

[52]The *Su Wen* prescribes needling this point to a depth of two *cun*, and *Qian Jin* prescribes needling to a depth of three *cun*.

[53]Chap. 63, *Su Wen.*

[54]This chapter is derived from the *Zhen Jiu Ming Tang Zhi Yao.*

[55]Chap. 60, *Su Wen*

[56]This phrase is incomprehensible. Variant editions substitute "entering the elbow" for "in the forked free rib region". Both are incomprehensible.

[57]"*Qi Fu Lun*", *Su Wen*. The comment of the later editor is incorrect. The point is not on the same level as Turtledove Tail (*Jiu Wei, CV 15*). The *Tong Ren Jing, Sheng Ji Zong Lu,* and *Zi Sheng Jing* advocate thirty cones.

[58]This chapter is derived from the *Zhen Jiu Ming Tang Zhi Yao.*

[59]Chap. 59, *Su Wen*

[60]The *Su Wen* prescribes needle retention for three exhalations.

[61]The name of this point refers to the movement of the jaws when chewing and this action causes movement at the location of the point as well. Wiseman translates this point as Forehead Fullness.

[62]Wiseman translates this point as Gum Intersection.

[63]Wiseman translates this point as Sauce Receptacle.

[64]In some versions, this point is located with the mouth open.

[65]Chap. 58, *Su Wen.*

[66]This chapter is derived from the *Zhen Jiu Ming Tang Zhi Yao.*

[67]Chap. 59, *Su Wen*

[68]Chap. 58, *Su Wen*

[69]Wiseman translates this point as Upper Duct.

[70]Wiseman translates this point as Below the Joint.

[71]Chap. 63, *Su Wen*

[72]The *Zhen Jiu Da Cheng* states that pressure at this point causes pain in the ear.

[73]This chapter is derived from the *Zhen Jiu Ming Tang Zhi Yao.*

[74]In some versions the root of the tongue is mentioned as a landmark to describe the location of point *Lian Quan* (CV 23). In that case, the sentence should be rendered as follows: "*Lian Quan*...above the throat knot but under the root of the tongue..."

[75]Chap. 59, *Su Wen*

[76]Chap. 79, *Su Wen*

[77]Musculus sternocleidomastoideus

[78]This is the abbreviated title of the *Zhen Jiu Ming Tang Zhi Yao.*

[79]This chapter is derived from the *Zhen Jiu Ming Tang Zhi Yao.*

[80]*I.e.*, the superior angle of the scapular crest

[81]Chap. 59, *Su Wen*

[82]*I.e.*, the extremitas acromialis of the clavicula and spina scapula

[83]*I.e.*, the caput humeri and acromion

[84]*I.e.*, the spina scapulae

[85]Chap. 60, *Su Wen*

[86]The *Su Wen* states that needling into the depression at *Que Pen* causes an exterior drainage of lung qi, resulting in counterflow dyspnea and wheezing.

[87]There have been divided views over the ascription of *Nao Hui*, but, in modern times, it is generally ascribed to the hand *shao yang* channel.

[88]This chapter is derived from the *Zhen Jiu Ming Tang Zhi Yao.*

[89]Chap. 59, *Su Wen*

[90]This chapter is derived from the *Zhen Jiu Ming Tang Zhi Yao.*

[91]Wiseman translates these two points as Lively Center and Spirit Ruins respectively.

[92]This chapter is derived from the *Zhen Jiu Ming Tang Zhi Yao.*

[93]Chap. 59, *Su Wen*

[94]Wiseman translates this point as Roof.

[95]This chapter is derived from the *Zhen Jiu Ming Tang Zhi Yao.*

[96]Chap. 59, *Su Wen*

[97]"Treatise on Needling for Heat Diseases", Chap. 32, *Su Wen*

[98]Wiseman translates this point as Chest Village.

[99]Wiseman translates this as Food Hole.

[100]This chapter is derived from the *Zhen Jiu Ming Tang Zhi Yao.*

[101]Saber lumps are clusters of tubercular masses growing under the axilla or on the neck.

[102]Chap. 58, *Su Wen*

[103]This description of the location of *Da Bao* is hard to understand. The point, if three *cun* under *Yuan Ye*, cannot be located below the ninth rib.

[104]The word *jin* suggests the ribs are like the ridges or ruts in a road. Wiseman translates this point as Sinew Seat.

[105]Chap. 59, *Su Wen*

[106]This description of the location of Celestial Pool (*Tian Chi*) is puzzling, since a point one *cun* lateral to the breast cannot be straight under the axilla or at the ends of the free ribs.

[107]This chapter is derived from the *Zhen Jiu Ming Tang Zhi Yao.*

[108]This prohibition is unjustified.

[109]Chap. 59, *Su Wen*

[110]Lu Guang lived in the Kingdom of Wu during the period of the Three Kingdoms and was a chancellor of the Royal Medical Office of Wu. His main contribution to medicine was the compilation and collation of a number of medical classics, the most influential of which is the *Nan Jing Ji Zhu* (*Collection of Notes on the Classic of Difficult Issues*).

[111]The penetrating vessel is the *chong mai* or penetrating vessel. It is called the yin penetrating vessel because it irrigates all the yin channels.

[112]This chapter is derived from the *Zhen Jiu Ming Tang Zhi Yao.*

[113]Chap. 59, *Su Wen*

[114]Chap. 61, *Su Wen*

[115]The horizontal bone refers to the pubic bone. Wiseman calls this point Pubic Bone.

[116]This chapter is derived from the *Zhen Jiu Ming Tang Zhi Yao.*

[117]Chap. 59, *Su Wen*

[118]In some versions, the clause, "extension of the middle point of the foot *yang ming* channel" is inserted in this sentence. However, this is quite a vague reference.

[119]Chap. 61, *Su Wen*

[120]Chap. 52, *Su Wen*

[121]Chap. 60, *Su Wen*

[122]This chapter is derived from the *Zhen Jiu Ming Tang Zhi Yao.*

[123]Chap. 59, *Su Wen*

[124]It is understood below that a vessel starts or deviates from this point.

[125]This chapter is derived from the *Zhen Jiu Ming Tang Zhi Yao.*

[126]Chap. 59, *Su Wen*

[127]Nowadays, this location is incorrect. In modern times, it is located on the lower border of the free end of the twelfth rib.

[128]This chapter is derived from Chap. 1, Vol. 1, and Chap. 71, Vol. 10, *Ling Shu,* and the *Zhen Jiu Ming Tang Zhi Yao.*

[129]This implies the associated channels or their qi.

[130]*I.e.,* the three yin channels of the hand, namely, the hand *tai yin,* the hand *shao yin,* and the hand heart-governor or *jue yin*

[131]*I.e.,* the tendon of the biceps

[132]Chap. 58, *Su Wen*

[133]The underlying logic is that the *qi kou,* the juncture through which all the qi of the five viscera and the six bowels have to pass, is inhabited by the spirit-brightness, and, since it is a metal point, fire (*i.e.,* moxibustion) is bound to do harm to the spiritBlight.

[134]This sentence has been a challenge to researchers of Chinese medicine and there is no consensus as to its meaning.

[135]This chapter is a combination of parts of the *Zhen Jiu Ming Tang Zhi Yao* and Chap. 71, Vol. 10, *Ling Shu.*

[136]*I.e.,* tendon musculus flexoris carpiradialis and palmis longus

[137]This chapter is derived from the *Zhen Jiu Ming Tang Zhi Yao* and Chap. 71, Vol. 10, *Ling Shu.*

[138]This statement should not be taken literally. It only implies that cardiac problems cannot be cured by the transporting points of the heart channel but rather by those on the pericardium channel.

[139]*I.e., Shen Men* (Ht 7)

[140]This means repletion or superabundance of the channel qi.

[141]Chap. 79, *Su Wen*

[142]*I.e.,* the musculus triceps brachii and musculus coracobrachialis

[143]This chapter is derived from the *Zhen Jiu Ming Tang Zhi Yao.*

[144]*I.e.,* tendon M. extensoris pollicis longi and brevis

[145]The meaning of this clause is vague.

[146]*I.e.,* the extensor carpi radialis longus and brevis

[147]*I.e.,* the deltoid

[148]This chapter is derived from the *Zhen Jiu Ming Tang Zhi Yao.*

[149]This vessel is not identifiable, and this description is confusing even in Chinese.

[150]Chap. 59, *Su Wen*

[151]This chapter is derived from the *Zhen Jiu Ming Tang Zhi Yao.*

[152]Chap. 58, *Su Wen*

[153]*I.e.,* the medial process of the humerus

[154]This chapter is derived from the *Zhen Jiu Ming Tang Zhi Yao.*

[155]Chap. 58, *Su Wen*

[156]"*Bie zou shang yi cun.*" This obscure sentence implies that the foot *tai yin* and the foot *jue yin* join at a place eight *cun* above the medial malleolus and that Earth's Crux lies one *cun* above this spot.

[157]The fish belly in this context refers to the swelling of flesh on the thigh above the knee.

[158]*I.e.,* M.sartorius, M. gracilis and Rami cutanei medialis n. femoris

[159]"Treatise on the Three Positions & the Nine Indications", Chap. 20, *Su Wen*

[160]This point is commonly known as *Zu Wu Li* (Liv 10).

[161]This chapter is derived from the *Zhen Jiu Ming Tang Zhi Yao*.

[162]"Treatise on Needling for Lumbar Pain", Chap. 41, *Su Wen*

[163]Chap. 58, *Su Wen*

[164]A reliable interpretation for this sentence is unavailable, given it's context.

[165]I.e., the tendons semimembranosus and semitendinosus

[166]Some editions prescribe three cones, but the *Wai Tai Mi Yao* prescribes two cones.

[167]This is a forty-volume work compiled by Wang Tao in 752 A.D., a comprehensive collection of past formulas, thanks to which many valuable medical works of ancient times are preserved.

[168]This chapter is derived from the *Zhen Jiu Ming Tang Zhi Yao*.

[169]"Treatise on Points for Water and Heat Diseases", Chap. 61, *Su Wen*

[170]"The Treatise on Needling for Lumbar Pain", Chap. 41, *Su Wen*

[171]This implies *Fu Liu* (Ki 7) and *San Yin Jiao* (Sp 6) respectively.

[172]I.e., the tibia and M. flexoris digitorum longi

[173]These are the tendons semimembranosus and semitendinosus.

[174]This chapter is derived from the *Zhen Jiu Ming Tang Zhi Yao*.

[175]Chap. 58, *Su Wen*

[176]Because the term "lower ridge" can be interpreted in more than one way, the exact location of this depression is uncertain. Nowadays Bountiful Bulge is generally located one *cun* posterior to Ribbon Opening.

[177]This is commonly known simply as *Xia Ju Xu* (St 39).

[178]The *Su Wen* prescribes a depth of one *cun*, and *Tong Ren* prescribes a depth of five *fen*.

[179]Chap. 41, *Su Wen*

[180]This chapter is derived from the *Zhen Jiu Ming Tang Zhi Yao*.

[181]The *Su Wen*, *Tong Ren*, and *Zi Sheng Jing* say three *fen*.

[182]Chap. 58, *Su Wen*

[183]This suggests that it is necessary to locate the point by occluding the blood vessels along the route of the foot *yang ming* on the instep with pressure.

[184]Chap. 60, *Su Wen*

[185]This clause means that *Yang Jiao* and *Wai Qiu* form a line extending to the parting of the flesh through which all the three foot yang channels pass.

[186]This chapter is derived from the *Zhen Jiu Ming Tang Zhi Yao*.

[187]Chap. 58, *Su Wen*

[188]The base of the fifth metatarsal bone is commonly known as the *jing* or capital bone.

[189]Chap. 41, *Su Wen*

[190]This implies that the point pertains to both the yang linking vessel and the foot *tai yang*.

[191]I.e., the fibula and tendon calcaneus

[192]Since the point belongs to the yang motility vessel, it is quite reasonable to say that the point is between the *tai yang* and *shao yang*. This expression, however, may sound ridiculous if looked at from the modern view that the point belongs to the foot *tai yang*.

[193]The word *nao* usually means the upper arm, but the point has nothing to do with the arm. Therefore, the material in the brackets is incomprehensible.

[194]Chap. 60, *Su Wen*

[195]This note is found in the "*Ci Re Lun*" (Chap. 32) rather than in the "*Ci Yao Tong Lun*" (Chap. 41) in the *Su Wen*.

[196]This ascription is difficult to understand and suggests that there might be something wrong here. Note, however, that it is the associated point of the triple burner in the lower part of the body.

[197]This implies that *Wei Yang* is between the foot *tai yang* and *shao yang*.

[198]This point is commonly known as *Cheng Fu* (Bl 50).

[199]The word "body" must be mistaken for knee.

[200]In some variant versions the modern name *Cheng Fu* (Bl 50) is given, apparently in disagreement to the conventional nomenclature current at the times of Huang-fu Mi.

[201]It was believed that intentionally producing moxa sores was of some help in the treatment of certain kinds of diseases.

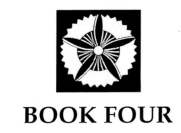

BOOK FOUR

Chapter One

Pulses (Part 1)[1]

(1)

Lei Gong asked:

The "*Wai Chuai*"[2] teaches that various subtle problems may be summed up in a single (concise) scheme. I am not familiar with this teaching. Would you explain it in a few words?

The Yellow Emperor answered:

The *cun kou* pulse reflects the interior while the *ren ying* the exterior. They are in mutual accord, coming and going synchronously, their amplitudes in proportion as if controlled by one thread. In spring and summer, the *ren ying* pulse is slightly larger, while in autumn and winter, it is the *cun kou* which is slightly larger. This is called normalcy.[3]

The *ren ying*, if twice as large as the *cun kou*, suggests disease in the *shao yang*; if thrice, disease in the *tai yang*; and if four times, disease in the *yang ming*. If there is overexuberance, this implies heat; if there is vacuity, this implies cold; if there is tension, this implies painful *bi*; and if (the pulse) is interrupted, this implies a disease of remittent nature.[4] Overexuberance requires drainage; vacuity requires supplementation; tenseness (in the pulse) requires treatment at the level of the borders of flesh;[5] interruption (in the pulse) requires pricking the blood connecting vessel in combina-

tion with the drinking of medication. A sunken (pulse) requires moxibustion; a case of neither overexuberance nor vacuity requires treating (the points of) the concerned channel. The last option is called channel needling (*jing ci*).

If the *ren ying* pulse is five times as large as the *cun kou*, this is called external barricade. External barricade is fatal (if the *ren ying*) is not only large but rapid. It is essential to carefully examine the condition in the context of its origins and branches and cold and heat in order to locate the affected viscus or bowel (before treating).

The *cun kou*, if twice as large as the *ren ying*, implies disease in the *jue yin*; if thrice, it implies disease in the *shao yin*; and if four times, it implies disease in the *tai yin*. Overexuberance implies distention and fullness, cold in the center, and normal appetite without ability to transform the food;[6] vacuity implies heat in the center, chyme-like stool and undigested food in the stool, shortage of qi, and change of urine color. An interrupted pulse implies intermittent pain. Overexuberance requires drainage; vacuity requires supplementation; tenseness (in the pulse) requires needling followed by moxibustion; and an interrupted (pulse) requires that one prick the blood connecting vessel followed by a regulating therapy ["draining therapy" in the *Tai Su (Primary Origination)*[7] {later editor}]; and a sinking pulse requires treatment exclusively by moxibustion. In case of a sunken pulse, there must be blood binding in the vessels, which causes static blood and cold blood; therefore, moxibustion is advisable. If the pulse is neither overexuberant nor vacuous, this condition requires treatment of (the points of) the concerned channel.

If the *cun kou* is five times as large as the *ren ying*, this is called internal blockade. Internal blockade is fatal if (the *cun kou*) is not only large but rapid. It is essential to carefully examine the condition within the context of its origins and ends and cold and heat in order to locate the affected viscus or bowel (prior to treatment).

Knowledge about the brook and rapids points is a prerequisite for mastery of the essentials (of acupuncture therapeutics). A large (pulse) is said to indicate overexuberance which requires treatment exclusively via drainage; a small (pulse) is said to indicate vacuity which requires treatment exclusively via supplementation. A tense (pulse) requires needling and moxibustion in combination with the drinking of medication. A sagging (pulse) requires treatment exclusively via moxibustion. A case of neither overexuberance nor vacuity requires treatment (of the points on) the concerned channel. The modality called channel treatment consists of the drinking of medication in addition to needling and moxibustion. An urgent pulse requires conducting therapy,[8] and an interrupted pulse ["large yet weak pulse" in a variant version {later editor}] requires quiet repose without exertion.[9]

(2)

The Yellow Emperor asked:

What are the indications of the progression or remission and the advance or decline of a disease?

Qi Bo answered:

The interior and the exterior may both serve as indicators. If upon palpation the *mai kou* feels slippery, small, tense, and deep, this indicates that the disease is deteriorating and is lingering in the center. If the qi of the *ren ying* feels large, tense, and floating, this indicates that the disease is deteriorating and lingering in the exterior. If

the *mai kou* is floating and slippery, this indicates an amelioration of the disease day by day; if the *ren ying* is deep and slippery, the disease diminishes day by day. A *cun kou* which is slippery and deep indicates (adverse) progress of the disease day by day which is lingering in the interior; while a *ren ying* which is felt slippery, exuberant, and floating demonstrates (adverse) progress of the disease which is lingering in the exterior. If the *ren ying* and the *qi kou* are both floating or sinking and equal to each other in the amount of qi they possess, the disease is difficult to treat. A disease in the viscus accompanied by a deep but large pulse is easy to cure, but (the outcome is) unfavorable if the pulse is small.[10]

A disease in the bowels accompanied by a pulse which is floating and large is easy to cure.[11]

A *ren ying* pulse which is exuberant and tense suggests cold damage, while a *cun kou* pulse which is exuberant and tense suggests food damage. If the pulse is slippery, large, interrupted, and long, the illness has invaded from the exterior and will manifest with symptoms of confused vision and confinement in orientation.[12] This is due to the concentration of yang (in yin), and it is amenable to regulating therapy.

(3)

The Yellow Emperor asked:

What is the pulse in normal people like?

Qi Bo answered:

For one exhalation the pulse beats twice, and for one inhalation, the pulse beats twice. For a whole process of respiration including the intermission between the exhalation and inhalation the pulse beat five times [questionable {later editor}].[13] This is the state in normal people. Normal people can be defined as those without disease. It is the common practice to compare (the pulses of) those without disease with those who suffer from illness. In as much as physicians are without disease, they can regulate their own respiration so as to measure their patient's pulses. If for a single exhalation the pulse beats once and for a single inhalation the pulse beats once again, this is called diminished qi. If for a single exhalation the pulse beats thrice, in an agitated way, and the skin at the cubit region[14] is hot, then a warm disease is indicated. If, however, the cubit region is not hot and the pulse is slippery, this suggests a wind disease. [Here the *Su Wen* reads, "if the pulse is choppy there is *bi*". {later editor}] If for a single exhalation the pulse beats more than four times, this portends death. If the pulse is expiring, (*i.e.,* stops arriving) this portends death. And, if the pulse beats at a varying rhythm and pace, this also portends death. Man relies on the stomach for qi, and, therefore, the stomach qi is the root of the pulse. For this reason, the absence of stomach qi is said to be an adverse condition and means death.[15]

(4)

In palpating the pulse and counting its beats, if there is no interruption in fifty beats, this indicates that all the five viscera are receiving qi. One interruption in forty beats indicates that qi is absent from one viscus. One interruption in thirty beats indicates that qi is absent from two viscera. One interruption in twenty beats indicates that qi is absent from three viscera. One interruption in ten beats indicates that qi is absent from four viscera and one interruption in less than ten beats indicates that qi is absent from all five viscera and (the patient's days) are numbered. An important comment on this matter may be found in the "*Zhong Shi*".[16] It states that no interruption for fifty beats is a normal state and demonstrates that the five viscera have a long life. A short life is indicated if the pulse beats at a variable pace and rhythm.[17]

(5)

The liver pulse is bowstring;[18] the heart pulse is hook-like;[19] the spleen pulse is belt-like;[20] the lung pulse is hair-like;[21] the kidney pulse is stone-like.[22]

(In its normal state) when the heart pulse arrives, it feels like a string of pearls or glossy jades.[23] If it feels like pearls fused together, pounding forcefully with small amplitude modulation, this portends disease. If it is first crooked and then straight, like the sensation of holding a crook girdle,[24] it portends death.[25]

When the lung pulse arrives, it appears like a falling elm seed, leisurely buoyed up in the air[26] and this is the normal (lung pulse). If it feels rough like touching a cock's feather, it portends disease. If it feels like something floating or hair being blown, this portends death.

When the liver pulse arrives, it feels gentle and long like holding the small end of a long pole. This is the normal (liver pulse). If it feels full, solid, and slippery like feeling a long pole, it portends disease. If it feels urgent and forceful like the string on a bow, this portends death.

When the spleen pulse arrives, it feels tender, moderate, and distinct, like a cock letting its feet down on the ground.[27] This is the normal (spleen pulse). If it feels solid, full, and rapid, like a cock lifting its feet,[27] this portends disease. If it feels hard and sharp like the beak of a bird or the spur of a cock, (as irregular) as a leak in a roof, and (as urgent as) flowing water, these conditions portend death.

When the kidney pulse arrives, it feels like a hook,[28] rippling energetically and felt hard upon pressure. This is the normal (kidney pulse). If it feels as if one is pulling a kudzu vine and very hard upon pressure, it portends disease. If it feels as if one were drawing a rope in a tug of war or (hard as a) pebble, this portends death.[29]

(In disease,) the spleen pulse, when vacuous and floating, may be confused with the lung pulse. The kidney pulse, when small and floating, may be confused with the spleen pulse, and the liver pulse, when urgent, deep, and dispersed, may be confused with the kidney pulse.

(6)

The Yellow Emperor asked:

Why does the appearance of the true visceral (pulse) mean death?

Qi Bo answered:

All five viscera rely upon qi from the stomach and, therefore, the stomach is the root of the five viscera. Since the visceral qi has no direct access to the hand *tai yin*,[30] (the visceral qi) can only reach (the hand *tai yin*) via the stomach qi. In this way, the five viscera make their appearance in the hand *tai yin* in their own prevailing seasons.[31] Therefore, if there is an overwhelming amount of evil qi, this debilitates the essential qi. In a serious case, the stomach qi is unable to accompany (the qi of the viscera) to the hand *tai yin*, thus leaving the true visceral qi exposed alone. The solitary appearance of the true visceral qi implies that disease has overwhelmed the viscera and, therefore, portends death.[32]

The spring pulse[33] reflects the liver. Associated with east and wood, spring is the season when every living thing begins to grow. Therefore, its (pulse) qi is gentle, light, vacuous, and slippery as well as straight and long and this is called a bow-string (pulse). A contrary display implies disease. If the (pulse) qi is solid and strong, this is said to indicate excess and that the disease is in the exterior. If (the pulse) qi appears vacuous and faint, this is said to indicate insufficiency and that the disease is in the center. Excess leads to irascibility, trance, dizziness, and madness, while insufficiency causes pain in the chest radiating to the back and the free rib region and fullness in the lateral costal region.

The summer pulse reflects the heart. Associated with the south and fire, summer is the season when every living thing flourishes. Its (pulse) qi arrives exuberantly but retreats in decline and is, therefore, called a hook-like pulse. A contrary display implies disease. If the (pulse) qi both arrives exuberantly and retreats exuberantly, it indicates that there is excess and that the disease is in the exterior, while if the (pulse) qi does not arrive exuberantly but rather it retreats exuberantly, this is said to indicate insufficiency and that the disease is in the interior. Excess leads to generalized

fever with pain in the skin which develops into a syndrome known as sapping[34] (*jin yin*, 浸淫), while insufficiency leads to vexation of the heart with coughing of foamy sputum above and qi leakage below.[35]

The autumn pulse reflects the lung. Associated with the west and metal, autumn is the season when every living thing matures and is harvested. Accordingly, its (pulse) qi appears light, vacuous, and floating, looming urgently, retreating dispersed. This is, therefore, called a superficial (pulse). A contrary display implies disease. If the (pulse) qi appears hairy with a hard core and vacuous sides, there is said to be excess and the disease is in the exterior. If the (pulse) qi appears hairy and faint, there is said to be insufficiency and the disease is in the interior. Excess leads to a counterflow of qi, pain in the back, and irascibility, while insufficiency causes dyspnea, cough with diminished qi, an ascension of qi with the coughing of blood, and loud rales.

The winter pulse reflects the kidney. Associated with the north and water, winter is the season when every living thing is collected and stored. Accordingly, its (pulse) qi is deep and soggy ["pounding" in the *Su Wen* {later editor}], and is, therefore, called a stone-like pulse. A contrary display implies disease. If the (pulse) qi is (hard like a) pebble, there is said to be excess and the disease is in the exterior. If the (pulse) qi retreats abruptly, there is said to be insufficiency and the disease is in the center. Excess leads to fatigue and listlessness, pain in the paravertebral vessels, diminished qi, and disinclination to talk, while insufficiency leads to a sensation of the heart being suspended as in hunger, coolness of the lateral abdomen, pain in the spine, lower abdominal fullness, and dark colored or yellowish urine.

The spleen pulse reflects earth. Spleen is a solitary viscus[36] and irrigates (the other viscera) on all four sides. It is auspicious (if the spleen pulse) cannot be seen, while on the contrary its appearance is an ill-omen.[37] If it appears like flooding water, there is said to be excess and the disease is in the exterior. If it is felt like the beak of a bird, there is said to be insufficiency and the disease is in the interior. Excess leads to inability to raise the limbs, while insufficiency leads to congestion in the nine portals, (a syndrome) called *zhong qiang* (重强).[38]

Chapter One

Pulses (Part 2)[39]

(1)

The appearance of the autumn pulse in spring, the winter pulse in summer, the spring pulse in long summer, the summer pulse in autumn, and the long summer pulse in winter suggest five types of incurable illnesses known as the five evils. All have the same prognosis; all are incurable and end in death.[40]

If the spring (pulse) reflects the stomach (qi)[41] with a slightly bowstring quality,[42] this is normal. A very wiry pulse with little of the stomach, however, suggests liver disease. (A spring pulse which is) solely wiry without stomach (qi) portends death. (A spring pulse characterized by) stomach (qi) and hair[43] portends disease occurring in autumn. While this pulse with much hair implies that disease is imminent.

The visceral trueness is dispersed in the liver, and the liver stores the qi (which nourishes) the sinew membrane.[44]

If the summer (pulse) reflects the stomach (qi) with a slight hook-like quality,[45] this is normal. A very hook-like (pulse) with little stomach (qi), however, suggests heart disease. (A summer pulse which is) completely hook-like without stomach (qi) portends death. (A summer pulse characterized by) stomach qi with a stone-like quality[46] portends a disease occurring in winter. If this pulse is very stone-like, this implies that disease is imminent. The visceral trueness opens into the heart, and the heart stores the qi (which nourishes) the blood vessels.[47]

If the long summer (pulse) reflects the stomach

(qi) and is slightly weak, this is normal. Little stomach (qi) with a great deal of weakness, however, suggests spleen disease. (A long summer pulse which is) completely belt-like with no stomach (qi)[48] portends death. Weakness with a stone-like quality portends disease occurring in winter, while this pulse with a very stone-like quality ["weakness" in the *Su Wen* {later editor}] implies that disease is imminent.

The visceral trueness moistens the spleen, and the spleen stores the qi (which nourishes) the flesh.[49]

If the autumn (pulse) reflects stomach (qi) with a slight hair-like quality this is normal. A very hair-like (pulse) with little stomach (qi), however, suggests lung disease. (An autumn pulse which is) solely hair-like with no stomach (qi) portends death. A hair-like (pulse) with a wiry quality portends disease occurring in the spring, while a very bowstring pulse implies that disease is imminent.[50]

The visceral trueness ascends to the lung which circulates the qi throughout the constructive and defensive, the yin and yang.

If the winter (pulse) reflects stomach (qi) with a slight stone-like quality, this is normal. (A pulse with) little stomach (qi) and a very stone-like quality suggests kidney disease. (A winter pulse which is) solely stone-like with no stomach (qi) portends death. A stone-like (pulse) which is hook-like portends disease occurring in summer, while a very hook-like (pulse) implies that disease is imminent.

The visceral trueness descends to the kidney where qi is stored for the marrow of the bone.

The major connecting vessel of the stomach is called the walled city (*xu li*, 虚里). It links up with the diaphragm and connects to the lung, emerging from below the left breast where it beats forcefully enough to rustle ones clothing, and it houses the ancestral qi of the pulse.[51] If (the walled city) beats energetically and urgently with interruptions, the disease is in the interior. If it beats slowly with interruptions and feels hard, there is accumulation. If it expires, this portends death.

If the stomach pulse is replete, this indicates distention, and if vacuous, this indicates diarrhea.

(2)

If the heart pulse pounds hard and long, this indicates illnesses such as retracted tongue and inability to speak. If it is soft and scattered, it indicates pure heat wasting thirst ["vexation" in the *Su Wen* {later editor}] which will cure itself.[52]

If the lung pulse pounds hard and long, it indicates illnesses such as spitting of blood. If it is soft and scattered, it indicates profuse spontaneous sweating which is difficult to overcome.[53]

If the liver pulse pounds hard and long and is not accompanied by a green-blue complexion, this indicates an impact injury inflicted in falling or fighting. In this case, there will be blood lodging below the lateral costal region causing counterflow dyspnea. If the liver pulse is soft and scattered with a brilliant complexion, this indicates spillage rheum. Spillage rheum occurs when one drinks a great deal of water while suffering from frantic thirst. This then spills into the flesh and skin outside the stomach and the intestines.[54]

If the stomach pulse pounds hard and long and is accompanied by a red complexion, this indicates a disease characterized by (pain) in the thigh as if it were about to break. If it is soft and scattered, this indicates food *bi*[55] and painful thigh.[56]

If the spleen pulse pounds hard and long and is accompanied by a yellow complexion, this indicates diminished qi. If it is soft and scattered and accompanied by a dull complexion, this indicates edema-like swelling of the foot and the lower leg.[57]

If the kidney pulse pounds hard and long and is accompanied by a reddish-yellow complexion, this indicates (pain) in the lumbar region as if it were about to break. If it is soft and scattered, this indicates a lack of blood which is difficult to overcome.[58]

The vessels are the mansion of the blood. If the (pulse) is long, the qi is in harmony. If the pulse is short, the qi is diseased.[59] If the (pulse) is rapid, there is heart vexation. If the (pulse) is large, a disease is progressing. If the upper pulse[60] is exuberant, the qi is elevated (*gao*, 高).[61] If the lower pulse[62] is exuberant, there is qi distention. If the (pulse) is interrupted, there is an exhaustion of qi. If the (pulse) is fine, the qi is diminished. If the (pulse) is choppy, there is heart pain. If the pulse surges with momentum like a gushing spring, the disease is shown to be progressing and becoming critical. If the pulse appears evasive, interrupted and flabby ["weak" in a variant version {later editor}] and if it retreats abruptly as when a string is broken, this portends death.

If the *cun kou* pulse is short as it strikes the palpating fingers, this indicates a headache. If the *cun kou* is long as it strikes the palpating fingers, this indicates pain in the lower leg. If the *cun kou* is deep and hard, this indicates disease in the center. If the *cun kou* is floating and exuberant, this is indicative of disease in the exterior. If the upper section of the *cun kou* (strikes the finger forcefully) and rapidly, this indicates pain in the shoulder and back. If the *cun kou* is tight, firm, and hard ["deep and firm" in the *Su Wen* {later editor}], this indicates painful accumulation lying transversely across the lateral costal region. If the *cun kou* is superficial and stirring ["deep and weak" in the *Su Wen* {later editor}], this indicates chills and fever. If the *cun kou* is exuberant, slippery, and hard, this indicates disease in the exterior. If the *cun kou* is small but replete and hard, this indicates disease in the interior. If the pulse is small, weak, and choppy, the disease is said to be chronic. If the pulse is superficial, slippery, replete, and large ["floating and rapid" in the *Su Wen* {later editor}], this indicates a new disease. If the illness is serious but the stomach qi is present (in the pulse) and in harmony, the illness is uncomplicated. If the pulse is urgent, this indicates *shan*, conglomeration, and pain in the lower abdomen. A slippery pulse indicates wind; a choppy pulse indicates *bi*; and an exuberant and tight pulse indicates distention. A slow and slippery pulse indicates heat in the center. If palpation of the *cun kou* shows it to be in accord with the four seasons[63], the illness is uncomplicated. If, however, the *cun kou* is not in accord with the four seasons, and no viscera are skipped over[64], this portends death.[65]

The *tai yang* pulse[66] should arrive surging, large. and long; the *shao yang* pulse[67] should arrive varying in rhythm and length; and the *yang ming* pulse[68] should arrive superficial and large but short.[69]

(3)

If there is surplus in the *jue yin*, the illness is characterized by yin *bi*,[70] while in the case of insufficiency, the illness is one of heat *bi*. If the pulse is slippery, this indicates fox-like *shan* wind,[71] whereas a choppy (pulse) indicates accumulation of qi ["accumulation inversion" in a variant version {later editor}] in the lower abdomen.

If there is surplus in the *shao yin*, the illness is characterized by skin *bi*[72] and craving papules, while an insufficiency is characterized by lung *bi*.[73] If the (pulse) is slippery, this is indicative of lung wind *shan*,[74] whereas a choppy (pulse) indicates an illness of accumulation and urination of blood.[75]

If there is surplus in the *tai yin*, the illness is characterized by muscle *bi* and cold in the center, while insufficiency is characterized by spleen *bi*.[76] If the pulse is slippery, this indicates spleen wind *shan*,[77] whereas a choppy (pulse) indicates an illness of accumulation and frequent fullness in the venter and the abdomen.[78]

If there is surplus in the *yang ming*, the illness is characterized by vessel *bi*[79] and frequent generalized fever, while insufficiency is characterized by heart *bi*.[80] If the (pulse) is slippery, this indicates heart wind *shan*, whereas a choppy (pulse) indicates illnesses of accumulation and susceptibility to fright.[81]

If there is a surplus in the *tai yang*, the illness is characterized by bone *bi*[82] and heaviness of the body, while insufficiency is characterized by kidney *bi*.[83] If the (pulse) is slippery, this indicates kidney wind *shan*, whereas a choppy (pulse) indi-

cates illnesses of accumulation and liability to head problems.[84]

If there is a surplus in the *shao yang*, the illness is characterized by sinew *bi*[85] with fullness in the lateral costal region, while insufficiency is characterized by liver *bi*.[86] If the (pulse) is slippery, this indicates liver wind *shan*, whereas a choppy (pulse) indicates a tendency to tense sinews and pain in the eye.[87]

(4)

Tai yin counterflow inversion is characterized by hypertonicity of the lower leg and heart pain radiating toward the abdomen. It is treated using the primary (channel points appropriate to) the illness.[88]

Shao yin counterflow inversion is characterized by vacuity fullness (*xu man*, 虚满) with vomiting above and clear-food diarrhea in the below.[89] It is treated using the primary (channel points appropriate to) the illness.

Jue yin counterflow inversion is characterized by spasms, lumbar pain, vacuity fullness, urinary block, and delirium. It is treated using the primary (channel points appropriate to) the illness.[90]

Counterflow in all three (foot) yin, causing an inability to urinate or defecate and cold hands and feet, results in death in three days.[91]

(Foot) *tai yang* counterflow inversion is characterized by sudden loss of consciousness, retching of blood, and frequent nosebleeding. It is treated using the primary (channel points appropriate to) the illness.[92]

(Foot) *shao yang* counterflow inversion is characterized by inhibition in the joints. Inhibition in the joints causes an inability to walk due to (debility) of the low back and in inability to turn the neck round. If the case is complicated by intestinal *yong*, it is incurable and, once susceptibility to fright develops, death ensues.

(Foot) *yang ming* counterflow inversion is characterized by dyspnea and cough, generalized fever, susceptibility to fright, nosebleeding, and retching of blood. It is incurable and, once susceptibility to fright develops, death ensues.

Hand *tai yin* counterflow inversion is characterized by vacuity fullness with cough, frequent retching, and foaming at the mouth. It is treated using the primary (channel points appropriate to) the illness.

Counterflow inversion of the hand heart-governor and the hand *shao yin* is characterized by heart pain affecting the throat. If this is complicated by a generalized fever it results in death. However, if there is no fever the condition is curable.

Hand *tai yang* counterflow inversion is characterized by deafness, lacrimation, and inability to turn the neck or to bend the lumbus either forward or backward. It is treated using the primary (channel points appropriate to) the illness.

Hand *yang ming* and *shao yang* counterflow inversion is characterized by throat *bi* and swelling and soreness of the throat. It is treated using the primary (channel points appropriate to) the illness.

(5)

If (the pulse) arrives quickly and retreats slowly, there is repletion above and vacuity below. This is characterized by inversion and madness. If (the pulse) arrives slowly but retreats quickly, there is vacuity above and repletion below. This is characterized by malignant wind (*e feng*, 恶风).[93] In the case of malignant wind stroke, it is the yang qi which receives (the damage). If the pulse is deep, fine, and rapid, *shao yin* inversion is indicated. If the pulse is not only deep, fine, and rapid but also scattered, then fever and chills are indicated. And if the pulse is floating and scattered, spinning collapse is indicated.[94]

Any pulse characterized by superficiality without agitation indicates (a disorder of) the yang, and hence heat. (A pulse) which is agitated indicates (a disease) in the hand.[95] Any pulse characterized by fineness and deepness indicates (a disorder of) the yin and hence pain in the bone. (A pulse) which is tranquil indicates (a disease) in the foot.[96] A rapid, stirring pulse which is intermittently interrupted is a pulse reflecting disease in the yang with the manifestations of swill diarrhea and blood in the stools. A choppy (pulse) indicates surplus in the yang qi; a slippery one indicates superabundance in the yin qi. A surplus of yang qi results in generalized fever with an absence of sweating, while superabundance of yin qi results in copious sweating with generalized cold. A surplus of both yin and yang leads to absence of sweat with generalized cold.

If one deduces the presence of an external disorder and finds an internal disorder rather than an external one, this indicates accumulations in the venter and abdomen. If one deduces the presence of an internal disorder and finds an external disorder rather than an internal one, this indicates heat in the center. If one deduces a disorder above and finds one below and not above, this indicates a cold back and feet. If one deduces a disorder below and yet finds one above and not below, this indicates headache and neck pain.[97]

If the pulse, even when pressed down to the bone, still exhibits a shortage of qi, this is indicative of pain in the lumbar spine and *bi* in the body.

Chapter One

Pulses (Part 3)[98]

(1)

The third yang is the avenue, the second yang is the streets, and the first yang is the liaison.[99] The third yang is the *tai yang*. If it presents itself at the hand *tai yin*[100] as wiry and floating rather than deep as expected, the specific conditions present in the case must be studied carefully and correctly assessed in keeping with the yin/yang principle. The second yang is the *yang ming*. If it presents itself at the hand *tai yin* as wiry, deep, and urgent rather than large and floating as expected, when heat appears, death is inevitable.[101]

The first yang is the *shao yang*. If it presents itself at the hand *tai yin* and the *ren ying* as continuously wiry, urgent, and suspended, this means that the *shao yang* is diseased.[102]

The third yin[103] is the governor of all the six channels.[104] If it presents itself at the (hand) *tai yin* as hidden and deep rather than floating as expected, there is emptiness in the upper (warmer) which extends to the heart.[105]

When the second yin[103] reaches the lung,[106] its qi returns to the urinary bladder, connecting externally with the spleen and the stomach.[107]

If the first yin[103] arrives alone, the channel is expiring and the qi is floating away. Therefore, the pulse will appear hook-like[108] and slippery, rather than full. In normal cases, the pulse peculiar to each of the five viscera should be accompanied by stomach qi, a pulse image of gentleness. If not, it is said to be left solitary.

The six pulses may present a yin (quality in the case of a yang disorder) or a yang (quality in the case of a yin disorder). Although this crossed-up display may be ascribed to the five viscera manifesting in an abnormal or complicated manner, it can nevertheless be understood in terms of yin and yang. That (pulse) which first appears is the host, while that (pulse) which appears later is the guest.[109]

The third yang is the father; the second yang is the guardian; the first yang is the coordinator. The third yin is the mother; the second yin is the feminine; the first yin is the sole envoy.[110]

(In the case of an abnormality in the channels of) the second yang and the first yin, the illness resides primarily within the *yang ming*, since it is restrained by the first yin. (In this case,) the pulse is soft and stirring, and the nine portals are all congested.[111]

(In the case of an abnormality in the channels of) the third yang and the first yin, the *tai yang* channel overwhelms and the first yin cannot resist, plunging the five viscera into internal disorder and provoking fright and panic externally.[112]

(In the case of an abnormality in the channels of) the second yin and the first yang, the illness lies in the lung.[113] (In this case,) the *shao yin* pulse is deep, the lung is overwhelmed and the spleen damaged, and consequently the four limbs are damaged externally.[113]

(In the case of an abnormality in) the mutual interaction between the second yin and the second yang, the illness lies in the kidney, giving rise to abusive speech, frenetic behavior, and madness which will develop into mania.[114]

(In the case of an abnormality in the channels of) the second yin and the first yang, the illness arises out of the kidney. In this case, the yin qi intrusively visits the heart, the cavities in the venter and below are blocked as if by dams, and the four limbs seem as if separated from the trunk.[115]

(In the case of an abnormality in the channels of) the first yin and the first yang, if the pulse appears interrupted and expiring, this indicates that the yin qi has invaded the heart. In this case, the disorder settles in no constant place, possibly above, possibly below, with the manifestations of inability to taste food, incessant diarrhea, and dry throat. The illness lies in the earth spleen.[116]

(In the case of an abnormality in the channels of) the second yang, the third yin and the consummate yin,[117] yin cannot approach the yang, while yang fails to inhibit yin, resulting in expiry of both yin and yang. If the pulse is floating, this indicates blood conglomeration; if it is deep, this indicates purulent decay.[118]

The coming of the third yang alone means the coming of the third yang (of the hand and foot) together.[119] The conspiracy assails (as drastically as) the storm, causing diseases of the head above and leakage below. The third yang is the consummate yang. When (the evil qi in) it builds up, it gives rise to fright, and the resultant disorder breaks out vehemently like roaring wind and thunder with all the nine portals blocked, the yang qi overflooding, and throat dry and congested. If it encroaches on yin, it causes erratic problems, settling in no fixed place, possibly above, possibly below. If it descends, there will be intestinal *pi*. If the third yang threatens the heart directly, there will be generalized heaviness with inability either to rise or to lie down and forced sitting posture. This is what is called the third yang disease.

(2)

The Yellow Emperor asked:

What causes variations of the pulses according to the four seasons?

Qi Bo answered:

Within the six directions,[120] all the changes in heaven and on earth find their reflection in yin and yang, for example the warmth in spring, the hot in summer, the wrath in autumn, and the fury in winter.[121] The pulse fluctuates in response to the changes in the four seasons. It is expected to respond like the compass[122] in spring, the square[123] in summer, the arm of a steelyard[124] in autumn, and the weight of a steelyard[125] in winter. Forty-five days after the Winter Solstice, yang qi begins to rise slightly, while yin qi begins to decline slightly. Forty-five days after the Summer Solstice, yin qi begins to rise slightly, while yang qi begins to decline slightly. The vicissitudes of yin and yang are regular, and the pulse changes are in agreement with these. If they do not agree, this reveals (the influence of) the (involved) part.[126] Since the part is known to be associated with a certain period (of the year), it is made possible to predict the date of death. Pulse examination is a subtle and delicate technique which entails painstaking study, and one should keep to the established criteria whose basis lies in yin and yang. Sound is analyzed in terms of the five notes, color in terms of the five phases, and the pulse in terms of yin and yang. According to the *dao* of pulse palpation, an empty mind and tranquil (spirit) are treasured (above all else).

In spring, the pulse is floating like a fish swimming on ripples. In summer, it beats in the skin like a flood or the fluorescence of living things. In autumn, it beats under the skin like insects bur-

rowing to lie dormant. And in winter, it lies against the bone like hibernating insects hidden in safety or gentlemen staying in their chambers. Knowledge of the internal (*i.e.*, viscera and bowels) enables one to locate (a disease) through pulse examination; knowledge of the exterior enables one to determine the origination and the termination (of the channel qi). The six (topics discussed above) are the essentials[127] of grasping the pulse.

(3)

A red complexion accompanied by a hard, forcefully pounding pulse implies a diagnosis of accumulated qi in the center often affecting the appetite. This is called heart *bi*. It results from an external condition. Preoccupation generates heart vacuity and, thus, the (external) evil is allowed to cause a problem.

A white complexion accompanied by a floating, forcefully pounding pulse indicates vacuity above and repletion below with symptoms of susceptibility to fright, accumulated qi in the chest, dyspnea, and weakness. This is collectively known as lung *bi* with chills and fever. This results from sexual intercourse while intoxicated.

A yellow complexion accompanied by a large, vacuous pulse indicates accumulated qi in the abdomen and inversion qi which is known as inversion *shan*. The same disease may occur in females. It results from being caught in a draft with sweat on the four limbs.[128]

A green-blue complexion accompanied by a long pulse flicking on both sides of the vessel indicates propping of the lateral costal region due to accumulated qi below the heart. This is known as liver *bi*. Like *shan*, it results from cold dampness. It is characterized by lumbar pain, cold feet, and headache ["tense vessels in the head" in a variant version. {later editor}]

A black complexion accompanied by a hard and large pulse indicates accumulated qi in the lower abdomen and the yin organs. This is known as kidney *bi*. It results from bathing in cool water and laying (down to sleep) while still wet.

(4)

A surplus of form qi (*xing qi,* 形氣)[129] and an insufficiency of vessel qi results in death. A surplus of vessel qi and an insufficiency of form qi portends survival. An equilibrium between form and qi[130] makes successful treatment possible. A weak yet slippery pulse demonstrates the presence of the stomach qi and the condition is said to be easily cured but calls for immediate treatment. This opportunity must not be allowed to pass. In the case of an imbalance between form and qi, the condition is said to be difficult to cure. A perished, sheenless complexion indicates an illness which is difficult to recover from. If the pulse is replete and hard, the condition is said to be intensifying. If the pulse is not in congruity with the seasons, the condition is said to be incurable. Incongruity of the pulse with the four seasons means that the lung pulse appears in spring, the kidney pulse appears in summer, the heart pulse appears in autumn, and the spleen pulse appears in winter and that they loom suspended and expiring, deep, and choppy.

Despite an absence of visceral form,[131] in the spring and summer the pulse may be deep and choppy. In the autumn and winter, the pulse may be floating and large. A heat disease may have a tranquil pulse. A case of diarrhea may be accompanied by a large pulse. Blood desertion may be accompanied by a replete pulse. An illness in the center may be accompanied by a hard, replete pulse. And an illness located in the exterior may be accompanied by a pulse which is not replete and hard. All these conditions suggest that the problem is difficult to treat. This is called incongruity with the four seasons (*ni si shi,* 逆四时).

(5)

The Yellow Emperor asked:

Please tell me the essentials of vacuity and repletion.

Qi Bo answered:

If the form appears replete when qi is replete or the form appears vacuous when qi is vacuous, this then is the normal state. The converse suggests disease. If grain is exuberant and the qi is exuberant[132] or, if grain is vacuous and the qi is vacuous, this is normal. The converse suggests disease. If the pulses are replete, the blood is replete and, if the vessels are vacuous, the blood is vacuous, this is normal. The converse suggests disease. When the qi is exuberant and the body is cold, or when the qi is vacuous and the body is hot, this is said to be aberrant (*fan,* 烦). When much grain is ingested and yet the qi is meager, this is said to be aberrant. When little grain is ingested and yet the qi is abundant, this too is said to be aberrant. When the pulse is exuberant and the blood is scant, this is said to be aberrant; yet when the pulse is small but the blood is abundant, this too is said to be aberrant. If the qi is exuberant and the body is cold, this is due to cold damage. If there is a vacuity of qi and the body is hot, this results from summer heat damage. Meager qi despite having ingested much grain results from blood desertion with dampness lodging in the lower of the body. Abundant qi despite having ingested little grain is due to evil in the stomach and the lung.[133] An abundance of blood with a small pulse is due to the drinking of center-heating liquid,[134] while meager blood with a large pulse is due to wind qi in the vessels and that it is impossible to take in liquid. All the above are (manifestations of) aberrations (in the state of the qi).

Now repletion is due to an invasion of (evil) qi, while vacuity is due to the departure of (the correct) qi.[135] Qi repletion is manifested by heat, while qi vacuity by cold. In treating repletion, the needle hole should be left open with the left hand (immediately after withdrawing the needle), whereas, in treating vacuity, the needle hole should be closed with the left hand (immediately after having extracted the needle).

(6)

A small pulse which is not accompanied by an ill complexion indicates a new disease. A pulse which is not ill but which is accompanied by an ill complexion indicates a chronic disease. If both the pulse and the complexion are ill, this too indicates a chronic disease, while if neither the pulse nor the complexion is ill this indicates a new disease. If the liver and the kidney pulses appear together accompanied by a somber red complexion, this is due to an impact injury and (swelling). Whether there is bleeding or not, (the condition) appears like dampness (illness) or water stroke.[136]

The inner (ulnar) aspect of the cubit region on both the arms reflects the lateral costal region, the outer (radial) aspect, the kidney, and the middle part represents the abdomen. Of the middle section of the cubit region on the left arm, the outer (radial) side represents the liver and the inner (ulnar) side, the diaphragm; on the right arm, the outer (radial) side represents the stomach and the inner (ulnar) side, the spleen. Of the upper section of the cubit region on the right arm, the outer (radial) side represents the lung and the inner (ulnar) side, the chest. On the left arm, the radial side represents the heart and the ulnar side, the center of the chest. The anterior aspect represents the anterior (of the body), while the posterior aspect, the posterior. The upper part represents the upper (part of the body), i.e., problems related to the chest, the throat, etc., while the lower part represents the lower,[137] i.e., problems related to the lower abdomen, the lumbus, the thigh, the knee, and the lower leg, etc. Coarse (skin) indicates an insufficiency of yin with superabundant yang, a syndrome called heat in the center.

(7)

Abdominal distention and generalized fever with a large ["small" in a variant version {later editor}] pulse is the first crisis (ni, 逆). Rumbling and fullness in the abdomen, cold limbs and diarrhea with a large pulse is the second crisis. Incessant bleeding with a large pulse is the third crisis. Urination of blood and desertion of the form with a small, forceful pulse is the fourth crisis. And coughing, desertion of the form and generalized fever with a small, racing pulse is the fifth crisis. If the above ever occur, death results in no more than fifteen days.

Enormous distention of the abdomen, cold extremities, emaciation, and severe diarrhea is the first crisis. Abdominal distention and hemafecia with a large and frequently interrupted pulse is the second crisis. Cough, urination of blood, and shedding of the formal flesh with a forcefully pounding pulse is the third crisis. Retching of blood and fullness of the chest affecting the back with a small, racing pulse is the fourth crisis. Cough, retching, abdominal distention, and swill diarrhea with pulse expiry is the fifth crisis. If the above ever occur, death results in one day.

If a practitioner is ignorant of these (patterns and blindly) proceeds with needling, this is said to be a contrary therapy (ni zhi, 逆治).

(8)

A heat condition accompanied by a tranquil pulse and an exuberant agitated pulse subsequent to diaphoresis is the first crisis. A case of diarrhea accompanied by a large, surging pulse is the second crisis. A case of fixed bi with cleavage of the major muscle masses and generalized fever and pulse expiry occurring on one side of the body is the third crisis. Licentiousness causing a whittling away of the form with generalized fever, a perished white complexion, or a severe case of defecation of clotted blood is the fourth crisis. And fever and chills causing a desertion of the form with a hard forceful pulse is the fifth crisis.[138]

(9)

The five repletions mean death, as do the five vacuities. An exuberant pulse, hot skin, abdominal distention, inability to urinate or defecate, and oppression with distorted vision are what are known as the five repletions. A fine pulse, cold skin, diminished qi, incontinence of urination and defecation, and inability to ingest food are what are called the five vacuities. If the diarrhea can be stopped by ingesting thin porridge into the stomach, the vacuity patient will survive. If (defecation is) disinhibited following diaphoresis, the repletion patient will survive. These are the indications (of the five repletions and the five vacuities).

(10)

A heart pulse which is full and large indicates epilepsy, clonic spasms, and hypertonicity of the sinews.

A liver pulse which is small and urgent indicates epilepsy, clonic spasms, and hypertonicity of the sinews.

A liver pulse which is deranged and fulminant indicates experience of fright and scare. However, even (if the condition is severe) and the pulse fails to appear or there is inability to speak, the illness can heal by itself.[139]

A kidney pulse which is small and urgent, a liver pulse which is small and urgent, or a heart pulse which is small and urgent indicate conglomeration if they do not beat forcefully.[140]

A kidney pulse which is large, urgent, and deep or a liver pulse which is large, urgent, and deep indicate *shan*.

If the liver and kidney pulses are both deep, stone water is indicated, while if they are both floating, wind water is indicated.[141] If they are both vacuous, death ensues, while if they are both small and bowstring, a susceptibility to fright will develop.

If the heart pulse pounds forcefully and is slippery and urgent, heart *shan* is indicated.

A lung pulse which is deep-lying and pounds forcefully indicates lung *shan*.

If the third yang[142] is urgent, conglomeration is indicated.

If the third yin[142] is urgent, *shan* is indicated.

If the second yin[142] is urgent, epilepsy and inversion are indicated. [*Shan* is indicated in a variant version. {later editor}]

If the second yang[143] is urgent, experience of fright may be indicated.

A spleen pulse which is deep but beats energetically indicates intestinal *pi* which will eventually heal on its own.

A liver pulse which is small and slow indicates intestinal *pi* which is easy to cure.

A kidney pulse which is small and deep and pounds forcefully indicates intestinal *pi* with defecation of blood. When warm blood and generalized fever develop, this leads to death.[144] Both heart and liver *pi* are characterized by defecation of blood. If the heart and the liver are both affected by the same illness, it is curable. A pulse which is small, deep, and choppy (in the heart and liver positions) indicates intestinal *pi*, and, when generalized fever occurs, death ensues. Severe fever [occurrence of fever in the *Su Wen* {later editor}] results in death in seven days.

If the stomach pulse is forceful and choppy when pressed deeply, if the stomach pulse is forceful and large when pressed lightly, or if the heart pulse is small, hard, and urgent, then there is obstruction (of qi and blood) resulting in hemilateral withering. If it occurs on the left side in males or the right side in females and the ability to speak and to move the tongue is preserved, then the condition is curable and recovery will be effected in thirty days. If it happens in the conformable side[145] with loss of voice, recovery will be effected in three years. If the victim is under twenty, death will occur in three years.[146]

If the pulse arrives forcefully and there is epistaxis and generalized fever, then death will occur.

If the pulse appears suspended, hook-like,[147] and floating, there is heat. [The *Su Wen* regards this as the normal pulse. {later editor}] If the pulse arrives forcefully, this is called sudden inversion (*bao jue*), and, in the case of sudden inversion, speech is beyond the patient.

If the pulse arrives rapidly, experience of violent fright is indicated, and (the patient) will recover in three or four days without treatment. If the pulse arrives superficially as overlapping waves and is as rapid as ten beats for a single breath, the channel qi is insufficient. Death comes ninety days after the first appearance of the pulse.

If the pulse arrives racing as the flaming of a woodfire, the heart essence is retrenched, and death comes with the drying of grass.[148]

If the pulse arrives like a bramble [the *Su Wen* says "like dispersed leaves" {later editor}], there is a vacuity of liver qi, and death comes with the falling of leaves from the tree.[149]

If the pulse arrives as a guest visiting a house, the house guest is likened to an obstructed vessel, beating off and on. In this case, the kidney qi is insufficient, and death comes with the blossoming and withering of the jujube flowers.[150]

If the pulse arrives like clay pellets, the stomach essence is insufficient, and death comes with the falling of the elm seeds.[151]

If the pulse arrives like the transverse branch of a tree, the gallbladder qi is insufficient, and death comes with the ripening of crops.[152]

If the pulse arrives like a tightened bowstring, the uterine essence is insufficient. If the patient is talkative, death comes with the coming of frost;[153] if the patient is not talkative, the disease is curable.[154]

If the pulse arrives like entangled brambles [the *Su Wen* says "like lacquer oil being filtered" {later editor}], these entangled brambles depict a pulse which beats here and there (in an indistinct way). Death will come thirty days after the first appearance of this pulse.

If the pulse arrives like bubbles, beating at the floating level of the vessel, the qi of the *tai yang* is insufficient with lack of flavor, and death comes with the budding of the leek flower.[155]

If the pulse arrives like decayed soil, (meaning) it is difficult to feel at a deep level, the muscular qi

is insufficient, and, if there is black complexion, death comes with the budding of the fleabane.[156]

If the pulse arrives as if suspended and detached, this suspended detachment depicts a pulse which is forceful when pressed lightly and is even larger and more forceful when pressed more deeply. In this case, the qi in the twelve associated points is insufficient, and death comes with the freezing of water.[157]

If the pulse arrives like a knife resting on its spine, this knife depicts a pulse as floatingly small and urgent, and harder and larger upon pressure. In this case, there is cold and heat ["stale, decayed things" in the *Su Wen* {later editor}] in the five viscera. If the cold and heat concentrate solely within the kidney, the patient is unable to sit up and he will die on the Beginning of Spring.[158]

If the pulse arrives like a small, slippery pill, [the *Su Wen* adds that "it is difficult to get a fix on"], this slippery pill reflects difficulty in feeling the pulse. In this case, the qi of the large intestine is insufficient, and death comes with the sprouting of the jujube leaves.[159]

If the pulse arrives like a pestle husking rice, the patient is susceptible to fright, reluctant to sit or sleep, but fond of standing all his ears, this implies an insufficiency of small intestine qi. In this case, death occurs in the last month of autumn.[160]

Chapter Two

Pathological Manifestation & Pulse Diagnosis (Part 1)[161]

(1)

The Yellow Emperor asked:

In what ways does evil qi strike the human body? Is there a rule concerning whether it strikes high or low?

Qi Bo answered:

The upper half of the body is subject to stroke by evil;[162] the lower half of the body, to stroke by dampness. When it strikes the yin, (evil qi) lodges in the bowels, and, when it strikes the yang, it lodges in the channels.[163]

The Yellow Emperor asked:

(Although the channels are distinguished) as either yin or yang with different names, they are of a kind. Meeting in the upper and the lower parts of the body, they connect with one another to form a ring-like circuit without an end. Now, evil may strike a person (anywhere). It may strike the yin or the yang, above or below, left or right. What accounts (for the behavior of this evil)?

Qi Bo answered:

All of the yang channels meet in the face. When a person's (channels) are in a state of vacuity, when one has recently exerted oneself, or when one has consumed hot beverage and food such that they have perspired and their interstices are open, then evil qi may strike the body. If it happens to strike the face, it descends along the *yang ming*. If it happens to strike the nape, it descends along the *tai yang*. If it happens to strike the cheek, it descends along the *shao yang*. If it happens to strike the breast, the back, or the lateral costal regions, it strikes the related channel. When it strikes the yin aspect, it typically starts in the forearm and the lower leg. The skin on the yin aspect of the forearm and lower leg is thin. Therefore, although both (the yang and yin aspects) are exposed to an attack of wind, the yin aspect alone is damaged.

The Yellow Emperor asked:

Does it then damage the (corresponding) viscus?

Qi Bo answered:

Once wind invades the body, it does not necessarily move to the viscus. The evil may enter the yin channels. If the visceral qi is replenished, the evil qi cannot enter and settle there and so it may rebound into the bowels. Because of this, only once (the evil qi) has struck the yang aspect may it become lodged in the channels, and only once it has struck the yin aspect may it become lodged in the bowels.

The Yellow Emperor asked:

On what occasions is evil capable of striking the viscera?

Qi Bo answered:

Fear and worry injure the heart. A cold body and cold drinks injure the lung. Because these two cold factors combine to influence the condition, both the interior and the exterior are damaged, causing the qi to counterflow and run upwards. If, in the case of a fall, foul blood becomes lodged in the interior or, in the case of violent fury, the qi ascends but cannot descend, then there will be an accumulation of (qi) in the lateral costal region, causing damage to the liver. Wounds inflicted in knocks and falls, sexual intercourse while intoxicated, or being caught in a draft while sweating damage the spleen. Strain inflicted in lifting weights, or overindulgence in sexual intercourse, or bathing while perspiring damages the kidney.

The Yellow Emperor asked:

What happens if wind strikes the five viscera?

Qi Bo answered:

Only when both yin and yang are affected can evil invade the viscus. From all the twelve channels with their three hundred and sixty-five points, the qi and blood ascend to the face and travel to the hollow portals. The essential yang qi ascends to the eyes and provides sight; the deviated qi[164] arrives in the ears and provides hearing; the ancestral qi emerges at the nose and provides the sense of smell; and the turbid qi emerges from the stomach below and then travels to the lips and tongue to provide them with the sense of taste. Because all the fluid and humor from qi rises to fume the face and because (the face) has thick skin and strong flesh, no matter how strong the heat or intense the cold, it cannot be affected.

When a vacuity evil[165] strikes the body, it produces (cold) shivering which shakes the body. When a regular evil[166] (*zheng xie*, 正邪) strikes the body, it causes but slight disorder. It may be seen first in the complexion but will not be expressed in the body where its presence is hardly perceivable, hardly tangible, hardly noticeable, and unobservable.

Complexion, pulse, and cubit skin correspond with one another and respond to one another without fail as does sound to the beating of a drum or shadow to form. These are the indications of the root and terminations, the root and leaf. When the root is dead, the leaves wither.[167]

So it follows then that a green-blue complexion will be accompanied by a wiry pulse; a red complexion by a hook-like pulse; a yellow complexion by an interrupted pulse; a white complexion by a hair pulse; and a black complexion by a stone-like pulse. If one observes a certain complexion and it is not accompanied by its (corresponding) pulse but rather by the pulse of its restraining phase, then this portends death. If (the complexion) is accompanied by the pulse of its engendering phase, this portends recovery.

The Yellow Emperor asked:

In what way can the various transformations of disease within the five viscera be determined?

Qi Bo answered:

First, the correspondences between the five complexions and the five pulses are established, and then disease can be differentiated.

The Yellow Emperor asked:

Having established the correspondences between the complexions and the pulses, how is (disease) then differentiated?

Qi Bo answered:

By ascertaining the slowness, urgency, largeness, smallness, slipperiness, and choppiness of the pulse, the nature of the disease may be established.

The Yellow Emperor asked:

How then are these characteristics (of the pulse) ascertained?

Qi Bo answered:

The pulse is urgent if the cubit skin is tense. The pulse is slow if the cubit skin is loose. The pulse is small if the cubit skin is thin with little qi. The pulse is large if the cubit skin is imposing. The pulse is deep if the cubit skin is sunken. The pulse is slippery if the cubit skin is slippery. The pulse is choppy if the cubit skin is rough. These variations (of the pulse and the cubit skin) may be either subtle or obvious. One who is skilled in examination of the cubit skin need not examine the pulse, while one skilled at examination of the pulse need not examine the complexion. Those who can synthesize (the above three modes) of examination are superior practitioners who will achieve nine successes in ten. Those who can execute two modes of examination are mediocre practitioners who will achieve seven successes in ten. And those who can execute one mode of examination are inferior practitioners who will achieve six successes in ten.

(2)

Cubit skin which is moist and brilliant ["slippery" in a variant version {later editor}], indicates wind. Weak cubit flesh[168] reflects listlessness and fatigue. Somnolence and shedding of flesh reflect fever and chills. [In a variant version here is added "which is incurable". {later editor}] Cubit skin which is rough indicates wind *bi*. Cubit skin which is as coarse as dry fish scales indicates water spillage rheum.

If the cubit skin is very cold and the pulse is small, diarrhea and diminished qi are indicated.

If the cubit skin is very hot and the pulse is exuberant and agitated, warm disease is indicated. If the pulse is exuberant and slippery, there will soon be perspiration ["the disease will be subdued" in a variant version. {later editor}] If the cubit skin and the hand feels as if it has been burned ["blazingly hot" in a variant version {later editor}] and there is fever followed by chills, this is called (alternating) cold and heat. If the cubit skin is first felt to be cold but upon prolonged contact feels hot, cold and heat are indicated as well. If the cubit skin is burning hot ["blazingly hot" in a variant version {later editor}] and the *ren ying* pulse is large, loss of blood is indicated. If the cubit skin is hard and imposing but the pulse is small, diminished qi is indicated, and, when vexation increases, death ensues [the *Mai Jing (Pulse Classic)* says that there is diminished qi if the cubit is more tense than the *ren ying*. {later editor}][169]

If only the elbow region is hot, heat above the waist is indicated. If only the region behind the elbow is hot, heat is indicated in the shoulder and the back. If only the region anterior to the elbow is hot, heat is indicated in the breast. If the region three or four *cun* below the back of the elbow is hot, worms in the intestines are indicated. If only the hands are hot, heat below the waist is indicated. If only the middle region of the forearm is hot, heat in the lumbus and the abdomen is indicated. If there is heat in the palms, heat in the abdomen is indicated. If there is cold in the palms, cold in the abdomen is indicated. And if green-blue veins are found in the white flesh of the fish's margin, cold in the stomach is indicated.

(3)

The Yellow Emperor asked:

What sort of disease is characterized by a very loose cubit skin region ["very loose and thin" in a variant version {later editor}] and yet tense sinews?

Qi Bo answered:

This is what is called papule sinews (*zhen jin*, 疹筋).[170] In the case of papule sinews, (the sinews) of the abdomen must be tense, and, if this is accompanied by a white or black complexion, the illness is very serious.

Chapter Two

Pathological Manifestation & Pulse Diagnosis (Part 2)[171]

The Yellow Emperor asked:

What kinds of disease do a slack, urgent, large, small, slippery, or choppy pulse each suggest?

Qi Bo answered:

An extremely urgent heart pulse suggests tugging and slackening, while a slightly urgent heart pulse suggests heart pain affecting the back with difficult ingestion.[172]

An extremely slack heart pulse suggests manic laughing, while a slightly slack heart pulse suggests deep-lying beam located vertically below the heart in addition to intermittent spitting of blood.[173]

An extremely large heart pulse suggests rales in the throat, while a slightly large heart pulse suggests heart *bi* affecting the back with frequent lacrimation.[174]

An extremely small heart pulse suggests frequent retching, while a slightly small heart pulse suggests pure heat wasting thirst.[175]

An extremely slippery heart pulse suggests constant thirst, while a slightly slippery heart pulse suggests heart *shan* affecting the umbilicus in addition to rumbling in the lower abdomen.[176]

An extremely choppy heart pulse suggests a loss of voice, while a slightly choppy heart pulse suggests blood spillage[177] and linking inversion, [the channels and connecting vessel referred to here are the yang linking and yin linking vessels {later editor}][178] ringing in the ear, and madness.[179]

An extremely urgent lung pulse suggests madness, while a slightly urgent lung pulse suggests cold and heat in the lung, fatigue and lassitude, spitting and coughing of blood affecting the lumbus, back, and chest, and, in some cases, nasal polyps with nasal congestion.[180]

An extremely slack lung pulse suggests frequent sweating, while a slightly slack lung pulse suggests atony and wind leakage[181] with incessant sweating below the head.[182]

An extremely large lung pulse suggests swelling of the lower leg, while a slightly large lung pulse suggests lung *bi* affecting the chest and back in addition to an aversion to sunlight.[183]

An extremely small lung pulse suggests diarrhea, while a slightly small lung pulse suggests pure heat wasting thirst.[184]

An extremely slippery lung pulse suggests inverted cup surging with an ascension of qi, while a slightly slippery lung pulse suggests bleeding in both the upper and lower parts of the body.[185]

An extremely choppy lung pulse suggests vomiting of blood, while a slightly choppy lung pulse suggests fistulae located in the neck and the axilla and a fondness of eating great quantities of things sour because the upper is unable to resist the lower.[186]

An extremely urgent liver pulse suggests offensive speech ["delirium" in a variant version {later editor}], while the slightly urgent liver pulse suggests fat qi[187] which lies, like a cup upside down, in the lateral costal region.[188]

An extremely slack liver pulse suggests frequent retching, while a slightly slack liver pulse suggests water conglomeration-blockage.[189]

An extremely large liver pulse suggests internal *yong* and frequent retching and bleeding, while a slightly large liver pulse suggests liver *bi*, genital retraction, and cough affecting the lower abdomen.[190]

An extremely small liver pulse suggests much drinking, while a slightly small liver pulse suggests pure heat wasting thirst.[191]

An extremely slippery liver pulse suggests *tui shan*, while a slightly slippery liver pulse suggests enuresis.[192]

An extremely choppy liver pulse suggests spillage rheum, while a slightly choppy liver pulse suggests tugging and slackening with hypertonicity of sinews.[193]

An extremely urgent spleen pulse suggests tugging and slackening, while a slightly urgent spleen pulse suggests diaphragmatic blockage characterized by ejection of food on ingestion and stools which are foamy.[194]

An extremely slack spleen pulse suggests atonic inversion, while a slightly slack spleen pulse suggests wind atony characterized by loss of use of the four limbs but a clear mind as if one were not ill.[195]

An extremely large spleen pulse suggests sudden loss of consciousness, while a slightly large spleen pulse suggests *shan* qi characterized by a big mass of pus and blood wrapped outside the stomach and intestines.[196]

An extremely small spleen pulse suggests cold and heat, while a slightly small spleen pulse suggests pure heat wasting thirst.[197]

An extremely slippery spleen pulse suggests *kui long*,[198] while a slightly slippery spleen pulse suggests roundworm toxins and hotness in the abdomen caused by tapeworms and pinworms.[199]

An extremely choppy spleen pulse suggests intestinal *tui* ["rectal festering" in a variant version {later editor}], while a slightly choppy spleen pulse suggests internal ulceration with frequent defecation of pus and blood.[200]

An extremely urgent kidney pulse suggests bone atony and madness, while a slightly urgent kidney pulse suggests running piglet and deep inversion[201] with loss of use of the feet and inability to urinate or defecate.[202]

An extremely slack kidney pulse suggests a spine (which is so painful it feels as if it were) fit to break, while a slightly slack kidney pulse suggests throughflux diarrhea. In the case of throughflux diarrhea, an inability to transform food occurs and so food is spit back up upon ingestion.[203]

An extremely large kidney pulse suggests impotence, while a slightly large kidney pulse suggests stone water. This is characterized by distending weight from the umbilicus down into the lower abdomen and extending up to the venter. It is fatal and cannot be cured.[204]

An extremely small kidney pulse suggests throughflux diarrhea, while a slightly small kidney pulse suggests pure heat wasting thirst.[205]

An extremely slippery kidney pulse suggests *kui long*, while a slightly slippery kidney pulse suggests bone atony characterized by an inability to get up when seated and blurred, dark dotted vision on attempting to rise.[206]

An extremely choppy kidney pulse suggests grand *yong*, while a slightly choppy kidney pulse suggests amenorrhea and persistent hemorrhoids.[207]

The Yellow Emperor asked:

What do the six types of pathologic (pulse) signify for acupuncture?

Qi Bo answered:

Any urgent (pulse) indicates much cold. Any slack (pulse) indicates much heat. Any large (pulse) indicates much qi with meager blood. Any small (pulse) indicates meager qi and meager blood. Any slippery pulse indicates exuberant yang qi with slight heat. Any choppy (pulse) indicates much blood but meager qi with slight cold. Accordingly, when needling in the case of an urgent (pulse, the needle) should be inserted deeply and retained for an extended period. When needling in the case of a slack (pulse, the needle) should be inserted shallowly and extracted quickly in order to dispel heat. When needling in the case of a large pulse, one should drain the qi slightly without causing blood to be let out. When needling in the case of a slippery pulse, the needle should be extracted quickly and inserted shallowly to drain yang qi and dispel heat. And when needling in the case of a choppy pulse, the needle should be aimed at the channel and retained long depending upon the favorable and unfavorable factors.[208]

(In the case of a choppy pulse, the points) should be massaged prior to insertion of the needle, and, after withdrawal, the holes should be pressed immediately to avoid bleeding so as to harmonize the channel. In the case of a small (pulse), since there is an insufficiency of yin and yang, form and qi, acupuncture is not indicated. Rather one should administer sweet medicinals in order to regulate (and harmonize the spleen and stomach qi).

The Yellow Emperor asked:

(It is my understanding that) the qi of the five viscera and six bowels submerges via the transporting points at the confluence points.[209] But what is the pathway for this submergence and what path does it follow once the qi has submerged?

Qi Bo answered:

(The qi submerges via) the network vessels of the yang channels (rather than the confluence points), and, after their submergence, they home to the bowels.

The Yellow Emperor asked:

Do the transporting points differ from the confluence points[210] in function?

Qi Bo answered:

The brook points cure the external channels, while the confluence points cure the internal bowels.

The Yellow Emperor asked:

How does one treat the internal bowels?

Qi Bo answered:

Select the confluence point.

The Yellow Emperor asked:

What are the names (of these confluence points)?

Qi Bo answered:

The confluence of the stomach is Three Li (*San Li*, St 36). That of the large intestine is the Upper Ridge of the Great Hollow (*Ju Xu Shang*, St 37). That of the small intestine is the Lower Ridge of the Great Hollow (*Ju Xu Xia*, St 39). That of the triple heater is Bend Yang (*Wei Yang*, Bl 39). That of the urinary bladder is Bend Middle (*Wei Zhong*, Bl 40). And that of the gallbladder is Yang Mound Spring (*Yang Ling Quan*, GB 34). [It is known that the confluence point of the large intestine is Pool at the Bend {*Qu Chi*, LI 11}; that of the small intestine is Lesser Sea {*Xiao Hai*, SI 8}; and that of the triple heater is Celestial Well {*Tian Jing*, TH 10}.[210] But now different affiliations are brought up. This is a treatment of older times. Another problem: It is also known that the Upper and the Lower Ridges of the Great Hollow[211] are classified as the uniting points of the foot *yang ming* with the large and small intestines. This is a different approach from that in which the stomach is said to have Three Li, the urinary bladder to have Bend Middle, and the gallbladder to have Yang Mound Spring as their confluence points. This latter approach regards the submerging places of the channels as the confluence points. Besides, here the triple heater is said to have Bend Yang as its confluence point. But Bend Yang is the lower assisting point of the triple heater, and nowhere else is it ascribed to the triple burner as its confluence point. {later editor}][212]

The Yellow Emperor asked:

How are (the confluence points) located?

Qi Bo answered:

To locate Three Li, lower the instep. For Great Hollow, lift the foot to locate it. For Bend Yang, bend (the leg halfway) to locate it. For Bend Middle, bend the knee to locate it. For Yang Mound Spring, straighten the leg while in a sitting position and behind this is Yang Mound Spring. Prior to treating the external channels, (the limbs) should be stretched.[213]

The Yellow Emperor asked:

Please tell me about (the indications) of diseases involving the six bowels.

Qi Bo answered:

Heat in the face indicates a foot *yang ming* disease. A blood connecting vessel found in the fish's margin indicates hand *yang ming* disease. If the vessels in the insteps are hard or sunken, this indicates foot *yang ming* disease since they are vessels of the stomach.

Chapter Three

Three Positions with Nine Indicators[214]

The Yellow Emperor asked:

What are the so-called three positions?

Qi Bo answered:

They are the upper position, the middle position, and the lower position. In each position, there are three indicators. These three indicators are the heaven, the earth, and the human.

The heaven of the upper position is the pulsating vessel on both temples.[215] The earth of the upper position is the pulsating vessel on both cheeks.[216] The human of the upper position is the pulsating vessel anterior to the auricles.[217]

The heaven of the middle position is the hand *tai yin*.[218] The earth of the middle position is the hand *yang ming*.[219] The human of the middle position is the hand *shao yin*.[220]

The heaven of the lower position is the foot *jue yin*.[221] The earth of the lower position is the foot *shao yin*.[222] The human of the lower position is the foot *tai yin*.[223]

In the lower position, heaven is reflected in the liver, earth is reflected in the kidney, and humanity is reflected in qi of the spleen and stomach.

In the middle position, heaven is reflected in the lung, the earth in the qi of the chest, and the human in the heart.

In the upper position, heaven is reflected in the qi of the corners of the head, the earth in the qi of the mouth and teeth, and the human in the qi of the ears and eyes.

The three positions contain three heavens, three earths and three humans, and, therefore, there are three times three or nine indicators in all. These nine indicators correspond with nine regions of the body which, in turn, correspond with the nine viscera. There are five spiritual viscera and four formal viscera which combine to form the nine viscera.[224] If the five viscera are overwhelmed, the complexion will appear perished, and such a perished complexion means death.

The Yellow Emperor asked:

How is (physical) examination carried out?

Qi Bo answered:

One must first evaluate the fatness or thinness of the form before vacuity and repletion can be regulated. If there is repletion, then it should be drained, and if there is vacuity, it should be supplemented. One should first remove any blood network vessels, and then one may administer regulating therapy. Whatever the nature of the disease, efforts should be directed to achieving the balance (between yin and yang).[225]

The Yellow Emperor asked:

What determines life or death?

Qi Bo answered;

A robust body with a fine pulse and diminished qi such that it is not enough to allow one to catch one's breath portends death. An emaciated body with a large pulse and abundant qi[226] in the chest portends death. Congruity between (bodily) configuration and qi portends life. Irregularities[227] are indicative of disease. If the nine indicators in the three positions are not in accord, this portends death. If the pulses above and below,[228] on the right and the left, all pound like pestles, this indicates that the problem is critical. If the pulses above and below, on the right and the left are not in accord and cannot be counted, this portends death. Although the indicators in the middle position alone present themselves normally, if they are out of sync with their corresponding viscera, this portends death. If the indicators in the middle position are diminished, this portends death. If the eyes are sunken, this portends death.[229]

The Yellow Emperor asked:

How can one know where a disease lies?

Qi Bo answered:

Of the nine indicators, if only one is small there is disease. If only one is large, there is disease. If only one is rapid, there is disease. If only one is slow, there is disease. If only one is hot there is disease.[230] If only one is cold, there is disease. And if only one is sunken, there is disease.

Holding the part five *cun* above the malleolus with the left hand, strike the malleolus with the right hand. If a sensation of worms wriggling is perceived more than five *cun* above the malleolus, then there is no disease. If the percussion conducts rapidly and is perceived as being unclear, there is disease. If the percussion is slow in coming to the left hand, there is disease. If the percussion can be perceived only at a distance of less than five *cun* or if no percussion can be perceived at all, this portends death.

Loss of flesh with a lack of mobility portends death.

When the pulses in the middle position beat at varying paces, this portends death. If the pulse is irregular and hook-like,[231] the disease lies in the network vessels.

The nine indicators should correspond with one another. They should behave as one (in pace and size) and should not be out of synchronization. If one is out of line with others, there is disease. If two are out of line, the disease is serious. If three are out of line, the disease is critical. What is referred to as being out of line directly implies disharmony. Further examination of the viscera allows one to know the course of death and life.

One must first have a knowledge of (the normal) channel pulses, and then one may have an understanding of diseased pulses. Once the true visceral pulse appears, the evil is overwhelming, and this portends death. If the qi of the foot *tai yang* expires, the feet are bereft of the ability to bend and stretch, and death comes with the upturning of the eyes.

The Yellow Emperor asked:

What do winter yin and summer yang signify?

Qi Bo answered:

If all pulses of the nine indicators are deep, fine, and expiring, this implies a yin (disease) which is associated with winter. In this case, death comes at midnight.[232] If all of them are exuberant, agitated, pounding, and rapid, this implies a yang (disease) which is associated with summer. In this case, death comes at midday.[232] In the case of cold and heat illness, death comes at the calm dawn watch.[232] In the case of heat stroke and heat disease, death comes at midday. In the case of wind disease, death comes at the sundown watch.[232] In the case of water disease, death comes at midnight. If the pulse beats at a variable rhythm and

pace, death comes at the watches of the day corresponding to the four seasons.[232] If the muscles of the body are shed, although the nine indicators may be normal, this situation still portends death. However, even though the seven signs[233] are evident, if the nine indicators are in congruence (with the four seasons), the illness may not be fatal. The reason why this condition may not be fatal is that the problem may be a wind qi disease or a gynecological (disorder) (*jing yue*, 经月).[234] These may appear to be characterized by the seven signs but, in fact, are not. Therefore, it is safe to say death will not occur. A disease with the seven signs in conjunction with a breakdown of the pulse portends death which will surely be accompanied by retching and belching.

It is necessary to inquire about the onset and the present condition of the disease. Then palpate the pulses, examining the channels and their network vessels in regard to their depth and superficiality, feeling them up and down along their pathways to distinguish counterflow from normalcy. A rapid pulse does not necessarily imply disease. However, a slow pulse does imply disease. (If the pulse) ceases in its coming and going, this portends death. If the skin is welded (to the flesh), this portends death.

The Yellow Emperor asked:

How is a curable disease treated?

Qi Bo answered:

For a channel disease, treat the channel. For a connecting vessel disease, treat the connecting vessel. [In the *Su Wen* "the connecting vessel" is preceded by the word "minute". {later editor}] For pain in the body, treat the channel and the connecting vessel. If the disorder is due to an uncommon evil, the vessel affected by the uncommon evil should be cross needled. If the disorder has lingered long, the body is thin, and the (evil) is implanted, needling should be performed at the joints. In the case of repletion above and vacuity below, it is necessary first to feel the channel along its route to ascertain where the vessel binds and to determine which are to be pricked and bled to free the flow of qi. If the pupils of the eyes are high, the *tai yang* is insufficient while upturned eyes indicate expiry of the *tai yang*. These are the essentials in the prognostication of life and death, and they should not be neglected.

Endnotes

[1] Part 1 is derived from Chap. 48, Vol. 8, *Ling Shu (Spiritual Pivot)*; Part 2 from Chap. 49, Vol. 8, *Ling Shu*; Part 3 from Chap. 18, *Su Wen (Basic Questions)*; Part 4 from Chap. 5, Vol. 2, *Ling Shu*; Part 5 from Chap. 18, 23, and 76, *Su Wen*; and Part 6 from Chap. 19, *Su Wen*.

[2] "Determination Based on External Signs", Chap. 45, Vol. 5, *Ling Shu*

[3] The *cun kou* belongs to the *tai yin* and reflects the circulation of qi in the viscera, and, as such, it reflects illnesses of the interior. The *ren ying* belongs to the *yang ming* and reflects the circulation of qi in the bowels, and, as such, it reflects illnesses in the exterior. They are both a product of the stomach qi, the two vessels have an interior/exterior relationship, and their circulation is synchronous with the respiration. Since there is an effulgence of yang qi in the spring and summer, the *ren ying* will be larger while the natural effulgence of yin qi in the autumn and winter accounts for the largeness of the *cun kou*.

[4] Various pulse patterns are implied in the use of terms such as exuberance and the like.

[5] A tense pulse suggests painful *bi*, which affects the muscles most. Accordingly the borders of flesh should be needled.

[6] Note that exuberance of yin rather than yang is meant, and consequently the syndrome depicted is readily understandable, which in a way can be regarded as a vacuity syndrome, but of yang .

[7] See note 6, Chap. 1, Book 1, present work.

[8] Conducting therapy simply means that the evil should be expelled.

[9] A tense pulse is indicative of cold, and, therefore, needling, moxibustion, and the administration of medicinals are indicated. A sagging pulse reflects cold strike, and, therefore, treatment via moxibustion is indicated. An urgent pulse indicates an evil exuberance and, therefore, requires conducting therapy. An interrupted pulse reflects a vacuity of qi and blood and, therefore, quiet repose is indicated.

[10] A slippery, small, and tense *cun kou* pulse reflects an exuberance of evil qi in the yin aspect, hence the illness is in the interior. A large, tense, and floating *ren ying* pulse indicates an evil exuberance in the yang aspect, hence the illness is in the exterior. A floating and slippery *cun kou* indicates a depletion of yang evil as the force of the illness diminishes. The same is true for a sinking and slippery *ren ying* pulse. A deep pulse is indicative of an illness which resides in the yin. However, a large pulse is indicative of the presence of spirit which facilitates an easy recovery. A deep fine pulse is indicative of a depletion of true yin and so represents a condition that is difficult to cure.

[11] A floating and large pulse is in accord with an illness of the bowels since both are yang conditions. If, however, the pulse is floating and small, this is not in accord with an illness of the bowels and represents a condition which is difficult to cure.

[12] Orientation in this context is synonymous with spirit. Confinement in orientation implies mental disorders such as ravings.

[13] Because the pulse beats, in fact, slightly more than two times with each inhalation and exhalation, it is said to beat five times in one whole cycle of respiration.

[14] According to the *Tai Su (Essentials)* the cubit skin is the skin in the area from Cubit Marsh (*Chi Ze*, Lu 5) to the wrist joint.

[15] If the pulse beats more than four times per exhalation, this portends death due to injury to the essence qi. If it is expiring, the true qi has been cut off and so this portends death. If it beats at an irregular rhythm and pace, the yin and yang have become chaotic and disordered, and, therefore, this portends death as well.

[16] "Zhong Shi (The Chapter on Consummate [Needling])", Chap. 9, *Su Wen*

[17] A short life might be thirty or forty years, and death is not necessarily imminent. It should be kept in mind, however, that an absence of qi from all of the five viscera is a very critical condition. A pulse which beats at a variable pace and rhythm implies a frequently interrupted pulse.

[18] Wiseman, *et al*, also translates this as wiry. Some textbooks give a straight and long pulse, but this is a gloss on the feeling of this pulse, not its name.

[19] Some textbooks call this a flooding pulse. It is a very ample pulse, looming or coming on forcefully, but retreating feebly, giving an impression of a hook. Besides, the name also suggests the hook-like shape of the heart.

[20]The term belt suggests flexibility or pliancy since the spleen pulse should be gentle and modifiable depending upon the seasons and able to blend with the other four visceral pulses.

[21]The name hair–like implies that the pulse feels as if one were touching soft hair, a feeling of lightness, floating, and vacuity.

[22]This implies a deep pulse.

[23]This description suggests the qualities of lubrication, fullness, and ampleness.

[24]This is a belt decorated with hook shaped ornaments, worn in ancient times. In feeling such a belt, one would perceive prominences followed by flatness, and this is what is suggested here.

[25]In this and the following four passages, two pathological pulse qualities are discussed for each viscera. The first pulse quality reflects a diminished amount of stomach qi, while the second reflects a complete lack of stomach qi and hence death. Arriving (*lai*) refers to the beating of the pulse. In some contexts, as in this and the following paragraphs, it reflects the entire process of the rising and falling of the pulse, while in others, it denotes only the rising aspect of the pulse.

[26]The description suggests a smooth, floating, tranquil pulse.

[27]This curious image illustrates Huang-fu Mi's meticulous observation of nature. When a chicken lets down its feet, its movement is seemingly leisurely, light, and peaceful, but in lifting its feet, it gives an abrupt and rapid jerk.

[28]Hook here implies that the kidney pulse is similar to the heart pulse.

[29]"Hard as a pebble" evokes the image of pebbles hitting the fingers as they palpate the pulse.

[30]This refers to the *qi kou* or *cun kou* pulse because it belongs to the hand *tai yin* channel.

[31]Spring is the season during which the liver prevails. Summer is the season during which the heart prevails. Autumn is the season during which the lung prevails. Winter is the season during which the kidney prevails. A distinctive pulse should appear only in a certain season in accordance with the prevailing interrelationships of the five phases. The kidney pulse, for instance, should make its appearance in winter rather than during other seasons.

[32]A distinctive pulse quality appears for each season. For example, during the winter, the kidney pulse with a stone-like quality predominates and during the summer, the heart pulse with a hook-like quality predominates. While this is the normal state of things, if there is no stomach qi manifesting as a moderating quality within the pulse, then the pulse cannot be considered normal. Only with the help of the stomach qi may the visceral qi present themselves normally within the *cun kou* pulse at the wrist.

The visceral qi and the true visceral qi should not be confused. The author uses the term visceral qi only within the context of the requirements for a normal pulse picture. The term true visceral qi is used to denote an abnormal situation relating to a specific diseased viscus.

[33]This refers to the pulse appearing in spring in normal cases. In other words, it is the liver pulse.

[34]The word sapping implies the idea of growing rampantly. In this case, the evil grows in an aggressive, threatening way, causing heat to pervade. There is, however, another interpretation of this term. Sapping may also refer to the outbreak of sores due to an effulgence of fire.

[35]*I.e.*, the passing of gas, or flatulence.

[36]It is so named because the spleen alone receives the turbid qi out of the viscera, and, unlike the other four viscera, it governs no particular season in the year.

[37]In normal cases, the spleen pulse should always "hide" within the other visceral pulses, moderating them or providing the background for other visceral pulse images.

[38]The term may be interpreted in a variety of ways. One is that because qi fails to travel around the body, the body becomes heavy (*zhong*) and rigid (*qiang*). Another interpretation says that, because the visceral qi is interposing or *chong*, (*chong* is a homograph of *zhong*), qi is put out of harmony. Still another possible interpretation holds that because evil begins to grow unchecked, this manifests as congestion of the nine portals.

[39]Part 1 is derived from Chap. 18, 23, and 17, *Su Wen*; Part 2 from Chap. 17, *Su Wen*; Part 3 from Chap. 18, *Su Wen*; Part 4 from Chap. 64, *Su Wen*; Part 5 from Chap. 45, *Su Wen*; and Part 6 from Chap. 17, *Su Wen*.

[40]Here again, the appearance of a pulse irregularity implies a lack of stomach qi. The five evils are the result of the visceral qi of a given season being overwhelmed by the qi of its controlling viscera.

[41]This is the stomach qi or, more exactly, its representation in the pulse which is expected to present a

mild, gentle picture. In the normal state in each season, the pulse image is expected to be peculiar to one of the four viscera, namely, the lung, liver, kidney, and heart, while each of the distinctive pulse images is supposed to have stomach qi as its background. The lack of stomach qi is indicative of serious problems. In summer, for example, it is normal for the pulse to be surging but only if it is mildly surging.

[42]This is the characteristic pulse image of the liver in the normal state.

[43]This is the characteristic pulse image of the lung in the normal state.

[44]Since the stomach is the root of all the viscera and the other bowels, its qi is justifiably called the true qi or the visceral trueness. Thus the visceral trueness is basically the stomach qi. This passage implies that the visceral trueness, or the stomach qi, is to be transported to the liver to be stored for nourishing the sinews. It is notable, however, that the similar term "true visceral (qi)", which means absence of stomach qi, suggests serious conditions.

[45]The characteristic pulse image of the heart in the normal state.

[46]The characteristic pulse image of the kidney in the normal state.

[47]A hook–like pulse with little stomach qi in the summer implies an exuberance of heart fire and a depletion of stomach qi. A completely hook–like summer pulse portends death because it implies that the stomach qi has expired. A summer pulse which is very stone–like implies that there is an arresting of fire and injury to water with an expiry of stomach qi, hence disease is imminent.

[48]This is the characteristic pulse image of the spleen in its normal state.

[49]A completely belt–like long summer pulse indicates a total lack of stomach qi and hence death. A very stone–like long summer pulse indicates a depletion of stomach qi and rebellion of water (kidney) against earth (spleen) and hence disease is imminent.

[50]An autumn pulse which is very wiry implies a depletion of stomach qi, and rebellion of wood (liver) against metal (lung).

[51]The walled city (xu li) is the place where the essence qi of water and grain transformed by the spleen and stomach meets the clear qi inhaled by the lungs. They gather here and form great qi (da qi) which is the source of the qi in the twelve channels. Anatomically, this is the region of the chest where one can feel the heart beating and in mod-

ern times the term is used to refer to the place where a physician places a stethoscope to listen to the heart. Xu li literally means village or small town, but was commonly used to refer to a much larger walled city. In the present context, xu li evokes an image of a bustling metropolis where various influences meet and intermingle.

[52]A long, hard heart pulse is due to an exuberance of evil which causes lingual retraction and inability to speak. A soft and scattered heart pulse indicates a restoration of stomach qi. The thirst is inconsequential.

[53]A long, hard lung pulse is due to fire evil overwhelming the lung causing spitting of blood. A soft, scattered lung pulse is indicative of lung vacuity with a lack of security of the skin and hair causing spontaneous sweating.

[54]A long, hard liver pulse without a green-blue complexion implies that the illness is not in the viscera and so must be due to trauma of some sort.

[55]This is characterized by heart pain and a distressed feeling on eating which can be relieved by vomiting.

[56]A long, hard stomach pulse with a red complexion is due to an exuberance of fire in the yang ming injuring the stomach channel and hence causing thigh pain. A soft and scattered stomach pulse is due to a vacuity of stomach qi which impairs the digestion.

[57]A long, hard spleen pulse with a yellow complexion is due to spleen vacuity and a failure to nourish the lung causing diminished qi. A soft, scattered spleen pulse with a dull complexion is due to a spleen vacuity and a failure to control water. In this case, water fails to circulate and thus there is edema.

[58]A long, hard kidney pulse with a reddish–yellow complexion is due to damp heat evil injuring the kidney, while a soft, scattered kidney pulse is due to a vacuity of blood and essence. Since this depletes the source, it is difficult to treat. In the above cases, in general, a hard, long pulse indicates a repletion pattern, while a soft, scattered pulse denotes some vacuity of the correct qi.

[59]The phrase "the qi is diseased" implies an insufficiency of qi.

[60]The cun section of the cun kou. There is, however, another interpretation that the upper pulse refers to the pulses in the upper part of the body, such as the ren ying.

[61]Elevation suggests a syndrome characterized by fullness and dyspnea.

[62]The *guan* and *chi* section of the *cun kou*. Refer to note 61.

[63]In spring, for example, the pulse is said to be in congruity to the season if it presents a wiry image.

[64]This refers to the transmission of disease. There is no skipping when a disease is transmitted in order of metal (lung), wood (liver), earth (spleen), water (kidney), fire (heart), and metal (lung). This is in order of the five phase inter-restraining cycle. If the disease transmits in the order of the five phase inter-engendering cycle, however, *i.e.*, heart (fire), spleen (earth), lung (metal), kidney (water), it is called skipping.

[65]A short *cun kou* pulse is due to an insufficiency of yang and this causes headache. A long *cun kou* pulse is due to an insufficiency of yin and this causes spasms in the legs. A deep and hard *cun kou* pulse is due to evil in the yin aspect and, therefore, the illness is in the interior. A floating, exuberant *cun kou* pulse is due to evil in the yang aspect and, therefore, the illness is in the exterior. An urgent *cun kou* pulse is due to an ascension of yang and so the illness is in the upper part of the body. A tight, wiry, hard, and replete *cun kou* pulse is due to an internal binding of yin evil. A floating *cun kou* is due to evil in the exterior giving rise to fever and chills. A flooding, slippery, and hard pulse is due to an exuberance of yang and thus the illness is external. A weak and choppy *cun kou* pulse is due to a vacuity of qi and blood and hence the illness is chronic. A floating, slippery, and strong *cun kou* pulse is due to a recent contraction of wind heat. If the *cun kou* pulse is tense and urgent, this is due to an accumulation of cold giving rise to *shan qi*. A slippery *cun kou* pulse is due to a yang evil such as wind illnesses. A choppy *cun kou* pulse is due to a yin evil such as *bi* illnesses. An exuberant, tense, and urgent *cun kou* pulse is due to an accumulation of cold qi resulting in abdominal fullness and distension. A relaxed and slippery *cun kou* pulse is due to heat evil in the spleen and stomach.

[66]*I.e.*, the pulse associated with the fifth and sixth months

[67]*I.e.*, the pulse associated with the first and second months

[68]*I.e.*, the pulse associated with the third and fourth months

[69]The *tai yang* is the great yang and associated with summer when the yang qi is exuberant in both humankind and in nature as a whole. This is justifiably reflected in an exuberant, surging, and long pulse. The *yang ming* is the stage of the approach but not quite the attainment of the zenith of yang associated with late spring and early summer. This is reflected in the pulse as floating, large, and short qualities. The *shao yang* is the inception of yang associated with the spring in which the remains of yin are still present. Since it is an unstable time where the yin is coming to an end and the yang is beginning to grow, this is reflected in an unstable pulse.

[70]This is a collective term for *bi* of yin nature, *e.g.*, cold *bi*, dampness *bi*.

[71]Here "wind" serves merely as an epithet. It does not add substantially to the meaning of "fox-like *shan*".

[72]Skin *bi* (*pi bi*) is a condition involving the skin characterized by papules, formication, and a dullness of sensitivity near to numbness. Craving papules (*yin zhen*) develop very quickly and are due to an internal accumulation of damp heat in combination with an external contraction of wind. They are characterized by raised papular patches accompanied by unbearable itching. In severe cases, there is abdominal pain, dyspnea, or even hemoptysis or hemafecia. The character *yin* implies addiction or craving, referring to the unsuppressible impulse to scratch.

[73]This is a syndrome characterized by vexation, fullness of the chest, panting and retching.

[74]This is *shan* induced by the external evil.

[75]*Shao yin* is ministerial fire. In this case, an exuberance of fire controls lung metal influencing the skin. An insufficiency of this fire allows for an invasion of dry evil and hence lung *bi*. A slippery, replete pulse indicates ministerial fire generating evil and overwhelming the lung. A choppy pulse is due to an inefficiency of heart blood which causes an accumulation in the channels and further causes the blood to become disordered resulting in hematuria.

[76]This is a syndrome characterized by lassitude, flabby limbs, cough, and vomiting of clear juice.

[77]The syndrome of spleen wind *shan* is characterized by swelling and prolapse of the genitals or rectum.

[78]A surplus in the *tai yin* implies repletion dampness and, because spleen earth governs the muscles, this dampness lodges there, resulting in muscular *bi*. Cold damp in the stomach and spleen results in cold in the center.

[79]This is a syndrome characterized by heat, including the extreme sensation of heat in the skin, abnormal complexion, and cracking of dried lips.

[80]This is a syndrome characterized by blocked blood vessels, vexation, pounding of the heart, fulminant counterflow of qi, panting, dry throat, frequent retching, and susceptibility to fright.

[81]The qi of *yang ming* is that of dry metal, and it is associated with the stomach and large intestine. A surplus of dry metal causes a vacuity in the blood vessels and a depletion of water resulting in vessel *bi*. An insufficiency of dry metal results in an exuberance of fire evil producing heart *bi*. A slippery pulse reflects a surplus of dry metal which bullies heart fire, producing heart wind *shan*. A choppy pulse implies blood stasis and an insufficiency of blood which fails to nourish the heart spirit, producing a susceptibility to fright.

[82]This is a syndrome characterized by painful, malformed bones, contraction of the muscles, and, in serious cases, atrophy of the muscles and a hunched back.

[83]As a syndrome, this is the late stage of bone *bi*.

[84]The qi of *tai yang* is that of cold water. It is associated with the kidneys and hence the bones. A surplus of cold water results in bone *bi*. A slippery pulse in this case indicates a wind cold evil creating renal wind *shan*, while a choppy pulse indicates accumulation in the kidneys.

[85]This is a syndrome of tense or rigid sinews, inhibited joints and spasms.

[86]This is a syndrome of sleep fraught with fright, much drinking, and frequent urination.

[87]The qi of *shao yang* is that of fire and it is associated internally with the liver which governs the sinew and resides in the lateral costal region. A surplus of *shao yang* fire qi is detrimental to the liver and results in sinew *bi*. A slippery pulse in this case implies wind heat evil injuring the liver while a choppy pulse implies liver stagnation which tenses the sinews and causes eye pain.

[88]This means that one should use those points on the affected channel known to be effective for the condition involved.

[89]The term vacuity fullness (*xu man*) refers to a subjective sense of emptiness and yet fullness one might have in the abdomen. It does not imply a specific state of vacuity or repletion. The stomach and the kidney are related. Therefore, a depletion of yang qi within *shao yin* can result in loss of transportation and transformation within the stomach and spleen and loss of control over ascent and descent.

[90]Since the *jue yin* governs the sinew, there will be back pain and spasms. If the liver insults earth, this will result in vacuity fullness. Since the liver channel circles the genitals, there may be urinary blockage. Since the liver stores the *hun*, a counterflow in the liver may disorder the spirit causing delirium.

[91]Counterflow of yin here refers to an exacerbation of yin and a depletion of yang. This causes cold hands and feet, and, when yin reaches its climax, death is inevitable. A statement later in the text in Book 7 asserts that the *yang ming* is the root of all life and exuberant in qi and blood. It can survive for three days and only then can death occur. It can, therefore, be hypothesized that death occurs in the above situation in three days because that is how long it takes to completely deplete the qi and blood.

[92]The foot *tai yang* ascends to the sides of the nose and inner canthi and connects with the kidney along the spine.

[93]*E feng*, i.e., pathogenic wind disorders

[94]A floating and scattered pulse is indicative of an insufficiency of qi and blood. This causes visual dizziness and collapse. Spinning refers to visual dizziness, while collapse implies falling down.

[95]This implies the three hand yang channels.

[96]This implies the three foot yin channels.

[97]If one expects to find a floating pulse because all the other signs point to an external condition and it turns out to be sinking in the foot position, this indicates an accumulation in the venter and abdomen. If one expects to find a sinking pulse because all the other signs point to an interior condition and, on the contrary, it is floating and rapid, this indicates heat in the center. If there is an illness above, one would expect it to be reflected in the upper aspects of the pulse. If, on the contrary, one feels the foot position of the pulse more strongly, this indicates an exuberance of yin, and thus there is cold back and feet. If there is an illness below, one would expect it to be reflected in the lower aspects of the pulse. If, on the contrary, one feels the *cun* position more strongly, this is indicative of an exuberance of yang above, and thus there is headache and neck pain. If the pulse is weak even when pressed to the bone, this implies a vacuity of kidney qi and, since the lumbar region is the mansion of the kidney, there will be back pain, etc.

[98]Part 1 is derived from Chap. 79 and 75, *Su Wen*; Part 2 from Chap. 17, *Su Wen*; Part 3 from Chap. 10, *Su Wen*; Part 4 from Chap. 19 and 80, *Su Wen*; Part 5 from Chap. 53, *Su Wen*; Part 6 from Chap. 17, *Su Wen*; Part 7 from Chap. 60, Vol. 9, *Ling Shu*; Part 8

from Chap. 61, Vol. 9, *Ling Shu*; Part 9 from Chap. 19, *Su Wen*; and Part 10 from Chap. 48, *Su Wen*.

[99]This figurative expression implies the fact that *tai yang*, the third yang, which governs the whole back, is the largest or longest of the three yang channels, that the *yang ming*, the second yang, which spreads in the upper and the lower of the front, connects the whole body, and that the *shao yang*, the first yang, which travels between the *tai yang* and *yang ming*, functions as a link.

[100]This implies the *cun kou* pulse which is on the route of the hand *tai yin* channel as the opening of qi.

[101]A wiry, deep, and urgent pulse is indicative of yin qi within a yang bowel. Such a manifestation of heat is indicative of the last burst of warmth from the waning yang and so death is inevitable.

[102]A *shao yang* pulse which is continuously wiry, urgent, and suspended indicates a pathogenic factor within the *shao yang*.

[103]The *tai yin* is the third yin; the *shao yin* the second yin; the *jue yin* the first yin.

[104]The six channels refer to the three yang and three yin hand and foot pairs.

[105]Emptiness in the upper warmer refers specifically to an insufficiency of lung qi which, in extending to the heart, injures the spirit.

[106]Here the lung refers specifically to the *cun kou* pulse.

[107]The second yin is the *shao yin* which circulates upward to the lung where it unites with the lung qi to descend and penetrate the urinary bladder and connect with the spleen and stomach.

[108]Refer to Chap. 1, Book 4 (present book), present work.

[109]The *tai yang* pulse is surging and long. The *yang ming* pulse is floating, large, and short. The *shao yang* pulse is in pace and rhythm with distinct intermissions. The *tai yin* is light and floating. The *shao yin* is soft, slippery, and long. Whichever comes first is the host, and what comes later is the guest. The guest/host relationship between affections is the same as that of the root and end.

[110]The foot *tai yang* is the longest of the yang channels, travelling from foot to head. As such, it is often referred to as the father or leader of the yang channels. The foot *yang ming* channel, aside from being quite a long vessel and travelling the anterior aspect of the body, is responsible for nourishing the entire body. As such, it is often referred to as the guardian or the defender. This idea of a guardian encompasses not only the function of

providing protection from external invasion but also the function of nursing in the context of promoting recuperation. The *shao yang* runs between the *tai yang* and the *yang ming*, travelling along the lateral aspect of the body. As such, it serves as a go–between or envoy.

The *Lei Jing (The Classified Classic)* provides another perspective on this: "*Tai yang* nourishes the channels and is, therefore, called the father. *Shao yin* relates to water and, since water is responsible for growth, it is called the mother. The envoy is said to communicate between the terminations and the beginnings, ending at the yin and developing from the yang. It is governed by the *jue yin* alone, so is therefore called the sole envoy.

[111]The second yang is the *yang ming* which relates to earth. The first yin is the *jue yin* which relates to wood, and wood controls earth. Thus, *yang ming* is the primary illness. The pulse is soft and stirring because the stomach qi is restrained by the control of the liver. The nine portals relate to the *yang ming*, and, if there is a lack of circulation of qi in a *yang ming* illness, then the portals become obstructed.

[112]The third yang governs the qi of cold and water. The first yin is the viscera of wind and wood as well as the dynamic for growth. When the qi of cold and water overwhelm the dynamic of growth causing restraint, the qi of the five viscera becomes chaotic. In the context of yang qi, essence nourishes the spirit. If the spirit is not nourished, this results in external symptoms of fright and panic.

[113]The second yin is the hand *shao yin*, the heart, which is fire, and the first yang, the foot *tai yang*, the gallbladder, which is wood. In the mutual affectation of these two, a soaring fire is burning to restrain metal, that is, the lung. On the other hand, since wood tends to overwhelm earth, the spleen (earth) is affected, too, in this case.

[114]The second yin is the kidney and relates to water, while the second yang is the stomach and relates to earth. According to five phase theory, earth should restrain water.

[115]According to the *Su Wen*: "The kidney is a yin viscera, and, therefore, the qi is also yin. The triple warmer is the mansion of fire which links internally with the three collectors and externally promotes free flow in the nine portals. Therefore, an illness of kidney water, being a fullness of yin, qi naturally ascends to the heart venter and influences all the portals, causing obstruction to arise there. The four extremities relate to stomach earth, and an exuberance of water insults earth,

causing them to feel as if separated from the trunk".

[116]The first yin is wood, and wood is the restraining phase of earth. This is a condition of an overexuberance of liver wood overwhelming earth.

[117]The consummate yin is the first yin, *i.e.*, the *jue yin*.

[118]The second yang is the stomach, the third yin is the lung, and the consummate yin is spleen earth. If all three are diseased, yin cannot enter yang and yang cannot reach yin. The pulse indicators are rather idiosyncratic. Ordinarily, a floating pulse indicates an external disorder, while a deep pulse indicates an internal disorder.

[119]The third yang of the hand and foot belongs to the urinary bladder and the small intestine which, in turn, are associated respectively with the kidney and the heart. These two viscera house true water and true fire. When both water and fire are disordered, the condition will be critical. Besides, the foot *tai yang*, the longest channel, govern the other yang vessels. Therefore, when the *tai yang* is diseased, all the other yang are surely involved.

[120]The six directions are east, west, south, north, the upper (heaven), and the lower (earth).

[121]Wrath and fury here are used to reflect different levels of intensity inherent in the yin qi in the autumn and winter respectively.

[122]A compass is an instrument for drawing and measuring circles; so it is used to describe a slippery, active, and smooth pulse image.

[123]A square is an instrument for drawing or measuring a square; so it is used to describe a flooding, full pulse image.

[124]The arm of a steelyard or hand–held Chinese scale is level, fluctuating slightly in weighing things; so it is used to describe a floating but tranquil pulse image.

[125]The weight of a steelyard is heavy, tending to descend; so it is used to describe a deep, steady pulse image.

[126]This refers to the related viscera.

[127]*I.e.*, the six essentials of pulse diagnosis are the responses of the pulse in the four seasons and the coordination of the pulses with the interior organs and the exterior reflections.

[128]According to the *Lei Jing*: "The pulse is large as a result of an exuberance of evil qi. (First) there is vacuity causing a vacuity of central qi. This vacuity of central qi impairs motility within the spleen, and thus there is an accumulation of qi within the abdomen. If the spleen is vacuous, wood overwhelms it and weakens it. There is no aversion to water (by wood), and the qi of both the liver and kidney counterflows upward. This is inversion qi." Another perspective is that any pathogen which causes cold limbs, mental disorders, or sudden collapse is referred to as inversion qi. Inversion *shan* is a counterflow of qi giving rise to abdominal and thoracic distension accompanied by periumbilical pain and warmth in the limbs, all of which were exacerbated by exposure to cold. In short, it is abdominal pain resulting from exposure to cold.

[129]Form is defined as the construction, the build, or body. Therefore, form qi is the appearance or look of a person, *i.e.*, the exhibition of their physical state.

[130]In the corresponding paragraph in the Chinese edition, the same characters are used in the same structure to denote "form qi" and "form and qi" (*xing qi*). This confusion can be accounted for by the fact that this paragraph is a combination of materials derived from different sources with little modification.

[131]Depending upon one's understanding, this group of words can be paraphrased in two different ways as follows. 1) Although there are no manifestations of disease in the viscera. . . 2) Provided that the visceral pulse fails to present a picture in congruence with the seasonal changes. . .

[132]Grain here is an abbreviation for grain qi, the essence derived from grain, and hence appetite or food intake.

[133]Eating little is the manifestation of an affected stomach, while much qi is capable of being interpretated as counterflow of qi, *e.g.*, panting. This reveals that the lung is diseased.

[134]*I.e.*, wine or the like

[135]It is understood that that which invades is the evil qi, while that which leaves is the true qi.

[136]Here blood stasis and vessel stagnation are implied. Stroke in this context means edema or a large scale swelling which is usually caused by dampness.

[137]When examining the cubit, "the upper" refers to the area near to the wrist, while "the lower" part refers to the area near to the elbow. This use of these terms is opposite to that in other places in this book.

[138]There is little connection between the three sets of

abnormalities outlined above. Both abdominal distension and generalized heat reflect an internal repletion of evil qi. A large pulse confirms this pattern. Abdominal rumbling, vacuity fullness, cold limbs, etc., are due to vacuity cold. The pulse should be vacuous or small but, on the contrary, is large. This is incongruous with this condition. Incessant bleeding should be accompanied by a scallion stalk pulse. When it is accompanied by a large pulse, it is incongruous with this condition. Coughing with blood in the stool and languishment is due to an inability of the correct to resist evil qi. A small pulse reflects a state of weakened correct qi, while a large pulse reflects an exuberance of evil qi. Cough and emaciation with generalized fever and a small, rapid pulse are due to a depletion of yin and an effulgence of fire. Although these patterns are critical, yin and yang are not yet exhausted. Death therefore comes in fifteen days.

Distension and enlarged abdomen with emaciation and severe diarrhea indicate a conquered spleen, while cold limbs indicate a desertion of yang. Abdominal distension with blood in the stool is an internal disease, and a large, occasionally expiring pulse indicates yang bordering on desertion. Cough and blood in the urine are a disease of both the qi and blood. A pounding pulse is a manifestation of the true visceral pulse. Vomiting of blood, thoracic fullness, and a small, rapid pulse indicate an exhaustion of the true yin or the true original qi. Cough, vomiting, abdominal distension, and diarrhea are an affliction of the three burners, and an expiring pulse reflects a desertion of the correct qi. All of the above are even more serious and are immediately fatal conditions.

Heat patterns should be accompanied by a large and flooding pulse. If, on the contrary, they are accompanied by a tranquil pulse, this reflects a yang condition with a yin pulse. Subsequent to sweating, the pulse should be tranquil. If, on the contrary, it is exuberant, large, and agitated, this implies a severance of the true yin. A patient with diarrhea should have a vacuous and weak pulse, and if, on the contrary, the pulse is large and flooding, this indicates a vacuity of the correct and an overwhelming of evil. A patient with *bi* with cleavage of the major muscle groups, generalized fever, and pulse expiry is suffering from a desertion of original qi. Licentious behavior leading to emaciation and generalized fever or defecation of clotted blood is a result of the perishing of yin. Chronic fever and chills causing a desertion of form with a hard, forceful pulse reflects a major injury to the spleen and stomach.

[139]The conditions, though seemingly critical, are not so serious because they are due to a violent fright or scare, which will be overcome easily and rapidly.

[140]A small, urgent pulse reveals severe cold, and a pulse not beating forcefully is indicative of stagnant blood, which is due to cold. Since blood stasis leads to conglomeration, one can safely diagnose the condition as conglomeration.

[141]Stone water is edema mainly confined to the lower abdomen, which feels very hard, accompanied by distending pain in the flanks. Wind water is a swelling starting first in the face and then spreading all over the body. It is accompanied by fever and aversion to wind.

[142]This includes, in order, the hand and foot *tai yang* (third yang) channels, the hand and foot *tai yin* (third yin) channels, and the hand and foot *shao yin* (second yin) channels.

[143]They include, in order, channels of the hand and foot *tai yang, tai yin, shao yin*, and *yang ming*.

[144]This refers to fever due to hot blood.

[145]Conformable means favorable. Hemilateral disease which occurs on the left side in females but on the right side in males is believed to be benign. But note that here the presence and absence of loss of voice is critical.

[146]Although the general prognosis for hemiplegia occurring on the left side in females and the right side in males is positive, the loss of voice indicates a profound level of severity. This condition, therefore, requires three years for recovery. For a person under twenty to contract hemiplegia there must have been a preexisting depletion of qi and blood, and so this condition in a young person cannot be compared to that of an old person. It is incurable and death occurs in three years.

[147]See Chap. 1, Book 4 (present book), present work.

[148]Grass dries in late autumn and early winter. Since winter is associated with water, from the point of view of the five phase cycle it is logical that heart (fire) disease becomes exacerbated when the grass dries up.

[149]Bramble implies roughness and harshness. Since leaves fall in autumn, a metal season, it is logical that a liver (wood) disease becomes critical when the tree leaves fall.

[150]The simile used here describes the irregular beats of the pulse, *i.e.*, long pauses followed by abrupt, forceful throbbing. The jujube blossom is seen in early summer.

[151]The simile used here describes a hard, short pulse. The elm seeds fall in later spring, and spring is a wood season which is believed to be unfavorable to stomach (earth) disease.

[152]The simile used here describes a hard, rigid pulse. Crops become ripe in autumn, a metal season which is believed to be unfavorable to spleen–gallbladder (wood) disease.

[153]The simile used here describes a tight, fine, and urgent pulse image. Talkativeness is a manifestation of yang vacuity. When cold weather arrives, yang is at its low ebb and yang vacuity will naturally become worse.

[154]Reticence or serenity reveals that the true yin of the kidney is preserved and the yang vacuity is not serious.

[155]The meaning of "lack of flavor" is incomprehensible here and leads one to suspect that something is missing in the text. The foot *tai yang* is a water channel because it matches the foot *shao yin*. The disease involving it should become worse in the earth season, the last month of summer, when the leek begins to bloom.

[156]Decayed soil is characterized by looseness, and this simile is employed to describe a limp pulse image. Muscular qi is synonymous with spleen qi. Fleabane buds in spring.

[157]These twelve points are the back *shu* points associated with the five viscera and six bowels.

[158]The condition of cold and hot in the five viscera primarily affects the kidney. There is repletion of yang and a depletion of yin. Since the lumbar region is the abode of the kidney, when there is a depletion of kidney yin, the patient cannot sit up. The Beginning of Spring (an astrological name for one of the Twenty-Four Nodes of Qi) is a time when there is an exuberance of yang and the yin is depleted. This further aggravates the condition and is fatal.

[159]Since the large intestine is a metal bowel and the jujube sprouts new leaves in summer, a fire season, it is natural that the large intestine may suffer when the jujube is sprouting leaves.

[160]The phrase, "standing all his ears", is a colloquialism describing someone who is in a nervous state, always on watch, fearing that other people are speaking ill of him, and is ever suspicious.

[161]Part 1 is derived from Chap. 4, Vol. 1, *Ling Shu*; Part 2 from Chap. 74, Vol. 11, *Ling Shu*; and Part 3 from Chap. 47, *Su Wen*.

[162]Evil here refers to evils resulting from heaven, namely those of wind, cold, summer heat, and rain.

[163]Yin and yang here refer to the yin (medial) aspect and the yang (lateral) aspect of the limbs.

[164]This refers to the qi which branches off from the main current towards the eyes.

[165]This refers to the wind evil arising out of the irregular weather change.

[166]*I.e.*, the wind evil arising in normal weather

[167]The terms roots and terminations, roots and leaves are full of meanings, including interior/exterior relationships, relationships between the correct and evil qi, and cause and effect relationships.

[168]*I.e.*, cubit skin as defined above in note 14

[169]This quotation can be found in Chap. 1, Vol. 4, the *Mai Jing (The Pulse Classic)* by Wang Shu-he. But the statement in the *Mai Jing* is a little different from the quotation. It reads as follows: "If the cubit skin is tense and the *ren ying* pulse is small, death is prognosticated in the case of diminished qi and white complexion."

[170]In ancient times the character *zhen* referred to swellings.

[171]This whole chapter is derived from Chap. 4, Vol. 1, *Ling Shu*.

[172]A very urgent heart pulse is due to wind cold in the blood vessels influencing the sinews causing spasms. If the heart pulse is only slightly urgent, this indicates slight cold causing cardiac pain which radiates to the back.

[173]A very slack pulse is due to a dispersal of spirit causing mania, while the deep lying beam associated with a slightly slack pulse is due to an accumulation of qi in the abdomen.

[174]A very large heart pulse is due to an ascension of fire into the throat which causes rales.

[175]A small heart pulse is due to a vacuity of yang which causes stomach cold and a counterflow of stomach qi and thus retching. Pure heat wasting thirst with a slightly small heart pulse is associated with a vacuity of yin and depletion of fluids.

[176]A very slippery heart pulse is due to an exuberance of yang and blood heat which causes constant thirst, while a slightly slippery heart pulse is due to heat below causing cardiac *shan*.

[177]Blood spillage refers to illnesses characterized by blood loss.

[178]Here linking refers to the four extremities, *i.e.*, the two hands and the two feet. Linking inversion (*wei jue*) refers to chilling of the extremities due to a stagnation of qi and blood.

[179]A very choppy heart pulse is due to stasis of qi and blood above causing loss of voice, while the symptoms associated with a slightly choppy heart pulse are due to an internal stagnation of qi and blood damaging the blood network vessels.

[180]A very urgent lung pulse is due to an exuberance of evil wind with wood overwhelming metal which causes madness, while the symptoms associated with a slightly urgent pulse are due to wind cold harassing the lung causing conflict between the correct qi and the evil and inhibiting the circulation of lung qi.

[181]This is a syndrome due to wind invasion after drinking wine which consists of profuse perspiration on exertion, aversion to wind, loss of ability to perform work, and panting.

[182]A very slack lung pulse is due to extreme heat in the lung which causes frequent perspiration, while the symptoms associated with a slightly slack lung pulse are due to lung heat scorching the lobes of the lung and a binding of yang. This lung heat also moves toward the exterior, forcing the intestines open resulting in wind leakage.

[183]A very large lung pulse is due to heart fire scorching the lung which injures the true yin and fluids, thus causing swelling in the leg. The symptoms associated with a slightly large lung pulse are due to lung heat which produces *bi* or creates an effulgence of fire which injures the yin, causing photophobia.

[184]A very small lung pulse is due to a vacuity of lung qi which results in the clear yang sinking below and insecurity of the large intestine. Pure heat wasting thirst with a slightly small lung pulse is due to a dual depletion of metal and water such that there is an insufficiency of water generation at its source.

[185]An extremely slippery pulse is due to repletion heat causing counterflow ascension of qi with asthma and inverted cup surging, while bleeding associated with a slightly slippery pulse is associated with hot qi causing a spillage of blood both above and below.

[186]An extremely choppy lung pulse is due to blood stasis impairing circulation which causes vomiting of blood, while the symptoms associated with a slightly choppy lung pulse are associated with depressive qi stasis creating a repletion of lung

metal above which overcontrols liver wood below. The craving for sour foods is an attempt to offset the liver vacuity.

[187]See Chap. 2, Book 8.

[188]A very urgent liver pulse is due to an exuberance of liver qi which causes delirium and anger, while a slightly urgent liver pulse is due to an accumulation of qi in the lateral costal region which is called fat qi.

[189]A very slack liver pulse is due to liver heat which causes a counterflow ascent of liver qi surging into the throat precipitating frequent retching, while a slightly slack liver pulse is due to liver heat injuring earth, causing an inability to control water and, therefore, a chronic accumulation of water.

[190]A very large liver pulse is due to liver heat and an exuberance of hot evil qi which binds internally to produce internal *yong*, or becomes depressed and counterflows upward to produce retching. A slightly large liver pulse is due to liver *bi*. Because the liver channel pours into the lung above and into the genitals below, so an ascending counterflow produces cough, while a descending counterflow produces genital retraction.

[191]Since the liver governs the blood, if the liver pulse is very small, this implies a great vacuity of blood and yin producing great thirst, while if it is only slightly small, this implies a vacuity of yin and blood dryness which engenders pure heat wasting thirst.

[192]A very choppy liver pulse is due to heat obstructing the yin aspect of the liver channel which produces *tui shan*, while a slightly slippery liver pulse reflects an unrestrained yin vacuity producing enuresis.

[193]A very choppy liver pulse implies a depletion stasis of qi and blood with dampness spilling into the extremities and spillage rheum, while a slightly choppy liver pulse implies an insufficiency of qi and blood whereby the sinews are not being nourished and moistened and thus become hypertonic.

[194]A very urgent spleen pulse is due to a cold spleen which has contracted wind, allowing liver wood to overwhelm earth and producing tugging and slackening in the extremities. A slightly urgent spleen pulse is due to cold injuring the spleen and impairing movement and transportation.

[195] A very slack spleen pulse is due to spleen heat. Since the spleen governs the muscles, when it contracts heat this causes atonic inversion. A slightly slack spleen pulse implies that wind evil is in the channels causing paralysis but not in the viscera, and so the mind is not affected.

[196] A very large spleen pulse is due to an exuberance of yang qi and a desertion of yin qi producing collapse. A slightly large spleen pulse is due to a binding of spleen qi producing *pi* in the form of a mass of blood and pus outside of the stomach and intestines.

[197] A very small spleen pulse is due to an insufficiency of yang qi in the middle warmer giving rise to cold and heat, while a slightly small spleen pulse is due to a diminution of qi and blood causing vacuity heat and thus pure heat wasting thirst.

[198] Also known as *kui long shan*, this is a syndrome characterized by swelling or ulceration in the pelvis or the lower abdomen which affects urination. It is a pattern like the urinary block.

[199] A very slippery spleen pulse is due to repletion heat and since the *tai yin* vessel is united with the ancestral sinew (*i.e.*, the penis), this results in *kui long* or urinary inhibition. A slightly slippery spleen pulse reflects damp heat in the spleen. This damp heat steams and fulminates and is conducive to the growth of parasites and heat in the abdomen.

[200] A very choppy spleen pulse is due to qi stasis and cold blood. This causes a prolapse in the large intestine resulting in *shan.* A slightly choppy spleen pulse simply reflects internal ulceration blood and pus in the stool. Intestinal *tui* is rectal prolapse, and, in women, includes vaginal discharge, too.

[201] Deep inversion refers to a syndrome of heaviness and cold of the feet and legs, and, in a serious case, loss of the use of the legs caused by descent of kidney yin.

[202] A very urgent kidney pulse is due to an invasion of cold evil into the bone which gives rise to emaciation, bone atony, and madness. A slightly urgent kidney pulse is due to kidney cold. This evil qi counterflows upward causing running piglet. Since the kidney yang is insufficient, there is deep inversion, and the qi fails to circulate downward so that the sinews fail to contract. Thus, the lower orifices become inhibited.

[203] Since the governing vessel rules the spine, a very slack kidney pulse reflects slackness in the spine and the feeling as if the spine were about to snap. A slightly slack kidney pulse is due to a depletion of life gate fire causing throughflux diarrhea.

[204] A very large kidney pulse is due to a vacuity of yin and an effulgence of fire which causes impotence. A slightly large kidney pulse is due to water not transforming into qi and accumulating as stone water below the umbilicus.

[205] A very small kidney pulse is due to severe weakness of kidney qi and a failure of control of the lower warmer, while a slightly small kidney pulse is due to a depletion of true qi which engenders pure heat wasting thirst.

[206] A very slippery kidney pulse is due to a heat evil which obstructs the small intestine and causes swelling and enlargement of the testicles.

[207] A very choppy kidney pulse is due to a stasis of qi and blood thus producing grand *yong*. A slightly choppy kidney pulse is due to a lack of circulation of qi and blood causing menstrual blockage in women and hemorrhoids.

[208] The favorable and unfavorable factors referred to here may be interpreted in two ways. First, they may refer to basic supplementation and draining techniques applied by manipulating the needle either with or against the flow of the channel. However, in this case, there is little point in specifying such a technique vis à vis the choppy pulse in particular since it holds true in all cases.

Another interpretation is that a choppy pulse often indicates a critical situation of a dual depletion of qi and blood which requires careful treatment. According to this reading, favorable and unfavorable factors can be easily understood as mitigating influences reflecting the degree of severity of the illness, such as the degree of agreement between the pulse quality and the pattern, etc.

[209] In this context the "*ying shu*" refers to the five transporting points as a whole, all of which are located below the elbow in the arms and the knees in the legs. We have, therefore, translated *ying shu* simply as the "transporting points."

[210] It is well known that each yang channel, whether of the hand or foot, is possessed of a confluence point among the transporting points. However, the three hand yang channels, *i.e.*, the triple

heater, the large intestine, and the small intestine vessels, each have a confluence point located below the knee on the leg in addition to that in the arm. In other words, the confluence points discussed in this chapter, which are said to be effective for bowel disorders, are all located below the knee. It is notable that as to the yang channels of the foot, there is nothing unusual about their confluence points and that in Chap. 33 and 35, for the sake of convenience in translation, Upper and Lower Great Hollow (St 37 and St 39) are called the uniting points of the large and small intestine vessel with the stomach vessel, while Bend Yang (Bl 39) is called the lower assisting point of the triple heater.

[211]I.e., *Shang Ju Xu* (St 37) and *Xia Ju Xu* (St 39)

[212]It should be noted that the confluence point of the large intestine is also said to be Pool at the Bend (*Qu Chi, LI 11*). The uniting point of the small intestine is also said to be Lesser Sea (*Xiao Hai*, SI 8). And that of the triple heater is Celestial Well (*Tian Jing*, TH 10).

[213]This means that the limbs should be stretched as in a series of warm–up exercises. No specific technique is given.

[214]This chapter is derived from Chap. 20, *Su Wen*.

[215]This is in the neighborhood of Forehead Fullness (*Han Yan*, GB 4) and Head Corner (*Tou Wei*, St 8) belonging to the foot *tai yang* and foot *yang ming* respectively.

[216]This is in the neighborhood of Great Reception (*Da Ying*, St 5), belonging to the foot *yang ming*.

[217]This is in the neighborhood of Great Bone Hole (*He Liao*, LI 19), belonging to the hand *tai yang*, hand *shao yang* and the foot *shao yang*.

[218]This is the *cun kou*, in the neighborhood of Channel Ditch (*Jing Qu*, Lu 8).

[219]This is in the neighborhood of Union Valley (*He Gu*, LI 4), the pulse of the large intestine.

[220]This is in the neighborhood of Spirit Gate (*Shen Men*, Ht 7), the pulse of the heart.

[221]This is in the neighborhood of Five Li (*Wu Li*, Liv 10) in males but of Supreme Surge (*Tai Chong*, Liv 3) in females, the pulse of the liver.

[222]This is in the neighborhood of Great Ravine (*Tai Xi*, Ki 3), the pulse of the kidney.

[223]This is in the neighborhood of Winnower's Gate (*Ji Men*, Sp 11), the pulse of the spleen. But to examine the stomach qi, the pulse located at Surging Yang (*Chong Yang*, St 42) in the instep is used.

[224]The five spiritual viscera are the liver (storing the ethereal soul), the heart (storing the spirit), the spleen (storing the reflection), the lung (storing the corporeal soul or *po*) and the kidney (storing the will). The four form viscera are the corner of the head, the ears and eyes, the mouth with teeth, and the chest.

[225]One should observe the fatness or thinness of the patient so as to decide how deep to needle. Blood stasis, as evinced by the presence of blood network vessels, must be removed via bleeding techniques prior to directly treating vacuity and repletion.

[226]Abundant qi often refers to a condition of rapid breathing or gasping as in asthma.

[227]Irregularities here can be interpreted in two different ways: 1) the pulse beating at no regular rhythm or pace, or a pulse with an irregularly varying size; 2) any unpredictable incongruity between form and qi.

[228]The pulses above and below refer to the *ren ying* and pedal pulses as well as *cun kou* pulse.

[229]An individual with a robust body should have a vigorous pulse or there is an incongruity which is always an unfavorable circumstance. A fine pulse reflects a depletion of qi and blood, while the severely diminished qi reflects an extreme vacuity of lung qi, all of which contribute to inevitable death. A thin body with a large pulse is again an incongruity, and an abundance of qi in the chest manifesting as thoracic fullness and difficulty breathing reflects an extreme vacuity of visceral qi and a failure of the qi to descend. A forcefully pounding pulse always indicates the advance of a disease process as the evil progresses in a menacing manner. The eyes are the locale where the essence qi from the viscera gathers, and, when they are sunken, they reflect an exhaustion of essence qi. The indicators of the middle region reflect the center which is the bodily pivot. When these are weaker than those in other regions, the central qi is expiring and death is imminent.

230In terms of pulse diagnosis, a hot pulse is slippery, while a cold pulse is tense.

231See Chap. 1, present volume.

232This passage implies a series of correspondences:

Cold & Heat	Heat Stroke & Heart Disease	Wind Disease	Water Disease
Calm Dawn Watch (3-5 AM)	Midday (11 AM-1 PM)	Sundown Watch (5-7 PM)	Midnight (11 PM-1 AM)
Spring, Liver	Summer, Heart	Autumn, Lung	Winter, Kidney

The spleen has no specific season to which it is related but flourishes for a certain period within each of the four seasons. In this context, it is associated with all four seasons and watches rather than one. The watches are *Chen* (B5 7–9 a.m.), *Xu* (B11 7–9 p.m.), *Chou* (B2 1–3 a.m.) and *Wei* (B8 1–3 p.m.). That is to say, in the case of a pulse beating at varying pace and rhythm, death comes in the above four watches.

233There has been some dispute over this reference to the seven signs. One school holds that the seven signs are the seven bad quality pulses: the small, large, rapid, retarded, hot, cold or sunken pulses. Another approach is that they are the deep, fine, and expiring pulse, the exuberant, agitated, pounding, and rapid pulse, cold and heat, heat stroke, wind disease, water disease, and the expiry of the spleen qi in the four seasons.

234The characters *jing yue* on initial reading seem simply to refer to gynecological disorder. However, they may also be interpreted as chronic malady. Which is correct is open to the judgement of the reader.

In wind diseases the pulse tends to be large while in menstrual disorders the pulse tends to be small and slight and although these are congruent with the seven signs and indeed indicate illness, they are not death pulses.

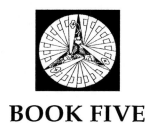

BOOK FIVE

Chapter One

Prohibitions of Acumoxatherapy (Part 1)[1]

(1)

The Yellow Emperor asked:

The qi of each of the four seasons has a different nature, and hundreds of diseases arise and all have a fixed location. In terms of the way of moxibustion and needling, what aspects are the most precious?

Qi Bo answered:

Because the qi of each of the four seasons influences (a different part of the body during each season), the (correct selection of) points of qi are the most precious in the way of moxibustion and needling.

Therefore, during the spring one should needle the network vessels[2] and the brook point, which are located (on or) between the channels in the partings of the flesh. In a serious (illness, the insertion of the needle) should be deep and for a minor (illness,) it should be shallow.[3]

The *Su Wen (Basic Questions)* states that, in spring, the dispersed points located in the parting of the flesh should be pricked and (the pricking) should be stopped once blood is let out. It adds that spring is a season when wood begins to prevail, and the liver qi begins to generate. This liver qi is impetuous and its wind[4] is swift. (On the other hand,) since the channels are submerged and the qi is scant, it is unable to penetrate and enter (the channels). Therefore, one should select the network vessels in the parting of the flesh.[5]

The *Jiu Juan (Ninefold Volume)* states that, in the spring, one should needle the brook points. This position is in accord (with the above statement) and is quite correct. (The *Jiu Juan*) also says that, in spring, the network vessels should be selected in the treatment of cutaneous problems. It also states that, in the spring, disorders of the channels (are treated by) selection of the blood vessels in the parting of the flesh. These statements are all in agreement.

It also states (in the *Su Wen*) that essentially in the spring, qi exists within the channels.[6]

In summer, one should select the rapids points and the minute network vessels at the surface of the flesh and skin (for treatment).[7]

(The *Jiu Juan*) also states that, in the summer, one should needle the rapids points. These two statements agree with one another and are quite correct. In long summer, one should needle the stream points. (The *Jiu Juan*) also says that, in summer, one should select the exuberant rapids points[8] and the minute network vessels in the parting of the flesh, and one should insert the needle no deeper than the skin. (And in another place,) the *Jiu Juan* adds that, in summer, one should select the points at the border between the flesh to treat the muscles. These statements are essentially in accord.

The *Su Wen* states that, in summer, one should needle the points of the network vessels and to cease (needling) once bleeding occurs. It explains that, during the summer, fire begins to prevail, the heart qi begins to grow, the vessels are thin, and the qi is feeble. The yang qi floods ["becomes lodged" in a variant version {later editor}], and blood warms the interstices which have access to the channels in the interior. Therefore one should select the exuberant channel at the parting of the flesh, and mere perforation of the skin is sufficient to remove the disease, since the evil resides at a shallow level. That which is referred to here as the exuberant channel is (the affected) yang channel.[9]

The two teachings (of the *Su Wen* and *Jiu Juan*) are in essential agreement. (The *Su Wen*) also says that, the summer qi lies within the minute network vessels, while the long summer qi lies within the muscles.

In autumn, one should needle the confluence points and the remaining details are the same as those techniques used in the spring. In autumn one may select the rapids points as well. However, when evil qi has become lodged within the bowels, one should select the confluence points.

The *Su Wen* states that, in autumn, the skin should be pricked through the border of flesh, and this is applicable to the upper and the lower alike.[10] It also states that autumn is the season when metal begins to prevail, the lung astringes and suppresses, and metal is about to overwhelm fire. Therefore, the yang qi exists in the confluence points. (During this season,) yin is at the initial stage of triumph and damp qi is beginning to assault the body. Because yin qi is not yet exuberant and is unable to penetrate deeply, the rapids points are selected to drain yin evil, while the confluence points are selected to evacuate yang evil. Since yang qi is beginning to decline, one selects the confluence points. This approach is applicable to the treatment of (pathological) changes in early autumn. It also explains that the autumn qi lies within the skin and that the interstices are closing then. (The *Jiu Juan*) adds that, in autumn, one should select the qi opening[11] to

treat the sinew vessels. This statement differs from the one above.[12]

In winter, one should select the well and rapids points in the border between flesh, and one should insert (the needle) deeply and retain it. (The *Jiu Juan*) also says that, in winter, one should select the well and the brook points. The *Su Wen* states that, in winter, one should select the rapids crevice[13] (for needling) in order to penetrate the border of flesh. In serious cases, (the needles should be inserted) directly into the affected area, while in slight cases, they should be inserted with a dispersing technique.[14] The rapids crevice and the rapids point mean essentially the same thing. (The *Jiu Juan*) also states that winter is the season when water begins to prevail, the kidney is just closing down, yang qi is in decline, and yin qi is luxuriant.[15]

The great yang[16] lies deeply and the other yang channels have consequently departed.[17] Therefore, one should select the well points to descend the counterflow of yin (qi) and select the spring points to free the flow of yang qi ["to replenish yang qi" in a variant version. {later editor}]

(The *Su Wen*) also states that, if the well and the rapids points are selected in winter, nosebleeds will not occur in the spring. This is said to be the treatment of choice for (pathological) changes occurring in late winter.

(The *Su Wen*) also explains that the winter qi lies within in the bone marrow. It also states that, in the winter, one should select the well points and, when a disease involves a viscus, one should also select the well points. These two opinions are consistent and hold good.

(The *Jiu Juan*) also states that, during the winter, one should select the stream points to treat (disorders of) the bone marrow and the five viscera. As for (the treatment of) the five viscera, the selection of the (stream) points is questionable.[18]

(2)

In the spring, if one needles (those points) prescribed for treatment during the summertime, the (blood) vessels become chaotic and the qi debilitated. This allows (evils) to sap the bone marrow. Rather than curing illness, it will cause a person to suffer from poor appetite and diminished qi. In the spring, if one needles (those points) prescribed for treatment during the autumn, this will cause spasms of the sinew and counterflow of qi which will cycle round and produce a cough. Rather than curing illness, this will cause susceptibility to fright with cries instead.[19]

In the spring, if one needles (those points) prescribed for treatment during the winter, this will cause evil qi to become lodged in the viscera resulting in abdominal distension. Rather than curing illness, it will result in talkativeness instead.[20]

In the summer, if one needles (those points) prescribed for treatment during the spring, rather than curing illness, this will cause a person to suffer from fatigue and lassitude instead. In the summer, if one needles (those points) prescribed for treatment in the autumn, rather than curing the disease, this will cause a person to suffer from a sense of oppression in his heart, muteness, and apprehension as if one feared arrest. In the summer, if one needles (those points) prescribed for treatment during the winter, rather than curing illness, this will cause diminished qi and occasional irascibility instead.[21]

In the autumn, if one needles (those points) prescribed for treatment during the spring, rather than curing illness, this will cause apprehension and such forgetfulness that the moment one arises to act, one is at a loss about what to do. In the autumn, if one needles (those points) prescribed for treatment in the summer, rather than curing the disease, this will cause somnolence and sleep fraught with dreams [occurring after the Beginning of Autumn. {later editor}] In the autumn, if one needles (those points) prescribed for treatment in the winter, rather than curing the disease, this will cause occasional shivering with cold instead.[22]

In the winter, if one needles (those points) pre-scribed for treatment in the spring, rather than curing the disease, this will cause a person to desire to lie down but be unable to sleep, and, if he does fall asleep, to dream of strange visages [occurring after the middle of the twelfth month {later editor}] instead. In the winter, if one needles (those points) prescribed for treatment during the summer, rather than curing the disease, this will cause the qi to ascend and cause the development of various kinds of *bi* instead. In the winter, if one needles (those points) prescribed for needling during the autumn, rather than curing the disease, this will cause constant thirst instead.[23]

(3)

The yang[24] of the foot is the lesser yang within yin,[25] while the yin[26] of the foot is the great yin within yin.[27] The yang[24] of the hand is the great yang within yang.[28] The yin[26] of the hand is the lesser yin within yang.[27]

In the first, second, and third months, a person's qi is on the left side, and the yang (channels) of the left foot are not to be needled (during this period). In the fourth, fifth, and sixth months, a person's qi is on the right side, and the yang (channels) of the right foot are not to be needled (during this period). In the seventh, eighth, and ninth months, a person's qi is on the right side and the yin (channels) of the right foot are not to be needled (during this period). And in the tenth, eleventh, and twelfth months a person's qi is on the left side, and the yin (channels) of the left foot are not to be needled (during this period).[29]

(4)

"*Ci Fa* (Needling Strategies)"[30] states that no needling therapy may be employed to treat intense heat.[31] No needling therapy may be employed to treat prodigious sweating. No needling therapy may be employed to treat a deranged pulse. And no needling therapy may be employed to treat an incongruity between a disease and the pulse. The superior practitioner first needles a disease before it arises. He will then needle a disease before it is fully developed. And he will finally needle a disease as it is on the wane. (On the contrary,) an inferior practitioner elects to needle a disease just as it is launching its assault or just as it is running rampant, or he will needle a disease which is incongruous with the pulse. (The "*Ci Fa*") also states that, in the case of a disease running rampant, no attempt should be made to thwart it and that treating a disease which is on the wane is a sure means to success. It follows that a superior practitioner prefers to treat a disease before it arises rather than treating a disease which has already arisen.

During periods of severe cold, one should not needle. However, during periods of intensely hot weather, one need not hesitate (to perform acupuncture). When the moon is waxing, do not administer draining therapy, and, when the moon is full, do not administer supplementation. When the moon is completely empty (*i.e.*, there is a new moon), one should not treat at all.[32]

(5)

Do not receive needling treatment immediately after sexual intercourse, and do not engage in sexual intercourse immediately after having been needled. Do not receive needling treatment while in a violent rage, and do not become angry immediately after having been needled. Do not receive needling treatment when overworked, and do not labor immediately after having been needled. Do not receive needling treatment while intoxicated, and do not become intoxicated immediately after having been needled. Do not receive needling treatment when having overeaten, and do not overeat immediately after having been needled. Do not receive needling treatment when very hungry, and do not go hungry immediately after having been needled. Do not receive needling treatment while thirsty, and do not become thirsty immediately after having been needled. If one has arrived in a cart, one must lay down to rest for about the time it takes to eat a meal before being needled. If one has arrived on foot, one must sit and rest for about the time it takes to walk ten *li* before being needled. If one is terribly frightened or scared, one must quiet one's qi before being needled.[33]

These prohibitions apply in cases where a deranged pulse and dissipated qi have resulted in disharmony of defensive and constructive (qi) and where the channel qi flows chaotically.

Needling (in defiance) of the above warnings leads a yang disease deep into the yin, while a yin disease exits (outward) and produces a (new) yang disease, thus compounding the evil. If the mediocre practitioner acts in ignorance, this is referred to as mangling the body. This results in soreness and pain accompanied by fatigue, consumption of the bone marrow, failure of fluid transformation, and desertion of the five flavors which is referred to as loss of qi.[34]

(6)

The Yellow Emperor asked:

Please tell me about how to determine the (appropriate) depth for needle insertion.

Qi Bo answered:

When needling the bone, avoid injuring the sinew. When needling the sinew, avoid injuring the flesh. When needling the flesh, avoid injuring the vessel. And when needling the vessel, avoid injuring the skin. When needling the skin, avoid injuring the flesh. When needling the flesh, avoid injuring the sinew. When needling the sinew, avoid injuring the bone.

The Yellow Emperor asked:

I still do not understand. Please provide a more detailed account.

Qi Bo answered:

In order to needle the bone without injury to the sinew, the needle should pass through the sinew and depart without (damage) to the depth of the bone. In order to needle the sinew without injury to the flesh, the needle should reach the flesh and depart without (damage) to the depth of the sinew. In order to needle the flesh without injury to the vessels, the needle should reach the vessel and depart without (damage) to the depth of the flesh. In order to needle the vessels without injury to the skin, the needle should reach the skin and depart without (damage) to the depth of the vessel.[35]

Needling the skin without injury to the flesh implies that the disease lies within the skin and that the needle should penetrate the skin only without striking the flesh. Needling the flesh without injury to the sinew implies that (the needle) should pass through the flesh (but not) strike the sinew. Needling the sinew without injury to the bone implies that (the needle) should pass through the sinew but not strike the bone. (Violation of) these axioms is referred to as acting in a contrary manner.

(7)

If a needle strikes the heart, death will occur in a day accompanied by symptoms of belching. If a needle strikes the lung, death will occur in three days accompanied by the symptom of coughing. If a needle strikes the liver, death will occur in five days accompanied by the symptom of yawning. [The *Su Wen* says "talkativeness." {later editor}] If a needle strikes the spleen, death will occur in fifteen days [the *Su Wen* says "ten days"; a variant version says "five days" {later editor}], the symptom of which is swallowing. If a needle strikes the kidney, death will occur in three days [the *Su Wen* says "six days"; a variant version says "seven days" {later editor}] accompanied by the symptom of sneezing. If a needle strikes the gallbladder, death will occur in one and a half days accompanied by the symptom of retching. If a needle strikes the diaphragm and damages the center, although the disease appears to be cured, death will come in one year. When needling the instep, if one strikes the major vessel there and causes incessant bleeding, this will eventually result in death. When needling the medial aspect of the thigh, if one strikes the major vessel, this causes incessant bleeding and, eventually, death. When needling the face, if one strikes the flowing vessels,[36] this will unfortunately result in blindness. When needling Guest Host Person (*Ke Zhu Ren*, GB 3),[37] if (the needle) penetrates too deeply

and strikes the vessel there, this results in leakage[38] and deafness. When needling the head at Brain Door (*Nao Hu*, GV 17), if (the needle) enters the brain, this causes instant death. When needling the (area around) the knee cap, if fluid emerges, this results in lameness. If one needles the vessel below the tongue too deeply, this causes incessant bleeding leading to loss of voice. When needling the arm along the *tai yin* vessel, if a copious amount of blood emerges, this results in immediate death. When needling the network vessels spread throughout the foot,[39] if one strikes a (blood) vessel and the blood is not let out, this will result in swelling. If (there is already kidney vacuity) and one needles the foot *shao yin* vessel, this may give rise to a dual vacuity and hemorrhage which results in the tongue having difficulty in articulation. When needling the Cleft Center (*Xi Zhong*),[40] if one strikes a major vessel, this causes a sudden loss of consciousness and a perished complexion. When needling the breast, if (the needle) penetrates too deeply and strikes a lung, this results in counterflow dyspnea and (compels one to adopt a) supine posture in order to breathe. When needling the Qi Thoroughfare (*Qi Chong*, St 30), if one strikes a (blood) vessel, there will be swelling of the groin if the blood is not let out. If one needles the elbow too deeply, the qi will be led internally, causing inability to bend or stretch (the elbow). When needling the intervertebral joints of the spine, if one strikes the marrow, this will result in a hunched back. If one needles the point three *cun* below (the groin) on the yin (i.e., medial) aspect of the thigh too deeply, this causes a person to suffer from enuresis. In needling the breast, if one strikes the nipple, this results in rooted corrosive swelling (of the breast).[41]

When needling between the ribs below the axilla, if (the needle) penetrates too deeply, this causes a person to suffer from cough. When needling the supraclavicular fossa, if (the needle) is inserted too deeply, this results in a drainage of qi, causing a person to suffer from counterflow dyspnea and cough. When needling the lower abdomen, if one strikes the urinary bladder, this results in a spillage of urine which leads to fullness in the lower abdomen. When needling the fish's margin of the hand, if (the needle) penetrates too deeply, this causes swelling. When needling the calf, if (the needle) penetrates too deeply, this causes swelling. When needling the depression in the orbit of the eye, if (the needle) strikes a (blood vessel), this causes leakage[42] and blindness. When needling the joints, if one strikes fluid which pours out, this will result in an inability to bend or stretch them.

Chapter One

Prohibitions of Acumoxatherapy (Part 2)[43]

(1)

The Yellow Emperor asked:

Please discuss the essentials of needling.

Qi Bo answered:

Because disease may be either superficial or deep, the insertion of the needle should be accordingly shallow or deep, each (insertion) within measure and not exceeding its appropriate depth. (Needling) too (deeply) results in internal injury, while needling to an inadequate depth gives rise to external gatherings. In the event of such external gatherings, evils are thus provided (with the opportunity to invade). Needling either too shallowly or too deeply is the insidious culprit responsible for internal damage to the five viscera which will, over time, engender major illness. It is said that disease may lodge in the fine hair and interstices, in the skin, in the muscles, in the vessels, in the sinews, in the bones or in the marrow. Therefore, when needling the fine hair and interstices, one must not injure the skin. If the skin is injured, the lung will be affected internally. If the lung is affected, there will be illnesses in the autumn such as warm *nue*, heat inversion, and shuddering with cold. In needling the skin, one must not injure the flesh. If the flesh is injured, the spleen will be affected internally. If the spleen is affected, in the seventy-two days of the four season-months[44] there will be abdominal distention, vexation, and no desire to eat. In needling the flesh, one must not injure the vessels. If the vessels are injured, the heart will be affected internally. If the heart is affected, there will be heart pain in summer. In needling the vessels, one must not injure the sinews. If the sinews are injured, the liver will be affected internally. If the liver is affected, there will be diseases such as heat disease and slack sinews in the spring. In needling the sinews, one must not injure the bones. If the bones are injured, the kidney is affected internally. If the kidney is affected, there will be distention and pain in the lumbus in the winter. In needling the bones, one must not injure the marrow. If the marrow is injured, there will be aching pain and weakness in the lower leg, fatigue and lassitude, and inability to move about.

(2)

Spirit Court (*Shen Ting*, GV 24) is prohibited to needling. Upper Pass (*Shang Guan*, GB 3) may not be needled deeply. ["Deep needle insertion causes deafness." {later editor}] Small Lu (*Lu Xi*, TH 19) may not be needled to cause copious bleeding. The left corner of the head[45] may not be needled with prolonged retention. Needling Man's Prognosis (*Ren Ying*, St 9) too deeply will kill a person. Cloud Gate (*Yun Men*, Lu 2) may not be needled deeply. ["Deep needle insertion causes counterflow dyspnea and inability to ingest food." {later editor}] The center of the navel[46] is prohibited to needling. Five Li (*Wu Li*, Liv 10) may not be needled. Crouching Rabbit (*Fu Tu*, St 32) may not be needled. [{In the discussion} regarding this point[47] (the author) prescribes a needle insertion of five *fen*. {later editor}] Three Yang Connecting (*San Yang Luo*, TH 8) may not be needled. Recover Flow (*Fu Liu*, Ki 7) may not be needled to cause copious bleeding. Sinew Support (*Cheng Jin*, Bl 56) may not be needled. Blazing Valley (*Ran Gu*, Ki 2) may not be needled to cause copious bleeding. Breast Center (*Ru Zhong*, St 17) may not be needled. Turtledove Tail (*Jiu Wei*, CV 15) may not be needled. The above points are prohibited to needling.[48]

Head Corner (*Tou Wei*, St 8) is prohibited to moxibustion. Light Guard (*Cheng Guang*, Bl 6) may not be moxaed. Brain Door (*Nao Hu*, GV 17) may not be moxaed. Wind Mansion (*Feng Fu*, GV 16) may not be moxaed. Loss of Voice Gate (*Yin Men*, GV 15) may not be moxaed. [Moxibustion may cause loss of voice. {later editor}] Lower Pass (*Xia Guan*, St 7) may not be moxaed if there is wax in the ear. Ear Gate (*Er Men*, TH 21) may not be moxaed if there is pus and ear wax in the ear. Man's Prognosis (*Ren Ying*, St 9) may not be moxaed. Silk Bamboo Hole (*Si Zhu Kong*, TH 23) may not be moxaed. [Moxibustion may cause an unfortunate narrowing of the eyes or blindness. {later editor}] Tear Container (*Cheng Qi*, St 1) may not be moxaed. Spinal Center (*Ji Zhong*, GV 6) may not be moxaed. [Moxibustion may cause hunched back. {later editor}] White Ring Shu (*Bai Huan Shu*, Bl 30) may not be moxaed. Center of the Nipple (*Ru Zhong*, St 17) may not be moxaed. Stone Door (*Shi Men*, CV 5) may not be moxaed in females. Qi Thoroughfare (*Qi Jie*, St 30) may not be moxaed. [Moxibustion may cause an unfortunate difficulty in breathing. {later editor}] Armpit Abyss (*Yuan Ye*, GB 22) may not be moxaed. [Moxibustion may cause an unfortunate corrosive swelling. {later editor}] Channel Ditch (*Jing Qu*, Lu 8) may not be moxaed. [Moxibustion may impair a person's spirit. {later editor}] Turtledove Tail (*Jiu Wei*, CV 15) may not be moxaed. Yin Market (*Yin Shi*, St 33) may not be moxaed. Yang Pass (*Yang Guan*, GV 3) may not be moxaed. Celestial Storehouse (*Tian Fu*, Lu 3) may not be moxaed. [Moxibustion may cause counterflow breathing. {later editor}] Crouching Rabbit (*Fu Tu*, St 32) may not be moxaed. Earth Fivefold Convergence (*Di Wu Hui*, GB 42) may not be moxaed. [Moxibustion may make the body thin. {later editor}] Spasm Vessel (*Qi Mai*, TH 18) may not be moxaed. The above points are contraindicated to moxibustion.

(3)

The key in needling is to strike the point of qi while not striking the juncture between the muscle and the bone. The sensation of hitting the point of qi is like walking on an open street, but striking the juncture between the muscle and the bone causes nothing but pain in the skin.[49]

Inappropriate application of draining and supplementing therapies will only aggravate the disease. If one (inadvertently) strikes the sinew, that sinew will become slack and the evil qi will not be expelled. Where that (evil qi) contends with the true (qi), it will wreak havoc and not depart. On the contrary, (the evil qi will penetrate) even further into the interior. Indiscreet application of the needle will only make the situation worse.

(4)

As for the principle of needling, supplementation and drainage must not exceed their appropriate measure, and, in the case of an incongruity between the illness and the pulse, needles should not be used. The manifestation of the first deprivation (*duo*, 夺) is emaciated flesh. The second deprivation (is the condition of the body) following a great loss of blood. The third deprivation is (the condition of the body) following a great loss of sweat. The fourth deprivation is (the condition of the body) following violent diarrhea. And the fifth deprivation is the postpartum state or (the conditions) following great amounts of blood loss. None of these states may be drained.

(5)

The Yellow Emperor asked:

Since a needle can kill a living person, can it also raise the dead?

Qi Bo answered:

(No. While a needle) can kill a living person, it cannot raise the dead. Humans receive their qi from grain, and it is the stomach which the grain (first) pours into. The stomach is a sea of grain and water, qi and blood. Just as the seas spread clouds and rain under heaven, the stomach distributes qi and blood through canals, and these canals are the major network vessels of the five viscera and the six bowels. Contrary use of retrenching therapies at these vessels will consume (the qi and blood).

Take, for instance, (the point) Five Li (*Wu Li*, LI

13). If an offensive manipulation is applied here, (the visceral qi) is deterred half way. (The qi of one viscus) can sustain five (such assaults), and five of these assaults mean exhaustion of the visceral qi. Therefore, five times five, i.e., twenty-five, mistreatments in succession deplete all of the transporting qi. This is known as retrenchment of natural qi. It follows that (due to malpractice of this kind) the patient may return home (from the physician) to die if the needle has been inserted shallowly or (the physician) will send him to his death on the spot if the needle has been inserted deeply.

The Yellow Emperor said:

Please pass these prohibitions for acupuncture on to future generations.

Chapter Two

The Nine Types of Needles, the Nine Affections, the Twelve Needling Manipulations, the Five Needling Methods, & the Five Evils[50]

(1)

The Yellow Emperor asked:

How is it that there have come to be nine needles?

Qi Bo answered:

The nine needles relate to the numerical system of heaven and earth. The numerical system of heaven and earth begins at one and finishes with nine. For this reason, one relates to heaven; two relates to earth; three relates to humankind; four relates to the four seasons; five relates to the five tones; six relates to the six pitch bamboo pipes;[51] seven relates to the seven stars;[52] eight relates to the eight winds; and nine relates to the nine regions.[53]

(2)

The Yellow Emperor asked:

How do the (nine) needles relate to the nine numbers?

Qi Bo answered:

The number one pertains to heaven, and heaven is yang. Of the five viscera, the one corresponding to heaven is the lung. The lung is the canopy of the viscera and bowels. The skin is associated with the lung and hence with a person's yang. Therefore, in treating (the skin), the arrowhead needle (chan) is employed.

The arrowhead needle is based upon the cloth needle ["towel" in a variant version {later editor}] needle which abruptly becomes pointed half a cun from the tip and is one cun and six fen in length. Because it has a big head with a pointed end, it will not penetrate deeply (into the body) and lets only the yang qi out. For this reason, it is suitable for treatment of heat in the head and trunk. Accordingly, it is said that, in the case of cutaneous problems with no fixed location, the arrowhead needle should be chosen (and manipulated at the location of the) disease. If the skin is white, however, it may not be used.[54]

The number two pertains to earth and earth is the soil. In the human body it is the flesh which corresponds to the soil. Therefore, in treating (the flesh), the tubular needle (yuan) is employed. The tubular needle is based upon the wadding needle. It has a cylindrical body, a round end like a (small) egg, and is one cun and six fen in length. It is used to drain the qi in the partings of the flesh, and, although it will not injure a person's flesh, it is capable of evacuating evil qi. Accordingly, it is said that, when a disease lies in the parting of the flesh, the tubular needle should be chosen.

The number three pertains to humankind. In the human body, it is the blood vessels which foster growth. Therefore, to treat (the vessels), the blunt (di) needle is employed.

The blunt needle is based upon (the shape of) broomcorn millet. It has a large body and a round end like broomcorn millet and is three cun and five fen in length. It presses the vessel without sinking deeply into it in order to access the qi yet drives out only the evil qi. Accordingly, it is said that, for diseases within the vessels and diminished qi, supplementation should be applied with the blunt needle, needling the well and brook points.[55]

The number four pertains to the four seasons. When a person, after having been struck by one of the winds of the eight directions and four seasons, develops a chronic illness where the evil has invaded and penetrated the channels and network vessels, then (this condition) is treated by the sharp (feng) needle.

The sharp needle is based upon the wadding needle. It has a cylindrical body and a pointed end of three blades and is one cun and six fen in length. It is used to drain heat and let out blood to dissipate and drain chronic diseases. Accordingly, it is said that, if the disease is securely housed within the five viscera, the sharp needle should be selected and draining (technique applied) to the well and brook points according to the seasons.[56]

The number five pertains to the five tones. The five tones are situated between winter and summer, and between zi and wu.[57] When yin becomes separated from yang, cold and heat contend with one another, and these two qi are in conflict, then yong and swelling [the Ling Shu says "yong and pus"] develop. Therefore in the treatment (of this kind of disorder), the sword (pi) needle is applied. The sword needle is based upon a sword. It has a sharp end like a sword and is two and a half fen wide and four cun long. It is used to remove serious purulent sores via bleeding techniques. Accordingly, it is said that one should select the sword needle in the case of serious purulent sores.

The number six pertains to the six pitches. These pitches serve as the regulators of yin and yang in the four seasons and correspond to the twelve channels. In the case of a visitation of a vacuity evil into the channels and network vessels resulting in fulminant bi, the round-sharp needle (yuan li) is used to treat this condition.

The round-sharp needle is based upon a yak hair which has a round tip and a body which is slightly thicker at the middle. It is one cun and six fen in length and is used to remove yong and swelling as well as the fulminant bi. Some people describe it as having a yak hair-like tip with a slightly enlarged end and a smaller body to facilitate deep insertions. Accordingly, it is said that one should select the round-sharp needle in the case of fulminant bi qi.

The number seven pertains to the (seven) stars. These stars are likened to the seven portals[58] in humans. When an evil has invaded the channels and become lodged in the network vessels resulting in painful bi, the filiform needle (hao) is selected for treatment.

The filiform needle is based upon the shape of a fine hair. It is one cun and six fen in length and has a sharp tip like the proboscis of the gadfly. (The needle) should be inserted slowly, twirled gently, and retained for a long duration in order to conduct the correct qi and to expel a true evil. After extraction of the needle, (the patient) should rest. It is primarily used to treat painful bi in the network vessels. Accordingly, it is said that one should employ the filiform needle in the case of enduring pain due to bi qi.

The number eight pertains to wind. Wind relates to the eight joints (of the thigh and humerus).[59] When vacuity winds from the eight directions injure the body and lodge deep in the bone fissures, intervertebral joints, and partings of the flesh causing deep bi, the long (chang) needle is selected for treatment.

The long needle, developed from the shoe needle, is seven cun long with a thin body and sharp end. It is suitable for removal of deep-lying evils and longstanding bi. Accordingly, it is said that one should employ the long needle for disease in the center.

The number nine pertains to the nine regions. These regions relate to the regions of the body delineated by the bones. When a vacuity wind injures a person or when a rampant evil spills over, as in a wind water (disease) pattern, hindering the passage (of true qi) through the major joints of the body, the large (da) needle is selected for treatment.

The large needle, developed from the sharp needle ["blunt needle" in a variant version {later editor}] has a slightly round tip and is four *cun* in length. It is used to drain evil qi from the interior and exterior which prohibits passage of the great qi through the articulations. Accordingly, it is said that one should employ the large needle when water swelling prohibits the passage (of qi) through the joints.[60]

(3)

The choice of these standardized needles is totally important in needling treatment. Each of the nine types of needle has its own use. Whether they be long or short, large or small, they each have their specific applications. If used inappropriately, the illness cannot be removed. If the illness is shallow and one needles deeply, this will only injure the healthy flesh and cause *yong* in the skin. On the other hand, if the illness is deep but one employs a shallow needle insertion, the disease qi will not be drained. On the contrary, this will result in grand purulence. If a disease is mild and a large needle is used, this will drain the qi too rapidly, ultimately causing further harm. If the disease is a major one and a small needle is used, the (evil) qi will not be drained off and this too will result in failure. The most appropriate manner of needling is to apply major drainage in the case of a major (illness) and to avoid drastic (therapies) in the case of minor illnesses. Having now spoken of the potential errors (in needling), please let me speak on the applications (of acupuncture).[61]

There are nine needling (methods) corresponding to the nine affections. The first is called transport needling (*shu ci*). Transport needling consists of needling the various brook and rapids points and the visceral points.[62] The second is called distant needling (*dao ci*, 道刺). In distant needling, if the disease is in the upper (part of the body), one selects points in the lower (part of the body), needling the *shu* transport points (appropriate to the disorder) on the bowel channels. The third is

channel needling (*jing ci*) where one pricks the places of binding in the network vessels and the channel routes of the major channels. The fourth is connecting vessel needling (*luo ci*) where one pricks the blood vessels of the small network vessels.[63] The fifth is parting needling (*fen ci*). In parting needling, one punctures at the separations of the flesh. The sixth is major drainage needling (*da xie ci*) [a variant version calls this "great needling" {later editor}] which consists of lancing areas of great purulence with a sword needle.[64] The seventh is hair needling (*hao ci*). Hair needling consists of puncturing the skin in cases of superficial *bi*. The eighth is grand needling (*ju ci*). Grand needling consists of (treating) the right side for (diseases) of the left, (or treating) the left for disease of the right. The ninth is fire needling (*cui ci*). Fire needling consists of using a red-hot needle to treat *bi* qi.

There are twelve needling manipulations (*jie*) corresponding to the twelve channels:

The first is paired needling (*ou ci*). Paired needling is characterized by inserting (two needles) with the hands in the patient's heart region and in the opposite region of the back. (The needles) should be inserted directly into the painful areas, one needle in the front and another needle in back. This is effective in the treatment of heart *bi*. The needles should be inserted obliquely (to avoid hitting the heart).

The second is reciprocal needling (*bao ci*). Reciprocal needling is effective for migratory pain which moves up and down and is characterized by the insertion of a needle directly (into the painful place. While the needle is retained,) the left hand of the practitioner palpates the affected area, and then, upon removing the needle, he re-inserts it (at a newly found painful place).

The third is extensive needling (*hui ci*). Extensive needling is characterized by the perpendicular insertion of a needle into an affected area which is then (repeatedly) lifted and thrust forward and backward. It relaxes sinew tension in the treatment of sinew *bi*.[65]

The fourth is uniform needling (*qi ci*). Uniform

needling is characterized by the insertion of one needle directly (into the affected area) and two others on either side. It is effective in the treatment of localized, small (-sized accumulations of) deep lying cold qi [the *Ling Shu* says "hot qi"]. It is also called tri(lateral) needling (*san ci*). This tri(lateral) needling is effective for the treatment of small accumulations of deep-lying *bi* qi.

The fifth is elevated needling (*yang ci*). Elevated needling is characterized by the insertion of a single needle into the center (of an affected area) followed by the insertion of (needles) at each of the four sides (around the affected area), all of which are shallow. This treats extensive chills and fever.

The sixth is direct (subcutaneous) needling (*zhi zhen ci*). Direct (subcutaneous) needling is characterized by drawing up the skin and inserting the needle (obliquely) along it. It is effective for the treatment of shallow-lying cold qi.

The seventh is dredging needling (*shu ci*). Dredging needling is characterized by the (rapid) perpendicular insertion and removal of a small number of needles which are inserted deeply. It is effective for the treatment of an exuberance of qi with heat.

The eighth is short needling (*duan ci*). This is a needle technique for (the treatment of) bone *bi*. It is characterized by a gentle shaking of the needle as it is inserted deeply to the bone. It is then (repeatedly) lifted and thrust to rub against the bone.

The ninth is superficial needling (*fu ci*). Superficial needling is characterized by the oblique insertion of the needle to a shallow depth. This manipulation treats sinews which are tense and cold.

The tenth is yin needling (*yin ci*).[66] It is characterized by needling both the right and the left sides of the body. This treats cold inversion due to cold in the center, and the point selected is posterior to the medial malleolus in the (foot) *shao yin* channel.[67]

The eleventh is adjacent needling (*pang ci*).

Adjacent needling is characterized by the insertion of one needle directly (into the affected area) while another is inserted obliquely adjacent to it. This treats long-standing fixed *bi*.

The twelfth is assisting needling (*zan ci*). Assisting needling is characterized by the (rapid), perpendicular insertion and removal of numerous needles to a shallow depth to let out blood. This treats *yong* and swelling.

In puncturing a place where the vessel lies deep and cannot be seen, caution should be taken to insert the needle gently and retain it long enough to empty the vessel. Those places where the vessel qi is shallow should not be needled (in an impetuous manner. Before) insertion of the needle, one should press the vessel aside to prevent the essence from escaping and to ensure that the evil qi alone is driven out. As for that which is termed the tri(lateral) insertion for promotion of grain qi (*i.e.*, the correct qi), one first inserts the needle shallowly, barely penetrating the skin in order to drive out yang evil. Next, one needles to drive out yin evil by (inserting the needle) slightly deeper to penetrate the skin and the flesh but not penetrating the parting of the flesh. Finally, one needles still deeper, penetrating the parting of the flesh to promote the emergence of the grain qi. The *Ci Fa* (Needling Strategies)[68] states: "The insertion of the needle is at first shallow to drive the qi of the yang evil [*Ling Shu* states "to drive out the evil qi and cause the blood qi to arrive"], then deeper to (expel) the qi of the yin evil, and finally as deep as is allowed, down (to access) the grain qi." This conveys the same idea. [This is given in order to explain the statement that tri(lateral) insertion of the needle is to meet the qi, which is found in a later chapter, "Consummate Needling".[69] {later editor}]

An acupuncturist who is not acquainted with the phases of the year,[70] the waxing and waning of qi and blood (within these phases), and the etiologies of vacuity and repletion is not a superior practitioner.

There are five needling techniques corresponding to the five viscera. The first is half needling (*ban ci*). Half needling is characterized by the shallow insertion and rapid withdrawal of the needle such that the needle does not injure the flesh. (This technique) resembles pulling a hair from the head ["as if pulling hair" in a variant version {later editor}] and is used in case of skin qi. (This technique) corresponds to the lung.

The second is leopard spot needling (*bao wen ci*). Leopard spot needling is characterized by the pricking of the vessels on either side, in front, and behind (an affected area) in order to release the blood of the network vessels. This (technique is done with a number of needles) and corresponds to the heart.

The third is articular needling (*guan ci*). Articular needling is characterized by the needling of each extremity of a given sinew (close to a joint or articulation). It is used for sinew *bi*. Caution should be taken against inducing any bleeding during this procedure. This (technique) corresponds to the liver.

The fourth is valley union needling (*he ci*). It is also called deep source needling (*yuan ci*) or forking needling (*qi ci*). Valley union needling is characterized by the insertion (of a single needle in the middle) accompanied by one on either side (such that it forms the figure of a) claw of a cock. The needles are all inserted into the partings of the flesh, and this technique is used for muscle *bi*. This (technique) corresponds to the spleen.[71]

The fifth is transport needling (*shu ci*).[72] Transport needling is characterized by the perpendicular, (rapid) insertion and extraction of a needle which is inserted deeply to the bone and is used for bony *bi*. This (technique) corresponds to the kidney.

(4)

The Yellow Emperor asked:

Since needling can (cure) the five evils, what then are the five evils?

Qi Bo answered:

The diseases, gathering *yong*,[73] major (qi)[74] and minor (qi),[75] and heat and cold are the five evils.

In needling a *yong* pathogen ["a sword needle is used". {later editor}] (The practitioner) should avoid taking offensive action against the leading edge (of the evil) and wait patiently for it to develop.[76] If there is as yet no purulence, other methods (of treatment) may be tried. Once (the evil) is deprived (of its lodging), it will disperse and eventually disappear. ["When *yong* occurs in any of the yin or yang channels, related channel points should be chosen and drained." {later editor}]

In needling a major evil, ["a sharp needle is used" {later editor}] to gradually diminish (the evil) by means of draining and whittling away at the surplus ["in order to boost the vacuity condition". {later editor}] (This modality) aims toward striking (the evil) directly. (Treatment should continue) until there is no observable anomaly within the muscle and the true has been restored to normal. ["The needle should be inserted into the parting of the flesh in the yang channel." {later editor}]

In needling a small evil ["a tubular needle is used" {later editor}] to gradually enhance (the correct qi) and to supplement insufficiency so as to render (the evil) harmless. Based on correct evaluation of the location of the disharmony, offensive measures should then be taken to attack the evil before it approaches. In this way, (the true qi) far and near will be able to find its way back, and (the evil qi) cannot invade from the exterior and circulate (within the channels). Thus it expires of its own accord. ["Insertion of the needle in the border of the flesh is required." {later editor}]

In needling a heat evil ["the arrowhead needle is used" {later editor}] to dissipate and cool (this evil. The evil) is then forced out with no means of return, thus nullifying the illness. The pathways must be opened and the gates must be unrestricted so as to expel the evil. Thus, the disease will be overcome.

In needling a cold evil ["a filiform needle is used"

{later editor}] to gradually warm (the cold). It should be inserted slowly and removed rapidly in order to access the spirit. While the gates are closed, the qi cannot be dispersed, thus allowing vacuity and repletion to become regulated and the true qi to be preserved.[77]

Chapter Three

Cross Needling[78]

The Yellow Emperor asked:

What is cross needling?

Qi Bo answered:

When an evil invades the body, it first settles in the skin and hair. If it becomes lodged there and is not eliminated, it will then penetrate deeper and settle in the minute network vessels. If it becomes lodged there and is not eliminated, it will then penetrate deeper and settle in the network vessels. If it becomes lodged there and is not eliminated, it will penetrate deeper and settle in the channels. In this way, it connects internally to the five viscera and disperses in the stomach and the intestines, affecting both yin and yang and damaging the five viscera. This is the course of evil invasion, beginning in the skin and hair and ultimately penetrating the five viscera in the final stage. In conditions such as these, (points on the affected primary) channel must be treated.

Now, an evil, having invaded the skin and hair, may enter and settle in the minute network vessels. If it becomes lodged there and is not eliminated and, due to some obstruction, cannot penetrate into the (primary) channel, (the evil) will then spill over into a major connecting vessel (i.e., one of the fifteen network vessels), giving rise to unusual diseases.

Once an evil has invaded the major network vessels, it may pour from the left side into the right or pour from the right side into the left. It may

flow up and down, from side to side, interfering with the channels and spreading into the four extremities. Despite its migratory nature, (the evil) qi does not involve the transporting points of the channels. (The technique used to treat such a condition) is called cross needling.

The Yellow Emperor asked:

Because this is a technique for treating the left side for a problem on the right or the right side for a problem on the left, in what ways does it differ from grand needling?

Qi Bo answered:

Once an evil has invaded the channel, if there is an exuberance on the left side, the illness will be on the right, and, if there is an exuberance on the right side, the illness will be on the left. It is also likely that, in the case of a migratory illness, the vessel on the right may have become diseased even before the pain on the left has completely subsided. In this case, grand needling is required to hit the (primary) channel as opposed to the connecting vessel. As for diseases of the connecting vessel, which are different from that of the channel in the location of pain, it is natural that a different method (i.e., cross needling,) should be employed. ["Grand needling is applied to the channel while cross needling to the connecting vessel." {later editor}][79]

The Yellow Emperor asked:

How is cross needling applied?

Qi Bo answered:

An evil invasion of the connecting vessel of the foot *shao yin* may cause a person to suffer from sudden heart pain with fulminant distention and propping fullness of the chest and the lateral costal region. If there is no accumulation, then one should needle in front of Burning Valley (*Ran Gu*, Ki 2) to let out blood. After about the time it takes to eat a meal, (the problem will) be relieved. For afflictions on the left, treat the right side, and for afflictions on the right, treat the left side. If the illness is recent, (even if refractory,) it will be relieved in five days.[80]

An evil invasion of the connecting vessel of the hand *shao yang* may cause a person to suffer from throat *bi*, retracted tongue, dry mouth, vexation of the heart, pain in the posterior aspect of the arm, and an inability to lift the hand to the head. (One should, therefore,) needle the point on the finger next to the small (finger) which is located the distance of a leek leaf above the corner of the nail.[81] One treatment is sufficient. A strong patient will be cured on the spot, and an old one will recover before long. For afflictions on the left, select the point on the right, and for afflictions on the right, select the point on the left. If the illness is recent, (even if refractory), it will be relieved in several days.

An evil invasion of the connecting vessel of the foot *jue yin* may cause a person to suffer from sudden *shan* with violent pain. (One should, therefore,) needle the point on the large toe at the juncture of the nail and the flesh.[82] One treatment is sufficient. A male will be cured on the spot and a female will recover before long. For afflictions on the left, select the point on the right, and for afflictions on the right, select the point on the left.[83]

An evil invasion of the connecting vessel of the foot *tai yang* may cause a person to suffer from head and neck pain as well as shoulder pain. (One should, therefore,) needle the small toe at the juncture between the nail and the flesh.[84] One treatment is sufficient to effect an immediate cure. If not, then one must needle the point below the lateral malleolus[85] three times. For afflictions on the left, select the point on the right, and for afflictions on the right, select the point on the left. In about the time it takes to eat a meal, (the patient) will recover.

An evil invasion of the connecting vessel of the hand *yang ming* may cause a person to suffer from qi fullness of the chest, rapid dyspneic breathing, propping fullness of the lateral costal region, and heat in the chest. (One should, therefore,) needle the finger next to the thumb at a point the dis-

tance of a leek leaf from the corner of the nail.[86] One treatment is sufficient. For afflictions on the left, select the point on the right, and for afflictions on the right, select the point on the left. In about the time it takes to eat a meal, (the patient) will recover.

An evil invasion of the palm and the lower part of the forearm may result in an inability to bend (the wrist. One should, therefore,) needle the region proximal to the styloid process, having first selected tender points by digital palpation. The number (of punctures) is determined by the waxing and waning of the moon. As the moon waxes, (one should add one needling per day counting from the appearance of the new moon, *i.e.*,) one puncture on the first day, two punctures on the second day, fifteen punctures on the fifteenth day, but fourteen punctures on the sixteenth day, etc.[87]

An evil invasion of the yang motility vessel may cause a person to suffer from pain in the eye originating from the inner canthus. (One should then) needle the point half a *cun* below the lateral malleolus,[88] two punctures per point. For afflictions on the right, select the point on the left, and for afflictions on the left, select the point on the right. In about the time it takes to walk ten *li*, (the patient) will recover.

If a person falls down and is knocked about, then foul blood will become lodged in the interior, causing fullness and distention of the abdomen and inability to urinate or defecate. It is then necessary, first of all, to drink disinhibiting medicinals. [The *Tai Su* states "One must drink blood cracking decoctions to disinhibit and expel (the stasis)."] This is (due to simultaneous) injury to the (foot) *jue yin* vessel above and injury to the (foot) *shao yin* connecting vessel below. (One must then) prick the blood vessel in front of Blazing Valley (*Ran Gu*, Ki 2) and below the medial malleolus, as well pricking the instep at the major beating vessel.[89] If no effect is achieved, (one must) needle the three hairs region,[90] one puncture per point. The moment blood is observed, recovery is effected. For afflictions on the left, select the point on the right, and for afflictions on the right, select the point on the left. In the case of a tendency to fright, melancholy, and sadness, needle the above formula.

An evil invasion of the connecting vessel of the hand *yang ming* may cause a person to suffer from deafness or occasional inability to hear. (One should then) needle the finger next to the thumb at a point the distance of leek leaf from the corner of the nail,[91] one puncture per point, and hearing may be restored on the spot. If not, then needle the middle finger at the juncture between the nail and the flesh,[92] and hearing will certainly be restored on the spot. If one cannot even occasionally hear (*i.e.*, there is a complete loss of hearing), then needling is not allowed. In the case of a sensation of wind blowing in the ear, this formula may also be needled. For afflictions on the left side, select the point on the right, and for afflictions on the right, select the point on the left.

(To treat) migratory *bi* with no fixed location, (locate) a place in the parting of the flesh which is painful and needle it. The number (of punctures) is determined by the waxing and waning of the moon. The acupuncturist should base the number of punctures on the state of exuberance or exhaustion of the qi.[93]

Needling more than the number of punctures (prescribed) daily may lead to desertion of qi (of the body), while (needling) less than the daily number will not drain off (the evil). For afflictions on the left side, needle the points on the right, and for afflictions on the right, needle the points on the left. If the problem persists, the needling technique may be repeated, using the waxing and waning of the moon to determine the number of punctures. As the moon waxes one puncture on day one, two punctures on day two, the number increasing to fifteen on the fifteenth day, and then fourteen on the sixteenth day, the number (of punctures) decreasing with the days.

An evil invasion of the connecting vessel of the foot *yang ming* [The *Su Wen* says, "the foot *yang ming* channel". Wang Bing[94] agrees with the *Su Wen*, explaining that after crossing each other in the face, the left and right routes of the channel run contralaterally, and it is reasonable to speak of the channel in relation to disease when dealing specifically with cross needling and the like. {later editor}][95] may cause a person to suffer from runny snivel nosebleeding and cold in the upper teeth. (One should then) needle the toe next to the large one at the juncture of the nail and the flesh,[96] one puncture per point. For afflictions on the left, select the point on the right, and for afflictions on the right, select the point on the left.

An evil invasion of the connecting vessel of the foot *shao yang* may cause a person to suffer from pain in the lateral costal region with difficult breathing, cough, and spontaneous sweating. (One should then) needle the toe next to the small one at the juncture of the nail and the flesh,[97] one puncture per point. The difficult breathing will be checked on the spot; the sweating will be checked on the spot. In the case of cough, warm clothes and (warm) food should be provided, and, in one day, the patient will have recovered. For afflictions on the left side, needle the point on the right, and for afflictions on the right side, needle the point on the left. The disorder will be relieved on the spot. If not, then repeat the needling formula.

An evil invasion of the connecting vessel of the foot *shao yin* may cause a person to suffer from sore throat, inability to ingest food, a tendency to become angry for no reason, and an ascension of qi to the diaphragm. (One should then) needle the connecting vessel in the center of the sole,[98] three punctures per treatment, six needling (treatments) in all and (following these treatments the patient will) recover on the spot. For afflictions on the left side, needle the point on the right, and for afflictions on the right side, needle the point on the left.

An evil invasion of the connecting vessel of the foot *tai yin* may cause a person to suffer from lumbar pain influencing the low and lateral abdomen and inability to breathe in the supine posture. (One should then) needle the sacral joint which is located at the paravertebral muscle at the iliac crest. This is Lumbar Shu (*Yao Shu*, Bl

34).[99] The waxing and waning of the moon determines the number of punctures. Once the points have been needled (and the needles removed), the condition will be relieved. For afflictions on the left, needle the point on the right, and for afflictions on the right, needle the point on the left.

An evil invasion of the connecting vessel of the foot *tai yang* may cause a person to suffer from generalized stiffness with rigidity of the back producing a dragging pain in the lateral costal region, even extending to the heart region in the interior. Needling should start from the nape and proceed down the spine, puncturing the places found to be painful by pressing the paravertebral (sinews) with the hands in a rapid manipulation. By puncturing three points, the patient will recover on the spot.[100]

An evil invasion of the connecting vessel of the foot *shao yang* may cause a person to suffer from enduring pain in the hip joint with an inability to lift the thigh. (One should then) needle the hip joint[101] with a filiform needle, and, in the case of cold, the needle should be retained. The waxing and waning of the moon determines the number of punctures. There will be immediate recovery.

Whenever a (primary) channel (is diseased), needle it. If no disease can be found along the course (of the channel), then cross needling should be administered.

In the case of deafness, needle the hand *yang ming*.[102] If no effect is achieved, needle the point on the channel in front of the auricle.[103]

In the case of tooth decay, needle the hand *yang ming* and there will be an immediate recovery. If not, needle the point where the (hand *yang ming*) channel enters the teeth, and there will be an immediate recovery.[104]

An evil invasion of the region of the five viscera may cause illnesses such as dragging pain along the vessel which comes and goes. On the vessel observed to be diseased, cross needle the nail of a related finger or toe[105] and prick the (affected) vessel so that blood emerges, one treatment every other day. If one needling does not resolve the problem, five treatments are sufficient.[106]

Abnormal transmutation (*mou zhuan*, 缪传)[107] may affect the upper teeth, with cold and pain in the teeth and the lips. Locate the vessels on the back of the hand and bleed them, then needle the foot *yang ming* at the nail of the middle toe.[108] In addition, needle the finger next to the thumb at the nail, one puncture at each point, and the problem will be immediately relieved. For afflictions on the left side, select the points on the right, and for afflictions on the right, select the points on the left.

In the case of swelling in the throat with inability to swallow or spit, cross needle the area anterior to Burning Valley (*Ran Gu*, KI 2) and bleed it. The problem will be immediately cured. For afflictions on the left side, select the points on the right, and for afflictions on the right side, select points on the left. [The above passage beginning with "swelling in the throat" and containing 29 (Chinese) characters is located within the passage beginning with "If the invasion of the connecting vessel of the foot *shao yin*..." in the edition of the *Su Wen* with Wang Bing's annotations.]

An evil may invade the network vessels of the hand and foot *shao yin* and *tai yin* ["tai yang" in a variant version {later editor}] and the foot *yang ming*. All five of these network vessels meet in the ear and connect with the left corner of the head. (Such an evil) may cause the five network vessels to become exhausted, resulting in a syndrome characterized by the normal beating of the pulses throughout the body although the patient is unconscious and in a deathlike state. This is called deathlike inversion. (In this case,) needle the point on the medial aspect of the large toe the distance of a leek leaf from the corner of the nail.[109] Next, needle the center of the sole.[110] Then needle the middle toe at the (lateral corner of) the nail.[111] Then needle the radial aspect of the thumb at a point the distance of a leek leaf from the corner of the nail.[112] Finally, needle the hand *shao yin* at the point at the end of the styloid process (of the radius).[113] Each point is punctured once, and an immediate cure will be effected. [The *Su Wen*'s inclusion of the hand heart governor in the needling prescription is mistaken. {later editor}] If not, blow into the ears through a bamboo pipe. Then cut one square *cun* of hair from the left corner of (the patient's) head and burn it to ash. Instruct the patient to drink wine with this ash. If the patient does not imbibe, then force it down. The patient will recover immediately (upon swallowing this ash).

In practicing (cross) needling, it is necessary to examine the channels by palpating along their pathways so as to determine their state of vacuity or repletion. Then a (specific) regulating therapy may be administered. (If a treatment) fails to regulate (the condition), channel needling may be administered. Pain without disease in the channel may be treated by cross needling. If a blood connecting vessel (*i.e.*, a varicosity) is ever observed in a cutaneous region, remove the blood completely. These are the essentials of cross needling.

Chapter Four

Needling Techniques[114]

(1)

The essentials of needling are easy to explain but difficult to master in practice. The mediocre practitioner abides by the form, but the superior abides by the spirit. Oh, spirit, the guest passes with it through the same door![115] Without a study of the illness, how can one understand it's source? The most essential aspect of needling is the speed (of manipulation). The mediocre (physician) abides by the passes,[116] while the superior (physician) abides by the (qi) dynamic. The (qi) dynamic confines its activity to the holes,[117] and, within the holes this dynamic remains composed, quiet, and delicate. (The sensation of qi around the needle) is difficult to experience, and its retreat is difficult to trace.[118] Those who have mastered this dynamic will never let slip a good opportunity to hit the target with their arrow.[119] Those unacquainted with this dynamic and those who are not familiar with the mechanism just draw their bow without knowing how to timely let fly their arrow. An understanding of the comings and goings (of qi) makes it possible for the needle to meet the qi. The mediocre (physician) is in the dark (when it comes to this subtle dynamic). Such miraculous knowledge is the sole province of the superior physician. The retreating is classified as the negative, and onflow as the positive. So long as it is based on a knowledge of the negative and the positive, unfailing treatment is guaranteed. A head-on attack (*ying*, 迎) will never fail to lead to vacuity,[120] whereas tracking (*sui*, 随) will surely contribute to repletion.[121] The use of either head-on attack or tracking to restore harmonization presupposes a correct assessment (of the problem at hand). What is discussed above comprises all the essentials of needling techniques.[122]

Whenever using needles, vacuity should be replenished, fullness should be drained, stagnation and stasis should be eliminated, and prevalence of evil should be evacuated. The *Da Yao (The Great Outlines)*[123] states that slow insertion in combination with rapid extraction replenishes, while rapid insertion in combination with slow extraction evacuates. Repletion and vacuity (*i.e.*, the presence or absence of channel qi) is so subtly manifest that it escapes perception. One must study which (evils have arrived) most recently and which are older in deciding whether or not to retain (the needles). One must study vacuity and repletion in deciding whether or not the patient will lose or gain. As for the mysteries of vacuity and repletion, the nine types of needle are most miraculous (in influencing the channel qi) and, when supplementing or draining, (the most appropriate) needle (technique) should be employed.

Drainage may be defined as head-on attack. Head-on attack means (rapid) insertion (of the needle) while twisting to enlarge the hole and (slowly) extracting it so as to discharge the (evil) qi. If (the points) are pressed following extraction of the needle, this is called penetrating warmth, and the blood will not be dispersed and qi will not depart.[124]

Supplementation may be defined as tracking.

Tracking implies (insertion of the needle) in a seemingly casual way, very gently as if nothing were being done, like the biting of the mosquito. After retention, the needle should be withdrawn quickly, like an arrow is leaving the bowstring and the left hand should coordinate with the right hand (to close the needle hole immediately after the extraction). In this way, qi is stopped from escaping, and, with the outer gate shut, the center qi is replenished. No static blood, however, should be allowed to be left behind and, if ever discovered, it must be removed promptly.

In manipulating the needle, a steady (hand) is of key importance. One should locate the correct point and must not insert the needle (off the point) to the left or right. A wondrous (result) hangs on the breath of an autumn hair.[125] The practitioner must concentrate on the patient and closely examine his blood vessels if he is to avoid mishap. Before puncturing, it is necessary to carefully observe the spirit of the patient's eyes and the region above the eyebrows. Only by unwavering concentration may one know whether a disease has lingered or disappeared. In pricking blood vessels, one should prick those transverse vessels around a channel point which look conspicuously full and feel comparatively hard.

Of the (evil) qi that has invaded the vessels, the evil qi[126] exists above, the turbid qi[127] exists in the middle, and the clear qi[128] exists below. Therefore, needling the sunken vessels[129] allows the evil qi to exit, and needling at the middle vessel[130] allows the turbid qi to exit. However, needle insertion which is unduly deep will push the evil deeper and aggravate the illness. It is, therefore, said that the skin, the flesh, the sinews, and the vessels are located in different places and that each disease lodges in a (different part of the body). Each kind of needle has a specific use, each has a different shape (and size), and each should be chosen to their best utility. One must not replenish repletion, nor evacuate vacuity. This will only further deplete an insufficiency or boost a surplus, compounding the problem and causing the disease to progress. (Unwarranted attack of) the five vessels[131] causes death, and (unwarranted attack of) the three vessels[132] caus-

es debility. Retrenchment of yin leads to inversion, and retrenchment of yang leads to mania. These are the hazards of needling.

(2)

The Yellow Emperor asked:

I have learned a great deal from you about the nine needles and wish to sum this up with a precis. Pray let me summarize this account, and please lend me your ear. You may stop me when you hear anything absurd and throw light on the problem. I would like this material to be passed on forever so that later generations may avoid the same mistakes. And I will impart it to whomever is worthy but keep it a secret from the unworthy.

Qi Bo answered:

I am ready to listen with pleasure to what your enlightened Majesty will say.

The Yellow Emperor said:

One of the principles in employing acupuncture is that one be well informed regarding the specific conditions of (bodily) form and the qi (of the five viscera and the six bowels) both above and below. (One should understand) the specific conditions of the left and the right, of yin and yang, of the interior and the exterior. (One should be informed regarding) the amounts of blood and qi, the negative and positive flows (of the channels), and the exits, entrances, and meetings (of the channel qi). Based on all this, attack must always be directed at that which is excessive. One must know how to unravel entanglements, how to replenish vacuity, and how to evacuate repletion of the qi both above and below. One must be acquainted with the four seas and examine their locations. One must examine the various points of a channel which are subject to cold, heat, rain, or dew. (All of these must be scrutinized in order to) regulate the qi. Clarity as to the courses of the channels and their branched network vessels yields an understanding of their anastomoses.[133]

In the face of cold contending with heat, skill is

required to reunite and regulate them. When vacuity borders on repletion, one must know how to identify and adjust them. In the case of lack of regulation between the left and the right sides, take hold and circulate it (via cross needling techniques). If one is conscious of that which is unfavorable or favorable, one may determine whether a case is treatable. When neither yin or yang is aberrant, a practitioner must then know that recovery will occur. In examining the root and the branch and studying cold and heat, the location of the evil may be determined and there will be no error in ten thousand needlings. In understanding the nine needles, the way of acupuncture is realized.

One must have a clear understanding regarding the five transporting points and be well informed regarding the slow and rapid (manipulation of the needle in the supplementing and draining therapies). One must also know the bending and stretching postures (prescribed in locating various points),[134] and all this knowledge should be systematic.

When speaking of yin and yang, one must be able to associate them with the five phases. The five viscera and the six bowels each store something. The four seasons and eight winds are ultimately understood in terms of yin and yang, and each of these manifests itself in a specific area (of the face) on which the various regions of color represent the five viscera and the six bowels. Detection of painful places on the left or the right, above or below results in an understanding of the cold and heat (nature of the condition) and an understanding of which channel is affected. Examination of the cold, warmth, slipperiness, and coarseness of the skin of the cubit region yields an understanding of what is plaguing the patient. Examination of what is above and below the diaphragm[135] yields an understanding of the state of the qi there.

Based on the above knowledge, the practitioner will select as few points as possible. He will insert the needles somewhat deeply and then retain them, and he will know how slowly the needles should be inserted.[136]

In the case of intense heat above, bear it down. If (it) develops from below to above, conduct it outward. The pain which manifests first is the one which should be treated first.

If there is intense cold in the exterior, retain the needle for supplementation (of the yang). If it has entered the center, drain it via the confluence point. If acupuncture does not help the situation, moxibustion is indicated.

If the qi is insufficient above, promote and propagate it (upward). If the qi is insufficient below, accumulate it by tracking the qi and retaining the needle. If yin and yang are both vacuous, the use of fire[137] is indicated.

If there is inversion with severe cold accompanied by sunken vessels along the borders of the bones where the cold extends to the knee, select Three Li (San Li, St 36) below the knee. When cold becomes lodged along the yin network vessels and has entered the interior, push it to promote circulation. When the channel is sunken, fire is indicated, and, if there is a binding in the connecting vessel which is hard and tense, fire may be used to treat it. If one contracts a baffling ailment, treat the points below the two motility vessels.[138] The selection of the yang (motility channels) in males and the yin (motility channels) in females[139] is prohibited by proficient practitioners. This concludes the discussion of (the principles of) acupuncture.

(3)

Whenever needling, vacuity should be replenished and fullness should be drained. Whoever adapts the laws of heaven and earth (to treat) according to the conditions and movements (of normal and abnormal qi within the body) will achieve success (as promptly) as the echo responds to the sound and (as surely) as the shadow follows the figure. This way is not one of ghost or god but one of perfect mastery (of the essentials of acupuncture).

The key to proper needling is to first attend to one's own spirit. In this way, the condition of the five viscera and the nine indicators are made clear and only then may the needle be inserted.

The manifestations ["absence" in the *Su Wen* {later editor}] of the various pulses and the expressions ["absence" in the *Su Wen* {later editor}] of the various omens (must be analyzed in an integrated manner) in conjunction with the compatibility between the interior and the exterior to avoid a form-biased diagnosis.[140] Moreover, unless the comings and goings (of the qi and blood) are made clearly known, one cannot treat people.

The essence of treating vacuity/repletion is that, in the case of the five vacuities, one must avoid acting rashly, and, in the case of the five repletions,[141] one must avoid acting too late. When opportunity presents itself, there is no time to lose. With one's hands in action, the practitioner is single-minded, seeing to it that the shining needle is moved steadily.[142]

One should remain calm and intent at all times, observing the response to the needle and awaiting the arrival of the qi. (The response of qi) is said to be mysterious, subtle, and without form. The appearance (of qi) is like the soaring of flocks of birds or swaying of millet in the fields, which, though perceptible, cannot be discerned. Retaining (the needle) is like lying with a bow fully drawn, ready to shoot, and extracting it is like letting the arrow fly. In needling vacuity, there must be replenishment, and, in needling repletion, (the evil) must be evacuated. Once the channel qi has arrived, the opportunity should by no means be missed. The depth of insertion requires careful calculation and, regardless of whether the condition is old or new, single-mindedness is required. As if perched above a fathomless abyss with one's hand grasping a tiger, (when holding a needle) the spirit must not be distracted by anything.

(4)

The Yellow Emperor asked:

I would like to hear (what parts of the body) are prohibited to acupuncture.

Qi Bo answered:

The viscera are vital areas and, as such, one should not fail to examine them. The liver develops on the left side, the lung is stored on the right,[143] and the heart is situated at the exterior. The kidney manages the interior, the spleen is at the service (of the viscera). The stomach is the marketplace. The parents[144] reside above the diaphragm. The heart of the will lies beside the seventh (thoracic) vertebra.[145] [The *Su Wen* says "small heart". {later editor}] Compliance with (needling prohibitions in these areas) brings happiness, while violation of them brings about calamity.

(5)

In applying drainage, the square[146] ["the compass" in the *Su Wen* {later editor}] must be employed. The point should be pressed while the needle is twisted so as to move the qi. The insertion should be performed rapidly and the needle extracted slowly so as to allow the evil qi to exit. The tip of the needle is inserted against the direction of channel flow. The hole should be enlarged in the process of withdrawing the needle so as to allow the (evil) qi to exit more quickly.

In applying supplementation, the compass ["the square" in the *Su Wen* {later editor}] must be employed. It is necessary first to feel the skin to expose the gate and then to spread the adjacent areas with the left hand while the right hand presses the skin. The needle should be twisted gently and thrust in slowly, all the while keeping the end of the needle perpendicular. The practitioner should remain calm and quiet and unremittingly focused. (The needle) is retained for a short time and, once the qi has arrived, it is extracted rapidly. (After withdrawal of the needle,) one must press the skin, shutting the outer gate so as to preserve the true qi. The key in applying acupuncture is never to forget to nurture the spirit (of the patient).

(6)

In applying drainage, the qi (of the patient) must

be at high tide, the moon must be full, the day warm, and the body quiet. The needle should be inserted upon (the patient's) inhalation. During the succeeding inhalation, the needle should be manipulated, and then, with the following exhalation, one should slowly draw it out.

Supplementation means conduction, and conduction implies movement. One must needle the brook (ying) points[147] (in all cases) and the extraction of the needle should be performed upon inhalation. One must examine the fatness and thinness of the form and the exuberance and diminution of construction and defensive as well as blood and qi. Blood and qi are (the mansion of) a person's spirit, and, as such, they must be carefully nourished.

Oh formal diagnosis, it requires no visual examination. By palpating the places of pain [the *Su Wen* says "after inquiry into the illness" {later editor}] and searching the channels, a clear picture of the case is formed. On the other hand, if no pain is found, it is possible that no understanding of the condition may be obtained. For this reason, (this examination method) is called formal.[148]

Oh spiritual diagnosis, it does not require the ears to listen. With eyes bright, an open mind and discernment, a clear picture presents itself. Although he is unable to express it in words, the examiner alone among all his colleagues sees clearly. The picture seems to him like the evening star, outstandingly bright, or (the sun) revealed from behind the clouds scattered by wind. For this reason, (the examination method) is called spiritual and is executed based on the three positions with the nine indicators. It has nothing to do with (the theory of) the nine types of needle.[149]

(7)

If the qi does not arrive when one is needled, regardless of the number (of respirations), the needle should be manipulated until its arrival. Only then may the needle be extracted, and no further needling is required. Each of the needles have their own specific use, each has a distinct shape, and each is effective for specified cases. The key issue in needling is to ensure that the qi

arrives and has an effect. This effect is said to be like wind scattering the clouds to reveal the clear sky. This concludes the principles of needling.

The juncture-crosses (*jie zhi jiao*, 节之交) constitute three hundred and sixty-five meeting points. If one has a knowledge of the essential (acupoints,[150] their implications may be revealed) in a single sentence and that is the end of it. However, if one has no knowledge of these essential (acupoints), one's discussion will be muddled and endless. That which is referred to as the juncture (*jie*) implies the exit and entrance of spirit qi as it circulates. It does not imply the junctures of the skin, flesh, sinews or bone.

Observe the complexion and examine the eyes so as to comprehend the dissipation and concentration (of evils within the body). Examine the form and listen to sound so as to discriminate evil qi from the correct.[151]

The right hand controls the insertion of the needle, while the left hand holds it and guides it. Only when the qi has arrived may (the needle) be removed.

Whenever administering acupuncture, one must first observe whether the vessel qi is in a state of intensity or ease. Then one may treat disease. If the qi of the five viscera is expiring in the interior, replenishment of the exterior will result in what is called dual exhaustion (*chong jie*). Dual exhaustion is assuredly fatal, and in this case, death comes quietly. This is due to mistaken treatment whereby the practitioner selects (points) which run counter to the qi of the viscera and vessels, such as those points in the axilla and bosom.[152]

If the qi of the five viscera is expiring in the exterior and the acupuncturist mistakenly replenishes the interior, this results in what is called counterflow inversion. Counterflow inversion is sure to result in death, and in this case, death is accompanied by agitation. This is due to treatment in which points are mistakenly selected at the extremities.[153]

As for the adverse effects of needling, if one has

struck (the disease) and yet delayed in removing (the needle), this results in leakage of essence. If one has not struck (the disease) and yet extracts the needle, this results in stagnation of qi. Leakage of semen aggravates the condition and causes the body to languish, while stagnation of qi generates *yong* and open sores.

(8)

In administering acupuncture, one must always be serious. In treating swelling, shake the needle; but in channel needling, do not shake it. These are the essential principles of needling.

In needling any hot (disease, one should manipulate the needle) as if one's hand were touching hot water.[154] In needling clear cold (*han qing*[155] disease, one should manipulate the needle) as if one were reluctant to take leave (of one dear and near).[156] In needling a vacuity condition, one must perform a supplementing manipulation when the channel qi is in retreat, and in needling repletion, one must perform a draining manipulation as the channel qi appears.

Upper Gate (*Shang Guan*, TH 3) should be needled with the (patient's) mouth open rather than shut, while Lower Gate (*Xia Guan*, St 7) (should be needled) with the (patient's) mouth shut rather than open. Calf's Nose (*Du Bi*, St 35) should be needled with (the patient's knee) bent rather than extended, while Inner Gate (*Nei Guan*, Per 6) should be needled with (the patient's elbow) extended rather than bent.

When disease is located high up and in the interior, select Yin Mound Spring (*Yin Ling Quan*, Sp 9) and when disease is located high up but in the exterior, select Yang Mound Spring (*Yang Ling Quan*, GB 34). When the yin phase suffers from a yang disease, select Three Li (*San Li*, St 36) below the knee. This should be strictly adhered to without any negligence. (Moreover,) needling may be discontinued only once the qi has arrived, and, if the qi should refuse to come, repeated needling is indicated.

Chapter Five

Consummate Needling[157]

All of the issues concerning needling are dealt with in a comprehensive way in the (chapter of the *Spiritual Pivot* called) "Consummate Needling (*Zhong Shi*)."[158] In order to have a clear understanding of consummate (needling), one must realize that the five viscera constitute a frame of reference, while yin and yang are the (basic) criteria for classification (of all things). Yin governs the viscera, whereas yang governs the bowels.[159]

The yang receives qi from the four limbs, and the yin from the five viscera. Drainage implies meeting (the flow of qi) head-on, while supplementation implies tracking (the flow of qi). Understanding how to apply meeting and following techniques, one will (be skillful) in the methodology of harmonizing qi, although this presupposes a familiarization with yin and yang. The five viscera belong to yin, and the six bowels to yang. Pray let me give an account of consummation in respect of the laws of heaven.

Consummate (needling) requires the utilization of the channels as the frame of reference. By palpation of the *mai kou* and *ren ying* pulses, one may determine whether there is a surplus or insufficiency of yin and yang or whether they are balanced or unbalanced. Such mastery of universal laws is called consummation.

Those who are considered normal are without disease. Those who are without disease are characterized by a congruity of their *mai kou* and *ren ying* pulses with the four seasons and by congruity (between the pulses) in the upper and lower parts of the body which are synchronous with one another.

In a normal person, the pulses of the six channels are neither bound up nor stirring. The root and the end[160] are joined with one another and work in concordance with one another in both cold and hot weather. And the form of the flesh is in good proportion to the blood and qi.[161]

If there is diminished qi, the *mai kou* and *ren ying* pulses are diminished, not matching their prescribed measurement. Then both yin and yang are insufficient.[162]

In this case, when yang is supplemented, yin will be exhausted, and when yin is drained, yang deserts. Accordingly, sweet tasting medicinals should be administered, and one may not drink harsh (*i.e.*, purgative) formulas. In addition to this, moxibustion is forbidden. If the disorder does not improve and one subsequently employs drainage, the qi of the five viscera are bound to break down.

If the *ren ying* pulse is twice as exuberant (as normal), the disease lies in the foot *shao yang*. (But) if it is twice as exuberant and there is agitation, the disease lies in the hand *shao yang*. If the *ren ying* pulse is thrice as exuberant (as normal), the disease lies in the foot *tai yang*. If it is twice as exuberant and there is agitation, the disease lies in the hand *tai yang*. If the *ren ying* pulse is four times as exuberant (as normal), the disease lies in the foot *yang ming*. (But) if it is four times as exuberant and there is agitation, the disease lies in the hand *yang ming*. If the *ren ying* pulse is five times as exuberant (as normal) and if it is large and rapid, this is called spillover of yang (*yi yang*) which is a type of external repulsion.[163]

If the *mai kou* pulse is twice as exuberant (as normal), the disease lies in the foot *jue yin*. (But) if it is twice as large and there is agitation, the disease lies in the hand heart-governor. If the *mai kou* pulse is three times as exuberant (as normal), the disease lies in the foot *shao yin*. (But) if it is three times as exuberant and there is agitation, the disease lies in the hand *shao yin*. If the *mai kou* pulse is four times as exuberant (as normal), the disease lies in the foot *tai yin*. (But) if it is four times as exuberant and there is agitation, the disease lies in the hand *tai yin*. If the *mai kou* pulse is five times as exuberant (as normal) and is, in addition, large and rapid, this is called spillover of yin (*yi yin*) which is a type of internal blockade.[164]

A case (of internal obstruction) characterized by discommunication (between yin and yang) is ter-

minal and cannot be cured. If the *ren ying* and the *mai kou* pulse are both five times as exuberant (as normal), this is called blockade repulsion (*guan ge*).[165] In the case of blockade repulsion one's days are numbered.

If the *ren ying* pulse is twice as exuberant (as normal), drain the foot *shao yang* and supplement foot *jue yin*, draining the (foot *shao yang*) twice as much as the (foot *jue yin*) is supplemented once a day.[166]

(Treatment must be preceded) by palpation and examination of (the two pulses). If they are agitated, treat the upper (*i.e.*, channels of the hand)[167] until qi is restored to harmony.

If the *ren ying* pulse is three times as exuberant (as normal), drain the foot *tai yang* and supplement the foot *shao yin*, draining (the foot *tai yang*) twice as much as (the foot *shao yin*) is supplemented, once every other day. (Treatment must be preceded) by palpation and examination of (the two pulses). If they are found to be agitated, treat the upper (arm channels) until qi is restored to harmony.

If the *ren ying* pulse is four times as exuberant (as normal), drain the foot *yang ming* and supplement the foot *tai yin*, draining (the foot *yang ming*) twice as much as (the foot *tai yin*) is supplemented, twice daily. (Treatment must be preceded by) palpation and examination (of the two pulses). If they are agitated, treat the upper (part of the body) until qi is restored to harmony.

If the *mai kou* pulse is twice as exuberant (as normal), drain the foot *jue yin* and supplement the foot *shao yang*, supplementing (the foot *jue yin*) twice as much as (the foot *shao yang*) is drained, once daily. (Treatment must be preceded by) palpation and examination of (the two pulses) and must continue until qi is restored to harmony.[168] If the pulses are agitated, treat the upper (part of the body).

If the *mai kou* pulse is thrice as exuberant (as normal), drain the foot *shao yin* and supplement the foot *tai yang*, supplementing (the foot *tai yang*) twice as much as (the foot *shao yin*) is drained, once every other day. (Treatment must be preceded by) palpation and examination of (the two pulses) and must continue until the qi is restored to harmony. If the pulses are agitated, treat the upper (part of the body).

If the *mai kou* pulse is four times as exuberant (as normal), drain the foot *tai yin* and supplement the foot *yang ming*, supplementing (the foot *yang ming*) twice as much as (the foot *tai yin*) is drained, twice daily. (Treatment must be preceded by) palpation of (the two pulses) and must continue until the qi is restored to harmony. If the pulses are found to be agitated, treat the upper (part of the body). The reason treatment may be administered twice a day is that the *tai yin* governs the stomach and is particularly rich in grain qi. Therefore, it may be administered twice a day.

If the *ren ying* and the *mai kou* pulses are both five times or more [the *Ling Shu* says "four times" {later editor}] as exuberant (as normal), this is called spillover of yin and yang (*yin yang ju yi*). In this case, stoppage (created by a spillover of yin and yang) obstructs the blood vessels and the qi, unable to circulate (normally), floods the interior, causing internal damage to the five viscera. In this instance, if moxibustion is administered, it will only serve to transmute the condition into other problems.

A basic principle of needling (is to continue treatment) until the qi is harmonized and only then may it be discontinued. Supplementation of yin accompanied by drainage of yang renders the (patient's) voice resonant and makes his hearing and eyesight acute. The converse of this inhibits the flow of blood and qi.[169]

That which is said to be the (therapeutic) effect of the arrival of the qi is manifest in the vacuity of the pulse once drainage has been administered. This evacuation is expressed by a pulse which remains large but which is not as hard. If, however, the pulse remains large and becomes still harder, although (the patient) may express relief, the illness has not been reduced in the least.

Supplementation results in a replenishing (of the channels). This replenishment is manifest in a pulse which is just as large as previously but has become harder. If the pulse remains as large as before but becomes no harder, although the patient may express relief, the illness has not been reduced in the least.

If one supplements, there is sure to be replenishment, while if one drains, there is sure to be evacuation. Although the illness may not appear to have been diminished following acupuncture, it will indeed have been mollified. One must first become familiar with the development of illness within the twelve channels and only then may the implications of consummation be imparted. Yin and yang must not be confused with one another, and one must not deviate in (the treatment of) vacuity and repletion. Only in this way may one treat the channel (to cure the disease).[170]

Whenever needling any (of the illnesses) indicated (for treatment with acupuncture), it is necessary to employ the triple needling method[171] to attain the grain qi. Promiscuous blending of the evil and true qi dislocates yin and yang, reverses the normal flow, transposes the superficial and the deep-lying, and renders the pulse incongruous to the four seasons. As a consequence of this, (the evil qi) becomes lodged, permeating and sapping (the true qi), and, therefore, (this evil) must be punctured so as to drive it out. Upon initial insertion of the needle, the yang evil is expelled. Upon subsequent insertion of the needle, the yin evil exits. And upon the third insertion of the needle, the grain qi is drawn out, bringing the treatment to a close. The so-called arrival of the grain qi implies that supplementation has replenished (the channel) and drainage has evacuated (the channel). Thus one may know that the grain qi has been attained.[172]

Once the evil qi has been removed, despite a failure to regulate yin and yang, the disease will display signs of improvement. This is why it is said that supplementation is sure to replenish, while drainage is sure to evacuate, and that, although the disease may not appear to have diminished following acupuncture, it will have indeed been mollified. [This passage seems to offer an explanation about what is discussed in the third chapter. {later editor}]

If yang is exuberant and yin is vacuous,[173] one must first supplement yin and then drain yang in order to harmonize them. If yin is exuberant while yang is vacuous, one must first supplement yang and then drain yin in order to harmonize them.

The three vessels[174] pulse around the large toe, and their state of repletion and vacuity should be examined. Draining vacuity is doubling vacuity, and doubling vacuity only aggravates the illness. (Prior to) needling such a condition, the pulsing of the vessels must be palpated. If they are pounding, replete, and racing, then drainage is justified. If they are vacuous and slow, supplementation is justified. Contrary treatment will only aggravate the illness. The three beating vessels are located as follows: The *yang ming* lies above, the *jue yin* lies in the middle, and the *shao yin* lies below.[175]

The points on the bosom govern the bosom, while the points on the back govern the back.[176] In the case of vacuity syndromes involving the shoulder and the upper arm, select the upper points. In the case of double tongue, lance the tongue column[177] with a sword needle.[178]

If the hand is contracted and unable to stretch, the illness lies in the sinew, while if it is stretched and unable to contract, the problem lies in the bone. (In illnesses of the) bone, one should treat the bone, while in (illnesses of the) sinews, one should treat the sinews.

Where (a condition) is only just becoming replete, supplementation[179] must be administered. The needle should be inserted deeply and the punctured hole is not immediately pressed (after the extraction of the needle) so as to allow maximal expulsion of evil qi.

Where (a condition) is only just becoming vacuous, one must needle shallowly in order to nurse the vessel, and the punctured hole should be pressed immediately (after the extraction of the needle) in order to prevent the evil qi from penetrating.

The evil qi appears tense and urgent, while the grain qi feels gentle and quiet.[180]

If the pulse is replete, needle deeply to drain the (evil) qi, but if the pulse is vacuous, needle shallowly to prevent the essential qi from escaping so as to nourish the vessel while allowing only the evil qi to escape.

When needling any sort of pain, the needle must be inserted deeply. This is because all kinds of pain are accompanied by a replete pulse.

For illnesses from the waist up, the hand *tai yin* and the hand *yang ming* are effective, but for problems from the waist down, the foot *tai yin* and the foot *yang ming* are effective.

For illnesses in the lower (part of the body), select points above, but for illnesses in the upper (part of the body), select points below.[181]

For illnesses in the head, select points in the foot, but for illnesses in the lumbus, select points in the popliteal fossa. When a disease is generated in the head, there will be heavy headedness. When it is generated in the hand, there will be heaviness of the arm. And when it is generated in the foot, there will be heaviness of the foot. To treat such illnesses, first needle the place where the illness begins.

The spring qi lies within the fine hair; the summer qi lies within the skin; the autumn qi lies within the border of the flesh; and the winter qi lies within the sinews and bones.[182] When needling (seasonal) illnesses, each should be treated with reference to its depths in the four seasons. In needling a fat person, (the depth of the needle insertion) should be similar to that (of an average person) in autumn and winter. To treat a thin person, (the depth of the needle insertion) should be similar to that (of an average person) in spring and summer.

Pain disorders are yin in nature, and pain which

is difficult to locate by palpation is also yin. These must be needled deeply. Itching is yang in nature and should be needled shallowly. Diseases located in the upper (part of the body) are yang in nature, while those located in the lower (part of the body) are yin.

If a disease originates in a yin (channel), one must first treat the yin (channel) and then treat the yang (channel). If a disease originates in a yang (channel), one must first treat the yang (channel) and then treat the yin (channel).

In a chronic disease, the evil qi has penetrated deeply. When needling such an illness, the needle must be inserted deeply and retained for a long period of time with treatment administered once every other day. Priority must be given to the regulation of the left or the right[183] and the removal of (stagnant blood) within the blood vessels.[184] This completes the discussion of the principles of needling.

Whenever administering needling techniques, one must (first) examine the bodily form and its qi. If neither form nor qi has deserted, [the *Tai Su* states, "if neither form nor flesh has deserted"] then, in the case of diminished qi and an agitated, rapid pulse, one must administer cross needling in order to retrieve the (true) qi which has been dispersed and to dissipate the concentration of (evil) qi. (Prior to needling, the practitioner should) retire to a quiet place and commune with his spirit with doors and windows shut. (The practitioner's) ethereal and corporeal souls must not be scattered, his mind must be focused, and his essence qi undivided. Undistracted by human sounds, he must marshal his essence, concentrate his mind, and direct his will entirely toward needling.

(In this way, the practitioner may skillfully practice) shallow insertion while retaining the needle or gentle, superficial insertion so as to successfully conduct the patient's spirit and finish the treatment with the arrival of qi. Deeper insertion for females and shallower insertion for males is the proper way to firmly restrain (the escape of true qi) and to prevent the evil (qi) from penetrating. This is called security of qi.[185]

Chapter Six

Natural Needling, Abnormality & Normality[186]

(1)

The Yellow Emperor asked:

Please tell me about the principles of natural needling.

Qi Bo answered:

The utilization of natural (needling) may be illustrated by the bursting of a dam and the drainage of its water into an abyss. This requires little (outside) force and yet the water is disposed of. In excavating a key spot from which to launch a charge, the channels can then flow freely no matter how impregnable (the illness is). This (analogy) is said to relate to the smoothness or choppiness of the qi, the clarity or turbidity of the blood, and the abnormal or normal circulation (of both the qi and blood).[187]

The Yellow Emperor asked:

Are there rules (for treatment) in relation to whether a person's complexion is dark or light and whether one is fat or thin, young or old?[188]

Qi Bo answered:

Those in the prime of life and of strong build have abundant blood and qi with solid and strong skin. Therefore, when they are affected by an evil, they should be needled by means of deep insertion and retention of the needle. This holds true for fat persons (as well). Those with broad shoulders, axillae and napes, thin flesh, thick skin, dark complexions, and drooping lips have black, turbid blood and choppy qi and move slowly. They are not enterprising and generous in nature. In needling such a person, the needle should be inserted deeply and retained to the maximum degree possible.

The Yellow Emperor asked:

How are thin people needled?

Qi Bo answered:

Those thin individuals having thin skin with little color, lean flesh, thin lips, and soft voice have thin blood and slippery qi. Consequently, their qi is liable to desertion and their blood is subject to damage. In needling them, the needle should be inserted shallowly and extracted rapidly.[189]

The Yellow Emperor asked:

How are average people needled?

Qi Bo answered:

Specific modalities should be administered based on whether their complexion is white or black. Those with a well-proportioned build and who are possessed of integrity in character have blood and qi which are in harmony. In needling them, do not deviate from the average measurements.

The Yellow Emperor asked:

How are those in their prime of life and those with strong bones needled?

Qi Bo answered:

They are possessed of strong muscles, mobile joints, and sturdy bones. If these individuals behave in a serious manner, their qi is choppy and their blood is turbid. In needling such a person, the needle should be inserted deeply and retained to the maximum degree possible. However, if they behave in a rash manner, then their qi is slippery and their blood thin, and the needle should be inserted shallowly and extracted rapidly.

The Yellow Emperor asked:

How are infants needled?

Qi Bo answered:

Infants have fragile flesh, meager blood, and

weak qi. Therefore, a hair(like) needle should be employed in needling them. This is inserted shallowly and extracted rapidly. (Treatment may be administered) once every other day.

The Yellow Emperor asked:[190]

What does bursting the dam and conducting the water into the abyss mean (in terms of acupuncture)?

Qi Bo answered:

(In an individual with) thin blood and slippery qi, rapid drainage may exhaust the qi.

The Yellow Emperor asked:

What does the saying "excavating at the key parts from which to launch a charge" mean (in terms of acupuncture)?

Qi Bo answered:

(In an individual with) turbid blood and choppy qi, rapid drainage promotes the free flow of qi.

(2)

The Yellow Emperor asked:

Abnormality or normality within the context of the five types of form and the measurements of the channels and network vessels are all established with reference to ordinary laborers. Those who have delicacies for their daily meals [the *Jiu Xu (Nine Hills)* says, "gentlemen who have meat for their daily meals" {later editor}] have slender bodies, weak skin and flesh, and swift, fierce, and slippery blood and qi. How can they be treated in the same way as ordinary laborers?

Qi Bo answered:

How can the flavor of meat and refined millet be compared to that of beans and bean leaves? If there is slippery qi, the needle must be extracted rapidly, but if there is choppy qi, it must be done slowly. If the qi is swift and fierce, the needle used must be small and inserted shallowly, but if the qi is choppy, it must be large and inserted deeply. Deep insertion implies retention, while shallow insertion necessitates rapid extraction. In treating a poorly clad laborer, the needle must be inserted deeply and retained, whereas in treating a noble or an official, the needle must be inserted gently and slowly since their qi is swift, fierce, and slippery.

The Yellow Emperor asked:

What is (the correct approach) to abnormality and normality of form and qi (in relation to acupuncture)?

Qi Bo answered:

An insufficiency of form qi with a surplus of diseased qi indicates that the evil is overwhelming (the correct qi) and, subsequently, warrants prompt drainage. A surplus of form qi with an insufficiency of diseased qi calls for prompt supplementation. An insufficiency of form qi with an insufficiency of diseased qi demonstrates that yin and yang are both insufficient, and, consequently, excludes acupuncture as a treatment. If the patient is needled, this will cause a double insufficiency (*chong bu zu*). Such a double insufficiency will result in exhaustion of both yin and yang, consumption of both blood and qi, vacuity of the five viscera, and wilting of the sinews, the bones, and the marrow. (This complication) is fatal to the old, and even the robust cannot overcome it. A surplus of form qi with a surplus of diseased qi is called a surplus of both yin and yang, and it warrants prompt drainage of the evil to regulate vacuity and repletion. Therefore, it is said that surplus requires drainage, while insufficiency requires supplementation.[191]

It is stated that if, when needling, one is unaware of the abnormality and normality (of form and qi) or (is unaware) of the degree of conflict between the true and evil (qi), this (invariably) results in inappropriate application of supplementation to treat repletion. This is the cause of spillage of yin and yang, spillage of blood and qi, bloating of the stomach and the intestines, internal distention of the lung and the liver, and dislocation of yin and yang. If vacuity is treated by drainage, the channels will become empty, blood and qi will become exhausted, the stomach and the intestines will become shriveled, the skin will become thin and adhered (to the flesh), and the hair and the interstice will be scorched.[192] The (patient's) days are numbered.

It is stated that, in the administration of acupuncture, the knowledge of how to regulate (yin and yang) is essential. Once yin and yang are well regulated, the essential qi is bountiful, form and qi are united, and the spirit is stored in the interior.

It is stated that the superior practitioner pacifies the qi; a mediocre practitioner is capable of plunging the channels into disorder; and an inferior practitioner cannot but cause the qi to expire and endanger life itself. This warning should not be ignored. One must first examine the (clinical) changes of the five viscera, the congruity between the five pulses,[193] the vacuity and repletion of the channels, and the tenderness and coarseness of the skin, and only then may acupuncture be administered.

Chapter Seven

External Assessment, and Suspending & Stopping the Needle in Puncturing[194]

(1)

The Yellow Emperor asked:

Now (the use of) the nine needles represents a degree of exquisite finesse on the microcosmic level and grandiose magnificence on the macrocosmic level. There is no end to its mysteries, and its implications are boundless. It is my understanding that (the application of the nine needles) is in congruence with the way of heaven, is analogous to human affairs, and is in correspondence with the changes of the four seasons. I would like to know whether all the (subtle and abstruse) problems concerned can be generalized within one principle?

Qi Bo answered:

As for all of these theories, can one not combine all of their complexities, such as the size (of the needle) and the depth (of its insertion), with a single principle? The distant is used to acquire knowledge about the interior via the exterior. That which is close-up is used to acquire knowledge about the exterior via the interior. They are said to be embraced by yin and yang and as boundless as heaven and earth.[195]

(2)

The Yellow Emperor asked:

When is it necessary to suspend and arrest needling?[196]

Qi Bo answered:

One must first be fully aware of the roots and ends of the twelve channels, the cold and heat of the skin, and the exuberance, diminution, slipperiness, and choppiness of the pulses. A pulse which is slippery and exuberant indicates a gradual disease process. A pulse which is vacuous and fine indicates a longstanding illness. And a pulse which is large and choppy indicates painful *bi*. If yin and yang are both impaired, the disease will be difficult to treat. If heat is found in the roots or the ends,[197] both above and below, this indicates that the disease has not yet resolved. If the heat has abated, this indicates the disease is resolving. In grasping the cubit skin, observe the hardness and fragility, the size, the slipperiness and coarseness, the cold and hotness, and the dryness and dampness of the flesh. In examining the five colors of the eyes, the conditions of the five viscera can be detected, and this, therefore, determines death and life. In examining the blood vessels, observe the five colors (of the complexion) so as to ascertain cold and heat, *bi* and pain.

The Yellow Emperor asked:

I still have no idea about suspending and arresting needling.

Qi Bo answered:

The principle of performing acupuncture is to be serious and earnest, quiet and calm. One must first understand vacuity and repletion in order to determine the applicability of rapid or slow needling techniques. While the left hand holds the bone, the right hand should feel (the area being needled) and make sure that the needle is not stuck in the flesh. Drainage demands straight needling, while supplementation must be followed by closure of the skin (hole). The needle should be twisted to conduct the qi so as to prevent evil qi from sapping (the correct qi) while at the same time accommodating the true qi.[198]

The Yellow Emperor asked:

What is meant by smoothing the skin and opening the interstices (prior to needle insertion)?

Qi Bo answered:

While the left hand is palpating the parting of the flesh and spreading the skin, the needle is inserted gently, slowly, and perpendicularly so that the spirit is not dispersed and yet the evil can be driven out.

Endnotes

[1]Part 1 is derived from Chap. 19, Vol. 4, *Ling Shu (Spiritual Pivot)*; Part 2 from Chap. 2, Vol. 1, *Ling Shu*, and Chap. 16, 61, and 64, *Su Wen (Basic Questions)*; Part 3 from Chap. 16, *Su Wen*; Part 4 from Chap. 41, Vol. 7, *Ling Shu*; Part 5 from Chap. 55, Vol. 8, *Ling Shu* and Chap. 26, *Su Wen*; Part 6 from Chap. 9, Vol. 2, *Ling Shu*; Part 7 from Chap. 51, *Su Wen*; and Part 8 from Chap. 52, *Su Wen*.

[2]Here, network vessels imply the grand or major network vessels. They are also defined as branches named after important points, for instance, Large Goblet (*Da Zhong*, Ki 4) and Woodworm Canal (*Li Gou*, Liv 5). For details, see Chap. 2, Book 2, present work.

[3]Despite the structure of the first sentence as it is literally rendered above, it is the network vessels which are located between the channels and not the brook points. In the spring, the *shao yang* is predominant

and the yang qi is ascendent. The network vessels lie superficially, and the qi at the brook points is slight. These are both qualities corresponding to spring.

[4]This implies problems such as tugging and slackening which are windy in nature and develop very swiftly.

[5]Even the *Nei Jing (The Yellow Emperor's Classic of Internal Medicine)* itself is inconsistent as to how the dispersed points are defined, and later scholars are even more divided. Since the point here is that one needles shallowly in the spring, the dispersed points may be understood as superficial points on the connecting channel.

[6]Given the inconsistencies within the *Nei Jing* itself on this issue, Huang–fu Mi is here making a comparison of statements from the *Su Wen* and the *Ling Shu*.

[7]The exuberance of the rapids points and the superficiality of the minute network vessels both correspond to summer when yang is exuberant and most exterior. Therefore, one needles these areas shallowly at the surface of the flesh and skin.

[8]This means the rapids points of the three yang channels.

[9]The channels to be selected are either the *tai yang, yang ming,* or *shao yang.* The reference to the parting of the flesh here refers to the relatively shallow depth of these channels.

[10]This means the hand and foot channels.

[11]The confluence is where the visceral qi submerges. Therefore, the so-called qi opening here means the confluence point of the hand *tai yin,* i.e., Cubit Marsh (*Chi Ze,* Lu 5).

[12]The lung here reflects the metal/autumnal quality of astringency in general. During the metal phase, yang qi is on the decline, having retreated to the confluence points, and yin qi is in ascendancy in the human body.

[13]The crevice means the deep hole.

[14]This implies that the needles inserted should be arranged around the affected part and manipulated gently.

[15]The kidney is the true yin. They are responsible for shutting and storage, *i.e.,* the manufacture of qi in modern parlance, and, in this context, their functions are becoming dormant.

[16]I.e., the foot *tai yang*

[17]In this context, the words "lies deeply" and "departed" refer to a reduction in function of the channel qi

and should not be taken literally in the sense of the channels themselves being located deeper.

[18]The above seasonal needling techniques are all based upon the depth and location of evil qi within the body. For instance, since the yang qi floats to the exterior in the spring and summer, evils reside shallowly. Thus, deep needling is not indicated. In the spring, one selects the brook points and the network vessels. And in the summer, one selects the rapids points and the minute network vessels, and, during this time, one should also needle in the borders between the flesh.

[19]Needling summer points in the spring injures the heart qi, therefore causing the blood vessels to become chaotic. Not only is the illness not cured, but heart fire becomes debilitated and fails to nourish stomach earth via the ten stems generation cycle, thus resulting in poor appetite and diminished qi. Needling autumn points in the spring injures the lung qi, and, since liver wood fails to receive the qi of autumn via the five phases control cycle, sinew spasms and counterflow of liver qi result. This ultimately produces cough. Susceptibility to fright is the result of damage to the liver, while crying is a result of damage to the lung.

[20]Some sources say laughter. This is possibly a typographical error.

[21]Needling spring points in the summer injures the liver which then fails to nourish the sinews and the person becomes fatigued. Needling autumn points in the summer injures the lung which results in oppression in the ears and muteness. This damage to the mother (the lung) also causes illness in the son (the kidney) in the form of apprehension. Needling winter points in the summer injures the kidneys. A vacuity of kidney essence with a failure to transform qi results in diminished qi. If water fails to moisten wood, there will also be irascibility.

[22]Needling spring points in the autumn injures the liver which causes the heart to lose its mother, resulting in an insufficiency of spirit qi, forgetfulness, etc. Needling summer points in the autumn injures the heart qi, so that heart fire fails to generate earth and somnolence results. The heart cannot store the spirit and, therefore, there is frequent dreaming. Needling winter points in the autumn injures the kidney so that the kidney cannot store and qi and blood are scattered. This results in occasional shivering.

[23]Needling spring points in the winter injures the liver which then fails to store the *hun,* causing the spirit and *hun* to become chaotic. This results in an individual desiring to lay down but being unable to sleep or, having fallen asleep, to see odd visages.

Needling summer points in the winter injures the qi of the blood vessels due to the relationship of the vessels with the heart. Damage to the blood vessels causes a counterflow of qi and allows the simultaneous invasion of external evils into the vessels resulting in *bi* patterns. Needling autumn points in the winter injures the lung and damage to the mother causes illness in the son (*i.e.*, the kidney). This manifests as a depletion of kidney water resulting in constant thirst.

[24] *I.e.*, the yang channels on the lateral or the posterior aspect

[25] *I.e.*, the part below the waist

[26] *I.e.*, the yin channels in the medial or the anterior aspect

[27] *I.e.*, the part above the waist

[28] *I.e.*, the vessel running to the eyes

[29] The association of the location of the channel qi with a given month is as follows:
Month 1, left foot *shao yang*
Month 2, left foot *tai yang*
Month 3, left foot *yang ming*
Month 4, right foot *yang ming*
Month 5, right foot *tai yang*
Month 6, right foot *shao yang*
Month 7, right foot *shao yin*
Month 8, right foot *tai yin*
Month 9, right foot *jue yin*
Month 10, left foot *jue yin*
Month 11, left foot *tai yin*
Month 12, left foot *shao yin*

[30] This chapter supposedly from the *Su Wen* is missing and cannot be found in any of the extant versions published in history. Thanks to the efforts of many generations of researchers, it has been recovered. It is included in some editions brought out in recent years in the mainland. It is arranged as the seventy–second chapter in the *Huang Di Nei Jing Su Wen with Translation in Contemporary Chinese and Commentaries*, ed. by Medical Classics Office of Nanjing College of Traditional Chinese Medicine, published by Shanghai Science & Technology Press, 1981.

[31] This refers to an exuberance of heat or fire.

[32] One must not needle during periods of intense cold because the circulation of qi and blood is sluggish and the defensive qi lies deeply. During periods of intense heat, the blood circulates freely and the defensive qi is superficial, so there are no proscriptions against needling.

[33] In general, all of the above conditions result in a state of chaotic qi making acupuncture therapy inappropriate.

[34] Because the five flavors from the five grains supply the fuel for generating and sustaining qi, when there is a desertion of these flavors and they no longer provide nourishment, then the qi will be lost.

[35] This means that in needling illnesses of the bones, for instance, the needle should penetrate deeply to the level of the bones. If the needle only reaches the level of the sinews and fails to reach the level of the bones, this will cause the illness to become lodged in the sinews as well, thus injuring the sinews. This dynamic holds true for needling on every level of tissue.

[36] The flowing vessel indicates the blood vessels flowing into the eyes.

[37] Commonly known as Upper Pass (*Shang Guan*, GB 3)

[38] Discharge of pus from the ears.

[39] Specifically the scattered vessels around Burning Valley (*Ran Gu*, Ki 2), in a depression anterior to the medial malleolus.

[40] Another name for Bend Middle (*Wei Zhong*, Bl 40)

[41] Corrosion in this context refers to a severe, persistent swelling located inside the breast which causes putrefaction internally and the exudation of pus externally.

[42] Leakage refers to constant lacrimation.

[43] Part 1 is derived from Chap. 50, *Su Wen*; Part 2 from unknown source; Part 3 from Chap. 4, Vol. 1, *Ling Shu*; Part 4 from Chap. 61, Vol. 9, *Ling Shu*; and Part 5 from Chap. 60, Vol. 9, *Ling Shu*.

[44] Because the spleen does not correspond to a specific season, it "borrows" the last eighteen days from the last month of each season, *i.e.*, the third, the sixth, the ninth, and the twelfth months. It prevails during these seventy–two days.

[45] *I.e.*, Head Corner (*Tou Wei*, St 8) on the left side

[46] *I.e.*, Spirit Gate (*Shen Que*, CV 8)

[47] The point appears in Book 3 of this text, which is the list of points, their locations, and needling methods. See page 109 for this reference.

[48] The points listed are not all prohibited to needling even in this passage. The points particularly mentioned as contraindicated to bleeding, for instance, do allow needling.

[49] When walking on an open street, one is unfettered

and moves freely with no obstruction. When one strikes the point of qi in this manner, there is no obstruction and so there is no pain.

[50]Part 1 is derived from Chap. 78, Vol. 12, *Ling Shu*; Part 2 from Chap. 78, Vol. 12 and Chap. 7, Vol. 2, *Ling Shu*; Part 3 from Chap. 7, Vol. 2, *Ling Shu*; and Part 4 from Chap. 75, Vol. 11, *Ling Shu*.

[51]See Chap. 9, Book 1, present volume.

[52]This may refer to the plow.

[53]When applied to heaven, the nine regions refer to the nine divisions of space. When applied to the country, they refer to the nine counties in ancient China. When applied to the human body, they refer to the nine areas of the body, namely, the head, the breast, the throat, the hand, the foot, the lumbus, and the lateral costal regions.

[54]The characters *chan ci* may be rendered either as cloth or coin needle. In ancient China, certain types of ancient coins were shaped like arrowheads. This needle is indicated for illnesses of the skin without a fixed location. This is indicative of actively circulating fire qi. White skin indicates the absence of fire or yang, and, therefore, the use of this needle is not indicated.

[55]In pressing the vessel without sinking deeply, the blunt needle allows for the drainage of evil qi while preventing it from actually entering the blood vessel.

[56]The qi resides in the liver in the spring, the heart in the summer, the spleen in the long summer, the lung in the autumn, and the kidney in the winter. The implication of this sentence is that points should be needled on the channel appropriate to the season.

[57]In the Diagram of Nine Palaces, No. 1 is placed in the north which corresponds to winter and *zi* in the twelve earthly branches, while No. 9 is in the south which corresponds to summer and *wu* in the twelve earthly branches. And No. 5 is in the middle of the line between No. 1 and No. 9, that is, between winter and summer, *zi* and *wu*.

[58]The underlying logic is that the stars are high up in the sky and the seven portals, *i.e.*, the mouth, the two ears, the two nostrils and the two eyes, are likewise high up in the body. For this reason, the stars and the portals are linked together.

[59]This implies that the qi and blood run quickly like the wind through the joints which are their thoroughfares.

[60]Great qi in this context means the correct qi. However, it may also sometimes refer to an immense evil qi.

[61]Standardized needles (*guan ci*) are needles of an officially prescribed shape and size. Grand purulence simply denotes great quantities of pus.

[62]*I.e.*, the five transporting points below the knee and the elbow on the five visceral channels.

[63]These are pathologically visible blood vessels, such as spider nevi and large and small varicosities. In other words, they are visible blood vessels where there should not normally be any or blood vessels which are abnormally engorged and prominent.

[64]This is essentially the practice of lancing suppurative boils and lesions.

[65]Sinew *bi* implies hypertonicity, spasm, and contraction of the sinews.

[66]Yin needling in this context implies cold, and this technique is so named in reference to its treatment of cold evil.

[67]*I.e.*, Great Ravine (*Tai Xi*, Ki 3)

[68]This is a long lost work.

[69]Chap. 6, Book 5, present work

[70]According to the five movements/six qi theory, one of the six qi *i.e.*, wind, cold, summerheat, dampness, dryness, and fire, is extraordinarily active in each season. This is called visitation (guest) qi.

[71]In valley union needling, once *de qi* is attained with deep insertion, the needle is then withdrawn to the skin layer. It is then reinserted in another direction at the same point.

[72]The characters *shu ci* rendered here as transport needling are the same as those used above for dredging needling. Since they denote different techniques, we have applied different English words.

[73]Gathering *yong* (*chi yong*) is a binding accumulation of pathogenic qi causing *yong* and swelling.

[74]*I.e.*, overwhelming evil qi or repletion evil

[75]*I.e.*, shortage of correct qi or vacuity evil

[76]This means that draining therapy may not be prescribed at the fulminant stage of *yong*. The leading edge of the evil refers to fulminant swelling which has not yet suppurated. At this stage, it should not be drained or lanced.

[77]The gates referred to in this passage are the needle holes. These should be gently rubbed following extraction of the needle.

[78]This chapter is derived from Chap. 63, *Su Wen*.

[79]This passage differentiates between cross needling and grand needling. Both techniques involve needling one side of the body to treat illnesses in the other. Grand needling, however, is a technique for needling the primary channels in the treatment of evils within those primary channels. Cross needling is a technique for needling the network vessels and is used to treat evils lodged within the network vessels.

[80]Propping fullness is a subjective sense of fullness and upward pressure on the diaphragm. Accumulations here refer to masses which are often accompanied by hardness and pain.

[81]*I.e.*, Passage Hub (*Guan Chong*, TH 1)

[82]*I.e.*, Great Metropolis (*Da Dun*, Liv 1)

[83]The *Tai Su* states: "*Shan* pain is a yin illness. In females, the yin qi cannot overcome the yang. Therefore they recover before long (as opposed to immediately)."

[84]*I.e.*, Extreme Yin (*Zhi Yin*, Bl 67)

[85]*I.e.*, Metal Gate (*Jin Men*, Bl 63)

[86]*I.e.*, Shang Yang (*Shang Yang*, LI 1)

[87]The number of punctures may mean either the accumulated number of treatments at the same point or the number of points selected in one treatment.

The number of punctures refers to the number of different points which may be needled at a given time. As the moon waxes, the number of needlings is increased. However, as it begins to wane, the number of needlings that are allowed decreases. This technique applies only to the network vessels. Although an acupoint is specified for needling, it is the connecting vessel which is actually being treated, and the vessel itself is discerned by its prominent or abnormal color. The author specifies punctures rather than acupoints because they are not established acupoints *per se* but *ah shi* points surrounding an orthodox point.

[88]*I.e.*, Extending Vessel (*Shen Mai*, Bl 62)

[89]*I.e.*, Supreme Surge (*Tai Chong*, Liv 3)

[90]*I.e.*, Large Pile (*Da Dun*, Liv 1)

[91]*I.e.*, Shang Yang (*Shang Yang*, LI 1)

[92]*I.e.*, Central Hub (*Zhong Chong*, Per 9)

[93]The state of the qi here may refer to either the correct qi or the evil qi.

[94]See note 35, Chap. 4, Book 1, present work.

[95]The argument advanced by the later editor is specious and most modern researchers agree that the character for channel in the *Su Wen* is a typographical error.

[96]*I.e.*, Severe Mouth (*Li Dui*, St 45)

[97]*I.e.*, Portal Yin (*Zu Qiao Yin*, GB 44)

[98]*I.e.*, Gushing Spring (*Yong Quan*, Ki 1)

[99]Note that the point is Lower Bone Hole (*Xia Liao*, Bl 34) rather than the commonly known Lumbar Shu (*Yao Shu*, GV 21). It is suspected that the mistaken placement of Lumbar Shu must have been the work of some unidentified careless editor(s).

[100]Actually, the points to be needled are the painful spots lateral to the vertebrae. These are the so-called *Hua Tuo Jia Ji* points.

[101]*I.e.*, Jumping Round (*Huan Tiao*, GB 30)

[102]*I.e.*, Shang Yang (*Shang Yang*, LI 1)

[103]*I.e.*, Auditory Convergence (*Ting Hui*, GB 2)

[104]No specific point is defined here. The channel is needled at the point where it enters the teeth.

[105]The well points of the twelve channels are indicated.

[106]This is a general statement regarding any visceral disharmony producing symptoms along its related channel.

One should needle the *jing* points of the affected vessel, and, in the case of blood stasis in the network vessels, the affected connecting vessel should be bled at some other point.

[107]This is the transmission of disease in a manner not in accordance with the five phase cycle.

[108]*I.e.*, Severe Mouth (*Li Dui*, St 45)

[109]*I.e.*, Yin White (*Yin Bai*, Sp 1)

[110]*I.e.*, Gushing Spring (*Yong Quan*, Ki 1)

[111]*I.e.*, Severe Mouth (*Li Dui*, St 45)

[112]*I.e.*, Lesser Shang (*Shao Shang*, Lu 11)

[113]*I.e.*, Spirit Gate (*Shen Men*, Ht 7)

[114]Part 1 is derived from Chap. 38, Vol. 6, *Ling Shu*; Part 2 from Chap. 5, Vol. 2, *Ling Shu*.

[115]Form here refers to the apparent signs and symptoms. Spirit here implies the true qi or correct qi and the guest implies evil qi. The door refers to the coming and going or the waxing and waning of the correct and evil qi.

[116]This implies that the mediocre physician selects the points below the elbow and knee.

[117]*I.e.*, points on the channels

[118]This line implies that it is not permissible to apply supplementation when the evil qi is at high tide or to apply drainage when the evil is gone and the true qi is vacuous.

[119]This implies that one must access the qi in a timely fashion.

[120]This means that the intent of evacuation is realized.

[121]This means that the intent of replenishment is realized.

[122]The spiritual (or true) qi and evil qi come and go together, and concentration is required to discern them. The dynamic or change of qi acts only inside the hole of the acupoint, and this dynamic is exceedingly delicate and subtle. Therefore, careful discernment is required.

Head–on attack and tracking have a number of different connotations. Head–on attack implies draining the child; tracking implies supplementing the mother. The needling of a yang illness when the constructive and defensive circulate in the yang division is referred to as head–on attack, while the needling of a yin illness when the constructive and the defensive circulate in the yin aspect is referred to as tracking. Slow insertion and rapid extraction of the needle constitutes supplementation and is called tracking, while the reverse constitutes drainage and is called head–on attack.

[123]An ancient medical work, now missing.

[124]Depending on one's interpretation, this sentence may also be rendered in a quite different way: Extracting the needle with a hand pressing the point leads to inner warmth. Note that blood here means static or malignant blood and qi means evil qi.

[125]The Chinese often liken fineness, thinness, and the like to hair grown in autumn.

[126]Here evil qi is referred to in a narrow sense, that is, a wind evil which tends to reside in the upper part of the body.

[127]Here, turbid qi refers to evil qi or the accumulated turbid grain qi caused by dietary irregularities.

[128]*I.e.*, cool, damp qi

[129]The term "sunken vessels" implies the points located in depressions between the sinews or in the bone fissures. They are all located at superficial places on the body.

[130]This refers to the confluence point of the foot *yang ming*, Leg Three Li (*Zu San Li*, St 36). It never fails to provide a cure for diseases in the center.

[131]This refers to points on the channels of the five viscera.

[132]This refers to points on the three hand and foot yang channels or of the bowels.

[133]Being informed regarding conditions of the bodily form refers to whether one is fat or thin, and being informed as to the condition of the qi refers to vacuity or repletion.

[134]The phrase is interpreted by some scholars of Chinese medicine as follows: "the turns and bends, the exits and entrances of the channels."

[135]This refers to the five viscera and the six bowels.

[136]This appears to imply a vacuity condition since few needles are used, they are inserted slowly and deeply, and they are retained. Nevertheless, the above passage may be read as pertaining to both vacuity and repletion. Many eminent acupuncturists, such as Dou Mo (1196–1280), author of *Zhen Jiu Zhi Nan* (*A Guide to Acupuncture*), have instructed that the needle be inserted both slowly and gently as a matter of general principle so as to avoid causing the needle to stick and cause unnecessary pain.

[137]*I.e.*, moxibustion

[138]*I.e.*, Extending Vessel (*Shen Mai*, Bl 62) for the yang motility vessel and Shining Sea (*Zhao Hai*, Ki 6) for the yin motility vessel

[139]In males, the yin motility vessel, *i.e.*, Shining Sea, should be needled, while in females, the yang motility vessel, *i.e.*, Extending Vessel, is prescribed.

[140]The form, *i.e.*, symptoms or pathological changes, should not take precedence over the overall *gestalt* of the patient and the compatibility between the interior and the exterior.

[141]See Chap. 3, Book 4, present work.

[142]This refers to the steady, smooth manipulation of the needle without jerking or trembling.

[143]This refers specifically to the qi of the liver and lung.

[144]*.e.*, the heart and the lung

[145]*I.e.*, the kidney

[146]There is no firm consensus regarding this reference to square and compasses. It is safe to say, however, that they refer to manipulations of drainage or supplementation rather than to types of needle.

[147]Here the brook points are used in an all–inclusive sense, implying all the important points of a channel. Another interpretation is that *rong* refers to the constructive qi rather than the brook points. In that case, puncturing the constructive means insertion of the needle to the level of the blood.

[148]Formal diagnosis in this context implies diagnosis by palpation alone and does not involve visual examination.

[149]Spiritual diagnosis is achieved through the examiner's spirit–mind which reveals the true condition of the patient. The dark of evening and the clouds refer figuratively to confusing or baffling symptoms. This passage implies an intuitively based evaluation of the patient's condition.

[150]The essential acupoints are the five *shu* points, *i.e.*, the well, brook, rapids, stream, and confluence points.

[151]This may also be read: "Examine the form and listen to sound so as to discriminate a vacuity evil from a true evil."

[152]The state of intensity or ease within the vessel qi includes its state of vacuity or repletion and the severity of the illness. The *Lei Jing (The Classified Classic)* states, "the five viscera expiring in the interior implies a vacuity of yin and, in replenishing the exterior, one may mistakenly boost the yang. If one boosts the yang, this further damages the yin, resulting in dual repletion." In this case, the *chi kou* pulse is floating and vacuous and there is no strength when pressed. This indicates treatment to supplement the yin. However, if for instance one mistakenly selects the points of the yang channels, this will cause a further exuberance of yang qi to the detriment of the yin. The axilla and bosom are regions where the vessels of the viscera exit to the limbs, and, in the case of internal expiry of visceral qi, needling these points guides and drains the qi to the exterior, thus further agitating the exhaustion of yin.

[153]The *Lei Jing* states, "An expiry of visceral qi in the exterior is a yang vacuity. If one replenishes the interior, one mistakenly supplements the yin. Assisting the yin further exhausts the yang." If one selects the rapids points on the extremities and retains the needles in order to supplement the yin, this causes an exuberance of yin and a further depletion of yang. Such a condition precipitates a counterflow chill in the four extremities which is called inversion counterflow.

[154]This phrase suggests shallow insertion and rapid extraction of the needle.

[155]This implies a condition of yin cold stagnation.

[156]This phrase suggests deep insertion of the needle, patiently waiting for the arrival of qi, and slow extraction of the needle.

[157]This entire chapter is derived from Chap. 9, Vol. 2, *Ling Shu*.

[158]Chap. 5, Vol. 2, *Ling Shu*. In the present chapter the term "consummate" sometimes is referred to as the title of Chap. 5 of *Ling Shu* but sometimes as the concept of generalization or total knowledge. The term literally means the origination and termination or the commencement and ending.

[159]The five viscera constitute the basis for understanding everything concerning human life, while yin and yang constitute the broader framework for this understanding.

[160]The root here implies the internal organs, *i.e.*, the five viscera and the six bowels, while the end implies the form or body.

[161]See Chap. 16, Book 1, present work for a discussion of the relationship between the form of the flesh and the qi and the blood. For instance, a fat person with a sheenless complexion is possessed of a surplus of qi but an insufficiency of blood.

[162]This implies that the pulse is short, scant, and lacking strength and does not match the normal pulse.

[163]The *Tai Su (Essentials)* states that when the *ren ying* pulse is four times as exuberant (as normal) and is large and rapid, the yang qi is exuberant and spills outward. This repels the yin qi which is then unable to exit outward and is, therefore, called external repulsion.

[164]The *Tai Su* states: "When the yin qi is four times as exuberant as the yang and the *mai kou* is large and rapid, the yin qi is exuberant and spills inward, obstructing the penetration of the yang qi. This is called internal blockade." It should be understood that one rarely sees a *ren ying* pulse that is three or four times as exuberant as the normal in clinical practice. If one does, this is representative of a critical condition and the patient will most likely be hospitalized.

[165]According to the *Lei Jing*, this condition implies a complete disconnection of yin and yang.

[166]Most scholars feel that this is a reference to the duration of time the various needle techniques are applied.

[167]In this paragraph, the upper refers to the relevant channels on the hand, specifically the *shao yang* and hand *jue yin*.

[168]This phrase is ambiguous but probably means that the needling should continue until the qi is restored to harmony as evidenced by palpation of the pulse.

[169]The passages above detail the means by which one may determine the degree of vacuity and repletion in a condition based upon the exuberance or depletion of the *ren ying* and *mai kou* pulses. A *ren ying* pulse which is more exuberant than normal is indicative of an illness which lies within the yang channels. This is a condition in which there is an exuberance of yang accompanied by a vacuity of yin, and, as such, one should drain the yang and supplement the yin. A *mai kou* pulse which is more exuberant than normal is indicative of an illness which lies within the yin channels. This is a condition in which there is an exuberance of yin accompanied by a vacuity of yang, and, as such, one should drain the yin and supplement the yang. The pathomechanism here is nothing more than a lack of regulation between yin and yang, and therapy should be geared toward the regulation and harmonization of the tendencies of yin and yang to be either exuberant or vacuous.

[170]Depending on one's understanding, the sentence can be rendered in quite another way: "The channel must be treated if neither yin nor yang is prevalent over the other and there is no predominance of either vacuity or repletion."

This means that, if the channel is to be treated, neither yin nor yang or vacuity nor repletion should be stronger. For example, if yin is so vacuous that it borders on expiry, while yang is only a little vacuous or may even be normal or replete, then the channel should not be needled to address this condition. This is solitary yang lacking yin.

[171]This is a method of inserting the needle in three stages to induce the qi. More precisely, first penetrate the skin, then the flesh, and finally the parting of the flesh.

[172]The initial insertion implies a shallow insertion of the needle into the skin layer so as to allow the expulsion of yang pathogens. The subsequent insertion implies inserting the needle deeper into layers of the muscle and flesh, guiding the pathogen outward from the yin aspect. With the third insertion the needle is inserted into the border of the flesh to attain the grain qi. Techniques for supplementation or drainage are administered, and the needle is then removed.

There are no major commentaries which specifi-

cally define how long the needle is to be retained at each layer. The duration of time the needle is retained at each layer is dependent upon the attainment of qi at that layer or the amount of time it takes to manipulate the needle at that layer. For instance, the channel qi must be attained (*de qi*) before the needle may be inserted more deeply. Another technique specifies that, when the needle is inserted into heaven (the subcutaneous layer), it is twisted a certain number of times before being thrust into the human level (the flesh).

[173]In this passage, yang is referred to as the *ren ying* pulse, which is located higher, and yin as the *mai kou* or qi opening pulse, which is located in a lower place. The same interpretation of the two terms applies in other similar contexts in the present passage.

[174]The three vessels belong respectively to the foot *yang ming*, the foot *shao yin*, and the foot *jue yin* because all of these three channels originate in the neighborhood of the big toe.

[175]The vessels are 1) from Severe Mouth (*Li Dui*, St 45) to Thoroughfare Yang (*Chong Yang*, St 42); 2) from Large Pile (*Da Dun*, Liv 1) to Supreme Surge (*Tai Chong*, Liv 3); 3) from Gushing Spring (*Yong Quan*, K 1) to Great Ravine (*Tai Xi*, Ki 3).

[176]The bosom is referred to as the yin channels or rather, diseases involving the yin channels. The back is referred to as the yang channels or rather, diseases involving the yang channels.

[177]I.e., the major sublingual sinew

[178]The double tongue is a condition in which a smaller tongue grows beneath the tongue. This is, in actuality, a tongue–like swelling.

[179]Supplementation in this sentence appears to be a typographical error. The translators suspect something is missing from the paragraph.

[180]This is a description of the sensation of needling. The sentence can be paraphrased as follows: When the evil qi turns up, it will give one a tense and urgent sensation, but if the grain qi makes its appearance, one will experience a gentle and quiet sensation.

This sentence may also be read, "(If upon needling), the evil qi arrives, (there will be a sense of) tension and urgency (below the needle), while if the grain qi arrives, (there will be a sense of) gentleness and quietude."

[181]This statement should not be considered as contradictory to the preceding one, which is confined to an explanation of the selection of points.

Because the hand and foot *yang ming* and *tai yin* are interconnected, disease involving the hand *yang ming* in the upper part of the body can be cured by treating the foot *yang ming* or the foot *tai yin* in the lower part of the body.

The selection of points below in the treatment of an illness in the upper part of the body is called distant needling, while the selection of points below for an illness in the lower part of the body is called close needling. Both needling techniques are in wide use and are applicable in different cases.

[182]From the next sentence, it is obvious that the spring qi, etc., are referred to as the evil qi or disease in a season.

[183]This implies that cross or channel needling should be chosen.

[184]This implies bloodletting to expel static blood from the network vessels.

[185]Hua Shou offers another interpretation of this passage: "(If, for an extended period of time, the channel qi fails to arrive,) one should insert the needle more deeply and retain it there when treating males or lift it to a more shallow level and retain it there when treating females. In this way the qi will soon be obtained."

[186]Part 1 is derived from Chap. 38, Vol. 6, *Ling Shu*; Part 2 from Chap. 5, Vol. 2, *Ling Shu*.

[187]This passage is rather abstruse. The metaphor here is that of a dam which has been breached at a strategic place causing the entire structure to fall, allowing the water to surge away. One need not attempt to tear down the entire dam oneself. One need only exert enough force to create a small breach if it is located in the correct spot. By the same token, a skillfully crafted therapy need only exert a small influence to have a significant impact on a disease. To further complicate matters, there are similar expressions elsewhere in the text which, in a different context, have somewhat different meanings and implications.

[188]In this context, the lightness or darkness of the skin refer to overall complexion as opposed to any variables related to race.

[189]Slippery qi in this context implies that the qi circulates smoothly and freely.

[190]Many Chinese medical scholars have pointed out that this paragraph might have been a part of the first passage in this chapter. In that case, the passage would read in a more coherent manner.

[191]Diseased qi here implies an evil occurring on the level of the channel qi.

[192]In other words, the pores and glands will become dried up as the understandable result of an exhaustion of blood, and death will occur before long.

[193]*I.e.*, the pulses reflecting the five viscera

[194]Part 1 is derived from Chap. 45, Vol. 7, *Ling Shu*; Part 2 from Chap. 71, Vol. 10, *Ling Shu*.

[195]The assessment of the state of the exterior based on a knowledge of the state of the interior is called "close up" (*jin*). The converse is called "distant" (*yuan*) and an example of this is the ability of a skilled physician to predict signs and symptoms in a patient if he knows the state of vacuity or repletion of the viscera and bowels.

[196]The meaning of suspending and stopping is a little confusing. Some Chinese medical scholars interpret these as cessation of needle manipulation during the process of puncture because of the arrival or absence of qi, while others give the explanation that some cases do not allow acupuncture or need suspension for a time. It seems that Qi Bo's answer does not touch either of these presumed topics.

[197]Roots here refer to the chest and abdomen, while ends refer to the four limbs.

[198]The left hand is of primary importance in needling technique. Hold the bone under the point with the left hand to stabilize the skin and flesh and to ensure an accurate location of the acupoint. Palpate up and down the channel, focusing on the point to be needled so as to accelerate the arrival of qi. Drainage is employed to draw out evil qi. Therefore, straight needling clears a path for its departure. In this context, straight implies rapid extraction as well as a perpendicular insertion.

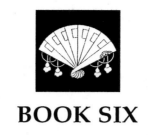

BOOK SIX

Chapter One

Great Treatise on the Eight Orientations, Eight Vacuities, and Eight Winds[1]

(1)

The Yellow Emperor asked:

In a given year, everyone may contract the same disease. What kind of qi is responsible for this?

Shao Shi answered:

This concerns reflections of the eight orientations, of which the Winter Solstice is usually counted as the starting day. The wind arriving from the south is called vacuity wind, and is a bandit which harms people. If it starts up at midnight when tens of thousands of people are sleeping and protected from it, then the year will scarcely see disease in people. If it starts up during the day when tens of thousands of people are relaxed and fatigued and are all struck by (such) evil wind, then many people will contract disease.[2]

Vacuity evils may intrude upon the bone without finding an (immediate) expression externally. With the Beginning of Spring, yang qi begins to effuse in a major way, and the interstices are open. If the wind blows from the west on the day of the Beginning of Spring and tens of thousands of people are all struck by (such) vacuity wind, then the two evils contend, and channel qi is bound and overridden. Being caught in the wind and overtaken by rain are called encountering annual dew. When weather in the year is favorable with little bandit wind, few people will suffer from disease and death, while in a year abundant in bandit wind and evil qi with untimely cold and warmth, a great many people suffer from disease and death.[3]

The Yellow Emperor asked:

What is the cost of the (various) evil vacuity winds and how are they determined?

Shao Shi answered:

On the day of the new moon of the first month,[4] if the wind comes from the west and is strong, it is called white bone. It will bring disasters to the country and cause many deaths. On the day of the new moon of the first month, if a northwest wind blows during the calm dawn watch, many people will suffer from disease, as many as three people in ten. On the day of the new moon of the first month, if a north wind blows at the midday watch,[5] many people will die ["from disease" in a variant version {later editor}] in summer. On the day of the new moon of the first month, if there is a north wind at the calm dawn, many people will die in the spring. On the day of the new moon of the first month, if there is a north wind in the evening, many people will die in the autumn. On the day of the new moon of the first month, if the weather is mild and windless, the people will be free from disease. But, if there is intense cold and fierce wind, many people will suffer from disease. If

193

the *chou* day of the second month is windless, a great many people will suffer from cardiac and abdominal disease. If the *xu* day of the third month is not warm, many people will suffer from cold and heat disease. If on the *si* day of the fourth month there is no summerheat, many people will suffer from jaundice. If the *shen* day of the tenth month is not cold, many people will suffer sudden deaths.[6, 7]

All of these so-called winds (are capable of) demolishing houses, pulling up trees, raising sand and stones, making the fine hair (of the people) stand on end and forcing the interstices open.

(2)

Wind coming from an antagonistic direction or from afar is called vacuity wind. It is a bandit wind which harms people and is capable of killing. (People) must watch out for this vacuity wind and carefully shelter themselves from it. Sheltering oneself from this evil is as good as escaping from stone arrows. Then the evil can do no harm.[8]

Wind coming from the south is called great enfeebling wind. Insofar as it hurts people, it settles internally in the heart and lodges externally in the vessels, its qi being capable of giving rise to heat.

Wind coming from the southwest is called intriguing wind (*mou feng*, 某风). Insofar as it hurts people, it settles internally in the spleen and lodges externally in the muscle, its qi being capable of giving rise to weakness.

Wind coming from the west is called unyielding wind (*gang feng*, 刚风). Insofar as it hurts people, it settles internally in the lung and lodges externally in the skin, its qi being capable of giving rise to dryness.

Wind coming from the northwest is called breaking wind. Insofar as it hurts people, it settles internally in the small intestine and lodges externally in the hand *tai yang* vessel. If the vessel expires, there is diarrhea; if the vessel is blocked,

there is binding and flow stoppage, often giving rise to sudden death.

Wind coming from the north is called great unyielding wind. Insofar as it hurts people, it settles internally in the kidney and lodges externally in the bones and paravertebral sinews in the shoulder and the upper back, its qi being capable of giving rise to cold.

Wind coming from the northeast is called ferocious wind. Insofar as it hurts people, it settles internally in the large intestine and lodges externally under the bones below the lateral costal region and axilla and in the limb joints.

Wind coming from the east is called infant wind. Insofar as it hurts people, it settles internally in the liver and lodges externally in the juncture between the sinews and the bone, its qi being capable of giving rise to dampness.

Wind coming from the southeast is called enfeebling wind. Insofar as it hurts people, it settles internally in the stomach and lodges externally in the muscles, its qi being capable of giving rise to generalized heaviness.[9]

All the above eight winds come from the home of vacuity, and it is because of this that they can cause illness in people. If three vacuities conspire, they will cause sudden disease and sudden death. Two vacuities with one repletion cause rain-dew cold and heat, or atony if (the body) is attacked by rainy and damp environments. For that reason the sage shelters from the evil as if sheltering from stone arrows. In the presence of three vacuities, evil wind may strike people unilaterally, and then sudden collapse and hemilateral withering are caused.[10]

(3)

The Yellow Emperor asked:

The eight winds in the four seasons strike people because of the strength of cold and summerheat. Cold causes the skin to be tense and the interstices to shut, while summerheat slackens the skin and opens the interstices. In invading (the body), must bandit wind and evil qi rely on the help of the wind evil of the eight orientations in order to harm a person?[11]

Shao Shi answered:

The bandit wind and the evil qi may strike a person at any time. However, when (the interstices) are open, (wind and evil qi) can penetrate deeply, and, when these are in the interior, they may cause very serious disorders, afflicting people suddenly and acutely. (On the other hand, if the interstices) are closed, although (bandit wind and evil qi) can still penetrate, they become lodged shallowly, afflicting people with diseases which progress slowly.[12]

The Yellow Emperor asked:

Even though the temperature is moderate and the interstices are not open, a sudden disease may arise. What is the cause of this?

Shao Shi answered:

Even though people live an uneventful life, their interstices open and shut and are slack and tense regularly. This is because human beings react to (the changes of) heaven and earth and respond to the sun and the moon. For this reason, when the moon is full and, consequently, the western sea is at high tide, people are brimming with blood and qi, their muscles and flesh are full, their skin is compact, their hair is strong, their interstices are closed, and smoky grime covers their bodies. At such a time, even if a bandit wind does attack, it penetrates shallowly and is unable to go deeply. When the moon is waning to the close and, consequently, the eastern sea is at high tide, people experience a vacuity of blood and qi, their defensive qi is gone, their form is left alone, their muscles and flesh are diminished, their skin is slack, their interstices are open, their hair is thin, and the smoky grime has fallen off. At such a time, if a bandit wind attacks, it will penetrate deeply and afflict people suddenly and acutely.[13]

The Yellow Emperor asked:

Some people die a sudden death. What kind of evil causes this?

Shao Shi answered:

Under the influence of the three vacuities, death comes abruptly. Under the influence of the three repletions, evil is incapable of hurting people. The declining year, the waning moon and perturbation of the four seasons when people's qi is lacking and short and bandit wind and evil qi are liable to hurt people are called the three vacuities. If ignorant of these three vacuities, a practitioner will be a poor (physician). Under the influence of a booming year, with a full moon and fair weather in the four seasons, even if bandit winds and evil qi are present, they can do no harm.[14]

Chapter Two

Great Treatise on the Favorable & Unfavorable (Conditions), Root & Branch of Disease, Physiographic Characteristics, and Configurations & Orientations[15, 16]

(1)

The Yellow Emperor asked:

Could you explain how to treat the people and oneself?

Qi Bo answered:

Whether treating people or oneself, treating this or treating that, treating the small or treating the great, treating the country or treating one's family, a therapy which runs counter to the predilection (of the patient) can never succeed. Only in complying with this can one expect success. It follows that just as one should enquire about the customs of whatever (strange) land one comes to, so one should ask patients about their predilections before one treats them.[17]

The Yellow Emperor asked:

What are the relationships between such predilections and disease?

Qi Bo answered:

Center heat wasting thirst displays a predilection for cold. With cold in the center, there is a predilection for heat. Heat in the stomach disperses grain, causing people to experience a sensation of a suspended heart, constant hunger, and heat in the skin above the navel. Heat in the intestines causes yellow, chyme-like stools and cold in the skin below the navel. Cold in the stomach causes abdominal distention. Cold in the intestines causes intestinal rumbling and swill diarrhea. Cold in the stomach with heat in the intestines causes distention and diarrhea as well, while heat in the stomach with cold in the intestines produces rapid hunger, lower abdominal pain, and distention.[18]

The Yellow Emperor asked:

Suppose the stomach desires cold drinks while the intestines desire hot liquids. These two desires are counter to each other. How are they treated then?

Qi Bo answered:

In spring and summer, the branch should be treated prior to the root, while in autumn and winter, the root should be treated prior to the branch.[19]

The Yellow Emperor asked:

What can be done about predilections that run counter to (the nature of a disease)?

Qi Bo answered:

Those with such predilections should be fed and clothed as they desire, being kept moderately cold or warm. (A predilection for) cold can be satisfied to a certain degree but not by icy cold, while (a predilection for) heat can be satisfied to a

certain degree but not to the extent that sweating should be induced. As regards food and drinks, these can be prepared hot but not burning hot; they can be prepared cold but not freezing cold. The qi is sustained by moderate cold and warm and, (as a result,) evil is warded away.[20]

(2)

If first there is a disease and then there is counterflow, then treat the root. If first there is counterflow and then disease, then treat the root as well. If first there is cold and this engenders a disease, then treat the root. If first there is a disease and this engenders cold, then treat the root as well. If first there is heat and this engenders a disease, then treat the root. If first there is a disease and this engenders heat, then treat the root as well. If first there is heat and this engenders fullness in the center, then treat the branch. If first there is disease and then diarrhea, then treat the root. If first there is diarrhea and this then engenders a disease, then treat the root: that is, first regulate (the diarrhea) and then treat the other disease. If first there is a disease and then fullness of the center, treat the branch. If first there is center fullness and then vexation of the heart, then treat the root. Regardless of whether the patient is possessed of a visiting or intrinsic qi, the branch should be treated in the case of inhibited urination and defecation, but the root should be treated in the case of disinhibited urination and defecation. If a disease arises with surplus, (it should be determined as) the root as against the branch, and one should first treat the root and then treat the branch. If a disease arises with insufficiency, (it should be determined as) the branch as against the root, and one should first treat the branch and then treat the root. It is necessary to carefully assess the degrees of severity before regulating (vacuity and repletion accordingly). Slight problems can be handled simultaneously, but severe problems must be dealt with separately. If inhibited urination and defecation precede and result in another disease, the root should be treated.[21]

(3)

In the east, which is the coastal region beside the

water, the people eat fish and are fond of salt. Fish causes people to suffer from heat in the center, and salt overwhelms the blood. (For this reason,) the people there are black with loose interstices and, (therefore,) subject to grossness. To treat them, the stone needle is appropriate.

In the west, where water and soil are hard and rigid, the people live on fresh delicacies and are fat. For that reason, evil is unable to harm their physiques. Diseases are generated internally. To treat them, toxic medicinals are appropriate.[22]

In the north, where the wind is cold and ice is biting, the people like living in the open and having milk foods. (As a result) their viscera are cold, causing disease. To treat them, moxibustion is appropriate.

In the south, where the land lies low, the water and the soil are soft, and fog and dew are heavy. The people there are fond of sour and feed on fermented food. As a result, they have dense interstices and red complexions. They are subject to illnesses of spasmodic *bi*. To treat them, the tiny needle is appropriate.[23]

In the central region, where the ground is level and damp and heaven and earth produce things in great quantities, the people live on miscellaneous foods without the need to toil and are, therefore, subject to atonic inversion and cold and heat. To treat them, cultivation of qi and massage are appropriate.

For the above reasons, the sage has a command of various methods which enable him to treat (any case) in an appropriate way.

(4)

As a result of gratified form and tormented orientation, disease is engendered in the vessels and should be treated by acupuncture and moxibustion. As a result of tormented form and gratified orientation, disease is engendered in the sinews and should be treated by ironing and conduction. As a result of gratified form and orientation, disease is engendered in the muscles and should be

treated with (metal) or stone needles. As a result of tormented form and orientation, diseases are engendered which are characterized by depletion and exhaustion, and these should be treated with sweet medicinals. As a result of the form repeatedly experiencing fright and alarm (causing) stoppage in the channels and network vessels, diseases are engendered which are characterized by insensitivity. These should be treated by massage and medicinal wines. The above are called five form/orientation (patterns of disease). It is, therefore, said that, in needling the *yang ming*, blood and qi may be emitted. In needling the *tai yang*, blood may be emitted but not qi. In needling the *shao yang*, qi may be emitted but do not emit blood. And in needling the *tai yin*, blood may be emitted but not qi. In needling the *shao yin*, qi may be emitted but not blood. And in needling the *jue yin*, blood may be emitted but not qi.[24]

Chapter Three

Great Treatise on the Five Viscera & Six Bowels, Vacuity & Repletion[25]

The Yellow Emperor asked:

It is stated in the *"Ci Fa (Needling Methodology)"*[26] that surplus should be drained and insufficiency should be supplemented. What does this signify?

Qi Bo answered:

Spirit may exist in a state of either surplus or insufficiency. Qi may exist in a state of either surplus or insufficiency. Blood may exist in a state of either surplus or insufficiency. Form may exist in a state of either surplus or insufficiency. And will may exist in a state of either surplus or insufficiency. The heart stores spirit. The lungs store qi. The liver stores blood. The spleen stores flesh. The kidneys store will. When will and mind expand, linking internally with the bone marrow, they become form. The passageways of the five viscera are the channels (and) canals through which blood and qi circulate. Once blood and qi are in disharmony, hundreds of diseases may be transmuted and generated. Therefore, the channels (and) canals must be attended to.

In terms of the spirit, surplus causes incessant laughing, while insufficiency causes worry ["sorrow" in the *Su Wen*; Wang Bing says, worry is used erroneously. {later editor}] (Suppose) the blood and qi have not yet merged (with evil) and the five viscera remain undisturbed. The evil may then intrude only upon the form, and chilling frigidity ["quivering as after a soaking" in the *Su Wen* {later editor}] may arise from the fine hair. (The evil) has not yet penetrated into the channels and the network vessels, and this is termed a slight disorder of the spirit. If the spirit exists in a state of surplus, drain the blood of the small network vessels. In bloodletting, (the needle) should not penetrate deeply or widen (the hole), nor should it strike a major channel. Thus the spirit and qi are balanced. If the spirit is insufficient, locate the vacuous vessel, press it to facilitate the arrival (of qi), and then needle it to harmonize the (blood and qi). Do not let out blood, nor should the qi be drained. One need only unblock the flow within the channel and this will cause the spirit and qi to be balanced.[27]

The Yellow Emperor asked:

How does one needle this minor disorder?

Qi Bo answered:

Practice prolonged massage and, when needling, do not widen the hole. Once the qi has moved to where there is insufficiency, spirit and qi are restored to normalcy.

In terms of the qi, surplus causes qi ascension dyspnea and coughing, while insufficiency causes respiration with diminished qi which, however, is uninhibited. (Suppose) the blood and qi have not yet merged, and the five viscera remain undisturbed. (The evil has only penetrated to the level of the skin) and this slight disorder of the skin is called slight leakage of white qi. A surplus (of qi) requires that one drain the channel canal without injuring the channel, letting out blood, or

draining qi. An insufficiency (of qi) requires supplementation of the channel canal without emitting qi.[28]

The Yellow Emperor asked:

How does one needle this minor disorder?

Qi Bo answered:

Practice prolonged massage, and then show (the patient) the needle, declaring, "I'm going to insert it very deeply." At this he must become nervous and, therefore, his essential qi is bound to lie deeply. Thus the evil qi cannot but disperse chaotically, unable to find a place for repose. (As a result,) the (evil) qi is discharged through the interstices and the true qi is secured.[29]

In terms of blood, a surplus causes irritability, while insufficiency causes sorrow[30] ["susceptibility to fright" in the *Su Wen* {later editor}]. (If) the blood and qi have not yet merged and the five viscera remain undisturbed, (the evil has only penetrated to the level of) the minute network vessels which spill outward, causing blood stasis in the channel. In the case of a surplus (of blood,) one should drain the exuberant channel by letting out its blood. In the case of an insufficiency, one should supplement the vacuous channel by pushing the needle into the vessel, retaining the needle until blood arrives and the pulse becomes large ["until the pulse is observed" in the *Su Wen*. {later editor}] Then the needle should be extracted immediately without letting any blood drain out.

The Yellow Emperor asked:

How is blood stasis needled?

Qi Bo answered:

Locate the blood connecting vessel and needle it to let out blood so that the foul blood will not penetrate the channel and cause (other) diseases.

In terms of the form, surplus causes abdominal distention and inhibited urination and defecation, while insufficiency causes loss of use of the four limbs. (If) blood and qi have not yet merged and the five viscera remain undisturbed, (the evil qi has only penetrated to the level of the flesh) and the ensuing vermicular (or wormlike) movement of the muscle and flesh is called slight wind. Surplus requires that one drain the yang vessels; insufficiency requires supplementation of the yang connecting vessel.[31]

The Yellow Emperor asked:

How does one needle this minor disorder?

Qi Bo answered:

Needle at the border of the flesh without striking the channel or injuring the connecting vessel so that the defensive qi is restored and the evil qi scattered.

In terms of will, a surplus results in abdominal distention and swill diarrhea, while an insufficiency results in inversion. (If) the blood and qi have not yet merged and the five viscera remain undisturbed, (the wind evil has penetrated to the level of the bones) and the bony articulations may be damaged. Surplus requires that one drain the *ran* sinew containing blood by bloodletting. Insufficiency requires supplementation at Return Flow (*Fu Liu*, Ki 7).[32]

The Yellow Emperor asked:

How does one needle when (blood and qi) have not yet merged?

Qi Bo answered:

Treat (the affected place) without striking the channel to remove the evil and effect an instant evacuation.[33]

The Yellow Emperor asked:

I wonder how the signs of vacuity and repletion are brought about?

Qi Bo answered:

When blood and qi have merged, then yin and yang are out of balance. The qi is chaotic in the defensive (layer) and blood counterflows in the channels. The blood and qi are separated, thus producing repletion in one (part of the body) and vacuity in another. If blood is merged with the yin while qi is merged with the yang, this results in fright mania. If blood is merged with the yang while qi is merged with the yin, this results in heat in the center. If blood is merged above while qi is merged below, this results in vexation and oppression of the heart and irascibility. If blood is merged below while qi is merged above, this results in chaos (*i.e.*, derangement) and forgetfulness ["poor memory" in the *Su Wen*. {later editor}]][34]

The Yellow Emperor asked:

If blood has merged in the yin, while qi (has merged) in the yang, so that blood and qi are separated, (then) which of them is replete and which is vacuous?

Qi Bo answered:

Blood and qi are fond of warmth and averse to cold. Therefore, when encountering cold they curdle and do not flow, but when warmed (the curdling) diffuses and departs. Hence, where qi is merged, there is blood vacuity, and where blood is merged, there is qi vacuity.[35]

The Yellow Emperor asked:

The human (body) possesses blood and qi. Merged blood is said to give rise to vacuity and merged qi (also) to vacuity. Is there no (possibility of) repletion?

Qi Bo answered:

Presence is repletion, while absence is vacuity. Therefore, wherever qi is merged, there is an absence of blood, and wherever blood is merged, there is an absence of qi. Now that blood and qi are separated, there is vacuity. Because all the network vessels and the minute network vessels pour ["are transported" in a variant version {later editor}] into the channels, when blood and qi are merged (in the same place), repletion ensues. If blood and qi are merged and rush upward, this results in grand inversion. This is inversion capable of producing sudden death. If the qi can be restored (to normalcy, the patient) will live. However, if (the qi) cannot be restored, the condition is fatal.[36]

The Yellow Emperor asked:

From what path does repletion come and from what path does vacuity come?

Qi Bo answered:

Yin and yang both have their own transporting and meeting points. The yang pours into the yin; the yin fills the exterior. When yin and yang are equally balanced ["balanced" in the *Su Wen* {later editor}] in replenishing form and keeping the nine indicators synchronous, one is referred to as a normal person (*ping ren*).[37] Evil may be generated in the yang or in the yin. Evil generated in the yang is the result of wind, rain, cold, and summerheat, while evil generated in the yin is the result of dietary and living (irregularities), yin and yang, and (inordinate) joy or anger.[38]

The Yellow Emperor asked:

How do wind and rain harm people?

Qi Bo answered:

In order for wind and rain to harm people, (their respective evils) must first intrude upon the skin and then transfer to the minute network vessels. Once the minute network vessels are filled up, they transfer to the network vessels. Once the network vessels fill up, they pour into the grand channel vessels. (Finally,) the blood and qi together with the evil qi settle in the parting of the flesh. Because the pulse is hard and large, this is called repletion. In repletion, (there may be a part that is) hard and full externally and does not allow pressure since pressure causes pain.

The Yellow Emperor asked:

How do cold and dampness harm people?

Qi Bo answered:

When cold and dampness strike people, the skin is contracted ["not contracted" in the *Su Wen* {later editor}], the muscles and flesh become hard and tense, the constructive blood stagnates, and the defensive qi departs. This is, therefore, called vacuity. In vacuity, the skin shrivels, the qi becomes diminished, and the blood stagnates. When pressure is applied, qi becomes replenished, producing warmth, and, as a result, (the patient) is made comfortable and freed from pain.[39]

The Yellow Emperor asked:

How is repletion generated in the yin?

Qi Bo answered:

Inordinate joy and anger cause yin qi to counterflow upward. This ascending counterflow results in vacuity below. When there is vacuity below, the yang moves here. This is reasonably said to be repletion.[40]

The Yellow Emperor asked:

How is vacuity generated in the yin?

Qi Bo answered:

Joy causes the qi to descend and sorrow causes the qi to disperse. In dispersing, the vessels are left empty and void. If cold food and drink are consumed, their cold qi stirs the viscera ["causes dual fullness" in a variant version. {later editor}] Consequently, blood becomes curdled and qi departs. This is, therefore, called vacuity.[41]

The Yellow Emperor asked:

Yang vacuity results in external cold; yin vacuity, in internal heat; yang exuberance, in external heat; and yin exuberance, in internal cold. I wonder what accounts for all this.

Qi Bo answered:

Yang receives qi from the upper burner to warm the skin and the parting of the flesh. Now, if cold exists externally, the upper burner stops flowing. Because of this stoppage of flow, cold alone is left lodging in the exterior, causing cold shuddering.

When there is taxation fatigue, the form qi is diminished and debilitated, the grain qi wanes, the upper burner becomes sluggish, and the lower burner ["the lower venter" in the *Su Wen* {later editor}] stops flowing. (Thus) the stomach qi becomes hot and steams the inside of the chest. Therefore, there is internal heat.[42]

When the upper burner is inhibited, the skin becomes compacted, the interstices are congested [the "sweat pores are congested" in the *Su Wen* {later editor}] and blocked, and the defensive qi is no longer able to drain outward. Therefore, external heat arises.[43]

When inversion qi counterflows upward, cold qi accumulates in the chest without draining. Because it is not drained, the warm qi departs. When cold alone becomes lodged here, the blood congeals and curdles. This congelation blocks the interstices, and the pulse becomes exuberant and large but choppy. There is, therefore, cold in the center.[44]

The Yellow Emperor asked:

Suppose yin and yang have merged together, blood and qi have merged together, and the disease has taken shape. How is this condition needled?

Qi Bo answered:

In needling this condition, take the channel canal, take blood on behalf of the constructive, take qi on behalf of the defensive, making use of the form. The seasonal disposition and the location (of the points to be needled) either in the upper or lower (body) determine the number (of needlings).[45]

The Yellow Emperor asked:

Suppose blood and qi have merged together, the disease has taken shape, and yin and yang are out of balance. How are drainage and supplementation performed?

Qi Bo answered:

To drain repletion, (one should) insert the needle till the qi becomes exuberant and the needle (should be) inserted simultaneously with the qi so as to open the gate as if disinhibiting a door. (One should) extract the needle simultaneously with the qi. (Thus) the essential qi is not injured and the evil qi is downborne. The outer gate is left unshut in order to expel the illness. (One should) shake (the needle) to widen its path as if clearing a road. This is known as grand drainage. It is necessary to press (the point before) extracting (the needle), and thus the great qi will be subjugated.[46]

The Yellow Emperor asked:

How is vacuity supplemented?

Qi Bo answered:

Hold the needle but do not push it in (for a while) so as to calm (the patient). Insert the needle with the exhalation, so that, while his qi is going out, the needle is going in. (Make certain that) the needle completely fills the hole, allowing the essence no way out. Just as (the essential qi) is replenished, extract the needle rapidly so that, while his qi is going in, the needle is extracted. This prevents heat from escaping. Then shut the gate, and the evil qi will be scattered and dispersed but the essential qi will be preserved. (It is essential) not to delay this movement until (the essential qi retreats). In this way, the qi at hand will not get lost and the distant qi will arrive. This is called pursuit (*zhui*, 追).[47]

The Yellow Emperor asked:

There are ten types of vacuity and repletion which are produced in the five viscera and their five respective channels. Within each of the twelve channels, hundreds of [the *Su Wen* adds "their own" {later editor}] diseases can be generated. Here, however, only the five viscera are under discussion. Because the twelve channel vessels connect with the three hundred and sixty-five articulations, when a joint becomes diseased, the channel vessel inevitably also becomes involved. All (of these illnesses) may be classified into vacuity or repletion. How then is this to be integrated?

Qi Bo answered:

The five viscera and six bowels stand in an interior/exterior relationship. The channels, the network vessels, the limbs, and the articulations may all engender vacuity and repletion. Based on the location of the disease, (one should) use an appropriate regulating therapy.[48]

If disease lies within the vessels, regulate the blood. If it is found in the blood, regulate the connecting vessel. If disease lies within the qi, regulate the defensive. If disease lies within the flesh, regulate the partings of the flesh. If disease is found within the sinews, regulate the sinews. If it is found in the bones, regulate the bones.

Surprise manipulation of the red-hot needle can be performed beneath (the diseased sinew) and the spasmodic area. For disease within the bone, perform red-hot needling and drug-ironing. For a disease of without knowing pain,[49] the two motility vessels are the best choices. Pain in the formal body in which none of the nine indicators appears abnormal is treated by cross needling. Disease on the left with a pathological pulse on the right is treated by grand needling. It is vital to examine the nine indicators carefully. This is the perfect *dao* of needling.[50]

Chapter Four

Great Treatise on Yin & Yang, Clearness & Turbidity, and Order/Discipline & Counterflow/Chaos[51]

The Yellow Emperor asked:

The twelve channels are differentiated into five phases and divided among the four seasons. What sorts of failures create chaos among them, and what kinds of gains makes them disciplined?

Qi Bo answered:

The five phases interact with each other in order and the four seasons supersede one another at a fixed rate. Order brings about discipline, while counterflow brings about chaos.

The Yellow Emperor asked:

What does it mean that order brings about discipline?

Qi Bo answered:

The channels are twelve in number and correspond to the twelve months. The twelve months are divided into four seasons. These four seasons are spring, summer, autumn, and winter, and (the nature of) their qi differs from one another. If constructive and defensive accompany each other, if yin and yang are in harmony, and if clearness and turbidity do not interfere with one another, then order is kept and discipline is maintained.[52]

The Yellow Emperor asked:

What does it mean that counterflow brings about chaos?

Qi Bo answered:

The clear qi lies within the yin, while the turbid qi lies within the yang. If the constructive qi follows the vessels but the defensive qi counterflows, the clear and the turbid interfere with one another. If this chaos occurs in the chest, this is called great grievance. If the chaotic qi occurs in the heart, this results in vexation of the heart, taciturnity, and an (inclination to) sit quietly with head bent down. If the chaos occurs in the lung, this results in asthmatic wheezing in either the supine and prostrate positions requiring that one press the hands against the chest to facilitate breathing. If the chaos occurs in the stomach and the intestines, this results in sudden turmoil (*i.e.*, cholera-like disease). If the chaos occurs in the arms and the legs, this results in counterflow frigidity of the limbs. If the chaos occurs in the head, this results in counterflow inversion headache ["heavy headedness" in a variant version {later editor}] and spinning collapse.[53]

If there is qi in the heart, take the rapids of the hand *shao yin* and the heart-governor. [54]

If there is qi in the lung, take the brook points of the hand *tai yin*[55] and the rapids of the foot *shao yin*.[56]

If there is qi in the stomach and the intestines, take the hand and foot *tai yin* and *yang ming*.[57] If (the evil qi) has not been eliminated, take Three Li (*San Li*, St 36).

If there is qi in the head, take Celestial Pillar (*Tian Zhu*, Bl 10) and Great Shuttle (*Da Shu*, Bl 11). If this does not cure it, take the brook and rapids points of the foot ["hand" in the *Ling Shu* {later editor}[58]] *tai yang*.[59]

If there is qi in the hand and the foot, first remove the blood vessel and then take the brooks and rapids of the *yang ming* and *shao yin*.[60]

Slow insertion and slow extraction (of the needle) is called conducting the qi, while draining and supplementing intangibly is called communicating essence. (This is indicated in cases of) neither surplus nor insufficiency where chaotic qi counterflows.[61]

Chapter Five

Great Treatise on Bandit Winds & Evil Qi During the Four Seasons[62]

(1)

The Yellow Emperor asked:

Several persons may walk or stand side by side who are of the same age and are wearing clothes of the same thickness. When they are caught in sudden, violent wind or storm, some may fall ill while others may not or all of them may die. Why is this?

Qi Bo answered:

In spring, a warm wind blows. During the summer, a yang wind blows. In the autumn a cool wind blows. And during winter, a cold wind blows. The winds of the four seasons each bring on diseases with varying manifestations. Those with yellow complexion, thin skin, and weak flesh cannot stand the vacuity wind of spring. Those with white complexion, thin skin, and weak flesh cannot stand the vacuity wind of summer. Those with green-blue complexion, thin skin, and weak flesh cannot stand the vacuity wind of autumn. Those with red complexion, thin skin, and weak flesh cannot stand the vacuity wind of winter.[63]

The Yellow Emperor asked:

Do those with black complexions not become diseased?

Qi Bo answered:

Those with black complexions, thick skin, and firm flesh are certainly free from damage by the winds of the four seasons, but those with thin skin, infirm flesh, and a variable complexion may become ill during long summer when a vacuity wind blows. Those with thick skin and firm muscles and flesh do not become ill even when long summer comes and a vacuity wind blows. Those with thick skin and firm muscles and flesh must contract dual cold, (sustaining damage) both internally and externally, and only then will they fall ill.

(2)

The Yellow Emperor asked:

203

If bandit wind and evil qi damage people, these factors will cause them to contract disease. Now, there are persons living well within the protection of screens and curtains who never step out of their chambers or cave dwellings, and yet they may suddenly become ill. What is the cause of this?

Qi Bo answered:

All of these have, at some time, been damaged by damp qi which hides inside the blood vessels and in the parting of the flesh. (This evil) has been retained for a long time without departing. (These people may have had accidents) such as falls, and the resulting foul blood has become lodged internally and not eliminated. When one experiences sudden, inordinate joy or anger, or undisciplined diet, or unseasonal temperature changes when the interstices are shut and blocked or wind cold strikes the opened (interstices, all these factors cause) blood and qi to become congealed and bound. (The new and old) evil conspire together and launch an attack. This results in cold *bi*. (Another possibility is that) existence of heat causes perspiration, and, while perspiring, (people) are then subjected to wind. Even though they have not been caught by a bandit wind and evil qi, (the trouble) must be initiated by an additive factor.[64]

The Yellow Emperor asked:

All that your honor has explained is apparent to the patient himself. Suppose one has never been caught in an evil wind and is free of such emotions as apprehension and fright but suddenly falls ill. Then what is the cause? Should it be ascribed to the work of a ghost or god?

Qi Bo answered:

In this case also, there must be an old evil which has never before been apparent. When the orientation is affected by antipathy or compassion, qi and blood become internally chaotic. Then these two qi join forces to cause oppression. The (evil)

that comes (from the past) is fine, invisible to the eye, and inaudible to the ear. Therefore, it seems like a ghost or god.

The Yellow Emperor asked:

How can recovery by means of supplication (*zhu you*, 祝由) be explained?

Qi Bo answered:

Sorcerers in the past knew methods for combating the hundreds of diseases, equipped with knowledge of their origins. Therefore, recovery might be effected through supplication.[65]

Chapter Six

Great Treatise on the Internal & External Examination of the Form (*i.e.*, Classifications of) the Old & Young, the Thin & Fat, and Serenity in the Morning but Worsening in the Night[66]

The Yellow Emperor asked:

People may be born stiff or flexible, weak or strong, short or tall, and with either a yin or yang (nature). Please tell me about these differences.

Qi Bo answered:

Within yin there is yang, and within yang there is yin. Careful examination and identification of yin and yang ensures the proper needling method, while (the ability to) detect the onset of a disease allows it to be needled in the right way. (It is important to) carefully consider every aspect of disease which, associated with the seasons, is related to the viscera and bowels internally as well as the sinews, bone, and skin externally. It follows that the interior contains yin and yang and the exterior also contains yin and yang. Internally, the five viscera are yin and the six bowels are yang. Externally, the sinews and the bone are yin, while the skin is yang.[67]

Therefore, it is said that when disease exists in the yin within the yin, the brooks and rapids of the yin (channels) should be needled. When disease exists in the yang within the yang, the confluences of the yang (channels) should be needled. When disease exists in the yin within the yang, the streams of the yin (channels) should be needled. When disease exists in the yang within the yin, the network vessels of the yang (channels) should be needled.[68]

Disease in the yang is called wind. Disease in the yin is called *bi*. And disease involving both the yin and yang is called wind *bi*. A tangible disease without pain is categorized as yang, whereas an intangible (disease) with pain is categorized as yin. An intangible (disease) with pain (indicates) that the yang is intact ["slack" in the *Jiu Xu* and the same hereafter {later editor}] but the yin is damaged. Promptly treat the yin without attacking the yang. A tangible (disease) without pain (indicates) that the yin is intact but the yang is damaged. Promptly treat the yang without attacking the yin. The stirring of both yin and yang with the irregular appearance and disappearance (of external signs), plus the symptom of vexation of the heart is called the prevalence of yin over yang. This is spoken of as a neither exterior nor interior (disorder. In this case,) the form will depart before long.[69]

The Yellow Emperor asked:

How are form and qi diseases prioritized, and what are the internal and external expressions (of these diseases)?

Qi Bo answered:

Wind and cold damage the form, while worry, fear, resentment, and anger damage qi. Qi may damage the viscera and hence produce disease in them. Cold may damage the form and find its expression in the form. Wind may damage the sinews and vessels, and it is in the sinews and vessels that it finds its expression. These are the internal and external expressions of the form and qi.[70]

The Yellow Emperor asked:

How are they needled?

Qi Bo answered:

A disease that is nine days old is terminated in three needlings; and a disease that is one month old is terminated in ten needlings. With diseases of longer or shorter durations, the same proportion (of time to needlings) holds. (To treat) an enduring *bi* which refuses to leave the body, locate the blood network vessels and remove all the blood from them.

The Yellow Emperor asked:

How difficult or easy is it to treat external and internal diseases?

Qi Bo answered:

If a disease arises first in the form but has not yet entered the viscera, the number of needlings is half that of the days of its duration. If a disease first arises in the viscera and then the form produces manifestations (*i.e.*, symptomology in the viscera), the number of needlings should be double that of the days of its duration. This is the proportion of the internal and the external diseases in terms of difficulty or ease (of treatment).

(2)

The Yellow Emperor asked:

How can one know whether a disease is one of the skin, muscles, blood, qi, sinews, or bones?

Qi Bo answered:

A color appearing between the eyebrows, thin and brilliant, indicates disease in the skin. Lips shaded green-blue, yellow, red, white, or black indicate disease in the muscles and flesh. Constructive qi that is sodden indicates disease in the blood and qi ["in the vessel" in the *Qian Jin Yi Fang (The Supplement to the Prescriptions Worth a Thousand Gold)* {later editor}]. Eyes colored green-blue, yellow, red, white, or black indicate disease in the sinews. Ears that are parched, desiccated, and grimy looking indicate disease in the bone.[71]

The Yellow Emperor asked:

What are formal diseases like? And how are they taken on?

Qi Bo answered:

The skin has regions, the flesh has columns, qi and blood have (channel) points, the sinews have binding (places), and the bones have accessories. The cutaneous region points are located in the four extremities. The fleshy columns are located between the partings of the flesh of the arms and the lower legs on the routes of the various yang (channels) and between the partings of the flesh on the route of the foot *shao yin*. Qi and blood have their points on the various network vessels which become exuberant and raised when qi and blood are retained and lodge there. The sinew (binding places lie along) neither the yin nor the yang (channels), nor to the left or the right (side). They are treated only insofar as they are (locally) diseased. The bone accessories are crevices between the bones where fluid is received to spill into the brain and the marrow.[72]

The Yellow Emperor asked:

How are they taken on?

Qi Bo answered:

The variety of diseases, whether they are floating or sinking, lying shallowly or deeply, is infinite even though each is located in a certain area. A mild disease requires shallow (needling), while a serious one, deep (needling). A mild disease requires fewer (points), while a serious one, more. Those who are able to regulate the qi according to these variances are superior practitioners.

The Yellow Emperor asked:

How are people, (no matter) whether fat or thin, small-sized or bulky, cold or warm, classified as to whether they are old, middle-aged, young, or children?

Qi Bo answered:

People fifty and over are old. Those thirty and over are middle-aged. Those eighteen and over are young. And those six and over are children.

The Yellow Emperor asked:

How are people classified in terms of fatness or thinness?

Qi Bo answered:

People are classified as oily, greasy, and fleshy.

The Yellow Emperor asked:

How are these types distinguished?

Qi Bo answered:

Those with tough muscular masses and replenished skin are (classified primarily as) oily. Those with muscular masses which are not tough and skin that is slack are greasy. And those in whom the skin and flesh cannot be separated are fleshy.

The Yellow Emperor asked:

How cold or warm are their bodies?

Qi Bo answered:

As for the greasy (type), those with tender flesh and coarse skin texture have a cold body, while those with fine skin texture have a hot body. As for the oily (type), those with tough flesh and fine skin texture have a hot (body temperature), while those with coarse skin texture have a low (body temperature). [As for the fleshy, there is no information given about their differences in temperature. {later editor}]

The Yellow Emperor asked:

What are the relationships between fatness or thinness and largeness or smallness (of the build)?

Qi Bo answered:

The greasy (type) are abundant in qi with slack skin and, therefore, are capable of a slack abdomen and drooping fat. The fleshy (type) have a bulky body of large volume. The oily (type) have a body that is compressed and small (of build).

The Yellow Emperor asked:

How much or little qi and blood do these three types possess?

Qi Bo answered:

The greasy (type) have an abundance of qi. Those who are abundant in qi are hot, and those who are hot can endure the cold. The fleshy have an abundance of blood. Those who are abundant in blood have a full form, and those who have a full form possess well-balanced (qi). The oily (type) have blood that is thin and qi that is meager and slippery. Therefore, they cannot grow bulky. The above distinguish these types from the general populace.

The Yellow Emperor asked:

What is the general populace like?

Qi Bo answered:

The majority of people possess no superfluous skin, flesh, or fat, nor do they have any superfluity of blood and qi. Accordingly, their forms are neither small nor large, with their various parts in good proportion to their trunk. (That is why) they are called the general populace.

The Yellow Emperor asked:

How are they treated?

Qi Bo answered:

One must first distinguish between three types, (determining) how much or little blood they have and how clear or turbid their qi is. Then (one can) regulate them. Their treatment should not deviate from the established standards (in regard to the types. The three types are) the greasy with a relaxed belly and drooping fat, the fleshy who have a large bulk both above and below, and the oily who have oil but possess a limited bulk.

(3)

The Yellow Emperor asked:

In most cases, patients tend to be serene in the morning, tranquil during the day, but worse in the evening and serious at night. What accounts for this?

Qi Bo answered:

In the spring there is birth; in the summer, growth; in the autumn, contraction; and in the winter, hibernation. These are the norms of qi, and humans correspond to these as well. A day and a night (together) can (also) be divided into the qi of the four seasons. The morning corresponds to spring; the noon corresponds to summer; the sundown corresponds to autumn; and the night corresponds to winter. In the morning the qi in humans begins to be generated while the ill qi declines. Therefore, mornings are serene. At noon, the qi in humans grows, and this growth prevails over evil. Thus there is tranquility. In the evening, the qi in humans begins to decline, and the evil qi begins to be generated. Thus there is an exacerbation (of the condition). At midnight the qi in humans has entered the viscera, and the evil qi takes exclusive possession of the body. Thus (the condition) becomes severe.[73]

The Yellow Emperor asked:

Why does the opposite sometimes happen?

Qi Bo answered:

This is because of an incongruity to seasonal qi (wherein) one single viscus rules the disease. In that case, the (condition) invariably becomes serious at the restraining phase of the qi of the viscus and ameliorates at the restrained phase.[74]

The Yellow Emperor asked:

How is this treated?

Qi Bo answered:

Acting in accordance with the heavenly phases ensures a desirable effect on the disease.[75] Whoever acts in accordance with (this principle) is a superior practitioner. Whoever acts counter to it is a poor practitioner.[76]

Chapter Seven

Great Treatise on Yin & Yang[77]

Yin is quiet and yang is restless. Yang is birth and yin is growing. Yang is killing and yin is storage. Yang transforms qi and yin gives shape. Extreme cold generates heat and extreme heat generates cold. The cold qi generates the turbid and the heat qi generates the clear. If clear qi exists below, this results in the generation of swill diarrhea. If turbid qi exists above, this results in distention. This is the contrary action of yin and yang and both the regressive and progressive courses of disease.[78]

The clear yang is the sky; the turbid yin the earth. The earthly qi ascends to form clouds, and the heavenly qi descends to form rain. Rain issues from the earthly qi, and clouds issue from the heavenly qi. It follows that the clear yang comes out through the upper portals, and the turbid yin through the lower portals. The clear yang effuses (through) the interstices, and the turbid yin penetrates the five viscera. The clear yang replenishes the four limbs, and the turbid yin gathers in the six bowels.[79]

Water is yin, and fire is yang. Yang is qi, and yin is flavor. Flavor is assimilated to form; form to qi; qi to essence; and essence to transformation. Essence feeds on qi, while form feeds on flavor. Transformation produces essence, and qi produces form. Flavor may bring damage to form, and qi to essence. Essence is transformed into qi which is subject to the damage by flavor.[80]

Yin flavor issues through the lower portals, and yang qi comes out through the upper portals. Flavor that is thick is yin, but when thin, it is the yang of the yin. Qi that is thick is yang, but when thin, it is the yin of the yang. Flavor that is thick results in diarrhea, but when thin, it promotes free flow. Qi that is thin becomes diffusive, but (qi) that is thick generates heat. Vigorous fire diminishes the qi, but a small fire invigorates the qi. Vigorous fire consumes the qi, but when qi is consumed, fire is diminished. Vigorous fire dissipates qi, but a small fire generates qi.

As for qi and flavor, acrid and sweet, being effusive and dissipating, are yang. Sour and bitter, being emetic and laxative, are yin. When yin prevails, yang becomes diseased; when yang prevails, yin becomes diseased. When yin is diseased, this results in heat; when yang is diseased this results in cold ["prevalence of yang means heat, while prevalence of yin means cold" in the *Su Wen*. {later editor}] Dual cold results in heat, while dual heat results in cold.[81]

Cold may damage form and heat may damage qi. Damaged qi gives rise to pain and damaged form gives rise to swelling. Therefore, when first there is pain and then swelling, it is the qi that has damaged the form. But when first there is swelling and then pain, the form has damaged the qi.[82]

A prevalence of wind results in stirring; prevalence of heat results in swelling; prevalence of dryness results in desiccation; a prevalence of cold results in puffiness; and a prevalence of dampness results in soft stool diarrhea. Heaven has the four seasons and the five phases for birth, growth, contraction, and storage as well as to generate cold, summerheat, dryness, dampness, and wind. People have the five viscera to transform the five qi to produce joy, anger, sorrow, worry, and fright. Joy and anger may damage the qi. Cold and summerheat may damage the form. Violent anger may damage the yin. Violent joy may damage the yang. When inversion qi circulates upwards, this fills the vessels and (spirit) will depart from the form. It is rightly said that inordinate joy and anger and excessive cold and summerheat render life insecure. Dual yin unavoidably grows into yang; dual yang unavoidably grows into yin. These are the transmutations of yin and yang.[83]

Yin lying internally is the guardian of yang; yang lying externally is in the service of yin. When yang prevails, the body becomes hot, the interstices shut, there is rough dyspneic breathing necessitating that one bend forward and backward (to facilitate respiration), and there is lack of perspiration accompanied by fever and dry teeth. When vexation, oppression, and abdominal distention develop, then death ensues. (Such patients) can endure the winter but not the summer. When yin prevails, the body becomes cold with sweating, constant generalized frigidity, and frequent shivering with cold. This cold causes inversion, and the inversion causes abdominal fullness and (eventually) death in turn. (Such patients) endure summer well but not winter. These are the transmutations resulting from the mutual retaliation between yin and yang and the signs and capacities of (the resulting) diseases.[84]

The Yellow Emperor asked:

How can these two be regulated?

Qi Bo answered:

If one has knowledge of the sevenfold reduction and the eightfold boost, then the two may be regulated. However, those ignorant of them become decrepit prematurely.[85]

The clear yang ascends to the heaven while the turbid yin returns to the earth. The heavenly qi accesses the lung. The earthly qi accesses the upper part of the esophagus (*yan*). The wind qi accesses the liver. The thunder qi accesses the heart. The grain qi accesses the spleen. And the rain qi accesses the kidney. The six channels are the rivers, while the stomach and the intestines are the seas. The nine portals are the qi of pouring water. Violent qi is like thunder, while the counterflow of qi is like yang. Therefore, if (one) treats without adopting the laws governing heaven or making use of the principles of earth, then this brings about disastrous consequences.[86]

Evil wind comes on as rapidly as a storm. Therefore, those skilled in (medical) treatment treat the skin and hair (first). Next they treat muscle and skin. Next they treat sinews and vessels. Next they treat the six bowels. And finally, they treat the five viscera. Once one must treat the five viscera, (the patient is) half alive and half dead.[87]

Therefore, heavenly evil qi, once contracted, harms the five viscera. Cold and heat from grain and water, once contracted, harm the six bowels. Earthly damp qi, once contracted, harms the skin, flesh, sinews, and vessels. For this reason, those skilled at needling are able to draw yin to yang and to draw yang to yin, to treat the left through the right, or to treat the right through the left. They come to realize (the conditions of) the patient by himself, realize the interior by the state of the exterior, and detect, by observing the mechanism of excess and insufficiency, problems from subtleties. (They) have (all this) at their command and never fail.[88]

Those skilled at examination study the complexion and palpate the pulses to first discriminate yin and yang and then discriminate the brilliant (color) from the turbid to determine the affected region. They then listen to the (patient's) breathing and voice to determine what the (nature of the) disease is. They then observe the weight and the steelyard and study the compass and the square to determine where the disease is generated. Finally, by observing floating and sinking, slipperiness and roughness of the cubit skin and the *cun kou* pulse, they determine where the disease lies. (Equipped with these skills,) they never fail in treatment and never make mistakes in diagnosing.[89]

It is rightly said that a disease that is just beginning can be needled and terminated, but if it is running rampant, one must wait until it has subdued to deal with it.

If it is light, (a disease) may be treated by upraising. If it is heavy, it can be treated by subtraction. If it is diminishing (nature), it can be treated by promotion.[90]

Insufficient form should be warmed with qi, and insufficient essence supplemented with flavor.[91] A (disease) located high (in the body) should be treated by overpassing (*yue*), and one located low (in the body) should be conducted to dry it up. Fullness in the center should be treated by draining the interior. If there is an evil, the form should be soaked by diaphoresis. If it is in the skin, it can be effused by diaphoresis. The impetuous and fierce should be subjugated by suppression, and repletion should be drained by dissipation.[92]

(It is necessary to) study yin and yang to distinguish the flexible from the rigid. A yang disease is treated through yin, and a yin disease through yang. (It is necessary to) determine (which is involved,) blood or qi, and then make them keep to their homes. It is required that blood repletion be treated by dredging, while qi vacuity, by dragging and conducting.[93]

(2)

Yang begins from the left; yin from the right. (The qi) in the old begins from above; that in the young from below. It follows that, in spring and summer, if (qi) is attributed to yang, there is life, but, if it is attributed to autumn and winter, there is death. Conversely (in autumn and winter,) if it is attributed to autumn and winter, there is life.[94]

Therefore, whether there is much or little qi, counterflow invariably gives rise to inversion. A surplus of qi may produce inversion, where a single qi goes upward without descending with cold inversion extending as high as the knees. The young die if they contract this in the autumn and winter, but the old survive if they contract this in the autumn and winter.[95]

If the qi ascends without descending, there is headache and madness. There is no yang anywhere to be searched out, (nor) is there yin ["nor is there yin to be sought anywhere" in the *Su Wen*. {later editor}] The five parts are all separated, presenting no (reliable) signs. (This situation) is likened to standing in the wilderness or lying in an empty house. There is nothing but a thread (of breath) that greets the eyes.[96]

(3)

A disease (contracted) in the three months of winter, if lethal, will inevitably kill when the grass and willows begin to grow leaves. If yin and yang are both expiring, (death) is expected in the first month of spring.

Disease (contracted) in the three months of winter, if subordinated to yang, will end in death at the end of spring ["at the beginning of spring" in the *Su Wen* {later editor}] if the pulse demonstrates fatal signs in the first month of spring.[97]

Disease contracted in the three months of spring is called yang killer. If yin and yang are both expiring, (death) is expected when the grass turns dry.[98]

Disease of consummate yin (contracted) in the three months of summer cannot last over ten days. If yin and yang cross, death is expected when water becomes still.[99]

Disease (contracted) in the three months of autumn, (though) all the three yang rise up, will heal of itself without the need to treat it. If yin and yang intermingle and blend, (the patient) is unable to sit down after standing or to stand up after sitting. If the third yang arrives alone, (death) is expected when water turns into stone. If the second yin arrives alone, (death) is expected when water is exuberant.[100]

Chapter Eight

Great Treatise on Dreams Produced by a Positive Evil Assailing the Interior[101]

The Yellow Emperor asked:

What happens when a rampant evil infiltrates (the body)?

Qi Bo answered:

When a positive evil has just assailed the interior from the outside, it has no fixed place to lodge and, instead, saps the viscera. If it still finds no fixed place to settle in, it travels together with the constructive and the defensive, soaring with the ethereal and corporeal souls to cause people to suffer from disturbed sleep and frequent dreams. Whenever the (evil) qi saps the bowels, superabundance arises in the external but insufficiency in the internal. If it saps the viscera, this causes surplus internally but insufficiency externally.[102]

The Yellow Emperor asked:

What form does surplus and insufficiency take?

Qi Bo answered:

With an exuberance of yin, one dreams of wading great waters and being fearful. With an exuberance of yang, one dreams of great fire and being burned. With an exuberance of both yin and yang, one dreams of violence, such as murder and intended injury. With an exuberance above, one dreams of flying. With exuberance below, one dreams of falling. After having overeaten, one dreams of offering; and when excessively hungry, one dreams of begging (for food). With exuberant liver qi, one has angry dreams. With exuberant lung qi, one dreams of crying, fear, or soaring. With exuberant heart qi, one dreams of joy and laughter and/or terror. With exuberant spleen qi, one dreams of singing and merriment, heaviness of the body, and inability to lift the hand and foot. With exuberant kidney qi, one dreams of fracture and separation of the lumbar spine. In the case of all of the above twelve exuberances, drain the (affected) place and recovery will immediately follow.

If inversion qi intrudes upon the heart, one dreams of hillocks with smoke and fire.[103] If it intrudes upon the lung, one dreams of soaring or of viewing metal tools and rarities. If it intrudes upon the liver, one dreams of wooded mountains and trees. If it intrudes upon the spleen, one dreams of hills, great lakes, and dilapidated houses in storms. If it intrudes upon the kidney, one dreams of facing an abyss and submerging in the water. If it intrudes upon the urinary bladder, one dreams of roaming. If it intrudes upon the stomach, one dreams of eating and drinking. If it intrudes upon the large intestine, one dreams of fields. If it intrudes upon the small intestine, one dreams of crowded townships or streets ["thoroughfares" in a variant version {later editor}]. If it intrudes upon the gallbladder, one dreams of fighting a suit in court or committing suicide by cutting the stomach open. If it intrudes upon the yin organ (i.e., the genitals), one dreams of sexual intercourse. If it intrudes upon the nape of the neck, one dreams of decapitation. If it intrudes upon the lower leg, one dreams of being incapable of moving a step forward and living in a deep cellar or expansive private park. If it intrudes upon the thigh and the upper arm, one dreams of protocols and obeisances. If it intrudes upon the urinary bladder and the rectum, one dreams of uninhibited urination and defecation.[104] In the case of the above fifteen insufficiencies, supplement the (affected) place and recovery will follow immediately.

Chapter Nine

Great Treatise on the Propensities of the Five Flavors & Diseases of the Five Viscera[105]

The Yellow Emperor asked:

Grain qi has five flavors. How do they penetrate

the five viscera and how are they discriminated?

Qi Bo answered:

The stomach is the sea of the five viscera and six bowels. Water and grain all enter the stomach, and the five viscera and six bowels are all endowed by the stomach. The five flavors each go toward where they are favored.

The sour grain flavor first penetrates the liver. The *Jiu Juan* also states that sourness enters the stomach, and, because its qi is astringing ["contracting" in a variant version {later editor}], it is unable to exit or enter (elsewhere). Since it cannot exit, it must remain in the stomach. Having been moderated and warmed in the stomach, it pours downward into the urinary bladder. The walls of the urinary bladder are thin and soft. Acted on by sourness, they shrink and curl, becoming constrained and blocked, causing a failure of circulation in the water passageways. This results in dribbling urinary blockage.[106]

The genitals are the place where the gathering sinews terminate and converge. For this reason, after it has entered the stomach, sourness penetrates the sinews.[107] The *Su Wen* states that sourness penetrates the sinews. Therefore, in sinew diseases, one must not eat much sour. The implications (of these statements) are in accord with one another. It also says that the liver desires acidity, but eating much sour makes the flesh callous and the lips out–turned, for wood prevails over earth. [The reference to wood–acridity is erroneous according to the *Jiu Juan*. {later editor}][108]

Bitterness first penetrates the heart. The *Jiu Juan* also states that after bitterness, the qi of which is dry and is capable of ejection and draining precipitation, has entered the stomach, no (other) qi of the five grains is able to restrain it. (Thereupon) it penetrates the lower venter. In the lower venter, all the passageways of the triple burner are thus shut, arresting their flow. As a result, qi changes to cause vomiting.

The teeth are the terminus of the bones. After it has entered the stomach, bitterness penetrates the bones and then returns to emerge (at the teeth). If the teeth become dark and loose, this invariably proves (that bitterness) has penetrated the bones.

Bitterness penetrates the heart, but now it is said to penetrate the bone. This is because water and fire interact upon each other, and the qi of the bone has access to the heart.[109]

The *Su Wen* states that bitterness penetrates the bone. Therefore, in bone diseases, one must not eat much bitter. The implications (of these statements) are in accord with one another. It also says that the heart desires sourness, but eating much bitter makes the skin withered and the hair fall off. This is because it is said that fire prevails over metal. [The reference to fire sourness is wrong according to the *Jiu Juan*. {later editor}][110]

Sweetness first penetrates the spleen. The *Jiu Juan* also states that once sweetness has entered the stomach, if its qi is so weak and meager that it fails to ascend to reach the upper burner, it must stay in the stomach together with the grain. Sweetness is capable of softening and moistening. When softened, the stomach becomes slack, and when it is slack, worms move about. The movement of worms causes people to suffer from oppression of the heart.

The qi (of sweetness) has access to the skin. Therefore, sweetness is said to penetrate the skin. The skin is the surplus of the flesh, and, although the skin is ascribed to the lung, it is linked with the flesh as one. For this reason, sweetness moistens the skin as well as the muscles and flesh.

The *Su Wen* states that sweetness penetrates the flesh, but in diseases of the flesh, one must not eat too much sweet. The implications (of these statements) are in accord with one another. It also states that eating a great deal of sweet makes the bones painful and the hair fall out. This is because it is said that earth prevails over water. [According to the *Jiu Juan*, this statement is not wrong. {later editor}]

Acridity first penetrates the lung. The *Jiu Juan* also states that once acridity has entered the stomach, its qi penetrates the upper burner. The upper burner receives various qi and operates the various yang. The qi of ginger and leek fumigates the constructive and defensive. If the constructive and defensive are constantly subjected to it, (the influence of leek and ginger) will be long retained below the heart, resulting in hollowed heart ["burning heart" in a variant version. {later editor}][111]

Acridity circulates with the qi and, therefore, once it has entered the stomach, it emerges along with the sweat. [The *Qian Jin* states that, "after it has entered the stomach, acridity drives the qi and emerges with it, and, as a result, qi becomes exuberant." {later editor}] The *Su Wen* states that acridity drives the qi, and (therefore,) in qi diseases, one must not eat too much acrid. The implications (of these statements) are in accord with one another. It also states that the lung desires bitterness, and eating much acrid makes the sinews tense and the nail desiccated. This is because it is said that metal prevails over wood. [The reference to the lung desiring bitterness is wrong according to the *Jiu Juan*. {later editor}][112]

Saltiness first penetrates the kidney. The *Jiu Juan* also states that once saltiness has entered the stomach, its qi ascends to the middle burner to pour into the various vessels. The vessels are where blood runs. When it meets with saltiness, blood congeals. When blood is congealed, the juice in the stomach must pour (into the vessels) to resolve the blood. When it pours out, the juice in the stomach becomes exhausted, and when it is exhausted, the passage of the throat becomes parched. As a result, the tongue becomes dry with constant thirst.

The blood vessels are the passageways of the middle burner. Therefore, saltiness penetrates the blood after it has entered the stomach. Saltiness first penetrates the kidney, but now it is said to penetrate blood. This is because the kidney is associated with the triple burner, and the blood vessels, though ascribed to the liver and the heart, are the passageways of the middle burner. Therefore, saltiness penetrates the blood after it has entered (the stomach).[113]

The *Su Wen* states that saltiness penetrates the blood, and in blood diseases, one must not eat too much salt. The implications (of these statements) are in accord with one another. It also states that eating a great deal of salt makes the vessels congeal and curdle, changing their color. This is because it is said that water prevails over fire. [Although both (statements) discuss the blood and vessels, their implications are different. {later editor}][114]

The grain qi circulates together with the constructive and defensive. When (it produces) movement in the fluid and humor, the constructive and defensive flow completely freely, and then it is transformed into wastes and conveyed downward step by step.[115]

The Yellow Emperor asked:

How does it circulate with the constructive and defensive?

Qi Bo answered:

Grain first enters the stomach. Its refined and purified aspect emerges from the stomach first into the upper and middle burners to irrigate the five viscera. It then leaves the two burners to travel along the routes of the constructive and defensive. The concentration of great qi does not circulate but accumulates in the chest and is called the sea of qi. It emerges through the lung, travelling along the throat, exiting with the exhalation, and entering with inhalation. The essential qi of heaven and earth is discharged and taken in approximately at a ratio of three to one. For this reason, if no grain is ingested, the qi will diminish in half a day and run short in a day.[116]

The Yellow Emperor asked:

Can you tell me what the five flavors of grains are?

Qi Bo answered:

Of the five grains, rice is sweet, flax ["red bean" in the *Su Wen* {later editor}] is sour, soybean is salty, wheat is bitter and millet is acrid. Of the five fruits, jujube is sweet, plum is sour, chestnut is salty, almond is bitter, and peach is acrid. Of the five animal (meats), beef is sweet, dog meat is sour, pork is salty, mutton is bitter, and chicken is acrid. Of the five vegetables, hollyhock is sweet, leek is sour, red bean leaf is salty, shallot is bitter, and scallion is acrid. Of the five colors, yellow has an affinity for sweetness, green–blue for sourness, black for saltiness, red for bitterness, and white for acridity.

For those with spleen disease, it is appropriate to eat rice, beef, jujube, and hollyhock. They are used because sweetness enters the spleen. For those with heart disease, it is appropriate to eat wheat, mutton, almond, and shallot. They are used because bitterness enters the heart. For those with kidney disease, it is appropriate to eat soybean, pork, chestnut, and redbean leaf. They are used because saltiness enters the kidney. For those with lung disease, it is appropriate to eat millet, chicken, peach, and scallion. They are used because acridity enters the lung. For those with liver disease it is appropriate to eat flax, dog meat, plum, and leek. They are used because sourness enters the liver. In liver disease, the use of acrid is prohibited. In heart disease, the use of salt is prohibited. In spleen disease, the use of sour is prohibited. In lung disease, the use of bitter is prohibited. And in kidney disease, the use of sweet is prohibited.

(2)

The liver is primarily treated through the foot *jue yin* and *shao yang*. The liver is bitter about tension, and sweetness can be eaten without delay to relax it. The heart is mainly treated through the hand *shao yin* and *tai yang*. The heart is bitter about slackness, and sourness can be eaten to contract it. The spleen is mainly treated through the foot *tai yin* and *yang ming*. The spleen is bitter about dampness, and bitterness can be eaten without delay to dry it. The lung is mainly treated through the hand *tai yin* and *yang ming*. The lung

is bitter about qi upward counterflow, and bitterness can be eaten without delay to drain it. The kidney is mainly treated through the foot *shao yin* and *tai yang*. The kidney is bitter about dryness, and acridity can be eaten to moisten it. (The above prescriptions are able to) open the interstices, bring over fluid and humor, and free the flow of the qi tunnels.[117]

Poisons (are eaten to) attack evils, the five grains (are eaten) as nourishments, the five fruits (are eaten) as aids, the five meats (are eaten) as boosters, and the five vegetables (are eaten) as supplements. (Different) qi and flavors administered in combination can replenish the essence and boost the qi. These five flavors may each bring specific benefits: acridity is dispersing, sourness is contracting, sweetness is slackening, bitterness is hardening, and saltiness is softening.

Liver disease (is characterized by) pain in the region of the free ribs radiating to the lateral lower abdomen and causes people to be irascible. In the case of (liver qi) vacuity, there is blurred vision, loss of hearing, and apprehension as if one feared arrest. Therefore, to treat it, one should take the channels of the liver, (*i.e.,*) the foot *jue yin* and *shao yang*. In the case of qi counterflow, there is headache, sore eyes, loss of hearing acuity, and swelling of the cheek. (To treat it,) take the blood (vessels).[118]

It is also stated that dizziness with blinking of the eyes, tremor of the head, heavy eyes, and deafness (are ascribed to) repletion above and vacuity below. The fault lies with the foot *shao yang* and *jue yin*, and, in the extreme, (the evil) may enter the liver.[119]

Heart disease (is characterized by) pain in the chest, propping fullness in the lateral costal regions, pain in the subaxillary regions, pain in the bosom, upper back, and border of the scapula, and pain in the inner aspect of the arm. In the case of (heart qi) vacuity, there is enlargement of the chest and abdomen and a dragging pain between the region of the free ribs and the lumbus. Take the channels of (the heart, *i.e.,*) the hand *shao yin* and *tai yang*, and the blood (vessel) under the tongue. If (extra) transmuted disease arises, prick the blood (vessel) at the popliteal fossa.[120]

It is also stated that pain in the chest with propping fullness and a dragging pain in the lumbar spine is impugned to the hand *shao yin* and *tai yang* [the *Su Wen* says that vexation of the heart and headache is a disease in the diaphragm, but the fault lies with the hand great yang and *shao yin*. {later editor}]

Spleen disease (is characterized by) generalized heaviness, a tendency to hunger, atonic muscles and flesh, debilitated feet, a tendency to tugging and slackening when walking, and pain in the soles of the feet. In the case of (spleen qi) vacuity, there is abdominal distention, rumbling of the intestines, swill diarrhea, and inability to transform food. Take the channels of the spleen, (i.e.,) the foot *tai yin* and the foot *yang ming* and the blood (vessels of) the foot *shao yin*.

It is also stated that, in the case of abdominal distention and (chest) fullness, propping fullness in the subaxillary and lateral costal regions, and inversion below and dashing upward are impugned to the foot *tai yin* and *yang ming*.[121]

Lung disease (is characterized by) counterflow qi dyspnea and cough, pain in the shoulder and upper back, sweating, hypertonicity of the sacro-coccygeal region, medial aspect of the thigh, and knee, and pain in all the hips, calves, and the lower leg (i.e., the shins) and feet. In the case of (lung qi) vacuity, there is diminished qi which is insufficient to allow one to catch one's breath, deafness and dry throat. Take the blood (vessels) lateral to the channels of the lung (i.e.,) the hand *tai yin* and foot *tai yang*, (the blood vessel) medial to the (foot) *jue yin*, and (the blood vessel of) the *shao yin*.

It is also stated that qi ascension coughing is a disease ["inversion" in the *Su Wen* {later editor}] in the chest, and is impugned to the hand *yang ming* and *tai yang*.

Kidney disease (is characterized by) abdominal distention, swelling and pain in the lower leg, coughing and dyspnea, generalized heaviness, sweating while asleep, and abhorrence of wind. In the case of (kidney qi) vacuity, there is pain in the chest, pain in the upper and lower abdomen, frigid inversion, and melancholy. Take the blood (vessels) of the channels of the kidney (i.e.,) the foot *shao yin*, and of the *tai yang*.

It is also stated that headache and madness (are due to) vacuity below and repletion above, that the fault lies with the foot *shao yin* and *tai yang*, and that, in the extreme, (evil) may enter the kidney.

Chapter Ten

Great Treatise on the Transmission of Disease Among the Five Viscera[122]

Disease in the liver will heal in summer. If it does not heal in the summer, it will become severe in autumn. If it does not end in death during the autumn, it will remain stable in winter and improve in spring.[123]

Disease in the liver will heal on *bing* and *ding* days.[124] If it does not heal on *bing* and *ding* days, it will worsen on the *geng* and *xin* days. If it does not worsen on *geng* and *xin* days ["if it does not end in death" in the *Su Wen*, the same hereafter {later editor}], it will remain stable on *ren* and *gui* days and improve on *jia* and *yi* days. One should avoid being caught in a draft.

Disease in the liver is serene during the calm dawn watch,[125] severe at the late afternoon watch, and tranquil during the midnight watch.

Disease in the heart will heal in long summer, and if it does not heal in the long summer, it will become severe in winter. If it does not end in death during the winter, it will remain stable in spring and improve in summer.

Disease in the heart will heal on *wu* and *ji* days, and if it does not heal on *wu* and *ji* days, it will worsen on *ren* and *gui* days. If it does not worsen on *ren* and *gui* days, it will remain stable on *jia* and *yi* days and improve on the *bing* and *ding* days. Warm clothing and hot food are prohibited.

Disease in the heart is serene during the midday watch, severe at the midnight watch, and tranquil during the calm dawn watch.

Disease in the spleen will heal in autumn. If it does not heal in the autumn, it will become severe in spring. If it does not end in death during the spring, it will remain stable in the summer and improve in long summer.

Disease in the spleen will heal on *geng* and *xin* days. If it does not heal on *geng* and *xin* days, it will worsen on *jia* and *yi* days. If it does not worsen on *jia* and *yi* days, it will remain stable on *bing* and *ding* days and improve on the *wu* and *ji* days. Warm clothing and damp living environments are prohibited. [It is said in the *Su Wen* that warm clothing, eating to satiation, living in a damp environment, and soaking wet clothing are prohibited. {later editor}]

Disease in the spleen is serene during the sun descent watch, severe at the calm dawn watch, ["sunrise watch" in the *Su Wen*, {later editor}] and tranquil during the midday watch.

Disease in the lung will heal in winter. If it does not heal in the winter, it will become severe in summer. If it does not end in death during the summer, it will remain stable in long summer and improve in autumn.

Disease in the lung will heal on the *ren* and *gui* days. If it does not heal on *ren* and *gui* days, it will worsen on the *bing* and *ding* days. If it does not worsen on *bing* and *ding* days, it will remain stable on *wu* and *ji* days and improve on *geng* and *xin* days. Thin clothing and cold food and drink are prohibited.

Disease in the lung is serene during the late after-noon watch, severe at the midday watch, and tranquil during the midnight watch.

Disease in the kidney will heal in spring. If it does not heal in the spring, it will become severe in long summer. If it does not end in death during the long summer, it will remain stable in autumn and improve in winter.

Disease in the kidney will heal on the *jia* and *yi* days. If it does not heal on *jia* and *yi* days, it will worsen on the *wu* and *ji* days. If it does not worsen on *wu* and *ji* days, it will remain stable on *geng* and *xin* days and improve on the *ren* and *gui* days. Fried and puffed food is prohibited, and hot food and warm clothing should be avoided. [It is said in the *Su Wen* that this prohibition of fried, puffed, hot food and warm clothing should not be violated. {later editor}]

Disease in the kidney is serene during the mid-night watch, severe at the watches corresponding to the four seasons, and tranquil during the late afternoon watch.[126]

Evil qi that has intruded upon the body is dependent on the inter-restraining relationship. On reaching the engendering phase, the condition is cured. On reaching the restrained phase, it becomes severe. On reaching the engendered phase, it remains stable. And it improves upon reaching its own phase.[127]

(2)

The kidney shifts cold to the spleen, giving rise to *yong* swelling and diminished qi. The spleen shifts cold to the liver, giving rise to *yong* swelling and hypertonicity of the sinews. The liver shifts cold to the heart, giving rise to mania and repel-lency in the center (*ge zhong,*膈中). The heart shifts cold to the lung, giving rise to lung wasting thirst. Lung wasting thirst (refers to) urinating twice as much water as one has consumed. It is fatal and cannot be treated. The lung shifts cold to the kid-ney, giving rise to gushing water. Gushing water is (a disorder in which) the abdomen does not feel firm. This is due to water qi intruding upon the large intestine, and it produces a gurgling sound with movement such as that emitted from a bag containing water. (One should) treat that which rules the lung. ["It is a disease of water" in the *Su Wen*. {later editor}][128]

The spleen shifts heat to the liver, giving rise to susceptibility to fright and nose-bleeding. The liver shifts heat to the heart, and this is fatal. The heart shifts heat to the lung which is transmuted into diaphragmatic wasting thirst. The lung shifts heat to the kidney which is transmuted into soft tetany. The kidney shifts heat to the spleen which is transmuted into vacuity intestinal *pi*. This is fatal and cannot be treated. The uterus shifts heat to the urinary bladder, giving rise to dribbling urinary block and urination of blood. The urinary bladder shifts heat to the small intestine, giving rise to intestinal stoppage, constipation with oral putrescence above. The small intestine shifts heat to the large intestine, giving rise to covert conglomeration (*fu jia*, 虙 瘕) and piles. The large intestine shifts heat to the stomach, giving rise to emaciation despite large food intake. This is referred to as food lassitude. The stomach shifts heat to the gallbladder, and this also is called food lassitude. The gallbladder shifts heat to the brain, giving rise to acrid nose nasal hollowing,[129] characterized by turbid snivel that runs incessantly. This may be transmuted into nosebleeding of filthy blood and heaviness of the eyes. (All the above) are a result of inversion.[130]

(3)

The five viscera (each) receive (evil) qi from the engendered (viscus) and transmit it on to the restrained (viscus). This (evil) qi settles in the engendering (viscus) and is fatal to the restrained (viscus). A disease leading to death must first be transmitted before reaching the restrained viscus and resulting in death. This (condition) is spoken of as the contrary movement of (evil) qi, and, therefore, this is fatal.[131]

The liver receives (evil) qi from the heart and transmits it to the spleen. This (evil) qi settles in the kidney and when it reaches the lung it ends in death. The heart receives (evil) qi from the spleen and transmits it to the lung. This (evil) qi settles in the liver, and when it reaches the kidney, it ends in death. The spleen receives (evil) qi from the lung and transmits it to the kidney. This (evil) qi settles in the heart, and when it reaches the liver, it ends in death. The lung receives (evil) qi from the kidney and transmits it to the liver. This (evil) qi settles in the spleen, and when it reaches the heart, it ends in death. The kidney receives (evil) qi from the liver and transmits it to the heart. This (evil) qi settles in the lung and when it reaches the spleen, it ends in death. All of these contrary (transmissions of evil qi) are fatal. Divide a day and night into five periods and one can tell whether the time of death will occur in the morning or in the evening.[132]

(4)

The Yellow Emperor asked:

I have learned the nine types of needle from Your Honor and have myself read about the various modalities. There is cultivation and conduction of qi, massage, moxibustion and ironing, acupuncture, red–hot needling, and drinking medication. (Should one) keep to one of them only or try to practice them all?

Qi Bo answered:

All of these modalities are suitable for one person or another, but not all of them should be tried on one single person.

The Yellow Emperor asked:

This means that if (one) keeps to one (principle) without straying, tens of thousands of things are all attainable. I have learned the essentials of yin and yang, the theory of vacuity and repletion, the troubles caused by overwhelming and (counter) transference, and what conditions are curable. I would like to learn of the transmutation of disease, the transmission of sapping (evil), and of vanquished and expired (true qi), all of which are incurable. Would you tell me about this?[133]

Qi Bo answered:

Your questions are quite to the point! In regard to the doctrines, (one who is) enlightened can be (as brilliant) as if awake at daybreak, while (one who is) puzzled can be (in the dark) as with eyes closed in the night. Receptivity and practice lead to the ultimate in spiritual attainment. If (one) has applied (all one has learned, one's) spirit will have full mastery. These spirit–enlightening doctrines, deserving of being committed to bamboo and silk, should not be limited to one's own offspring.[134]

The Yellow Emperor asked:

What is implied by being awake at daybreak?

Qi Bo answered:

When one is clear regarding (the condition of) yin and yang, it is as if one has solved a puzzle or become sober after being intoxicated.

The Yellow Emperor asked:

What is implied by eyes closed in the night?

Qi Bo answered:

(Evil) is silent, producing no sound, and obscure, having no shape. It breaks the hair, effuses the interstices, and plunges the righteous qi into tumult and commotion. This sapping evil runs wild and, transmitted through and lodged within the blood vessels, the great qi enters the viscera, causing abdominal pain and lower flux. It can result in death but never in survival.[135]

(5)

The Yellow Emperor asked:

What happens when the great qi has entered the viscera?

Qi Bo answered:

If a disease first develops in the heart, there will be cardiac pain. One day later, it reaches the lung, causing dyspnea and cough. Three days later, it reaches the liver, causing propping fullness in the (free) rib region. Five days later, it reaches the spleen, causing blockage and stoppage, generalized pain, and heaviness. If it is not cured within three days, the condition is fatal. This will occur during the midnight watch in winter or at the midday watch in summer.[136]

If a disease first develops in the lung, there will be dyspnea and cough. Three days later, it reaches the liver, causing propping fullness in the lateral costal region. One day later, it reaches the spleen, causing generalized pain and heaviness. And five days later, it reaches the stomach, causing distention. If it is not cured within ten days, death comes. This will occur during the sundown watch in winter or at the sunrise watch in summer.[137]

If a disease first develops in the liver, there will be headache and visual dizziness with pain in the lateral costal regions and propping fullness. One day later, it reaches the spleen, causing generalized pain and heaviness. Five days later, it reaches the stomach, causing abdominal distention. Three days later it reaches the kidney, causing pain in the lumbar spine, lower abdominal pain, and aching in the lower leg. If it is not cured within three days, death comes. This will occur during the sundown watch in winter or at the breakfast watch in summer.[138]

If a disease first develops in the spleen, there will be generalized pain and heaviness. One day later it reaches the stomach, causing abdominal distention. Two days later, it reaches the kidney, causing pain in the lateral lower abdomen and lumbar spine and aching in the lower legs. Three days later, it reaches the urinary bladder, causing pain in the paravertebral sinews of the back and urinary blockage. If it is not cured within ten days, death comes. This occurs during the serenity watch in winter or after breakfast in summer.

If a disease first develops in the stomach, there

will be distention and fullness. Five days later, it reaches the kidney, causing pain in the lateral lower abdomen and lumbar spine and aching of the lower legs. Three days later, it reaches the urinary bladder, causing pain in the paravertebral sinews at the back and urinary blockage. Five days later, it reaches the spleen, causing generalized pain and heaviness. If it is not cured within six days, death comes. This occurs during the midnight watch in winter or at the sundown watch in summer.

If a disease first develops in the kidney, there will be pain in the lateral lower abdomen and lumbar spine and aching in the lower legs. Three days later, it reaches the urinary bladder, causing pain in the paravertebral sinews of the back and urinary blockage. Three days later, it ascends to the heart, causing cardiac pain. Three days after, it reaches the small intestine, causing abdominal distention. If it is not cured within three days, death comes. This occurs at daybreak in winter or during the sundown watch in summer. [In the *Ling Shu* and the *Su Wen* the disease is said to reach the small intestine without mentioning the heart. This passage is a result of combined references to the above two books made by Huang-fu Shi-an. {later editor}]

If a disease first develops in the urinary bladder, there will be pain in the paravertebral sinews of the back and urinary blockage. Five days later, it reaches the kidney, causing lateral lower abdominal distention, pain in the lumbar spine, and aching in the lower legs. One day later, it reaches the small intestine, causing abdominal distention. Two days after, it reaches the spleen, causing generalized pain. If it is not cured within two days, death comes. This occurs during the cockcrow watch in winter or at the sun descent watch in summer.

Various diseases are transmitted in sequence. If they do so (in the above) order, they end (inevitably) in death on certain dates and should not be needled. If, however, (a disease) skips over one to three or even four viscera, this condition may be needled.[139]

Chapter Eleven

Great Treatise on Long Life & Premature Death as Diagnosed Through Examination of the Form, Disease Signs, and Whether or Not Pain Can Be Endured[140]

(1)

The Yellow Emperor asked:

Form may be slack or tense. Qi (may be) exuberant or diminished. The bone (may be) large or small. The flesh (may be) strong or fragile. The skin (may be) thick or thin. How are long life and premature death determined (based upon these factors)?[141]

Bo Gao answered:

If there is coordination between form and qi, one will live a long life, but if there is no such coordination, one will die prematurely. If there is a close fit (*xiang guo*, 相果) between the skin and the flesh, one will attain longevity, but if there is no such fit, one will die prematurely. If there is a prevalence of blood and qi and of the channels and the network vessels over form, one will live a long life, while if there is no such prevalence, one will die prematurely.[142]

The Yellow Emperor asked:

What does a slack or a tense form signify?

Bo Gao answered:

If the form is full and the skin slack, one will live a long life. If the form is full and the skin tense, one will die prematurely. A full form with a hard large pulse is a favorable (indication). A full form with a small, weak pulse means the qi is debilitated, and this debilitation is a dangerous condition. A full form with flat cheekbones means the kidney is small. This smallness signifies a premature death. A full form with major muscular masses that are solid and clearly outlined means the muscles are solid. This solidity signifies a long life. A full form with major muscular masses that are indistinctly outlined and lack solidity means the muscles are fragile. This fragility signifies a premature death. This is the way of heaven in which form is established and qi determined at birth. In examining (form and qi one may ascertain whether) one will live long or die prematurely. (One) must be clear about these factors and be capable of establishing form and determining qi (in a patient). Only then can one receive patients and ascertain whether they will die or live.[143]

The Yellow Emperor asked:

In establishing a prevalence of either form or qi over one another, how may a long life or a premature death be established?

Bo Gao answered:

In a normal person a prevalence of qi over form means they will live a long life. The diseased who shed flesh from their bodies will die if qi prevails over form. However, if form prevails over the qi, the condition is still critical.

(2)

The five viscera constitute the organs of the central (government). In a condition where the center is exuberant, the viscera full, the qi prevailing and there is fright damage, a voice that is as if it were coming from another room is due to dampness of the central qi. Speech that is faint and broken with long intermissions is due to a deprivation of qi. Slovenly dress and speaking nonsense regardless of whether one is dear or a distant (acquaintance) is a manifestation of deranged spirit light. A failure of the granaries to store is due to the gates failing in their assignment. Incessant flowing of the spring is due to the urinary bladder failing to store. Restoration (of the ability to perform one's) duties means survival; (long-lasting) dereliction of (one's) duties means death.[144]

The five viscera determine the strength of the body. The head is the dwelling place of bright essence. (Thus) inclination of the head with sunken eyes indicate impending deprivation of spirit. The upper back is the dwelling place (of those viscera lying within) the chest. When the upper back is bent with shoulders stooped, this indicates an impending breakdown (of the viscera) dwelling there. The lumbar region is the dwelling place of the kidney. Its inability to turn or rock indicates impending exhaustion of the kidney. The knees are the dwelling place of the sinews. Their inability to bend and stretch along with an arched back while walking indicates impending exhaustion of the sinews. The bones are the dwelling place of the marrow. An inability to stand for an extended period of time and an unsteady pace with a tremor while walking indicate impending exhaustion of the marrow. Restoration of strength means survival, while any (long–lasting) loss of strength is fatal.[145]

Qi Bo said:

In regard to any incongruity with the seasonal disposition, that which is in a state of surplus is essence, and that which is insufficient is wilting. When an extreme excess is expected, that which is insufficient is essence. When insufficiency is expected, that which is in a state of surplus is wilting. Incompatibility between yin and yang is a disease named barring and repulsion (guan ge).[146]

(3)

Those people with strong bones, forceful sinews, slack flesh, and thick skin endure pain (well), including pain produced (by metal and) stone needles as well as burning by fire. If they have a black complexion and well–developed ["beautiful" in a variant version {later editor}] skeleton in addition, they endure burning by fire still better. Those with solid flesh and thin skin do not endure the pain produced by (metal and) stone needles nor do they endure burning by fire. If their bodies are damaged to the same degree, those with much heat recover easily, while those with much cold recover with difficulty. Those with thick (walled) stomachs, black complexions, large bones, and fat flesh can overcome toxins, while those who are lean and possess thin (walled) stomachs cannot.[147]

Chapter Twelve

Great Treatise on the Waxing & Waning of Form & Qi[148]

(1)

The Yellow Emperor asked:

Can you tell me about the waxing and waning of qi?

Qi Bo answered:

At the age of ten ["sixteen" in a variant version {later editor}], humans have only just established their five viscera, and their blood and qi flow freely. Because their qi is located below, they are fond of running. At the age of twenty, their blood and qi are waxing and their muscles are growing (rapidly). So they tend to hurry. At the age of thirty, their five viscera have become ultimately established, their muscles and flesh are strong and solid, and their blood vessels are exuberant and full. Therefore, they are fond of walking at a slow pace. At the age of forty, their five viscera, six bowels, and twelve channel vessels are all in a state of major exuberance, in equilibrium and stability. Their interstices begin to open, their luxuriance and efflorescence begins to scale off, and the hair at their temples becomes gray. As (their blood and qi) are in a state of equilibrium and unshakability, they are fond of sitting. At the age of fifty, their liver qi begins to wane, the lobes of their liver become thinner, (the production of) gall begins to diminish, and their eye-sight becomes dim. At the age of sixty, their heart qi begins to wane and they become liable to worries and sadness. Because their blood and qi becomes listless and inert, they are fond of sleeping. At the

age of seventy, their spleen qi becomes vacuous and their skin desiccated. As a result, their four limbs lose their ability to lift. At the age of eighty, their lung qi begins to wane and their corporeal and ethereal souls have separated. As a result, their speech is often confused. At the age of ninety, their kidney qi is parched, their viscera become wilted and desiccated, and their channels and vessels become empty. Toward the age of one hundred, all their five viscera become vacuous, their spirit and qi have both departed, leaving the formal skeleton alone, and life comes to an end.[149]

(2)

In females, at seven years old their kidney qi is waxing, their teeth change, and their hair grows long. At two times seven, their celestial water (*tian gui*, 天癸) ["the celestial *gui*" in the *Su Wen* {later editor}] appears, their conception vessel flows freely, their great penetrating vessel is waxing, and their menses discharge regularly. As a result, they can bear a child. At the age of three times seven, their kidney qi is balanced and in equilibrium. Therefore, their true teeth[150] grow and (their body) grows to the maximum. At four times seven, their sinews and bones become strong, their hair has grown to its maximum, and their bodies are vigorous and sturdy. At five times seven, their *yang ming* vessel is on the wane, their face begins to become parched, and their hair begins to fall out. At six times seven, the three yang channels are on the wane above, their face is all parched, and their hair begins to turn gray. At seven times seven, their conception vessel becomes empty, their great penetrating vessel is diminished and scanty, their celestial water is exhausted, and their terrestrial tunnel is blocked. Consequently, their form becomes distorted and they can no longer bear children.[151]

In males, at eight years old their kidney qi is replete, their hair grows long, and their teeth change. At two times eight, their kidney qi waxes, their celestial water appears, their essential qi spills and drains, and their yin and yang come into harmony. As a result, they can father a child. At three times eight, their kidney qi is balanced and in equilibrium and their sinews and bones are strong and forceful. As a result, their true teeth grow and (their body) grows to the maximum. At four times eight, their sinews and bones become mighty and sturdy, and their muscles and flesh become full and solid. At five times eight, their kidney qi wanes, their hair begins to fall out and their teeth become dry. At six times eight, their yang qi is on the wane above, their face becomes parched, and their hair turns gray at the temples. At seven times eight, their liver qi is on the wane, their sinews are no longer able to act (in a flexible way), their celestial water becomes exhausted, their essence (i.e., semen) becomes scanty, their kidney qi is on the wane, and their formal bodies becomes extremely (decrepit). At eight times eight, their teeth and hair are gone. The kidney governs water, and receives and stores essence from the other viscera and the six bowels. Therefore, they are unable to discharge (essence) unless the five viscera are exuberant. Now their five viscera are all on the wane, their sinews and bones become listless and inert, and their celestial water comes to naught. As a result, their hair turns white at the temples, their bodies become heavy, their steps are awry, and they can no longer father a child.[152]

Endnotes

[1]Part 1 is derived from Chap. 79, Vol. 12, *Ling Shu (Spiritual Pivot)*; Part 2 from Chap. 77, Vol. 11, *Ling Shu*; and Part 3 from Chap. 79, Vol. 12, *Ling Shu*.

[2]The eight orientations are the Winter Solstice, Summer Solstice, Spring Equinox, Autumn Equinox, Beginning of Spring, Beginning of Summer, Beginning of Autumn, and Beginning of Winter. They fall on eight days which vary from year to year in the lunar calendar but can be calculated by a special method. They are also called eight transmissions because they each terminate a preceeding and begin a new period with a particular weather feature. The particular days they fall on and the characteristics of weather changes associated with them are believed to decide the weather and many other events, such as epidemics during the period they usher in.

[3]A vacuity evil may strike people without causing any trouble for the time being, but it will hide itself somewhere in the body. When a new evil strikes,

the old evil will conspire with it to cause illness this time. Then the channels are bound and the righteous qi within them is overridden once again by the evil qi. We see dew primarily in autumn, a season when every living thing is beginning to wither, therefore annual dew is a killer. Therefore, by analogy, if one is struck by wind and rain, one is encountering the killing dew.

[4]The first day of a month is called the new moon day.

[5]I.e., 3–5 a.m. and 11 a.m.–1 p.m. respectively

[6] In ancient China the twelve earthly branches were used to denote the dates in the month. However, they were usually employed in combination with the ten heavenly stems. *Chou* is B2; *xu* B11; *si* B6; *shen* B9. For details, see note 86, Chap. 9, Book 1, and parts of Chapter 10, Book 1, present work.

[7]This passage may be garbled since it differs in many places from the corresponding lines in the *Ling Shu*. These are given as follows for reference:

The Yellow Emperor asked:

What is the cost of the (various) evil vacuity winds and how are they determined?

Shao Shi answered:

On the day of the new moon of the first month, the supreme unity dwells in the celestial residence. If there is northwest wind without rain, many people will die. On the day of the new moon day of the first month, if there is north wind at the calm dawn watch, many people will die in the spring. On the day of the new moon of the first month, if there is a north wind at the calm dawn watch, many people will suffer from disease, as many as three people in ten. On the day of the new moon day of the first month, if there is a north wind at the midday watch, many people will die in the summer. On the day of the new moon of the first month, if there is a north wind in the evening, many people will die in the autumn. If north wind blows the whole day, six people in ten will contract severe disease and die. On the day of the new moon, the wind blowing from the south is called draft home. The wind blowing from the west is called white bone and brings disasters to the country and causes a great many deaths. On the day of the new moon of the first month, if there is a wind from the east demolishing houses and raising sand and stones, a great disaster will happen to the country. On the day of the new moon of the first month, if there is a wind from the southeast, the spring will see deaths. On the day of the new moon of the first month, if it is mild and windless, grains will be cheap and the people free from disease. If it is cold and windy, grains will be expensive and a great many people will suffer from disease. These are winds which decide the year and which may bring harm and damage to people. If it is windless on the *chou* day of the second month, a great many people will suffer from cardiac and abdominal disease. If it is not warm on the *xu* day of the third month, a great many people will suffer from cold and heat disease. If summerheat fails to come upon on the *si* day of the fourth month, a great many people will suffer from jaundice. If it is not cold on the *shen* day of the tenth month, a great many people will suffer sudden deaths.

The term Supreme Unity means the pole star. The celestial residence is the *gen* palace which is earth and is associated with the northeast. It is symbolic of the Beginning of Spring. Draft simply means the south.

[8]Antagonistic means opposite, while afar means from a great distance. Take, for instance, the eleventh month which is *zi* (S1) and is associated with the north. If a wind blows from *wu* (S7), *i.e.*, the south, which is exactly opposite to the appropriate direction of the given month, the way from *zi* to *wu* is longer than the distance to any other branch. Thus it is a vacuity wind.

[9]The above eight paragraphs come from Chap. 77, *Ling Shu*, where the nine palaces and the eight winds are discussed. See Chap. 10, Book 11, present work, for a discussion of the concepts involved.

Zhang Jing–yue explains in his *Lei Jing (The Classified Classic)*, "The south is the *li* fire palace, a quarter of exuberant heat. A wind from it must enfeeble (people) and is, therefore, called as great enfeebling wind. In relation to humans, the fire viscus corresponds to it. (Therefore,) it settles in the heart internally and lodges in the vessel externally, occasioning heat disease... The southwest is the *kun* earth palace, where the yin qi is just beginning to generate while the yang qi is still exuberant. (At the moment) yin and yang seem to be discussing their staying and departing. Therefore, the wind is called as intriguing wind. In relation to humans, the earth viscus corresponds to it. Therefore, it settles in the spleen in the internal and lodges in the muscles in the external. The spleen is averse to yin dampness. For that reason, the qi (of the wind) is capable of giving rise to weakness...The west is the *dui* metal palace. Metal qi is unyielding and strong. Therefore, the wind is called unyielding wind. In

relation to humans, the metal viscus corresponds to it. Therefore, it settles in the lung in the internal and lodges in the skin in the external. The northwest is the *qian* metal palace. Metal breaks and cuts. Therefore, the wind is called breaking wind. When a wind qi hurts people, a south (wind) finds expression in the upper (of the body), while a north (wind) in the lower (of the body). For that reason, the small intestine with the hand *tai yang* channel is subjected to disease (in the case). The small intestine...is a fire bowel in the lower burner. The metal in the west, however, is a depurating and killing qi, while the water in the north is a ruthless and savage qi. The combined qi of the north and west is most capable of felling the vital yang and, therefore, may cause people to die... The north is the *kan* water palace. Because its qi is cold, the wind is sweeping, and is, therefore, called great unyielding wind. In relation to humans, the water viscus corresponds to it. It settles in the kidney in the internal and lodges externally in the bones and the paravertebral sinews in the shoulder and upper back which are located on the route of the foot *tai yang* channel... The northeast is the *gen* earth palace. (At the moment,) the yin has not yet abated, while the harmonizing yang has not yet become exuberant. (This wind) is, therefore, called ferocious wind. In relation to humans, it hurts the large intestine... (Therefore, it affects) the regions under the bones below the lateral costal regions and axillae for they are adjacent to the large intestines. (It also affects) the limb joints since they are the places accessible to the hand *yang ming* channel... The east is the *zhen* wood palace, and the wind arising in the east is, therefore, called infant wind. In relation to humans, the wood viscus corresponds to it. Therefore, the disease settles in the liver and externally in the junctures between sinews and bones... The southeast is the *xun* wood palace. When qi is warm, wind is feeble, and, therefore, it is called enfeebling wind. In the southeast, dampness prevails, which under the help of wood rebels against earth. For that reason, insofar as it hurts people, it settles in the stomach internally and in the muscles and flesh externally. Its pathogenic qi is capable of giving rise to generalized heaviness."

[10]Wind from the home of vacuity is vacuity wind as explained earlier in this chapter. For further information about the three vacuities and three repletions, see the last paragraph of the present chapter. Rain-dew exposure cold and heat is a disease of cold and heat contracted on exposure to rain and wind.

[11]Wind evil of the eight orientations, *i.e.*, the eight winds means wind, prevailing in a given season.

In this sense it reflects normal weather change.

[12]The differentiation between bandit wind and the eight winds is of note. Bandit wind and evil qi refer to an untimely weather change which can happen any time in the four seasons, and possibly strike any part of the body. The eight winds, however, only occur on the eight orientations and cause definite patterns of disease.

[13]A note in the *Tai Su* says, "The sun is yang, while the moon is yin. The east sea is yang and the west sea is yin. The moon may be waxing and waning, and the seas may be void and replete. The moon is the yin essence, governing water. Therefore, with a full moon, the west sea is abundant, while with an invisible moon, the east sea becomes abundant, for when yin is diminishing, yang is exuberant." The *Lei Jing* explains smoky grime as "an oily layer. It is said to be like smoke because, with the blood replete and the body corpulent, it sticks to the skin as a defense of the exterior, while with blood vacuity it disappears."

[14]The declining year is also known as insufficient annual qi and is determined by an elaborate calculation of the five movements and the six qi. The annual qi, classified into five kinds, *i.e.*, metal, wood, water, fire, and earth, may be insufficient, surplus, and average or normal. Human qi corresponds to the moon, and these two wax and wane in step. For this reason, when the moon is waning, the qi in the body also wanes.

[15]Part 1 is derived from Chap. 29, Vol. 6, *Ling Shu*; Part 2 from Chap. 65, *Su Wen*; Part 3 from Chap. 12, Vol. 3, *Ling Shu*; and Part 4 from Chap. 24, *Su Wen*.

[16]The terms *ben* and *biao* are rendered here as root and branch respectively. It is of note, however, that in discussing channel pathways earlier in this work, these two terms have been rendered as origin and endpoint respectively to clarify their relationships with the *gen* and *jie*, or roots and terminations.

[17]Zhang Jing–yue explains in his *Lei Jing*, "Predilection is appropriateness. It encompasses living environments, tranquility and activity, yin and yang, cold and heat, temperament, smell and flavor."

[18]Center heat wasting thirst is middle burner pure heat wasting thirst. The center refers to the stomach and intestines.

[19]Zhang Jing–yue explains in the *Lei Jing*, "In spring and summer, qi manifests itself externally, so disease exists in the exterior. The exterior is the branch of the interior. It is therefore said that the branch is treated prior to the root. In autumn and winter, qi is hidden internally, so disease exists in the interior. The interior is the root of the exterior. It is therefore said that the root is treated prior to the branch."

[20]This paragraph can be understood in another way. It may assert that, in cold weather, such patients should be clothed moderately warmly, and, in summerheat, they should be clothed thinly and kept moderately cool. Food and drinks should never be too hot or too cold. There is still another understanding which is a combination of the preceding two. That is, this passage can be interpreted as a suggestion that one take into account both the patient's personal predilections and weather factors.

[21]If a disease results in counterflow, the disease is the root and should be treated first. If counterflow results in a disease, the counterflow is the root and should be treated first. If a cold disease results in a disease of another nature, the cold disease is the root and should be treated first. If a disease results in cold, the disease is the root and should be treated first. If a hot disease results in a disease of another nature, the heat disease is the root and should be treated first. If a disease results in heat, the disease is the root and should be treated first. If a disease of heat ensues in fullness in the center, the fullness is the branch but should be treated first, for this involves the stomach which is the root of all the viscera and bowels. If a disease results in diarrhea, the disease is the root and should be treated first. If diarrhea results in a disease of another nature, the diarrhea is the root and should be treated first. If disease results in center fullness, the fullness is the branch but should be treated first. If fullness in the center results in vexation, the fullness is the root and should be treated first. No matter whether there is a new external contraction of evil qi (*i.e.*, visiting or guest qi) or an old or inveterate disease (*i.e.*, intrinsic qi), inhibited urination and defecation, whenever they occur, must be treated first, even though they are the branch. This is because inhibition of urination and defecation is always an urgent condition. If a repletion pattern illness occurs, the repletion of evil qi is the root and other conditions are branches. In that case, the root should be treated first. If a disease characterized by insufficiency occurs, this insufficiency of the essential qi is the branch but should be treated first. Only afterwards can we turn to the cause of the disease which is the root.

There are different interpretations as to meaning of counterflow in this passage. Zhang Jing–yue asserts that it is counterflow of qi and blood. Wu Kun believes it to be counterflow retching. And Zhang Zhi–cong refers to it as counterflow inversion.

[22]Fresh delicacies refer to butter, milk, meat, and the like. The internal generation of diseases implies that diseases are caused by internal injuries, such as dietary irregularities, excessive sexual activity, and inordinate emotional disturbances. Toxic medicinals simply mean medicinals, since all medicines are somewhat toxic by nature.

[23]Tiny needle may be a collective term for various types of needles, but Wang Bing believes it to be the small type of needle.

[24]Physical toil is called tormented form, while distress by worry and thought is called tormented orientation. Freedom from worry and distressing thought is called gratified orientation, while an easy life is called gratified form. With gratified form but tormented orientation, the qi is blocked and blood is stagnated, and, therefore, the vessels are congested. The vessels need coursing, and moxibustion and needling accomplish this. Toil easily strains the sinews. Having contracted cold, the damaged sinews become tense, and having contracted heat, they become slack. Therefore, we should apply ironing to conduct the evil qi. An excessively comfortable life without work makes a person inert, and this damages the spleen. The spleen governs the muscles and flesh which, in this circumstance, are subjected to disease. When the flesh is diseased, the defensive qi is retarded, and, as a result, qi and blood are concentrated to produce pus. Stone needling is an ideal modality to remove purulence. When both the form and orientation are taxed too much, yin and yang are both damaged. To treat exhaustion of both yin and yang, the best choice is internal medication.

Emitting blood refers to bloodletting, while emitting qi refers to the administration of drastic draining manipulation. In Chap. 16, Book 1 of the present work, there is a detailed explanation of the quantities of blood and qi in each of the channels. This is the justification for the prescription of, for example, bloodletting or prohibition of it in needling a particular channel.

[25]This entire chapter is derived from Chap. 62, Su Wen.

[26]A long–lost acupuncture work.

[27]The sound that the heart issues is laughter, and the emotion it manifests is joy. A surplus spirit is surplus orientation or emotion, which causes incessant laughing. The heart stores spirit. When the spirit is insufficient, there is heart vacuity, and, as a result, the lungs, which ought to be restrained by the heart, rebel against it. Consequently, there is worry which is the orientation of the lungs.

The merging of blood or qi means that the evil qi, after striking the body, may concentrate in the blood or qi. The Su Wen Zhu Zheng Fa Wei (An Annotated Exposition on the Intricacies of the Basic Questions) explains the term vacuous vessel thus: "When the spirit is insufficient, certain network vessels are vacuous. Now it is necessary to treat the connecting vessel of the heart channel."

[28]This passage deals with the lung qi. Because the lung is metal which is associated with the color white, the lung qi is also known as white qi.

[29]The second sentence may be interpreted in quite a different way, giving the passage an entirely different meaning. This would read, "When needling, the practitioner must change (his mind)." In effect, this means the practitioner inserts the needle shallowly.

[30]I.e., sentimentality

[31]Jerking, tension, and hypertonicity are all ascribed to wind. Vermicular twitching (i.e., squirming movement), or sensations in the muscles and flesh, is also a wind disorder, but it is a mild one. Therefore, it is called slight wind. Because this is a problem involving the flesh which is governed by the spleen, the yang channel is the foot yang ming and the yang connecting vessel is the connecting vessel of the foot yang ming. Zhang Zhi–cong explains, "Needling to drain the channel serves the purpose of conducting (the evil) from the interior to the exterior, while needling to supplement the connecting vessel aims at conducting (the righteous) from the exterior to the interior."

[32]Will is stored in the kidney. A surplus of will may be interpreted as a surplus of kidney yin, which leads to failure of qi transformation, and hence to abdominal distention, etc. Insufficiency of will may refer to insufficiency of kidney yang which is responsible for frigidity and counterflow. The ran sinew containing blood means the blood vessel of the point Blazing Valley (Ran Gu, Ki 2). This is plausible since the author explicitly juxtaposes this place with Return Flow (Fu Liu, Ki 7).

[33]At this juncture, wind cold evil has intruded to the bone and the joints should be needled without delay. Evacuation should be understood in the context of the joints having been filled with wind cold prior to treatment and, following treatment, they are void or freed of the evil.

"Without hitting the channel" may be interpreted in quite a different way. It may be rendered as, "not letting the evil into the channel".

[34]The preceding paragraphs deal with five types of surplus and insufficiency when an evil has not yet

merged with the blood and qi. Whereas this paragraph treats vacuity and repletion when the evil qi has merged with the blood and qi.

When the qi merges with the yang, for example, it is understood that evil qi concentrates or gathers in the yang. When blood gathers in the yin, this is a condition of dual yin or superimposing yin. This leads to withdrawal. When qi gathers in the yang, this is a condition of dual or superimposing yang. This may cause mania. Blood gathering in the yang is a condition of yin lodging in the exterior, since blood can be considered to be yin while the exterior is considered as yang. Qi gathering in the yin is yang lodging in the interior, since qi is considered yang while the interior is yin. When the yang qi is trapped in the yin or the interior, it must be depressed to produce internal heat. The *Su Wen Jing Zhu Jie Jie (Annotations and Explanations on the Classic of the Basic Questions)* explains, "Blood is generated in the heart but stored in the liver. When blood is merged above, it must be exuberant (above) and qi must naturally be merged below, surging upward. Thus the heart and the liver are stirred, causing vexation, oppression, and irritability. If qi...is merged above, this means the qi keeps on ascending and blood is naturally merged below. Above is separated from below, causing dissipated and scattered essence and spirit. As a result, there is derangement and forgetfulness."

[35]The diffusion and departure of the curdling is understood as the resumption of the flowing of blood and qi. For a more thorough understanding of this entire paragraph, see the question and answer immediately below.

[36]If the qi is merged in the yang, there is an absence of blood there. If blood is merged in the yin, there is absence of qi there.

Zhang Jing–yue explains in his *Jing Yue Quan Shu (The Complete Works of [Zhang] Jing-yue)*, "When qi and blood are merged and rush upward, there is yin vacuity below and then the spirit is deprived of its root. This is a pattern of separation between yin and yang which may cause inversion collapse and hence death. (The ability of qi and blood) to restore to normal indicates a moderate case; inability indicates a severe case. This is what people call wind stroke of sudden collapse. It is also known as wind stroke due to congestion of phlegm fire in the upper (body)."

[37]*Ping* literally means balanced or level. A normal person (*ping ren*) is an individual whose yin and yang are in a state of balance.

[38]One should note the Chinese medical multi-meaning use of the same word in the same place. (For example) in this passage, yin and yang may denote three meanings: the yin and yang channels, the internal and external, and sexual intercourse. This is a characteristic of Chinese in general and of Chinese medicine in particular.

A note in the *Tai Su* explains, "The yin and yang vessels of the viscera and bowels all have divergent branches, and they communicate with one another through their transporting and meeting points. The foot *yang ming*, for example, branches off from the point Bountiful Bulge (*Feng Long*, St 40), diverging to the foot *tai yin*. Whereas the (foot) *tai yin* diverges from the point Offspring of Duke (*Gong Sun*, Sp 4) to the foot *yang ming*. This, therefore, is reasonably spoken of as (the yin filling) the external."

[39]Pressure here means massage.

[40]This paragraph focuses primarily on inordinate anger, and the word joy is, in effect, superfluous. Anger makes qi ascend and causes liver depression.

[41]In this case, descending qi means relaxed or slackened qi, as opposed to qi which is actually descending. This term should not be taken at face value. The *Su Wen* states, "Apprehension makes qi descend." Stirring the viscera implies that the cold qi contained in food damages the viscera and curdles the blood.

[42]Zhang Zhi–cong explains in *Su Wen Ji Zhu (Condensed Annotations on the Basic Questions)*, "Dietary (irregularities) and taxation fatigue damage the spleen which governs the muscles and flesh. As a result, the form qi is diminished. Water and grain, after having entered the stomach, are transported by the spleen qi. When the spleen fails to function, the grain qi wanes. When the upper burner is unable to dissipate the flavors of the grains and the lower burner is unable to receive the fluid from water and grain in the stomach, which is a yang bowel of heat, qi will be retained and stops flowing. As a result, hot qi steams the inside of the chest and turns into internal heat."

[43]Zhang Jing–yue explains, "The qi of the upper burner rules the yang phase. It follows that if there is external damage by cold evils, the upper burner stops flowing, the exterior of muscles are blocked, and the defensive qi is depressed and gathered. Because the defensive qi has nowhere to flow, it gives rise to external heat. This is what is meant by the statement that when people are damaged by cold, a disease arises of heat. This is a pattern of external contraction."

44Inverted qi is usually cold or yin in nature. Warm qi is yang qi. A large, exuberant pulse suggests exuberant cold qi in the internal, but since cold qi stagnates blood and qi, the pulse is choppy in addition. The center here refers to the chest rather than to the spleen/stomach as it often suggests.

The *Su Wen* and the *Tai Su* say vessels in place of interstices in this passage.

45To treat such conditions, it is necessary to needle the channel. If the problem involves the constructive, then treat the blood, and if the problem involves the defensive, then treat the qi. Patients vary in bulk, height, fatness, etc., and these variables must be taken into consideration when deciding the depth of the needle insertion and the duration of the retention of the needle. The reader should note that we insert "of needlings" after "the number" at the risk of limiting the meaning of the author. In fact, he may be referring to the number of the points chosen, the times of treatments, etc. Because of the open-endedness and ambiguity of this passage, we have rendered *si shi*, literally the four seasons, as seasonal disposition. Since even the waxing and waning of the moon should be taken into account when deciding the number of treatments, Huang-fu Mi may be using this term in a more general way.

46The reader should note that the author uses the word "qi" in this passage to refer to the breath.

To drain repletion, one should insert the needle when the qi becomes exuberant. In other words, push in the needle with the inhalation. This is done to leave a way for the evil qi to escape. One should withdraw the needle with the exhalation. After extraction, one should not press the needle hole, but, in the process of extracting, one should shake the needle to widen the hole in order to let the evil out. And, at the same time, we should press the point before extracting the needle. This is the so-called grand drainage. This needling method is effective for exuberant evil qi.

47To supplement, the needle inserted should not be shaken so that the needle is in close contact with the tissues around it in the hole. When the qi has reached its zenith, the needle should be rapidly withdrawn, and, after extraction, the hole should be pressed. The needle should be retained in the hole for a certain duration of time and not extracted till the qi is diminishing. Thus the qi that has arrived, *i.e.*, the qi at hand, is preserved, while the qi yet to come, *i.e.*, the distant qi, will not stop half way. Pursuit is another expression for supplementation.

48The five viscera are associated with the six bowels and are also related to the channels, network vessels, limbs, and joints. The vacuity or repletion of the viscera and bowels will find expression in the channels, etc. When one finds a disorder in the exterior, in a joint for example, this can be related to a viscus, and, in accordance with the vacuity or repletion of the viscus, an appropriate treatment plan can be constructed.

49This is pain without a fixed location.

50The term surprise manipulation of the red-hot needle is misleading. This process may sometimes involve simply warming an inserted needle to conduct heat inward. It does not necessarily require the rapid insertion or extraction of the needle as the word surprise suggests, nor is the needle necessarily red hot.

As for disease without knowing pain, Wu Kun explains, "This is a trouble of dampness *bi* with no cold. When dampness prevails, there arises *bi*; when cold prevails, there arises pain. Now, if it knows no pain, dampness *bi* is evident." This disease is one of insensitivity, but it is sometimes misinterpreted as a disease of migratory pain. The two motility vessels refer to Extending Vessel (*Shen Mai*, Bl 62) of the yang motility vessel and Shining Sea (*Zhao Hai*, Ki 6) of the yin motility vessel.

Cross needling and grand needling both require the selection of points contralateral to the diseased side. However, the former is performed on the network vessels, while the latter on the channels. See Chap. 4, Book 5, present work.

51This entire chapter is derived from Chap. 34, Vol. 6, *Ling Shu*.

52Seasonal qi refers to the characteristic weather change in a season which differs from one season to another. If people can adapt themselves to the seasonal qi and succeed in keeping their constructive and defensive flowing in an orderly manner, they will keep fit and healthy.

53The clear qi or the constructive should flow inside the vessels, which are yin. The turbid qi or the defensive should circulate outside the vessels which are yang. If the defensive qi counterflows, this engenders illness.

54*I.e.*, Spirit Door (*Shen Men*, Ht 7) and Great Mound (*Da Ling*, Per 7)
Apparently, the qi here refers to chaotic qi.

55*I.e.*, Fish Border (*Yu Ji*, Lu 10)

56*I.e.*, Great Ravine (*Tai Xi*, Ki 3)

[57]These are the rapids of the hand *tai yin*, *i.e.*, Great Abyss (*Tai Yuan*, Lu 9), the foot *tai yin*, *i.e.*, Supreme White (*Tai Bai*, Sp 3), the hand *yang ming*, *i.e.*, Third Space (*San Jian*, LI 3), and the foot *yang ming*, *i.e.*, Sunken Valley (*Xian Gu*, St 43).

[58]Currently extant versions of the *Ling Shu* also prescribe the foot *tai yang*.

[59]*I.e.*, Valley Passage (*Tong Gu*, Bl 66) and Bundle Bone (*Shu Gu*, Bl 65)

[60]This refers to the brooks and rapids of the hand and foot *yang ming* and *shao yin*, namely, Second Space (*Er Jian*, LI 2), Third Space (*San Jian*, LI 3), Armpit Gate (*Ye Men*, TH 2), Central Islet (*Zhong Zhu*, TH 3), Inner Court (*Nei Ting*, St 44), Sunken Valley (*Xian Gu*, St 43), Pinched Ravine (*Xia Xi*, GB 43), and Foot Overlooking Tears (*Zu Lin Qi*, GB 41).

[61]Supplementation is applicable to vacuity and requires slow insertion and rapid extraction of the needle. Drainage is performed in the case of repletion and is characterized by rapid insertion and slow extraction of the needle. The techniques of essence–communication and qi conduction are suitable for chaotic qi in the absence of notable vacuity or repletion. They are different from the needle techniques of drainage or supplementation. Conducting qi means normalizing chaotic qi, and communicating the essence implies that one is collecting the spirit or gathering the dispersed spirit together.

[62]Part 1 is derived from Chap. 50, Vol. 8, *Ling Shu*; Part 2 from Chap. 58, Vol. 9, *Ling Shu*.

[63]This passage implies five phase inter–restraining relationship. A yellow complexion with thin skin and weak flesh indicates insufficient spleen qi. This pertains to earth. Therefore, spring, which is ascribed to wood, is a challenge to this constitutional type. A white complexion with thin skin and weak flesh indicates insufficient lung qi, which is metal. Therefore, summer, which is ascribed to fire, is a challenge to this constitutional type. A green–blue complexion with thin skin and weak flesh indicates insufficient liver qi. This pertains to wood. Therefore, autumn, which is ascribed to metal, is a challenge to this constitutional type. And a red complexion with thin skin and weak flesh indicates insufficient heart qi. This pertains to fire. Therefore, winter, which is ascribed to water, is a challenge to this constitutional type.

[64]The last sentence implies that disease cannot arise in such people unless there is an old evil hidden in their bodies. Whatever its nature, this becomes exacerbated by a newly contracted evil.

[65]Wu Tang, a.k.a. Wu Ju–tong (1758–1863), the writer of the *Wen Bing Tiao Bian* (*Systematized Study on Warm Disease*), explains, "*Zhu* means telling, while *you* means the cause of disease. In current times some people equate sorcery to *zhu you* and include it as one of the thirteen departments. The *Nei Jing* (*Internal Classic*) asserts that one should not treat those who believe in witchcraft but not in medicine. How then can it be listed as one of the medical departments? To my mind, in treating all cases of internal damage, it is necessary to perform *zhu you*, giving a detailed account of the cause of the disease, (even) helping the patient to understand it, lest he should dare to disregard this aspect. It is necessary to go deep into the heart of those who have fallen in love, to familiarize oneself with the subtle feelings of the laborer and the passionate woman, and to straighten them in a roundabout way... This works miraculously." Based on this explanation, *zhu you* was a form of psychotherapy.

[66]Part 1 is derived from Chap. 6, Vol. 2, *Ling Shu*; Part 2 from Chap. 59, Vol. 9, *Ling Shu*; and Part 3 from Chap. 44, Vol. 7, *Ling Shu*.

[67]Zhang Jing–yue explains in his *Lei Jing*, "Stiffness and flexibility, weakness and strength, and short and tall height are all simply variations of yin and yang. When speaking of yin and yang, all people have some idea (of their meaning). When it comes to the statements that there is yin within yin and there is yang within yang, few people understand this. Therefore, it is necessary to carefully examine yin and yang before (one can) have the correct method of needling."

He continues, "By detecting the onset of disease, it is understood that (we) should determine whether (the disease) originates in the yin or starts in the yang. Then needling is warranted."

[68]Historically, numerous scholars of Chinese medicine, such as Ma Shi, Zhang Jing–yue, and Zhang Zhi–cong, have given their own varying explanations of this passage. They are summarized below:

Disease in the yin within yin is a disease of the five viscera manifesting in the sinews and bone. This is yin disease in a yin phase or channel and it requires that one needle the brooks and rapids of the yin channel, such as Fish Border (*Yu Ji*, Lu 10) and Supreme Abyss (*Tai Yuan*, Lu 9) of the lung channel, where the qi is not too exuberant.

Disease in the yang within yang is a disease of the bowels manifesting in the skin. This is yang disease in the yang phase or channel and it requires that one needle the confluences of the yang channels, such as Pool at the Bend (*Qu Chi*, LI 11) of the large intestine channel. The submerging place is the confluence, which still pertains to the yang phase. Needling here can prevent the evil from penetrating deeper.

Disease in the yin within yang is a disease of the bowels manifesting in the sinews and bone. This is yang disease in a yin phase or channel and it requires that one needle the streams of the yin channels such as Channel Ditch (*Jing Qu*, Lu 8) of the lung channel. The channel qi circulates here where the qi waxes. This is a case of a yang (exuberance) within yin (*i.e.*, a yin channel).

Disease in the yang within yin is a disease of the viscera manifesting in the skin. This is yin disease in a yang phase or channel and it requires that one needle the network vessels of the yang channels, such as Veering Passageway (*Pian Li*, LI 6) of the large intestine channel. These vessels are all superficial, and located in the yang phase.

[69]Disease in the yang is an external contraction of wind, cold, dampness, etc., with wind as the representative because it is the leader of all external evils. Disease in the yin is often characterized by a failure of qi and blood to flow. This is blockage and, therefore, is called *bi*.

Zhang Zhi–cong explains in his *Ling Shu Ji Zhu* (*Condensed Annotations on the Spiritual Pivot*), "What is called tangible are the visible forms of the skin, flesh, sinews, and bone. What is called the intangible is the qi of the five viscera and the bowels. A tangible disease without pain is an external disease and, as such, is yang. An intangible disease with pain is damaged qi giving pain." The abstruse language of these lines has often misled scholars of Chinese medicine to the interpretation that a disease with tangible forms or signs but without pain is a disease of a yang category; a disease with intangible forms of signs and pain is of a yin category; etc. This is an oversimplification.

One should note that when yin and yang are both affected, it is more justifiable to say that the disease lies both externally and internally. Such a case is fatal.

[70]Ma Shi explains in his *Ling Shu Zhu Zheng Fa Wei* (*An Annotated Exposition on the Intricacies of the Spiritual Pivot*), "Wind cold causes damage to the form of a person. Cold qi may damage the form, and then disease arises in the form which is expressed externally. Worry...damages the qi of a person. Therefore, the qi may damage the viscera, and then disease arises in the viscera which is expressed internally. When wind damages the sinews and vessels, (the illness) is expressed in the sinews and vessels. This is expressed as being between the interior and the exterior."

[71]The region between the eyebrows is the indicator of the lung which governs the skin, and a thin color shows a superficial disorder, *i.e.*, a skin disorder. The lips are associated with the spleen, and the latter governs muscles and flesh. For that reason, abnormal labial color indicates disease in the muscles and flesh. Ma Shi explains, "If we intend to detect whether there is disease in the blood and qi, we should observe (the state of) the constructive qi. (This is revealed by) intangible but copious perspiration soaking (the clothes) and shows a disease in the blood and qi." From this quotation, it is clear that sodden constructive qi means constant heavy sweating. The eyes are the portals of the liver, which governs the sinews. Therefore, an abnormal color in the eyes indicates sinew disease. The kidney, which governs the bone, opens into the ears. Therefore, the ears demonstrate the conditions of the bones.

[72]This passage explains what regions or points should be chosen to treat various external problems:

The defensive qi travels in the skin and is transported to the four extremities. Therefore, the four limbs are regions of the skin. Columns are supports, and the columns of flesh are the major masses of flesh. They are mostly seen in the arms and legs along the routes of the yang channels. The foot *shao yin* starts from the center of the sole, ascending along the posterior border of the medial malleolus, submerging at the heel, travelling upward into the calf, submerging at the hollow of the knee, proceeding up along the medial–posterior aspect of the thigh, and penetrating the hips. Along its route there are also fleshy columns. The bone accessories are simply the bony joints.

[73]Zhang Jing–yue explains in his *Lei Jing*, "Birth in spring is the upbearing of yang qi. Growth in summer is the yang qi becoming exuberant. Contraction in autumn is the downbearing of yang qi. Hibernation in winter is the yang qi lying deep. These norms of qi are spoken of as the yang qi." He continues, "The degree of seriousness (of disease) depends on the waxing and waning of the righteous qi and righteous qi means the yang qi."

[74]Since the four (or actually five) seasons are analogous to the periods of the day and match the five phases, a lung disease, for example, has its restrained phase in the morning and its restraining phase at noon. The logic is that the lung is metal, pertaining to autumn and hence the sundown period. Morning is spring, pertaining to wood, a phase

restrained by metal, *i.e.*, the lung. Therefore, the condition is better in the morning. Noon is fire, a phase restraining metal, and, therefore, lung disease advances at noon.

[75]The heavenly phases is a concept matching dates, periods of the day, the seasons, and the five viscera with the five phases. The five phase inter–restraining and inter–engendering relationship is the key.

[76]Ma Shi explains in his *Ling Shu Zhu Zheng Fa Wei*, "For example, a spleen disease cannot stand the morning wood. So (one should) supplement the spleen and drain the liver. Because the lung disease cannot stand the day fire, it is necessary to supplement the lung and drain the heart..." According to Ma Shi, compliance to or following the heavenly phases requires that we should perform supplementation and drainage according to the laws of the five phases.

[77]Part 1 is derived from Chap. 5, *Su Wen*; Part 2 from Chap. 80, *Su Wen*; and Part 3 from Chap. 79, *Su Wen*.

[78]Yin tends to be calm and quiet, while yang to move. Li Nian–wo explains in his *Nei Jing Zhi Yao (Essential Knowledge of the Inner Classic)*, "When in harmony, yang germinates, while yin, when in harmony, promotes maturity and bears fruit. This is what is meant by the statement that yang is birth while is yin growth. This is a state when yin and yang are in order. Yang, when hyperactive, burns and parches, while yin, when congealing, seals and blocks. This is what is meant by the statement that yang is killing while yin is storage. This is a state when yin and yang are in disorder." Because yang is ever moving, it tends to be dispersing and, therefore, transforms the intangible qi. Because yin is quiet, tending to congeal, it gives shape."

Zhang Jing–yue explains in his *Lei Jing*, "Yin being cold and yang hot is the correct qi of yin and yang. Extreme cold generating heat is yin transmuting into yang. Extreme heat generating cold is yang transmuting into yin...For example, when people are damaged by cold, they have a disease of heat. The original cold turns into heat. When internal heat goes to the extreme, there may, contrarily, arise cold shivering. This is original heat turning into cold. The law of yin and yang is that the extreme invariably turns (into its opposite)."

Ma Shi explains in his *Su Wen Zhu Zheng Fa Wei*, "Cold qi rules yin, while yin rules downward congelation and allows no dispersal. Therefore, it generates turbid qi. The hot qi rules yang, while

yang rules upbearing and allows no congelation. Therefore, it generates the clear qi."

Zhang Jing–yue explains in his *Lei Jing*, "The clear yang rules upbearing. When yang is debilitated below and is no longer able to upbear, this results in swill diarrhea. The turbid yin rules downbearing. When yin is retarded above and is no longer able to downbear, this results in distention...This is a fullness in the chest around the diaphragm."

[79]The upper portals are the eyes, ears, nose, and mouth, while the lower portals are the anus and the genitals. Zhang Zhi–cong explains in his *Su Wen Ji Zhu*, "The qi of the clear yang all have access to and meet in the interstices, while the essence–blood of the turbid yin penetrates the five viscera, since the viscera rule the storing of essence. The four limbs are the roots of the various yang (channels). The six bowels transform and convey things but do not store. The clear yang produced from food and drink goes to replenish the limbs, and the turbid substance (from food and drink) gathers in the six bowels."

[80]Ma Shi explains, "Assimilation means taking in from the outside. Flavor nourishes the form, while the form is activated by qi. Qi is brewed by essence, while essence is originally based on transformation."

The reader should note that this passage emphasizes the mutual interaction of many factors and that physiological and pathological processes vary with each of these factors. For example, flavor nourishes the form, but it is also capable of bringing damage to the form.

[81]A yin disease is debilitated or diminished yin, and when yin is diminished, yang must be exuberant. This accounts for heat generated in the context of a yin ailment. The converse is true of a yang disease.

[82]Li Nian–wo explains in his *Nei Jing Zhi Yao*, "Cold pertains to yin and form is also to yin. Therefore cold impairs form. Heat is yang and qi is also yang. Therefore, heat dissipates qi. Qi likes diffusion and free flow, and when damaged, it is congested and blocked, giving rise to pain. Form is substantial shape, and when damaged, (things) are retained and settle without being transformed, giving rise to swelling."

[83]Wind is constantly moving. So it causes tremors and stirring in the extremities or head. When heat prevails, the yang is depressed internally, causing blocked constructive and defensive. This congestion produces *yong* swelling. When cold prevails, the yang qi is no longer able to operate, causing

glomus and fullness which finally result in puffy swelling.

The five qi in humans are the qi of the five viscera, each of which rules an emotional change. Violent anger can be understood as the cause of damaged yin qi, while violent joy of damaged yang qi. Yao Zhi-an, however, explains in his *Su Wen Jing Zhu Jie Jie (Annotations and Explanations of the Classic of the Basic Questions)*, "Yin is blood, which is stored in the liver. The liver rules anger. In anger, the liver qi becomes tense and counterflows. This stirs the blood internally. In the extreme, there may arise vomiting of blood. Yang is qi. In cases of sudden and inordinate joy, the heart-spirit soars and the qi scatters."

[84]The signs and capacities of the diseases resulting from the transmutation of yin and yang simply imply the overall morphology of those diseases.

[85]There are a number of perspectives regarding the implications of the sevenfold reduction and eightfold boost, all of which are derived from Chap. 12, Book 6, present work, which in turn comes from Chap. 1, *Su Wen*.

Females undergo seven year cycles, while males undergo eight year cycles of physiological change in their lives. At two times seven, females begin menstruation. This is a reduction of blood. While at two times eight, males are full of essence and acquire the reproduction capability. This is a boost of life. Thus we have the concept of sevenfold reduction and eightfold boost.

Some scholars of Chinese medicine disagree with this interpretation. The outstanding Japanese scholar, Ni Wa (*Dan Bo Yuan-jian*), for example, takes a different approach in his *Su Wen Shi (A Conceptual [Understanding] of the Basic Questions)*. According to him, the sevenfold reduction is the threefold reduction from 5 times 7 to 4 times 7 in females plus the fourfold reduction from 5 times 8 to 8 times 8 in males. During these periods, the qi is on the decline. The eightfold boost is the fourfold boost from 1 times 7 to 4 times 7 in females plus the fourfold boost from 1 times 8 to 4 times 8 in males. During these periods, their qi is on the rise.

The fundamental idea of the paragraph is that health can be preserved only when one responds appropriately to one's physiological changes at different ages. It warns against disregarding the laws governing life.

[86]Zhang Jing–yue explains in his *Lei Jing*, "The heavenly qi is the clear qi and is referred to as the breathing qi. The earthly qi is the turbid qi and is referred to as the qi from food and drink. The clear qi has access to the five viscera, first entering the lung through the pharynx. The turbid qi has access to the six bowels, first entering the stomach through the opening of the esophagus.

Wind qi is ascribed to wood. It therefore travels to the wood viscus, *i.e.*, the liver. Thunder qi is fire. Therefore it communicates with the heart. Rain qi is water qi, and, as such, it moistens the kidney.

None of the nine portals are unrelated to water. The eyes have tears, the nose discharges snivel, and the mouth is full of saliva, to say nothing of the anus and urethra. Even the ears, which seem devoid of water, are constantly moistened by water qi to keep away dryness. One can justifiably say that all the nine portals are the places where the water qi pours." These passages may serve as a free translation of the relevant sentence in the text.

Violent qi is fury. In Chinese, the word qi is often used to express anger even in the common vernacular. It is like the thunder, capable of devastating the visceral qi. Counterflowing qi is an equal culprit like the yang, which here means the scorching sun. In Chinese, the sun is literally the great yang (*tai yang*).

[87]When the skin and hair is discussed as opposed to muscle and skin. for example, it refers to the superficial layer of the skin including the fine hairs.

[88]Wind cold penetrates from the superficial levels into the deeper levels, finally entering the five viscera. Dietary irregularities tend to affect the six bowels, since they are responsible for conveying and transforming food and drink. Wu Kun explains in his *Wu Zhu Su Wen (Wu [Kun's] Annotated Basic Questions)*, "The value of the five flavors is their neutrality and moderateness. When they are cold, yin prevails. When they are hot, yang prevails. When yang prevails, heat is generated. When yin prevails, cold is generated. Both conditions harm the stomach and the intestines."

According to a note in the *Tai Su*, drawing yin to yang and yang to yin implies that, if the liver *jue yin* channel is replete while the gallbladder *shao yang* channel is vacuous, one should drain the *jue yin* and supplement the *shao yang*. But, if there is repletion in the foot *shao yang* and vacuity in the foot *jue yin*, then one should drain the *shao yang* and supplement the *jue yin*.

Practitioners should be skilled at diagnosis. They can determine appropriate conditions and criteria, and, by using these, examine the patient and arrive at a correct diagnosis. They can also diagnose an internal condition by observing the external signs and foresee trouble before it has obviously manifested itself.

[89]In examination, it is necessary first to determine whether the disease is yin in nature or yang in nature. Yin and yang are the cornerstone of the Chinese medical diagnostic and therapeutic system. A clear and brilliant complexion indicates disease in the yang phase, while a turbid and dull complexion shows disease in the yin phase. By listening to the breathing and voice of the patient, information may be obtained regarding the specific symptoms of the illness. The pulse images are in keeping with the supersession of four seasons. For instance, the pulse is expected to react like a compass in spring, a square in summer, a steelyard in autumn, and a weight in winter. In other words, the pulse should be tender and moderate in spring, surging in summer, superficial in autumn, and deep in winter. Whether or not the pulse is in keeping with this law tells us which viscus is involved. One should note that the location of a disease may be different from the location of its generation. For example, a disease may be produced in the spleen, but it may affect the foot *tai yin* channel, the stomach, or the flesh. Finally, the passage from "locate the disease" to "in palpation" is characterized by a grammatic structure of old Chinese, when put into modern Chinese, it goes as follows: "...locate the disease by observing the floating and sinking qualities of the *cun kou* pulse and studying the slipperiness and roughness of the cubit skin...."

[90]Upraising implies diaphoresis. Subtraction implies the use of laxatives. Promotion means supplementation. Lightness implies that the disease is not serious and hence tends to lodge superficially. Therefore, the word light is a pun here, meaning not serious and not heavy. The case is similar with the word heaviness. It means that the disease is replete in nature, serious, and tending to be located in the lower part of the body. A diminishing disease is one of vacuity.

[91]The form is nourished by flavor, but flavor cannot be transformed without qi. For this reason, insufficient form should be supplemented by qi supplementing medicinals. Essence is transformed by qi, but derives from flavor. Hence insufficient essence should be supplemented by thickly flavored medicinals.

A disease located high in the body is one in the upper burner and requires overpassing, *i.e.*, ejection. A disease located low is one in the lower burner. In this case, one should free the stools and disinhibit urination. This is what is meant by conducting and drying up. The above two treatments are in conformity with the principle of following the natural tendency of the disease.

[92]If there is an evil, for instance an external contraction of wind cold, diaphoresis is indicated. However, another possible interpretation of this sentence which asserts that the body can be soaked with certain medicinals to promote sweat.

An impetuous and fierce evil is a sudden, fulminating evil qi. Suppressing it means to antagonize it by specifically treating its manifestations. Another interpretation of this sentence asserts that one should perform massage to drive the fulminating evil out.

[93]There are different interpretations regarding the flexible and rigid. The majority of scholars hold that the external yang evil is rigid, while the internal yin evil is flexible. Zhang Jing–yue, however, argues that patterns, pulses, flavors, etc. can all be classified as either flexible or rigid. On the whole, the two views differ little, since both maintain that the flexible is a yin disease, while the rigid is a yang one. Making blood and qi keep to their homes means tranquilizing or harmonizing the affected blood or qi, lest they become chaotic and interfere with one another.

Dragging and conducting is interpreted by Ma Shi as cultivation of qi, and most scholars accept this interpretation, but, in the present book, Huang–fu Mi gives a specific definition for *dao qi* (conducting qi) which is synonymous with dragging and conducting. He defines the conduction of qi as needling manipulation that is neither draining nor supplementing. Only this technique is applicable in a case of neither vacuity nor repletion.

[94]Yang qi ascends, beginning on the left side of the body. Yin qi descends, beginning on the right side. The old first experience decrepitude below. Their feet begin to feel heavy. Therefore, their qi starts from above. While the qi in the young first becomes exuberant below.

In the yang seasons of spring and summer, the yang qi should be flourishing. If, instead, the qi presents itself in a yin manner but depurating and downbearing as in autumn and winter, then this causes death. In autumn and winter, a reverse law governs life and death. The so–called yin or yang in the four seasons are reflected in every respect, including pulse quality and pattern. For instance, a slow pulse is yin, while a racing pulse is yang.

[95]It may seem that only exuberant qi is capable of counterflow, but, as a matter of fact, insufficient qi may counterflow as well. If yin qi is in a state of surplus and counterflowing upwards, yang qi will be trapped above, separating yin and yang. This is why frigidity extends from the feet up to the knees. Young people generally have an exuberance of yang qi, but if the yin is so exuberant as to produce such a serious case of frigidity, their yang qi must have become exhausted to an extreme degree, and the patient has little hope of survival. The case with the old is quite different. Their yang qi is meager, and moreover, autumn and winter are seasons characterized by an exuberance of yin qi. Therefore, a surplus of yin qi in old people in autumn and winter is not lethal.

[96]Here, qi means the yang qi and a counterflow of the yang qi results in headache, etc. Such a case is neither a yang pattern nor a yin pattern. In this case, all the five viscera are utterly separated from one another, and there are no signs for one to go by in determining the nature of the illness.

In the *Su Wen*, the last sentence reads: "There is nothing but a thread of breath and one cannot be expected to last for even one day." Because the writing of eye (*mu*) and day (*ri*) are very similar in Chinese, which of the two classics is right on this point remains to be determined.

[97]Winter is yin, and disease contracted in this season should be of a yin nature. If it manifests itself as a yang pattern, this is called subordination of yang.

In the current edition of the *Su Wen*, there is a similar expression on prognosing the date of death.

[98]A failure to nurture the body in autumn and winter leads to yin vacuity and yang exuberance. When spring comes with yang and becomes exuberant, disease arises and the yin qi cannot be restored to normal. For this reason, such a disease is called yang killer. It is in the autumn when the grass turns dry. Ma Shi, however, explains in his *Su Wen Zhu Zheng Fa Wei*, "Death is expected while the old grass is still dry and before the grass and willows begin to grow." According to him, death should come in early spring.

[99]Consummate yin is understood as an extremely serious disease of extreme yin or consummate yin, *i.e.*, the spleen. Zhang Jing–yue defines consummate yin here as the spleen and kidney. He explains in his *Lei Jing*, "The spleen and the kidney are both the consummate yin. The three months of summer are a season when yang is exuberant, but now the spleen and the kidney are

damaged to an extreme extent. Thus, the true yin is utterly vanquished. (The patient) cannot stand the dry weather and adverse qi and, therefore, dies within ten days."

The crossing of yin and yang is explained in Chap. 2, Book 7, present work. There it says, in effect, that a warm disease with sweating and relapse of fever immediately following sweating, the pulse consistently agitated and racing all the time, ravings, and inability to take in food is called crossing of yin and yang. Sweat is a yin–fluid, while fever is yang. Fever in spite of sweating is exuberant yang evil in combination with rampant yin evil, and this justifies the term. Wu Kun, however, defines it as a yin pulse in a yang pattern or a yang pulse in a yin pattern. Such a case ends in death in early autumn, since water becomes still in that period.

[100]The reader should first note that such words as rise and arrive often suggest the arising or contracting of evils. In autumn, the yin qi is turning exuberant. For that reason, even if it involves the three yang channels, the disease is mild and easy to cure. If both yin and yang are damaged and blood and qi both exhausted, the disease is serious. The third yang is the *tai yang* which is the leader of all the yang channels. If there is repletion in it, yang is superabundant, while yin is exhausted. When winter comes on with water turning into solid ice, the patient dies. The second yin is the *shao yin*, the consummate. If it is superabundant, this means solitary yin without yang. Then death occurs when the rainy season comes on.

[101]This whole chapter is derived from Chap. 43, Vol. 7, *Ling Shu*.

[102]A positive evil is an evil as distinguished from abnormal heavenly qi, *i.e.*, wind, cold, summer-heat, dryness, fire and dampness. As such, a positive evil may include emotional disturbances, hunger, taxation, etc. affecting the body and the heart such as appear in the text.

In some editions, in the last two sentences there is the word "dream." In that case, the last sentence, for example, should read as follows: "If it saps the viscera, people have dreams of surplus internally and insufficiency externally."

[103]The Chinese word *jue*, translated here as inversion, has many levels of meaning, but, in this context, simply implies an evil, specifically a vacuity evil.

[104]In the *Ling Shu*, there is no "uninhibited" before urination and defecation, and its absence may make the sentence more logical.

[105]Part 1 is a combination of parts of Chap. 56, Vol. 8 and Chap. 63, Vol. 9, *Ling Shu*, and Chap. 23 and Chap. 10, *Su Wen*; Part 2 is from Chap. 22 and Chap. 10, *Su Wen*.

[106]The part from "Having been moderated in the stomach" may be interpreted in another way as, "If the stomach is warm and harmonious".

[107]Sourness penetrates the liver which governs sinews. Therefore it also penetrates sinews.

[108]In currently extant editions of the *Su Wen*, the liver is said to favor sourness rather than acidity as pointed out by the unknown editor(s). The *Jiu Juan*, commonly known as the *Ling Shu*, and the *Su Wen* are identical in relation to the five flavors.

[109]Water refers to the kidney, while fire refers to the heart.

[110]In current editions of the *Su Wen*, the heart is said to favor bitterness rather than sourness as pointed out by the unknown editor(s). The *Jiu Juan*, commonly known as the *Ling Shu*, and the *Su Wen* are identical in relation to the five flavors.

[111]Hollowed heart means an empty sensation in the heart region caused by the dissipative influence of the acrid ginger and leek.

[112]In current editions of the *Su Wen*, the lung is said to favor acidity rather than bitterness as pointed out by the unknown editor(s).

[113]The middle burner receives qi and takes in juice to transform blood. Therefore, the blood vessels are the passageways for transporting the refined essence of the middle burner. Because saltiness enters the middle burner, blood is subject to saltiness.

[114]In this context, water means the kidney, while fire means the heart.

[115]The grain qi is first transformed into fluid and humor, and then circulates with the constructive and defensive.

[116]Great qi means the gathering qi.

The implications of this ratio of discharge and ingestion is subject to a number of different interpretations. Zhang Jing–yue and Ma Shi explain that the grain qi discharged through exhalation and the qi from heaven and earth, or air in modern terms taken in through inhalation are at a ratio of 3 to 1. A note in Chap. 2 of the *Tai Su* states that the ratio of the quantities of qi inhaled and exhaled is 3 to 1. In his *Ling Shu Ji Zhu*, Ren Gu-an offers his own idea regarding this ratio. He asserts that one refers to the intake of the five grains and that three refers to the three parts, *i.e.*, the wastes, fluid, and gathering qi that are derived from the five grains. If the last understanding is correct (this is, perhaps, the most probable explanation), then there is no problem regarding the ratio as a whole. However, there is a problem in terms of the whole to its parts, and the essential qi should be understood as the whole process of ingestion, digestion, and nourishing.

[117]The liver holds the office of general, its orientation is anger and its qi is impetuous. Being impetuous, it is liable to bring injury upon itself. For that reason it is said to be bitter about tension. This is a homophone in Chinese with impetuousness or urgency.

The heart produces blood and is the ruler over the whole body. It beats forever and is fraught with thought. Therefore, its blood is easily depleted. When it contracts disease, it becomes weak and slack.

The spleen is earth. If earth is insufficient, there is nothing to restrain water and dampness runs rampant. When dampness prevails, diarrhea results. With diarrhea, the spleen is ever more insufficient. Therefore, it is said to be easily tormented by dampness.

The lung governs qi. When qi counterflows, the lung is the first to suffer.

Sourness is appropriate to liver wood which engenders fire. Therefore, diseases of the heart which pertains to fire should be treated with sourness. A similar explanation based on five phase theory underlies bitterness prescribed for lung disease and acidity prescribed for kidney disease. Sweetness is moderating; so it is appropriate for impetuous qi of the liver. Bitterness is drying; so dampness disease of the spleen is best treated with bitterness. The last sentence may well have been added by some later and unknown editor(s).

[118]The liver is expressed as the emotion anger, opens into the eyes, and holds the office of general. Its channel travels through the lower abdomen, spreading over the lateral costal regions, and stands in an interior/exterior relationship with the foot *shao yang* which connects with the ears. This explains the symptoms described in the text above.

[119]Yao Zhi-an explains in his *Su Wen Jing Zhu Jie Jie*, "It is noted that heavy eyes and deafness are a disease of vacuity above. It is, however, only apparently a case of vacuity, since there is repletion

below. The two channels of the liver and gall-bladder are places where ministerial fire is accommodated. Therefore, when they counter-flow, surging upward, they cause heavy eyes and deafness... This disease, if not one of fire, is a pattern of depletion and detriment of essence and blood. This is vacuity both above and below. The reason why the classic determines that it is a case of repletion below is that heavy eyes and deafness are not purely a vacuity. It requires tracing to the liver and the gallbladder and does not allow only supplementation of the kidney."

[120]The hand *shao yin* heart channel starts from the heart in the chest, homing to the cardiac ligation, penetrating downward into the diaphragm, and connecting with the small intestine. Its divergent vessel deviates to Abyss Humor (*Yuan Ye*, GB 22), linking with the kidney. The hand *shao yang* stands in an interior/exterior relationship with the hand *shao yang* which travels along the arm, emerges from the shoulder joint, and wraps the scapula. All the above explain the symptoms described in the text.

Given the ambiguity of the Chinese, the last sentence may be understood and rendered in a number of different ways.

Wang Bing asserts that a transmuted disease refers to vomiting, and the blood vessel around the acupoint Yin Cleft (*Yin Xi*, Ht 6) should be pricked. Ma Shi interprets transmuted disease in a broad sense, saying, "What is meant by transmuted disease is any pattern arising in addition to the original." According to him, the point to needle is Yin Cleft. Gao Shi–zhong is of a different opinion. He explains in his *Su Wen Zhi Jie (Terse Explanations of the Basic Questions)*, "As far as transmuted disease is concerned, this implies that a disease starts in the channel of the pericardium, but now another disease is transmuted in the minute connecting vessel of the (foot) *tai yang*. It is, therefore, necessary to prick the Cleft Center, taking the blood vessel there. The Cleft Center is the point Bend Middle (*Wei Zhong*, Bl 40) of the foot *tai yang*." The reader should note that although we adopt the last approach, we do not necessarily think it is better than the others.

[121]Inversion below means cold qi retained below causing counterflow frigidity of limbs, while dashing upward refers to upward counterflow causing clouded head with oppression.

[122]Part 1 is derived from Chap. 22, *Su Wen*; Part 2 from Chap. 37, *Su Wen*; Part 3 from Chap. 19, *Su Wen*; Part 4 from Chap. 42, Vol. 7, *Ling Shu*; and Part 5 is a combination of parts of Chap. 65, *Su Wen* and

Chap. 42, Vol. 7, *Ling Shu*.

[123]This passage is based on five phase theory: Liver disease pertains to wood. Summer fire is engendered by wood, and so there is recovery. Autumn metal restrains wood, and so the illness advances. Winter water engenders wood, and so the illness is stable. Spring wood is the season pertaining to the illness, so once again there is improvement.

[124]See note 17-19, Chap. 2, Book 1, present work for an explanation of the ten heavenly stems and their five phase ascriptions vis à vis days of the calendar.

[125]See note 87, Chap. 9, Book 1, present work, for an explanation of the watches of the day and their five phase ascriptions.

[126]Here, the four seasons imply the months when the spleen reigns, *i.e.*, the 3rd, 6th, 9th, and 12th months. The watches corresponding to these are *Chen* (B5, 7-9 a.m.), *Xu* (B11, 7-9 p.m.), *Chou* (B2, 1-3 a.m.), and *Wei* (B8, 1-3 p.m.).

[127]See note 123 above, which is a comment on the first paragraph, present section.

[128]The following are quotations from the *Lei Jing* by Zhang Jing–yue explaining the genesis of the illnesses discussed above. "Both cold and heat are capable of producing *yong* and toxin. Heat leads to yang toxin, while cold to yin toxin. For the spleen governs the muscle and flesh, and when meeting with cold, qi gathers (in the muscles and flesh)...giving rise to swelling and *yong*. *Yong* is said to be blockage. The kidneys transmit the qi of cold water to its restraining phase in counter order, rebelling and aggressing against spleen earth. Consequently, this congestion causes water swelling...Diminished qi is due to exuberant cold which results in yang vacuity below. With yang vacuity, qi is incapable of being transformed.

"Insufficient heart fire is deprived of the ability to warm and nurture lung metal. The lung qi, if not warmed, is unable to convey or transform fluid and humor. This accounts for urination doubling drinking in terms of quantities of water. The lung is the mother of water. When water is lost to an excessive extent, the lung qi becomes desiccated, resulting in lung wasting thirst. Because the doors and gates fail to work, the fundamental origin is exhausted day by day. Consequently, the condition is fatal and cannot be treated.

"Gushing water is water coming from below as if from a gushing spring. Water is yin qi. Its root lies in the kidney, and its end in the lung. When the lung shifts cold to the kidney, then yang qi is not transformed below. The yang not being transformed, water floods, developing into an evil. It intrudes upon the large intestine because the large intestine is associated with the lung."

Treating that which rules the lung means treating a large intestine disease in the same way as one treats a lung disease.

[129]This refers to a spicy, acrid sensation in the nasal cavity.

[130]The liver is wind, and when heat is transmitted to it, wind and heat mutually exacerbate resulting in susceptibility to fright and nosebleeding. When the liver, which is wind as above mentioned, transmits heat to the heart, wind and fire mutually exacerbate to push yang to the extreme, resulting in expiry of the spirit. When the heart shifts heat to the lung, fire torments lung metal, consuming and impairing fluid and humor resulting in wasting thirst. When the lung shifts heat to the kidney, the true yin or kidney water is dried up, thus failing to nurture the sinews, and, consequently, soft tetany is caused. For a description of this ailment, see Chap. 6, Book 7, present work. If the kidney transmits heat to the spleen where dampness prevails, heat and dampness become entangled resulting in dysentery. If this is enduring, both the kidney and spleen are vanquished and death becomes a certainty.

All the patterns discussed in the text above are caused by the shifting of counterflow qi.

[131]Heart fire, for example, is the mother of spleen earth. Therefore, the heart receives evil qi from the spleen. The heart restrains lung metal. Therefore, it transmits the evil to the lung. The heart is the child of the liver, the wood viscus. Therefore, heart disease lodges in the liver. Because the heart is restrained by kidney water, heart disease ends in death when it is transmitted to the kidney. See the next paragraph which provides an example as illustration. This law concerns the days, months, and seasons as well, as far as they relate to five phase theory.

[132]Early morning is the time of liver wood. Noon is the time of heart fire. Afternoon is the time of spleen earth. Evening is the time of lung metal. And night is the time of kidney water.

[133]Ma Shi gives an explanation to the first sentence, saying, "If keeping to the general principle one makes a synthesized study of various therapies,

one will have a good command of them all. If one keeps to a general principle in the various therapies without missing it, then one is able to treat diseases of all kinds without error."

[134]Before the invention of paper, bamboo pieces and silk cloth were the materials used for writing. Therefore, bamboo and silk were often used as synonymous with books. The passage from "Receptivity" to "full mastery" may be interpretated in a different manner as follows: "Receptivity and practice, full concentration in learning, and thorough application of what is learned lead to perfect command of the doctrines."

[135]An equally plausible interpretation of the first sentence might read as follows: "One may be deaf to any sound and blind to any form." If one adopts such an understanding, then the topic of the second sentence remains the same, that being the transmission of evil qi or great qi throughout the body.

Lower flux implies loss of essence in the form of seminal emission and vaginal discharge.

[136]Zhang Jing–yue explains in his *Lei Jing*, "The midnight watch in winter months is a time when water is at climax, while the midday watch is a time when fire is at climax. The heart fire stands in awe of water, therefore death occurs in winter at the midnight watch. In summer death occurs at the midday watch because the yang evil is extremely hyperactive at this time. Extreme exhaustion is fatal as is extreme exuberance. Where there is overwhelming prevalence, there is overwhelming termination."

[137]This time of death may be explained in a number of different ways. The most plausible is that winter is cold water to which the lung has an aversion. The sundown watch is a time when lung metal should be exuberant, but, since the lung qi is impaired and cannot grow, life is put to an end. Cross–referencing the above passage with the next paragraph may be helpful. Summer is fire, which torments metal, and the sunrise watch is a time when the lung metal is at its nadir. Therefore, death occurs then.

[138]Zhang Jing–yue explains in his *Lei Jing*, "When wood is damaged, an overwhelming of metal constitutes a danger. This accounts for (the liver) in awe of the sundown watch in winter. If the liver starts a disease, the conditions deteriorate when wood turns rigid. This accounts for (the liver disease) standing in awe of the breakfast

watch in summer." One should note that the sun-down watch is a time when lung metal is exuberant, while the breakfast watch is a time when liver wood prevails.

[139]Given the limitations of the inter–restraining cycle, a disease can only skip over three viscera at the most before a fatal return to the viscera of its origin. Thus, the number four in the text is a redundancy. The transmission of disease is carried on in the order of the inter-restraining cycle of the five phases: liver wood→spleen earth→kidney water→heart fire→lung metal→liver wood. Skipping means jumping to a phase other than the next one in the cycle. There is, however, another interpretation which asserts that skipping over one viscus is transmitting disease in the order of the counter inter–engendering cycle, *e.g.*, kidney water (child)→lung metal (mother), etc. Skipping over two viscera is transmitting disease in the order of inter–engendering cycle, *e.g.*, kidney water (mother)→liver wood (child). Skipping over three viscera is transmitting disease in the order of the counter inter–restraining cycle, *e.g.*, kidney water (restrained)→spleen earth (restraining). In the source edition, the last sentence is omitted, and it is supplemented here in accordance with the *Su Wen*. Some archaic editions of the *Jia Yi Jing*, however, have retained it.

[140]Part 1 is derived from Chap. 6, Vol. 2, *Ling Shu*; Part 2 from Chap. 17, *Su Wen*; and Part 3 from Chap. 53, Vol. 8, *Ling Shu*.

[141]In this context, a premature death simply implies that one dies at an early age.

[142]Zhang Jing–yue explains in his *Lei Jing*, "The form accommodates the qi, while the qi replenishes the form. A particular form should be peculiar to a particular qi, and a particular qi should be peculiar to a particular form. Therefore, compatibility between the exterior and the interior suggests a long life. If one is strong and the other weak, the two are not coordinated and this means a premature death.

"The flesh is the interior of the skin, while the skin is the exterior of the flesh. Strong flesh with solid skin is said to be *xiang guo* (close fitting in our terms {tr.}); fragile flesh with loose skin is said to be not *xiang guo*. Given this condition of *xiang guo*, the qi is sure to accumulate, resulting in long life. However, if there is no such condition of *xiang guo*, the qi is easily lost, resulting in a premature death.

"Blood and qi, channels and network vessels are

the root in the interior, while formal body is the branches and leaves in the exterior. Prevalence of the root ensures longevity, while prevalence of branches and leaves dooms one to a short life."

[143]A full form implies a robust physique. The reference to the way of heaven implies that form and qi are established by the prenatal qi. Obviously, however, postnatal factors may influence the quality and quantity of both form and qi as well.

[144]Chest distention accompanied by panting is often referred to as exuberance in the center with fullness of the viscera. Fright damage implies kidney damage since the kidney is subject to damage by fright. A prevalence of qi implies an exuberance of evil qi. A voice as if coming from the next room refers to a dull and indistinct voice. Failure of the granaries to store reflects a dysfunction of the spleen/stomach. More precisely, this means frequent bowel movements or diarrhea. Failure of the gates are dysfunctions of the pylorus, the screen gate or ileocecal valve, and the anus. The spring is the urinary bladder, and its incessant flowing implies polyuria.

[145]Since the five viscera are the fundamental source of the strength of the body, this last sentence refers to restoration of normal function or protracted abnormal functions within the five viscera.

[146]This passage, read on its own, has been a challenge to scholars of Chinese medicine, and thus far, this arcane paragraph has no plausible interpretation. It is generally accepted that this passage has undergone some profound and probably unintentional tampering at some time in history.

[147]This paragraph is derived from Chap. 53, the *Ling Shu*, where the interlocutors are the Yellow Emperor and Shao Yu rather than Qi Bo.

[148]Part 1 is derived from Chap. 54, Vol. 8, *Ling Shu*; Part 2 from Chap. 1, *Su Wen*.

[149]This progression follows the inter–engendering cycle, *i.e.*, liver woodÆ heart fireÆ spleen earthÆ lung metalÆ kidney waterÆ, with liver wood as the starting phase.

[150]The reader might be inclined to conclude that the "true teeth" are simply the adult teeth. However, most commentators are in agreement that the true teeth refer to the wisdom teeth.

[151]Celestial water is also called celestial *gui* (*tian gui*). This concept is similar to that of sexual maturing

from the modern point of view. *Gui* is S10 and is ascribed to water in the nine palace diagram.

The great penetrating vessel is the penetrating vessel taken in combination with the foot *shao yin* channel. These two run together along the same route and are believed to be closely associated with sexual function.

The terrestrial tunnel is the vagina, and a blocked terrestrial tunnel implies amenorrhea or termination of menstruation.

[152]Many scholars assert that the part from "their celestial water becomes exhausted" to "extremely (decrepit)" should be moved to describe the age of sixty-four.

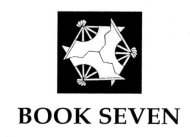

BOOK SEVEN

Chapter One

Cold Damage & Febrile Disease Due to Affliction of the Six Channels (Part 1)[1]

(1)

The Yellow Emperor asked:

Febrile disease, which is in the same category as cold damage, may result in survival or death. Why does death occur in six or seven days and yet recovery takes more than ten days?

Qi Bo answered:

The *tai yang* is in command of all the other yang. It links with Wind Mansion (*Feng Fu*, GV 16) and governs qi on behalf of all the yang (channels). When damaged by cold, people will contract febrile disease. This fever, however high, is not fatal. Those with disease due to dual affliction by cold will not necessarily escape from death.[2]

On the first day of cold damage, the *tai yang* is the recipient. Therefore, there is pain all along the nape of the neck and the lumbar spine ["pain in the head and the nape of the neck, and rigidity of the lumbar spine" in the *Su Wen*]. On the second day, the *yang ming* is the recipient. Since it governs the muscles and the vessel runs by either side of the nose and connects the eyes, (the symptoms of) generalized fever, pain in the eyes, a dry nose, and inability to sleep occur. On the third day, the *shao yang* is the recipient. Because it governs the bones, ["the gallbladder" in the *Su Wen*

{later editor}] and the vessel runs across the lateral costal regions and connects the ears, (the symptoms) of pain in the chest and lateral costal regions with deafness occur. When all the three yang ["the three yang channels and their network vessels" in the *Su Wen* {later editor}] are subjected to disease, which has not yet entered the bowels ["the viscera" in the *Su Wen* {later editor}], diaphoresis can effect recuperation.[3]

On the fourth day, the *tai yin* is the recipient. Since the *tai yin* vessel spreads over the stomach and connects with the throat, symptoms of abdominal fullness with dry throat occur. On the fifth day, the *shao yin* is the recipient. Since the *shao yin* vessel penetrates the kidney, connects with the lung, and links with the root of the tongue, symptoms of dry mouth and tongue with thirst occur. On the sixth day, the *jue yin* is the recipient. Since the *jue yin* vessel runs through the genitals and connects with the liver, symptoms of vexation and fullness with retracted testicles occur. When all the three yang and three yin as well as all the five viscera and six bowels are afflicted with disease, constructive and defensive cease to circulate, the five viscera become blocked, and death ensues.

If there is no dual affliction of cold, *tai yang* disease subsides on the seventh day and headache diminishes a little. *Yang ming* disease subsides on the eighth day and generalized fever diminishes a little. *Shao yang* disease subsides on the ninth day and deafness improves a little. *Tai yin* disease subsides on the tenth day and the abdomen returns to normal resulting in the restoration of appetite. *Shao yin* disease subsides on the eleventh day and thirst is quenched [also "disappearance of fullness" in the *Su Wen* {later editor}] and the tongue is no longer dry. *Jue yin* disease subsides on the twelfth day and the testicles become relaxed and the lower abdominal (fullness) diminishes a little. The great qi has departed, and the condition improves day by day.[4]

Treatment should be aimed at freeing the channel of the (affected) viscus. (In this way,) the disease will certainly subside day by day until it disappears. If (cold damage) has not yet lasted for three days, diaphoresis will cure it. If, however, it has lasted for three days (or more), draining precipitation will cure it.[5]

The Yellow Emperor asked:

What accounts for the residual (heat, *yi*, 遗) which occurs in some cases when a febrile disease has already been cured?

Qi Bo answered:

As for residual heat, when a fever is intense and the consumption of food is forced, this results in residual heat. In such cases, even when all the pathological conditions have been mitigated, some of the heat still remains hidden. When (this heat) encounters the grain qi, these two heats contend and unite with one another, and residual heat consequently results. To treat residual heat, (one should) examine vacuity and repletion and then regulate the positive and the negative (aspects of the condition). This (approach) promises an immediate recovery. Even when febrile disease has improved a little, eating meat may result in relapse and eating too much (of anything) results in residual heat. This is prohibited.[6]

In the case of dual affliction of cold, the *tai yang* and *shao yin* both become diseased on the first day, and symptoms of headache, a dry mouth, and vexation and fullness occur. On the second day, the *yang ming* and the *tai yin* both become diseased, and symptoms of abdominal fullness, generalized fever, no desire for food, and delirium occur. On the third day, the *shao yang* and *jue yin* both become diseased, and symptoms of deaf-

ness, retracted testicles, and inversion occur. In the case of inability to ingest (even) liquid food and loss of consciousness, death occurs on the sixth day.[7]

The Yellow Emperor asked:

When the five viscera are damaged, the six bowels are blocked, and the constructive and defensive cease to flow, why does death occur only after three days?

Qi Bo answered:

The *yang ming*, as the leader of the twelve channel vessels, has an exuberance of blood and qi. Therefore, it is not until three days after loss of consciousness that its qi runs out and death occurs.[8]

(2)

Liver febrile disease first manifests by yellowish urine, abdominal pain, somnolence, and generalized fever. When heat is locked in conflict (with the righteous qi), symptoms of raving, susceptibility to fright, fullness and pain in the chest [the word chest is absent in the *Su Wen* {later editor}] and lateral costal regions, fidgeting of the hands and feet, and disturbed sleep occur.[9]

Geng and *xin* days are characterized by deterioration. *Jia* and *yi* (days) are characterized by massive perspiration. If there is a counterflow of qi, death occurs on *geng* and *xin* days. (To treat this, it is necessary to) needle the foot *jue yin* and foot *shao yang*. Qi counterflow gives rise to headache with dizziness. This pain is due to the surging (of heat evil) along the channel into the head.[10]

Heart febrile disease is initially characterized by melancholy a number of days prior to the appearance of fever. When heat is locked in a conflict (with the righteous qi), symptoms of vexation and oppression of the heart [also "sudden heart pain" in the *Su Wen* {later editor}], frequent vomiting, headache, a red facial complexion, and absence of sweating occur.[11]

Ren and *gui* days are characterized by deterioration; *bing* and *ding* days by massive perspiration. If there is a qi counterflow, death occurs on *ren* and *gui* days. (To treat this, it is necessary to) needle the hand *shao yin* and the hand *tai yang*.[12]

Spleen febrile disease is initially characterized by heavy headedness followed by pain in the cheeks, vexation of the heart [the *Su Wen* adds the symptom of green-blue complexion of the forehead {later editor}], desire to vomit, and generalized fever. When heat is locked in a conflict (with the righteous qi), symptoms of pain in the lumbus with inability to bend it either forward or backward, abdominal distention, diarrhea, and pain in the submandibular region ["in the forehead" in a variant version {later editor}] occur.[13]

Jia and *yi* days are characterized by deterioration, *wu* and *ji* days by massive perspiration. If there is qi counterflow, death occurs on *jia* and *yi* days. (To treat this, it is necessary to) needle the foot *tai yin* and the foot *yang ming*.[14]

Lung febrile disease is initially characterized by inversion with shivering and, starting from the skin and hair, aversion to wind and cold, yellow tongue fur, and generalized fever. When heat is locked in a conflict (with the righteous qi), symptoms of dyspnea, cough, (migratory) pain travelling the chest, breasts, and upper back,[15] inability to breathe deeply, slight headache ["unbearable headache" in the *Su Wen* {later editor}], and cold after perspiration.[16]

Bing and *ding* days are characterized by deterioration; *geng* and *xin* days by massive perspiration. If there is qi counterflow, death occurs on *bing* and *ding* days. (To treat this, it is necessary to) needle the hand *tai yin* and hand *yang ming*. Once blood emerges, running in drops as big as beans, a cure is effected.

Kidney febrile disease is initially characterized by lumbar pain with aching in the lower legs, tormenting thirst, frequent drinking, and generalized fever. When heat is locked in a conflict (with the righteous qi), symptoms of pain and stiffness in the nape of the neck, aching and cold in the

lower legs, heat in the soles of the feet, and disinclination to talk occur, and, in the case of (qi) counterflow, there is pain in the nape with dizziness. [The *Su Wen* adds the symptoms of "a rolling sensation of the heart." {later editor}][17]

Wu and *ji* days are characterized by deterioration; *ren* and *gui* days by massive perspiration. If there is qi counterflow, death occurs on *wu* and *ji* days. (To treat this, it is necessary to) needle the foot *shao yin* and foot *tai yang*. In all the cases where perspiration is expected, sweat exits most copiously on the restraining days.[18]

(Just prior to the onset of) liver febrile disease, redness first appears on the left cheek. (Just prior to the onset of) heart febrile disease, redness first appears on the forehead. (Just prior to the onset of) spleen febrile disease, redness appears on the nose. (Just prior to the onset of) lung febrile disease, redness appears on the right cheek. (Just prior to the onset of) kidney febrile disease, redness appears on the chin.

If one needles before the disease actually arises (but) immediately upon discovering a red complexion, this is spoken of as prevention of disease (*zhi wei bing*, 治未病).[19] Febrile disease which manifests at the associated regions (in the face) will heal in due course. An inappropriate needling (treatment) delays recuperation for three cycles.[20] A dual inappropriate treatment is fatal.[21]

In the treatment of any type of febrile disease, cold water should be administered (to the patient) prior to needling. They should have on thin clothes and live in a cold environment. Once the body turns cold, recovery follows. If the illness is severe, the fifty-nine (points) for needling [22] are selected.[23]

For febrile disease initially characterized by pain and fullness in the chest and lateral costal region and fidgeting of the hands and feet, the foot *shao yang* should be needled while supplementing the foot *tai yin*. If the illness is severe, the fifty-nine (points) for needling are needled.[24]

For febrile disease initially characterized by generalized heaviness, pain in the bones, deafness, and heavy eyes, the *shao yin* should be needled. If the illness is severe, the fifty-nine (points) for needling are selected.[25]

For febrile disease initially characterized by dizziness and cloudedness, fever, and fullness in the chest and lateral costal regions, the foot *shao yin* and foot *shao yang* should be needled.[26]

As for the *tai yang* vessel, the appearance of a brilliant complexion in the zygomatic region indicates bone febrile disease. If the brilliance is not yet perished ["not yet crossed" in the *Su Wen*, same hereafter {later editor}], it will heal by itself when (the channel) has its day, provided perspiration is still possible. If the *jue yin* vessel vies for an appearance, death ensues, and it will occur in less than three days. This is because the febrile disease has already linked with the kidney.[27]

As for the *shao yang* channel, the appearance of a brilliant complexion on the cheeks indicate sinew febrile disease. If the brilliance has not yet perished, it will heal by itself when (the channel) has its day, provided perspiration is still possible. If the *shao yin* vessel vies for an appearance, death ensues.[28]

Of the qi points for febrile disease, the one located below the third vertebra[29] is the ruling (point for) heat in the chest. The one located below the fourth vertebra is the ruling (point for) heat in the diaphragm. The one located below the fifth vertebra is the ruling (point for) heat in the liver. The one located below the sixth vertebra is the ruling (point for) heat in the spleen. And the one located below the seventh vertebra is the ruling (point for) heat in the kidney. In the case of a brilliant complexion in the sacrococcygeal region, (a point) in the depression below the third vertebra in the nape of the neck (treats this condition). If (a brilliant complexion presents as) an adverse tendency from the cheek towards the zygomatic region, major conglomeration is indicated. (A brilliant complexion in) the mandibular region indicates abdominal fullness. (A brilliant complexion) lateral to the zygomatic region indicates

pain in the lateral costal region. (And a brilliant complexion appearing) on the cheek indicates (problems) above the diaphragm.[30]

(3)

If there is cold damage during the winter, warm disease will inevitably occur in the spring, while if there is summerheat damage inflicted in summer, this will inevitably result in *nue* disease in the autumn.

A (warm) problem developing from cold damage which arises before the summer solstice is considered a warm disease, while that arising after the summer solstice is considered a summerheat disease. In a summerheat condition, perspiration will be effusive and should not be checked. The sweat pores are what is known as the dark abode.

(4)

The Yellow Emperor asked:

The *Ci Jie (Needling Strategies)*[31] explains that disrobing[32] requires needling the curious points of the various yang (channels) which have no fixed locations. I would like hear about these at length.

Qi Bo answered:

This concerns a surplus of yang qi with an insufficiency of yin qi. An insufficiency of yin qi results in internal heat, while a surplus of yang qi results in external heat. When these two heats contend, the heat becomes as intense as a live charcoal held in the bosom, the clothes become so hot that the body dare not touch them, and the body becomes so hot that (one) dare not touch the mat. With the interstices shut and blocked, there is no perspiration, the tongue is parched, the lips become like pieces of dry, seasoned meat, and the throat is dry with desire for drinks.[33]

(To treat it,) take Celestial Storehouse (*Tian Fu*, Lu 3) and Great Shuttle (*Da Zhu*, Bl 11) thrice and needle Central Backbone (*Zhong Lu*, Bl 29)[34] to clear heat and supplement the hand and foot *tai yin* to induce sweat. Once the heat has departed and the sweat dried, the illness disappears as quickly as one disrobes.[35]

Ba Shi Yi Nan (Jing) (The Eighty-One Difficult Issues of the Nan Jing) explains that, in the case of yang vacuity with yin exuberance, recovery follows the emergence of perspiration, while precipitation results in instant death. (On the contrary,) in the case of yang exuberance with yin vacuity, death follows the onset of perspiration, while precipitation produces instant recovery. [This statement contradicts the relevant teachings of the classics. It is quite groundless and, therefore, cannot be abided by. {later editor}][36]

(5)

The Yellow Emperor asked:

Some people have heat in the four limbs due to exposure to wind cold and is like moxaing or like a fire. What is the cause?[37]

Qi Bo answered:

This is (due to) vacuity of yin qi with exuberance of yang qi in the patient, and heat in the four limbs which are yang conditions. While these two yang mutually promote one another, yin qi becomes all the more vacuous and meager. Thus meager water is unable to put out vigorous fire and, as a consequence, the yang qi overrides and predominates.

Overriding predomination of yang qi brings birth and growth to a stop. Solitary exuberance of yang qi brings about termination (of engendering and transformation). This is why heat becomes (as intense) as moxaing or like a fire once exposed to wind. In this case, the flesh of the patient becomes wasted and emaciated.[38]

The Yellow Emperor asked:

Some people experience uncommon febrile (diseases) without extraordinary heat but suffer from vexation and fullness. What is the cause?

Qi Bo answered:

Their yin qi is scant, while their yang qi is overwhelming. Therefore, there is heat with vexation and fullness.[39]

(6)

The Yellow Emperor asked:

Since the foot *tai yin* and *yang ming* stand in an interior/exterior relationship with one another and are the spleen and stomach vessels respectively, why do they produce different diseases?

Qi Bo answered:

The yin and yang differ in location, experience different (phases of) repletion and vacuity, and undergo variations in counterflow and conformity (*ni shun*, 逆顺). While (evil qi) intrudes via different ways, either from within or from without, and is transmitted with different tendencies. For that reason, there are different diseases.[40]

Yang is the heavenly qi, governing the exterior, while yin is the earthly qi, governing the interior. The yang track is a repletion track, while the yin track is a vacuity track. When thieving wind and vacuity evil attack, yang suffers and they invade the bowels. If there are dietary irregularities and irregular lifestyle from which yin suffers, (their evils) invade the viscera. When the bowels have been invaded, there is generalized fever with insomnia and asthmatic wheezing above. When the viscera have been invaded, there is distention and fullness and obstruction and blockage in the chest with swill diarrhea below. Overtime, this may develop into intestinal *pi*.[41]

The larynx controls the heavenly qi, while the upper end of the esophagus (*yan*, 咽)[42] controls the earthly qi. Therefore, yang is subject to wind qi, whereas yin is subject to damp qi. Yin qi travels first upward from the feet to the head and then turns downward to the tips of the fingers along the arms. Yang qi travels first upward from the hands to the head and then turns downward to the feet. Therefore, it is said that yang disease tends to turn downward upon reaching the upper extremity, whereas yin disease tends to turn upward upon reaching the upper extremity. For this reason it is the upper (part of the body) that first suffers from wind damage, and it is the lower (part of the body) that first suffers from damp damage.[43]

Chapter One

Cold Damage & Febrile Disease Due to Affliction of the Six Channels (Part 2)[44]

(1)

The Yellow Emperor asked:

What causes pain in febrile disease?

Qi Bo answered:

Febrile disease (affects) the yang vessels and, in this case, the three yang are all exuberant. If the *ren ying* (pulse) is twice as exuberant (as the *cun kou*, it indicates disease) in the *shao yang*. If (the *ren ying* pulse is) thrice as exuberant (as the *cun kou*, it indicates disease) in the *tai yang*. If (the *ren ying* pulse is) four times as exuberant (as the *cun kou*, it indicates disease) in the *yang ming*. Once a disease has entered the yin (vessels) from the yang, it will stay in the head and the abdomen, giving rise to abdominal distention and headache.[45]

(2)

The Yellow Emperor asked:

What is the cause of generalized fever disease where vexation and fullness remains unresolved in spite of sweating?

Qi Bo answered:

Sweating with generalized fever is due to wind, whereas sweating with unresolvable vexation and fullness is due to inversion. This disease is called wind inversion. Because the *tai yang* ["the great yang" in the *Su Wen* {later editor}] governs

qi on behalf of all the yang (channels), it is the first to suffer from evil. Since the *shao yin* stands in an interior/exterior relationship with the *tai yang*, when affected by heat (the *shao yin* follows the *tai yang*), and, when it follows upward, this results in inversion. The treatment is to needle both the exterior and the interior and to drink decoctions.[46]

The Yellow Emperor asked:

In (one type of) warm disease, there is perspiration which is immediately followed by recurrent heat and a pulse which is agitated and racing. (This disease) is not diminished by diaphoresis and is characterized by ravings and inability to ingest food. What is the name of this disease?

Qi Bo answered:

This is called yin/yang crossing and this crossing is fatal. Sweat in people is generated from grain, and grain produces essence. When there is crossing and contention of evil qi (with essence qi) in the bones and flesh producing perspiration, this should mean that the evil is retreating and the essence is triumphant. When the essence is victorious, the ability to eat ought to be restored and heat should not recur. A recurrence of heat is the evil qi, while sweat is the essence qi. Now heat, however, may recur immediately after perspiration. This indicates that the evil is overwhelming (the essence), while an inability to ingest deprives the essence of its means of recruitment. In the case of lingering heat, life may collapse in no time. When the pulse becomes agitated and racing after sweating, this means death. This is because, when the pulse does not react to perspiration in a congruous manner, this indicates (the essence) is unable to conquer disease. It is an evident (sign) of death. Ravings (reflect) the loss of orientation, and loss of orientation means death. Now that there are three (causes for) death without one (cause for) life, although (some degree of) recovery is seen, death is a certainty.[47]

(3)

If a wind disease is characterized by alternating

fever and chills and sweating with heat with several episodes occurring in a day, first prick the various network vessels in the partings of flesh. If alternating fever and chills (persist) despite perspiration, the needling should be performed every third day, and recovery can be expected in one hundred days.

(4)

The Yellow Emperor asked:

What is vacuity and (what is) repletion?

Qi Bo answered:

Exuberance of evil qi is repletion, while deprivation (*duo*) of essence qi is vacuity. Dual repletion is a disease of internal great heat. [The *Su Wen* states "is said to be a great heat disease." {later editor}] Hot qi and a full pulse are indications of dual repletion.[48]

The Yellow Emperor asked:

What is repletion of both the channels and the network vessels like?

Qi Bo answered:

Repletion of all the channels and network vessels is characterized by an urgent *cun kou* pulse and slackened cubit (skin. In this case,) both the channels and network vessels should be treated. It is said that a slippery (pulse) is a favorable indicator, while a choppy one is unfavorable. Vacuity and repletion are treated [the *Su Wen* states: "Vacuity and repletion are initiated {later editor}] in accordance with the concerned materials. It follows that when the five viscera, the bones, and the flesh are slippery and uninhibited, a long life is maintained.[49]

If cold qi ascends abruptly, the pulse is full and replete. (If the pulse) is not only replete but slippery, this is a favorable sign indicating survival. If replete but choppy, this is an unfavorable indicator, prognosticating death. (The physical body) may be full all over with an urgent, large, and

hard pulse and rough cubit skin. This is an incongruity. Such cases, given (the following) favorable indicators, may survive or, given (the following) unfavorable indicators, may be fatal. What is considered to be favorable are warm hands and feet, and what is considered to be unfavorable are cold hands and feet.[50]

The Yellow Emperor asked:

What is dual vacuity?

Qi Bo answered:

Pulse vacuity, qi vacuity, and cubit vacuity are called dual vacuity. What is called qi vacuity is characterized by erratic speech. Cubit vacuity is characterized by a timid and unsteady step. And pulse vacuity is characterized by a pulse not manifesting in accordance with its yin (character). In such a case, a slippery pulse indicates survival, while a choppy pulse foretells death.[51]

Qi vacuity is lung vacuity, and qi counterflow means cold feet. If this does not occur in its season (of restraint, the patient) may survive, but if it happens in its season (of restraint), the condition is fatal. This is true of the other viscera as well.[52] Those with a pulse which is replete and full, hands and feet which are cold, and a head which is hot ["headache" in a variant version {later editor}] may survive if it is spring or autumn but die if it is winter or summer.[53]

If the pulse is not only floating but choppy, and if there is generalized fever in addition to a choppy pulse, death is a certainty.[54]

If there is an insufficiency of connecting vessel qi but a surplus of channel qi, there will be a hot *mai kou* pulse with cold cubit (skin). This is unfavorable in autumn and winter, but favorable in spring and summer. (In that case, one should) treat that which is related to the disease.[55]

Vacuous channels but full network vessels with hot and full cubit (skin) and a cold and choppy *mai kou* are fatal if it is spring or summer but indicate survival if it is autumn and winter. In the case of full network vessels with vacuous channels, moxa the yin and needle the yang. In the case of full channels but vacuous network vessels, needle the yin and moxa the yang.[56]

The Yellow Emperor asked:

In autumn and winter, yin should not be forced to the extreme, while in spring and summer, yang should not be forced to the extreme. What is the meaning of this statement?

Qi Bo answered:

Not forcing yang to the extreme is a prohibition against repeatedly evacuating the *yang ming* during the spring and summer. Vacuity of the *yang ming* leads to mania. Not forcing yin to the extreme is a prohibition against repeatedly evacuating the *tai yin* during the autumn and winter. Vacuity of the *tai yin* leads to death.

During the spring, one should repeatedly treat the connecting vessel of the channel. During the summer, one should repeatedly treat the stream points. And during the autumn, one should repeatedly treat the six bowels. Because winter is characterized by blocking and shutting, medication is preferable to (metal and) stone needles (during this season). However, limiting (the use of metal) and stone needles is not spoken of in the cases of *yong* and *ju* (diseases).[57]

(5)

For a febrile disease which begins in the hands and arms, (one should) first take the hand *yang ming* and *tai yin*[58] to induce perspiration. For a febrile disease which begins in the head and face, (one should) first take the *tai yang* at the nape of the neck[59] to induce perspiration. For a febrile disease which begins in the feet and the lower legs, (one should) first take the foot *yang ming*[60] to induce perspiration.

The arm *tai yin*[61] ["*tai yang*" in the *Ling Shu*[62] {later editor}] is capable of inducing perspiration, and the foot *yang ming*[63] is capable of inducing perspiration. If a yin channel is taken and there is

excessive perspiration, it can be checked by taking a yang channel. While if a yang channel is taken and there is excessive perspiration, it can be checked by taking a yin channel. For shuddering with cold, chattering of the teeth, lack of perspiration, abdominal distention, vexation, and oppression, (one should) take the hand *tai yin*.[64]

(6)

On the third day of a febrile disease, if the *qi kou* is still tranquil but the *ren ying* is agitated, (one should) take the points of the various yang channels from among the fifty-nine needling (points) to drain the heat, induce perspiration, and replenish yin in order to supplement insufficiency.[65]

An intense generalized fever in which the yin and yang (pulses) are both tranquil should not be needled. However, so long as the condition allows needling, it should be administered without delay. Even though it may fail to promote perspiration, it will drain (the evil qi). It is always the existence of mortal signs which underlie the prohibition for needling.[66]

On the seventh or eighth day of a febrile disease, if the *mai kou* pulse is stirring and there is panting and dizziness, (one should) needle without delay. Perspiration will exit of its own accord. (One should) needle the thumb[67] shallowly.[68]

On the seventh or eighth day of a febrile disease, if the pulse is faint and small, and the patient has hematuria and a dry mouth, death occurs in one and a half days. If the pulse is regularly interrupted, death comes in one day.[69]

In a febrile disease, if successful diaphoresis is followed by an agitated ["exuberant" in a variant version {later editor}] pulse and there is dyspnea and recurrence of heat, needling ["shallow needling" in a variant version {later editor}] is of no use. If the dyspnea is violent, death is inevitable.[70]

On the seventh or eighth day of a febrile disease, if the pulse is not yet agitated, dispersed, or racing, perspiration will occur in three days. If perspiration does not occur within three days, death occurs in four (*i.e.*, the next) day. In the absence of perspiration, needling is of no use.[71]

If a febrile disease is first characterized by pain in the skin, nasal congestion, and puffiness of the face, (one should) treat at the level of the skin with the first type of needle,[72] choosing from the fifty-nine needling (points). In case of urticaria and dry nose, (one should) appeal to the skin on behalf of the lung. If this does not work, appeal to fire, fire being the heart.[73]

If a febrile disease is first characterized by rough (skin all over the) body, vexation with fever, vexation and oppression, and dry lips and throat, (one should) treat at the level of the vessels using the first type of needle, choosing from the fifty-nine needling (points). For febrile disease with distention of the skin, dry mouth, cold, and sweating, (one should) appeal to the vessel on behalf of the heart. If it does not work, appeal to water, water being the kidney.[74]

For a febrile disease with dry throat, copious drinking, susceptibility to fright, and disturbed sleep, (one should) treat at the level of the flesh using the sixth type of needle[75] and choosing from the fifty-nine needling (points). In the case of red ["green-blue" in the *Ling Shu* {later editor}] canthi, (one should) appeal to the flesh on behlaf of the spleen. If this does not work, appeal to wood, wood being the liver.[76]

For a febrile disease with pain in the chest and the lateral costal region ["green-blue facial complexion and pain in the chest"[77] in the *Ling Shu* {later editor}] and fidgeting of the hands and feet, (one should) treat between the sinews, puncturing the four extremities with the fourth type of needle.[78] In the case of sinew limpness and soaked eyes, (one should) appeal to the sinews on behalf of the liver. If this does not work, appeal to metal, metal being the lung.[79]

For a febrile disease with susceptibility to fright, tugging and slackening, and mania, (one should) treat at the level of the vessels, promptly draining the surplus (vessel) using the fourth type of needle. In the case of madness and loss of hair, (one should) appeal to the blood on behalf of the heart.

If this does not work, turn to water, water being the kidney.[80]

For a febrile disease with generalized heaviness, painful bones, deafness, and heavy eyes, (one should) needle at the level of the bone using the fourth type of needle and choosing from the fifty-nine needling (points). For bone disease with inability to ingest food, grinding of the teeth, and a green-blue cast to the auricles, (one should) appeal to the bone on behalf of the kidney. If this does not work, appeal to earth, earth being the spleen.[81]

Febrile disease with pain of indeterminate location, deafness, debility (of the four limbs), dry mouth, and in the presence of yang, intense heat or in the presence of yin, severe cold is due to heat in the marrow. It is fatal and cannot be treated.[82]

Febrile disease with headache, tense ["tugging" in a variant version {later editor}] vessels between the temples and the eyes, and frequent nosebleeding is known as inversion heat disease. (One should) treat this with the third type of needle[83] (in a manner) in accordance with surplus and insufficiency.[84]

For a febrile disease with cold and heat, piles, generalized heaviness, and heat in the intestines, (one should) treat using the fourth type of needle and the rapids[85] and points at the toes.[86] (One should then) appeal to the connecting vessel of the stomach for qi in order to acquire qi.[87]

For a febrile disease with urgent pain in the periumbilical region and fullness of the chest and lateral costal region, (one should) take Gushing Spring (*Yong Quan*, Ki 1) and Yin Mound Spring (*Yin Ling Quan*, Sp 9) and puncture Throat Interior (*Yi Li*, CV 23) with the fourth type of needle.

For a febrile disease in which sweating nonetheless occurs or with a favorable pulse indicative of diaphoresis, (one should) take Fish Border (*Yu Ji*, Lu 10), Great Abyss (*Tai Yuan*, Lu 9), Great Metropolis (*Da Du*, Sp 2), and Supreme White (*Tai Bai*, Sp 3). Drain them and the heat will depart; supplement them and there will be perspiration.

If there is excessive perspiration, (one should) take the transverse vessel above the medial malleolus[88] to check it.

In febrile disease, if upon diaphoresis, the pulse remains agitated and exuberant, this indicates that the yin vessels are at their nadir, and hence prognoses death. If diaphoresis occurs and the pulse becomes tranquil, (the patient) will survive.

In febrile disease, if the pulse remains continually agitated and exuberant and diaphoresis has not occurred, this indicates that the yang vessels are at their culminating point and hence foretells death. If the pulse is agitated and exuberant and, with the advent of diaphoresis, becomes tranquil, (the patient) will survive.[89]

For inversion with paravertebral pain, characterized by stiffness of the nape of the neck and the head, blurred vision, and rigidity of the lumbar spine, (one should) take the blood vessel of the foot *tai yang* in the popliteal fossa. In case of dry throat and hotness in the mouth as if glued, (one should) take the foot *shao yin*.[90] [This paragraph comes from the "*Ci Yao Tong Lun* (Treatise on Needling Lumbar Pain)" in the *Su Wen*,[91] and it is more proper to place it in a later place in the chapter. {later editor}][92]

There are nine mortal signs in febrile disease. First, lack of perspiration with redness in the zygomatic region is fatal. [The *Tai Su*[93] states, "if sweat does not emerge and the zygomatic region is red, death is certain because the (qi) cannot return." {later editor}] Second, diarrhea with severe abdominal fullness is fatal. Third, dim sight with persisting heat is fatal. Fourth, heat with abdominal fullness in the old and in infants is fatal. Fifth, lack of perspiration with retching of blood ["and blood in the stool" in the *Su Wen* {later editor}] is fatal. Sixth, erosion of the tongue root with persisting heat ends in death. Seventh, coughing with nosebleeding and lack of perspiration or perspiration which fails to reach the feet is fatal. Eighth, heat in the marrow is fatal. Ninth, fever with tetany is fatal. In fever with tetany, there is arched-back rigidity, tugging and slackening, clenched jaw, and grinding of the teeth.

These nine conditions may not be needled.[94]

The so-called fifty-nine needling (points) include a point on either side of the three fingers in each hand, totalling twelve in all;[95] a point between each of the five fingers, eight in all;[96] the same number in the feet;[97] three points on the head bilateral (to the midline of the head, beginning) one *cun* into the hairline, six in all;[98] five points in the hair, three *cun* bilateral to the midline of the head, ten in all;[99] one point anterior and one point posterior to the auricle, one point below the mouth, one point in the nape of the neck, six in all;[100] one point on the vertex, one point on the fontanel, one point on the (front and back) hairlines, solitary Ridge Spring (*Lian Quan*, CV 23), bilateral to Wind Pool (*Feng Chi*, GB 20) and bilateral to Celestial Pillar (*Tian Zhu*, Bl 10).[101] [This last point is absent from the original editions of the *Jia Yi Jing* and was subsequently added later based on its appearance in the *Ling Shu*. {later editor}]

The *Su Wen* states that there are fifty-nine points. There are (five points in each of the) five columns on the head,[102] and these columns are used to clear counterflow heat from the yang channels. As for Great Shuttle (*Da Zhu*, Bl 11), Bosom Point (*Yin Shu*, Lu 1), Empty Basin (*Que Pen*, St 12), and the back points,[103] these eight are used to drain heat ["yang" in a variant version {later editor}] in the chest. As for Qi Surge (*Qi Chong*, St 30), Three Li (*San Li*, St 36), the Upper and Lower Ridge of the Great Hollow (*Ju Xu Shang*, St 37 & *Xia Liang*, St 39), these eight are used to drain heat in the stomach. As for Cloud Gate (*Yun Men*, Lu 2), Collarbone (*Yu Gu*, LI 15), Bend Middle (*Wei Zhong*, BL 40), and Marrow Hollow (*Sui Kong*, Ki 11),[104] these eight points are used to drain heat in the four limbs. As for the points lateral to the five viscera associated points,[105] these ten are used to drain heat in the five viscera. All fifty-nine points are points for the treatment of heat. [Although the two classics[106] differ in this list, the points contained in both of them are important points for draining heat. {later editor}][107]

(7)

For cold in the head and brain ["cold and heat

with headache" in the *Qian Jin* {later editor}], runny snivel, and lacrimation, Spirit Court (*Shen Ting*, GV 24) is the ruling point.

For headache, generalized fever, nasal congestion, dyspnea and inhibited breathing, vexation and fullness, and lack of perspiration, Deviating Turn (*Qu Cha*, Bl 4) is the ruling point.

For headache, visual dizziness, pain in the eyes, rigidity of the neck, and a dragging (discomfort) between the chest and the flanks with inability to turn, Root Spirit (*Ben Shen*, GB 13) is the ruling point.[108]

For febrile disease with ["vexation and fullness" are added in the *Qian Jin* {later editor}] lack of perspiration, Upper Star (*Shang Xing*, GV 23) is the ruling point. It is necessary to first take Yi Xi (*Yi Xi*, Bl 45) and finally Celestial Window (*Tian You*, TH 16) and Wind Pool (*Feng Chi*, GB 20).

For febrile disease with lack of perspiration, tormenting retching, and vexation of the heart, Light Guard (*Cheng Guang*, Bl 6) is the ruling point.

For pain in and heaviness of the head and neck, collapse on attempting to stand up, nasal congestion, runny snivel nosebleeding, dyspnea, and inhibited breathing, Celestial Connection (*Tong Tian*, Bl 7) is the ruling point.

For aversion to wind of the head and nape of the neck, lack of perspiration, chilling inversion (*qi jue*), aversion to cold, retching and vomiting, a tense ocular ligation sending a dragging pain to the root of the nose, heavy headedness, and pain in the nape, Jade Pillow (*Yu Zhen*, Bl 9) is the ruling point.[109]

For frigidity in the cheeks ["ravings, grinding of the teeth and staring" in the *Qian Jin*[110] {later editor}], loss of eyesight, foaming at the mouth, lacrimation, and pain in the eyebrows, the ruling point is On the Verge of Tears (*Lin Qi*, GB 15).

For brain wind characterized by headache, aversion to wind and cold, runny snivel nosebleeding, nasal congestion, dyspnea, and inhibited

breathing, Spirit Support (*Cheng Ling*, GB 18) is the ruling point.

For headache with generalized fever producing stiffness ["pain" in a variant version {later editor}] in the mandibular regions, Brain Hollow (*Nao Kong*, GB 19) is the ruling point.

For wind stroke after drinking wine characterized by fever, dizziness with pain in the corners of the head ["in both eyes" in a variant version {later editor}], inability to ingest either drink or food, vexation and fullness, and retching and vomiting, Winding Valley (*Shuai Gu*, GB 8) ["Wind Gate {*Feng Men*, Bl 12}" in the *Qian Jin* {later editor}] is the ruling point.[111]

For stiffness of the nape of the neck, needle Loss of Voice Gate (*Yin Men*).[112]

For febrile disease with lack of perspiration, Celestial Pillar (*Tian Zhu*, Bl 10), Wind Pool (*Feng Chi*, GB 20), Shang Yang (*Shang Yang*, LI 1), Passage Hub (*Guan Chong*, TH 1), and Armpit Gate (*Ye Men*, TH 2) are the ruling points.

For pain in the nape of the neck with inability to turn the neck, tearing, copious eye mucous, runny snivel nosebleeding, redness and pain of the inner canthi, loss of hearing and visual acuity due to inverted qi, and throat fistula producing a dragging sensation in the neck with spasm and debility of the sinews, Wind Pool (*Feng Chi*, GB 20) is the ruling point.[113]

For cold damage with exuberant heat, vexation and retching, Great Hammer (*Da Zhui*, GV 14) is the ruling point.

For heavy headedness, heavy eyes, chilling inversion, cold and heat, stiffness of and inability to turn the neck, and lack of perspiration, Kiln Path (*Tao Dao*, GV 13) is the ruling point.[114]

For generalized fever with headache which is intermittent, Spirit Path (*Shen Dao*, GV 11) is the ruling point.

For splitting headache, fire-like generalized heat,

lack of perspiration, tugging and slackening ["headache" in the *Qian Jin* {later editor}], fever and chills, aversion to cold after sweating, abdominal urgency, and dragging pain between the lumbus and the abdomen, Life Gate (*Ming Men*, GV 4) is the ruling point.[115]

For pain in and inability to bend the neck either forward or backward, headache, shuddering with cold, tugging and slackening, flank fullness occurring with repletion of qi, cold qi in the paravertebral regions, lack of perspiration despite the presence of fever, and pain in the upper and lower back, Great Shuttle (*Da Zhu*, Bl 11) is the ruling point.[116]

For wind dizziness, headache, inhibited nose, frequent sneezing and running of clear snivel, Wind Gate (*Feng Men*, Bl 12) is the ruling point.[117]

For shivering with cold and frequent yawning and stretching, Diaphragm Shu (*Ge Shu*, Bl 17) is the ruling point.

For febrile disease with lack of perspiration, Upper Bone Hole (*Shang Liao*, Bl 31) and Collection Hole (*Kong Zui*, Lu 6) are the ruling points. [The *Qian Jin* explains, "the points induce diaphoresis. Either moxibustion or acupuncture works well for arm inversion and lack of perspiration febrile disease." {later editor}][118]

For hypertonicity around the shoulder and upper arm, chilling inversion, and aversion to cold, Po Door (*Po Hu*, Bl 42) is the ruling point.

For pain in the nape of the neck and the upper back sending a dragging (discomfort) to the front of the neck, Po Door is the ruling point.

For pain in the shoulder, fullness in the chest and abdomen, chilling inversion, and hypertonicity and rigidity of the spine and upper back, Spirit Hall (*Shen Tang*, Bl 44) is the ruling point.

For counterflow dyspnea, runny snivel nosebleeding, pain in the inner (medial) border of the scapula, inability to bend (the body) either forward or backward, and dragging pain and dis-

tention in the lower abdomen radiating from the lateral abdominal and free rib regions, Yi Xi (*Yi Xi*, Bl 45) is the ruling point.

For pain in the upper back with aversion to cold, rigidity of the spine with difficulty in bending either forward or backward, inability to ingest food, and retching and copious foamy vomiting, Diaphragm Shu (*Ge Shu*, Bl 17) ["Lumbar Yang Pass {*Yang Guan*, GV 3}" in the *Qian Jin* {later editor}] is the ruling point.[119]

For febrile disease with headache and generalized heaviness, Suspended Skull (*Xuan Lu*, GB 5) is the ruling point.

For distention and fullness in the chest and the lateral costal regions, pain in the upper back, aversion to wind and cold, inability to ingest, and retching and vomiting with inability to retain (food in the stomach), Hun Gate (*Hun Men*, Bl 47) is the ruling point.

For frequent sneezing, headache and generalized heat, Forehead Fullness (*Han Yan*, GB 4) is the ruling point.

For febrile disease with headache radiating to the outer canthi and producing tension extending to the submandibular region and teeth, vexation and fullness, lack of perspiration, red facial complexion, and pain in the skin, Suspended Skull (*Xuan Lu*, GB 5) is the ruling point.

For febrile disease with unilateral headache sending a dragging (discomfort) in the outer canthi, Suspended Tuft (*Xuan Li*, GB 6) is the ruling point.

For headache, pain in the pupils of the eyes with loss of eyesight, hypertonicity in the lateral aspects of the nape and inability to turn (the neck), Yang White (*Yang Bai*, GB 14) is the ruling point.

For head wind headache, runny snivel nosebleeding, pain in the eyebrows, frequent sneezing, eyes (painful) as if fit to burst from their sockets, sweating, cold and heat, red facial complexion, pain in the cheeks, inability to turn the cervical vertebrae, tense ocular ligation and tugging and slackening, Bamboo Gathering (*Zan Zhu*, Bl 2) is the ruling point.[120]

For cold and heat, chilling inversion, and chattering of the jaws, Nectar Receptacle (*Cheng Jiang*, CV 24) is the ruling point.

For generalized heat and pain, and pain in the chest and the lateral costal regions with inability to turn (the body), Skull Rest (*Lu Xi*, TH 19) is the ruling point.

For pain in the shoulder and the upper back, cold and heat, scrofulous lumps big and small wrapping the neck, presence of great qi, sudden deafness, qi clouding, loss of hearing and visual acuity, headache, pain in the submandibular region, tearing, nosebleeding, inhibited breathing, inability to detect fragrance from fetor, wind dizziness, and throat *bi*, Celestial Window (*Tian You*, TH 16) is the ruling point.[121]

For febrile disease with a rolling sensation below the heart, abdominal fullness with acute pain, trance and loss of consciousness, frigidity of the hands, fullness in the lower abdomen ["fullness in the heart region and the abdomen" in the *Qian Jin* {later editor}], tugging and slackening, heart pain, and qi fullness with inability to catch one's breath, Great Tower Gate (*Ju Que*, CV 14) is the ruling point.

For head dizziness and ache, generalized fever, and lack of perspiration, Upper Venter (*Shang Wan*, CV 13) is the ruling point.[122]

For generalized cold and heat, Yin Metropolis (*Yin Du*, Ki 19) is the ruling point.

For *nue* febrile disease with shuddering with cold and chattering of the jaws, abdominal distention, squinting and rale in the throat, Lesser Shang (*Shao Shang*, Lu 11) is the ruling point.

For cold inversion and heat (disease with) vexation of the heart, diminished qi which is insufficient to allow one to catch one's breath, genital dampness and itching, pain in the abdomen mak-

ing it impossible to ingest drink or food, hypertonicity of the elbows, propping fullness (of the chest), and parching dry throat with thirst, Fish Border (*Yu Ji*, Lu 10) is the ruling point.

Febrile disease characterized by shuddering with cold and chattering of the jaws, abdominal distention, impotence, cough producing a dragging (discomfort) in the testicles and causing urinary dribbling, is due to vacuity. If there is vacuity in the diaphragm, there will be a desire to retch upon ingestion, lack of perspiration despite the presence of generalized heat, frequent frothy eructation and vomiting, blood in the stools, cold and heat in the shoulder and upper back, ghostly complexion, and tearing. All of the above are due to vacuity. (For these conditions, one should) needle Fish Border (*Yu Ji*, Lu 10) with a supplementing (manipulation).[123]

For warm disease with generalized fever and lack of perspiration for above five days, (one should) needle Great Abyss (*Tai Yuan*, Lu 9) and retain the needle for a while before extracting it. If (the lack of perspiration) has not yet lasted for five days, the condition may not be needled.

For febrile disease first characterized by pain in the hands and arms and generalized fever at first, tugging and slackening, lockjaw, flaring of the nostrils, upturned eyes, sweat running like rolling pearls, hardness in the region three *cun* below the breasts, fullness in the region of the free rib, and palpitation, Broken Sequence (*Lie Que*, Lu 7) is the ruling point.[124]

Chapter One

Cold Damage & Febrile Disease Due to Affliction of the Six Channels (Part 3)[125]

For shivering with cold, tugging and slackening, inability to stretch the hands, coughing, turbid sputum, obstructed flow of qi, frequent retching, chattering of the jaws, lack of perspiration, vexation and fullness ["vexation of the heart and generalized pain" in the *Qian Jin* {later editor}], squinting, and violent nosebleeding, Cubit Marsh (*Chi Ze*, Lu 5) is the ruling point. If the left side is congested, needle the right. If the right side is congested, needle the left.[126]

For pain in the regions of the free ribs, vomiting above and diarrhea below, fullness in the chest with shortage of qi,and lack of perspiration, (one should) perform supplementation at the hand *tai yin* to induce (diaphoresis).

For febrile disease with heart vexation and heart oppression, lack of perspiration, heat in the palms, heart pain, fire-like generalized fever, vexation and fullness caused by sapping (evils), and pain in the root of the tongue, Central Hub (*Zhong Chong*, Per 9) ["Celestial Bone Hole {*Tian Liao*, TH 15}" in the *Qian Jin* {later editor}] is the ruling point.[127]

For febrile disease with heat, vexation and fullness with desire to retch and vomit, lack of perspiration in the first three days, apprehension, pain in the chest and lateral costal region with inability to turn over (the body), coughing, (panting and) fullness, reddish urine, blood in stools [the *Qian Jin* says "blood in the urine" {later editor}], incessant nosebleeding, retching and vomiting of blood, qi counterflow, incessant belching, sore throat, inability to ingest, constant thirst, putrefaction of the tongue body, hotness in the palms, and desire to retch, Palace of Toil (*Lao Gong*, Per 8) is the ruling point.

For febrile disease with vexation of the heart, lack of perspiration, hypertonicity of the elbows, swelling of the armpit, incessant laughing, pain in the heart region, reddening and yellowing of the eyes, urine which is blood (red), desire to retch, heat in the chest, melancholy and gloom, sighing, throat *bi*, dry throat, counterflow dyspnea, fire-like generalized fever, splitting headache, shortage of qi, and pain in the chest, Supreme Mound (*Tai Ling*)[128] is the ruling point.[129]

For febrile disease with heart vexation, frequent retching, and heat in the chest with faltering and stirring (of the heart), Intermediary Courier (*Jian Shi*, Per 5) is the ruling point.

For red facial complexion with heat in the skin, febrile disease with lack of perspiration, fever due to wind stroke, reddening and yellowing of the eyes, hypertonicity of the elbows, swelling of the armpits, and, in case of repletion, acute heart pain, and in case of vacuity, heart vexation, inactivity due to apprehension, and loss of orientation,[130] Inner Pass (*Nei Guan*, Per 6) is the ruling point.

For stirring and faltering of the heart, susceptibility to fright, generalized fever, vexation of the heart, a dry mouth, frigidity of the hands, qi counterflow, retching of blood ["agitation within the blood" in the *Qian Jin* {later editor}], intermittent tugging, a tendency to shake the head, a green-blue cast to the forehead, sweating confined to the region above the eyebrows, cold damage, and warm disease, Marsh at the Bend (*Qu Ze*, Per 3) is the ruling point.[131]

For somnolence, frequent spitting, pain and cold in the shoulder bones, runny snivel disorder with a red nose and copious blood, seeping sores breaking out on the face, generalized fever, throat *bi* with a sensation of a lump stuck in the throat, lesions of the canthi, sudden shivering with cold, and pain in the upper back, Second Space (*Er Jian*, LI 2) is the ruling point.[132]

For runny snivel nosebleeding, febrile disease with lack of perspiration, eye disorders, pain in the eyes preventing them from opening, headache, and decayed teeth, Union Valley (*He Gu*, LI 4) is the ruling point.[133]

For vexation of the heart in febrile disease, eye disorders, pain in the eyes with tearing, qi counterflow headache, fullness in the chest with inability to catch one's breath, febrile disease with intestinal *pi*, pain in the upper arm, elbow, and forearm, and, in the case of vacuity, qi obstruction and fullness, and inability to lift the shoulders, Yang Ravine (*Yang Xi*, LI 5) is the ruling point.

For cold damage with fever and chills, headache, retching, nosebleeding, and inability to lift the shoulders, Warm Dwelling (*Wen Liu*, LI 7) is the ruling point.

For cold damage with residual heat, Pool At the Bend (*Qu Chi*, LI 11) is the ruling point.

For headache and quivering with cold, Clear Cold Abyss (*Qing Leng Yuan*, TH 11) is the ruling point.

For headache and hypertonicity of the nape of the neck and the upper back, Dispersing Riverbed (*Xiao Luo*, TH 12) is the ruling point.

For shivering with cold, loss of use of the small fingers, fever and chills with lack of perspiration, headache, throat *bi*, curled tongue, heat around the small fingers, heat in the mouth, heart vexation, heart pain, pain in the inner aspect of the forearms and lateral costal regions, deafness, coughing, tugging and slackening, dry mouth, and pain in the nape with inability to look back, Lesser Marsh (*Shao Ze*, SI 1) is the ruling point.[134]

For shivering with cold, chills and fever, pain in the shoulders, upper arms, elbows, and forearms, spinning and ache of the head with inability to look back, vexation and fullness, generalized fever with aversion to cold, red, painful eyes, ulceration of the canthi, nebular screen generated (in the eye), acute pain, runny snivel nosebleeding, loss of hearing acuity, heavy, painful arms, hypertonicity of the elbows, scarred scabies, fullness of the chest sending a dragging (discomfort) to the upper arms, tearing with susceptibility to fright, stiffness of the neck, and generalized cold, Back Ravine (*Hou Xi*, SI 3) is the ruling point.[135]

For febrile disease with lack of perspiration, pain in the chest restricting respiration, swelling of the submandibular region, fever and chills, ringing in the ears, and deafness, Yang Union (*Yang Gu*, SI 5) is the ruling point.

For wind leakage with perspiration reaching down to the waist, rigidity of the neck with inability to look round or bend either forward or backward, slack shoulders and debilitated elbows, pain in the eyes, scarred scabies, warts, tugging and slackening, and spinning of the head with pain in the eyes, Yang Union (*Yang Gu*, SI 5) is the ruling point.[136]

For shivering with cold, fever and chills, swelling of the neck, and, in the case of repletion, spasms of the elbows with spinning and ache of the head as well as mania, and, in the case of vacuity, warts as small as scarred scabies, Branch to the Correct (*Zhi Zheng*, SI 7) is the ruling point.[137]

For wind dizziness with headache, Lesser Sea (*Xiao Hai*, SI 8) is the ruling point.

For panting, incessant nosebleeding in febrile disease, vexation of the heart, sentimentality, abdominal distention, counterflow breathing with hot breath, cold inside the lower legs, inability to lie down, fullness of qi in the chest with heat, violent diarrhea, forced supine posture to facilitate breathing, cold in the soles of the feet, oppression in the diaphragm, retching and vomiting, and no desire for drink or food, Sunken White (*Yin Bai*, Sp 1) is the ruling point.

For febrile disease with lack of perspiration, inversion with frigid hands and feet, violent diarrhea, and heart pain with abdominal distention, the pain being particularly intense in the heart but which is essentially a stomachache, Great Metropolis (*Da Du*, Sp 2) is the ruling point. Supreme White (*Tai Bai*, Sp 3) should be taken together with it. They are also the ruling points in treating abdominal distention, frequent retching, and vexation and oppression.[138]

For febrile disease first characterized by heavy headedness, pain in the forehead, vexation of the heart, and generalized fever, and then, when the heat comes into conflict (with the righteous qi), characterized by pain in and inability to bend the lumbus either forward or backward, abdominal fullness, intense pain in the submandibular regions, violent diarrhea, constant hungering without desire for food, frequent belching, heat in the center, frigid feet, abdominal distention with inability to transform food, a tendency toward retching, diarrhea with pus and blood in the stool, and tormenting and unproductive eructation, (one should) first take Three Li (*San Li*, St 36) and then Supreme White (*Tai Bai*, Sp 3) and Camphorwood Gate (*Zhang Men*, Liv 13) as the ruling points.[139]

For febrile disease with fullness, oppression, and inability to lie down [the *Qian Jin* gives, "inability to lie down, generalized heaviness and nonspecific pain in the bones" {later editor}], Supreme White (*Tai Bai*, Sp 3) is the ruling point.

In the case of heat in the center with diminished qi and inversion cold, moxibustion eliminates this heat ["moxibustion at Gushing Spring {*Yong Quan*, Ki 1} in the *Qian Jin* {later editor}]. For heart vexation, no desire for food, coughing with shortage of qi, frequent dyspnea, throat *bi*, generalized fever, dragging (discomfort) between the spine and the lateral costal regions, trance and poor memory, Gushing Spring is the ruling point.[140]

For febrile disease with heart vexation, cold and frigid feet, and profuse sweating, (one should) first take Burning Valley (*Ran Gu*, Ki 2), then Great Ravine (*Tai Xi*, Ki 3), and the moving vessel at the big toe. Supplementing (manipulation) should be performed first at all the points.[141]

For pain in the eyes producing a dragging (discomfort) in the canthi, pain in the lower abdomen at one side, hunched back ["arched spine" in a variant version {later editor}] with tugging and slackening, clouded vision, somnolence, Shining Sea (*Zhao Hai*, Ki 6) is the ruling point. (One should) drain the left yin motility vessel[142] and take the right *shao yin* point.[143] First needle the yin motility and then the *shao yin* point which is located at the pubic bone.[144]

For febrile disease with lack of perspiration, taciturnity and somnolence, yellowish urine, heat in the lower abdomen, sore throat, abdominal distention with swelling inside, drooling, and pricking heart pain, Great Ravine (*Tai Xi*, Ki 3) is the ruling point.

If cold in the hands and feet extends up to the joints, death occurs with the onset of dyspnea.[145] For febrile disease, needle Burning Valley (*Ran Gu*, Ki 2) ["Sunken Valley {*Xian Gu*, St 42}" in the *Qian Jin*. {later editor}] (With insertion of the needle,) a cold sensation begins in the feet, and once the cold has reached the knees, then the needle should be extracted.[146]

For frequent biting of the lips, frequent belching, pain and distention in the abdomen, and rumbling of the intestines, Sunken Valley (*Xian Gu*, St 43) is the ruling point.[147]

For febrile disease with lack of perspiration and heat and pain in the mouth, Surging Yang (*Chong Yang*, St 42) is the ruling point. It, too, is a ruling point for (the treatment of) pain in the venter and remittent cold and heat.[148]

For febrile disease with a lack of perspiration, frequent belching, abdominal distention and fullness, and heat in the stomach with delirium, Ravine Divide (*Jie Xi*, St 41) is the ruling point.

For inversion headache with water swelling of the face, vexation of the heart, manic spells with ghostly apparitions, incessant laughing such that one is overjoyed with happy events, and throat *bi* with loss of voice, Bountiful Bulge (*Feng Long*, St 40) is the ruling point.[149]

For yang inversion with shivering with cold, tightness of the lower abdomen, headache, pain in the lower legs, thighs and abdomen, pure heat wasting thirst, inhibited urination, and frequent retching, Three Li (*San Li*, St 36) is the ruling point.[150]

For lateral costal pain and counterflow coughing with inability to catch one's breath, Portal Yin (*Qiao Yin*, GB 44) is the ruling point. It is located at the juncture between the nail and the flesh of the fourth toe. For disorders of the right side, treat the (point) on the left. For disorders of the left, treat the (point) on the right. Immediate cure follows. If this is not the case, repeat the treatment.

For frigid hands and feet, vexatious ["vessel" in a variant version {later editor}] heat with lack of perspiration, cramps of the hands and arms, headache as if pricked by an awl, gradual development of generalized heaviness into inability to move, vexation of the heart exacerbated by movement, throat *bi*, curled tongue, dry mouth, pain in the inner aspect of the arms with inability to lift them to the head, and deafness with ringing in the ears, Portal Yin (*Qiao Yin*, GB 44) is the ruling point.[151]

For pain in the outer (*i.e.*, lateral) aspect of the knee, febrile disease with lack of perspiration, reddening and pain of the outer canthi, spinning of the head, pain in the submandibular regions, tearing on exposure to cold, deafness with ringing in the ears, profuse sweating, itching of the eyes, pain in the chest with inability to turn (the body) over, and migratory pain, Pinched Ravine (*Xia Xi*, GB 43) is the ruling point.[152]

For inversion causing counterflow frigidity of the limbs, panting, fullness of qi, wind causing generalized perspiration and frigidity, pain in the hips and upper thighs with inability to walk, and pain in the skin at the lateral aspects of the feet, On the Verge of Tears (*Lin Qi*, GB 41) is the ruling point.

For dim vision, quivering with cold, eye screen covering the pupil, lumbar and lateral costal pain, and aching and cramps of the foot, Hill Ruins (*Qiu Xu*, GB 40) is the ruling point.

For lassitude, generalized cold, diminished qi, aversion to the sight of people in the case of intense heat, and apprehensiveness, (one should) take Flying Yang (*Guang Yang*, GB 37), Severed Bone (*Ju Gu*, GB 38), and On the Verge of Tears (*Lin Qi*, GB 41) at the instep. Immediate cure follows. For aching and weakness of the shanks and febrile disease with lack of perspiration, these are also the ruling points.

For heavy headedness, nosebleeding, tugging and slackening, lack of perspiration, heart vexation, heat in the soles of the feet, reluctance to dress, pain in the nape of the neck, eye screen, inhibited nose,[153] and inhibited urination, Reaching Yin (*Zhi Yin*, Bl 67) is the ruling point.

For generalized aching pain, susceptibility to fright, tugging (of the sinews), and nosebleeding, Open Valley (*Tong Gu*, Bl 66) is the ruling point. For sudden disease of headache, generalized fever and pain, twitching of the muscles, deafness, aversion to wind, ulceration and reddening of the canthi, inability to turn the neck, pain in the hip joints, diarrhea, and intestinal *pi*, Bundle Bone (*Shu Gu*, Bl 65) is the ruling point.[154]

For incessant runny snivel nosebleeding, headache due to the gradual sapping (of the evil qi), white screen in the eye, tugging and slackening between the heel and the buttock, swelling and ache in the head, outpour diarrhea, (qi) surging up into the heart, reddening of the eye and ulcerating canthi with loss of eyesight, pain (of the eyes) starting from the inner canthi ["screen developing from the inner canthi" in the *Qian Jin* {later editor}], abdominal fullness, stiffness of the nape of the neck, inability to bend the lumbar spine either forward or backward, dizziness, heart pain affecting the shoulders and the upper back as if the heart were pressed against from the back, and generalized cold starting from the lower legs, Capital Bone (*Jing Gu*, Bl 64) is the ruling point.[155]

For cold below, lack of perspiration in febrile disease, generalized heaviness, and spinning and ache of the head due to qi counterflow, Flying Yang (*Fei Yang*, Bl 58) is the ruling point.

For runny snivel nosebleeding, pain in the upper and lower back, aching heaviness of the feet and calves with trembling and inability to support the body for long, splitting pain in the calves, hypertonicity of the feet and pain in the heels, spasms of the feet, abdominal pain provoking sore throat, difficult defecation, and abdominal distention, Mountain Support (*Cheng Shan*, Bl 57) is the ruling point.[156]

For febrile disease with paravertebral pain, Bend Middle (*Wei Zhong*, Bl 40) is the ruling point.

Chapter Two

Disease of the Foot *Yang Ming* Vessel Producing Fever & Manic Walking[157]

(1)

The Yellow Emperor asked:

In disease of the foot *yang ming* vessel, (the patient) is averse to (the presence of) people and fire, suffers from palpitations, becomes frightened at the sound of wood, and prefers solitude with doors and windows shut. Please tell me the reason for this.[158]

Qi Bo answered:

The *yang ming* is the vessel of the stomach, and the stomach is earth. If one becomes frightened upon hearing the sound of wood, this is earth being averse to wood. The *yang ming* governs muscles, and contains exuberant blood and qi. When evils intrude, this produces heat, and when the heat becomes intense, this produces an aversion to fire. Inversion of the *yang ming* produces dyspnea and oppression, while oppression itself results in aversion to (the presence of) people. In the wrestling between yin and yang, if yang becomes exhausted and yin becomes exuberant, (the patient) will prefer solitude with doors and windows shut [the lines from "When yin and yang wrestle" to the end of this paragraph are found in the "*Mai Jie Pian* (Explanation of the *Yang Ming* Vessels)", of the *Su Wen*[159] and were placed in the text by Shi-an. {later editor}]][160]

The Yellow Emperor asked:

Why is it that (those) with dyspnea sometimes survive and at other times those with dyspnea die?

Qi Bo answered:

Counterflow inversion involving the viscera results in death. However, if only the channels are involved, (the patient) will survive.[161]

The Yellow Emperor asked:

If the disease is serious, (the patient) runs about naked and is able to climb to heights singing or jump over walls and climb onto roofs even without anything to eat for days (on end). Why is it that what is beyond him in his normal state may be accomplished in a state of disease?

Qi Bo answered:

In contention between yin and yang, if the exteri-or merges with the yang (阴阳争而外并于阳) [the preceding eight characters also appear in the "*Mai Jie*" chapter of the *Su Wen* {later editor}], then the evil becomes exuberant and hence the four limbs become replenished. When replenished, (the limbs) enable (the patient) to climb to great heights and sing. Because heat is exuberant in the body, he therefore disrobes and desires to run about. Because yang has become exuberant, he raves and utters abusive words without regard to whom he is speaking.[162]

(2)

When great heat spreads throughout the body, there will be manic speech and confused vision and hearing. (One should) examine the foot *yang ming* and its major connecting vessel, and then supplement them in the case of vacuity, or drain them in the case of blood repletion. (With the patient) lying supine, (the practitioner) stands before his head, pressing the pulsating vessels in his neck with four fingers of both hands for a long time, then rolling and rubbing the area with the fingers down to the supraclavicular fossa. Initiate (this procedure) as described above again and again till heat has departed. This (technique) is what is called dispersing by pushing.[163]

(3)

For generalized fever, wild running, delirium, and claiming to see apparitions, tugging and slackening, Body Pillar (*Shen Zhu*, GV 12) is the ruling point.

For mania and raving, irritability, apprehension, aversion to fire, and frequent outbreaks of verbal abuse, Great Tower Gate (*Ju Que*, CV 14) is the ruling point.[164]

For febrile disease with lack of perspiration, runny snivel nosebleeding, dizziness, collapse from time to time, puffy swelling of the face, cold lower legs, insomnia, quivering with cold, aversion to (the presence of) people and the sound of wood, throat *bi*, decayed teeth, aversion to wind, inhibited nose, and susceptibility to fright, Severe Mouth (*Li Dui*, St 45) is the ruling point.

For inversion (frigidity) of the four limbs with oppression of the hands and feet causing one to hold them for long periods of time (to relieve the discomfort), for counterflow frigidity (of the four limbs) causing aching in the lower legs, abdominal distention with pain in the skin, frequent yawning and stretching, aversion to (the presence of) people and the sound of wood, quivering with cold and dragging pain in the throat, and for febrile disease with lack of perspiration, pain of the lower teeth, aversion to cold, eye tension, dyspnea with fullness (in the chest), shivering with cold, clenched jaw and deviated mouth, and no desire for food, Inner Court (*Nei Ting*, St 44) is the ruling point.[165]

For manic singing, raving, irritability, aversion to (the presence of) people and fire, and verbal abusing, Three Li (*San Li*, St 36) is the ruling point.

Chapter Three

Yin Debility Producing Heat Inversion, Yang Debility Producing Cold Inversion[166]

(1)

The Yellow Emperor asked:

What are cold and heat inversion?

Qi Bo answered:

When yang qi is debilitated below, this results in cold inversion. When yin qi is debilitated below, this results in heat inversion.[167]

The Yellow Emperor asked:

Why must heat inversion start from the soles of the feet?

Qi Bo answered:

The yang qi travels in the surface of the five toes of the feet, while the yin vessels gather in the soles, concentrating on its center. Therefore, when yang is victorious, heat is generated in the soles.[168]

The Yellow Emperor asked:

Why must cold inversion start from the five toes and extend up to the knee?

Qi Bo answered:

Yin qi originates within the five toes, gathering in the region below the knee and concentrating in the region above it. Therefore, when the yin qi becomes exuberant, cold extends from the five toes to the region above the knee. This kind of cold is engendered from within rather than from the outside.[169]

The Yellow Emperor asked:

What manner of negligence is responsible for cold inversion?

Qi Bo answered:

The *jue yin* is the gathering place of the various sinews ["the front yin is the place where the sinews gather" in the *Su Wen* {later editor}], and the meeting place of the *tai yin* and *yang ming* (as well).[170]

In spring and summer, yang qi is abundant but yin qi is diminished, while in autumn and winter, yin qi is exuberant but yang qi falls into decline. If one (counts) too much on one's strong constitution, one may rob oneself (of one's vitality) in autumn and winter. As a result, the qi below may ascend for a struggle, and unable to restore to its normal state, essence qi spills downward. This allows evil qi to ascend. With (evil) qi in the center ["because of the qi in the center" in the *Su Wen* {later editor}], the yang qi falls into a decline, becoming unable to percolate and manage the channels and network vessels. Thus yang qi is reduced day by day, leaving the yin qi alone and causing cold in the hands and feet.[171]

The Yellow Emperor asked:

How does heat inversion occur?

Qi Bo answered:

Once alcohol has entered the stomach, the network vessels become full, while the channel vessels become empty. The spleen governs the conveyance of fluid and humor on behalf of the stomach. When yin qi becomes vacuous, this allows yang qi to penetrate the spleen, and when penetrated by the yang qi, the stomach becomes disharmonious. When the stomach is in disharmony, the essence qi becomes exhausted, and when exhausted, the essence qi can no longer nurture the four limbs.[172]

Such a person will have repeatedly engaged in sexual intercourse while drunk or having overeaten. This allows the (alcoholic) qi to gather in the spleen where it cannot dissipate. This alcoholic qi becomes entangled in a conflict with the grain qi, resulting in heat throughout the body and (causing) heat in the interior and reddish urine. Because the alcoholic qi is exuberant, impetuous, and aggressive, the kidney qi becomes debilitated day by day. Because the yang qi alone is exuberant, there is heat in the hands and feet.[173]

The Yellow Emperor asked:

Inversion may cause a person to experience abdominal fullness or sudden loss of consciousness which may take from a half a day to a whole day to regain. Why is this the case?

Qi Bo answered:

When yin qi becomes exuberant above, it produces a vacuity below, and this vacuity below produces abdominal fullness. With the abdomen full [the *Su Wen* replaces abdominal fullness with "the yang qi becomes exuberant above" {later editor}], the lower qi also ascends to produce a counterflow of evil qi. With this counterflow, the yang qi becomes chaotic, resulting in loss of consciousness.[174]

In the case of inversion of the *tai yang*, there is

facial swelling, heavy headedness, inability of the feet to walk, and spells of spinning collapse.

In the case of inversion of the *yang ming*, there is madness, desire to run and shout, abdominal fullness with inability to lie down, a red facial complexion which feels hot, and confused vision and hearing.

In the case of inversion of the *shao yang*, there is sudden deafness, swelling and a feeling of heat in the cheeks, pain in the lateral costal regions, and inability to move the lower legs.

In the case of inversion of the *tai yin*, there is abdominal fullness and distention, inhibited defecation, no desire for food, retching on ingestion, and inability to lie down.

In the case of inversion of the *shao yin*, there is dry tongue, reddish urine, abdominal fullness, and heart pain.

In the case of inversion of the *jue yin*, there is lower abdominal swelling and pain, distention, inhibited urination and defecation, preference for lying down with the knees bent, retracted testicles, and a sense of heat in the medial aspect of the lower legs.[175]

Exuberance is treated by drainage; vacuity by supplementation. A case of neither exuberance nor vacuity is treated by taking the (affected) channel.[176]

(2)

Please let me explain the teaching on resolution. (Humans) interact with heaven and earth and (live) in accord with the four seasons. This reference of humanity to heaven and earth makes resolution possible. The dank moor below allows the cattail and reed to grow above. (In the same manner,) one may determine the amount of qi based upon the form.[177]

The manifestation of yin and yang are (winter) cold and summerheat respectively. During periods of hot weather, moisture ascends to form rain, and, therefore, the roots and stems (of plants) lack juice. During this time, the qi in humans is in the exterior. The skin is slack, the interstices are open, blood and qi are exuberant, profuse sweat is drained, and the skin is moisturized and brilliant.[178]

In cold weather the ground is frozen and water turns to ice. (During this time) the qi of humans is in the interior, the skin is compact, the interstices are shut, no sweat is drained, blood and qi are solid, and the skin is hard and rough. During this time, even a person who is proficient in hydro (engineering) is unable to free the flow of ice, and even a person who is skilled in drilling the ground is unable to dig through the frozen ground. (Similarly,) even one skilled in the use of needles is unable to treat counterflow (frigidity) of the four limbs. This is due to the congelation and binding of the blood vessels, which have become hardened such that (the blood) cannot come and go, nor can they be softened.[179]

Thus, those who promote the flow of water must wait for the weather to warm and for the ice to thaw, and those who are to drill the ground must wait for it to defrost. Only then will they succeed in drilling the ground. The vessels of people behave in a similar manner. In treating inversion, to regulate and harmonize the channels, one must first regulate and harmonize the channels by means of ironing and fire at the palm and armpit, the elbows and feet, and the nape of the neck and spine. Once the broad highways are unblocked, the blood vessels will begin to flow. Then (it is necessary to) examine the conditions of the illness. In the case of a slippery pulse, needle to level (the qi), and, in the case of a hard, tense pulse, needle to dredge (the vessel). Once the (inversion) qi has been led down, treatment may be stopped. This practice is known as untying (i.e., resolution of) bondage (jie jie, 解结).[180]

Those using needles aim at regulating the qi. The qi first gathers in the stomach in order to communicate with the constructive and defensive which will be made to flow in their respective pathway. The ancestral qi stays and gathers in the sea (of qi), the down-travelling part pouring into the qi thoroughfare and the uptravelling part pouring into the respiratory tracts. Therefore, when inversion occurs in the feet, the ancestral qi can no longer descend and the blood in the vessels congeals and stops flowing. Without the help of fire to regulate (this condition), needles are unable to treat it.[181]

The acupuncturist must first evaluate the state of vacuity and repletion of the channels and network vessels by palpating and stroking, pressing and percussing. Only when the (nature of) the affliction (within the vessels) has been identified may points be taken and (the needle) inserted.[182]

When the six channels are regulated, there is said to be no disease, and any disease (which does present itself) is said to heal on its own. There may be a channel blockage with repletion above and vacuity below. In this case, there must be a transverse connecting vessel somewhere which is exuberant and adheres to the grand channel, thus causing the blockage. Find and drain (this vessel) to unblock and dredge (the channel). This is what is called resolution of bondage.[183]

If there is cold above but heat below, (one should) first puncture the (foot) tai yang at the nape of the neck and retain the needle for a long time. After needling, (one should) iron the nape and the scapulae to lead the heat ["chill" in a variant version {later editor}] down to join with (the heat below), and then stop (the treatment). This is known as pushing to promote ascent. If there is heat above but cold below, (one should) discover the vacuous, sunken points on the channel and connecting vessel and treat these to lead the qi down completely. This is what is called conduction to promote descent.[184]

(3)

In needling heat inversion, retention of the needle can turn (heat) into cold. While to treat cold inversion, retention of the needle can turn (cold) into heat.[185]

Needling heat inversion (requires) two yang and one yin; needling cold inversion (requires) one yin and two yang. That which is referred to as two yin means that the yin is needled twice, and what is referred to as the two yang means that the yang is needled twice.[186]

For heat inversion, (one should) take the (foot) *tai yin* and *shao yang*, and for cold inversion, take the (foot) *yang ming* and *shao yin*, all at the feet and with retention of the needle.[187]

(4)

For inversion with fullness in the chest, swollen face, thickened lips,[188] sudden difficulty in enunciating, and, in the extreme, even loss of voice, take the foot *yang ming*.

For inversion with loss of voice due to (counterflow) qi penetrating the throat, cold hands and feet, and inhibited defecation, take the foot *shao yin*.[189]

For inversion with inflating distention of the abdomen, lavish cold qi, rumbling of the intestines, and difficult urination and defecation, take the foot *tai yin*.

(5)

For disease of counterflow inversion with sudden frigidity of the feet, a feeling in the chest as if it were about to burst, lancinating pain in the abdomen and the intestines, distention with inability to ingest food, and choppy pulses be they large or small, if (the trunk) is warm, take the foot *shao yin*, and, if (the trunk) is frigid, take the foot *yang ming*. The frigid (case) requires supplementation, while the warm (case) requires drainage.[190]

For counterflow inversion with abdominal fullness and distention, rumbling of the intestines, and fullness in the chest with inability to catch the breath, take (the points) in the two regions of the (free) ribs under the chest where movement may be felt when coughing and at the back points which produce some relief when pressure is applied.[191]

(6)

For inversion (frigidity) of the feet with counterflow dyspnea and frigidity extending from the soles to the knees, Gushing Spring (*Yong Quan*, Ki 1) is the ruling point.

Chapter Four

Contraction of Cold Dampness in Wind Stroke of the *Tai Yang* Producing Tetany[192, 193]

(1)

Tetany due to heat is characterized by arched-back rigidity, tugging and slackening, and clenched jaw and grinding of the teeth.[194]

Zhang Zhong-jing[195] states that a *tai yang* disease presenting with all of its typical signs is diagnosed as tetany if the body is stiff and (the nape and back) are rigid while the pulse is deep and slow. The tetany pulse appears when pressed as solid, bow-string, and tight all over. Hard tetany is a disease of fullness in the chest, clenched jaw, inability of the back to touch the mat in the (supine) lying posture, and hypertonicity of the feet. The patient must grind his teeth. The *tai yang* disease with fever and a deep, thin pulse is diagnosed as tetany. The tetany patient invariably has a deep pulse which is hard and tight all over. *Tai yang* disease with fever, lack of perspiration, and aversion to cold is diagnosed as hard tetany. *Tai yang* disease with fever, perspiration, and no aversion to cold is diagnosed as soft tetany.[196]

In tetany due to damp stroke to the *tai yang*, the pulse is deep, level down with the surrounding sinews. *Tai yang* disease with lack of perspiration, scant urine, qi surging up into the chest, and clenched jaw with inability to speak tends to present as hard tetany. Wind stroke of the *tai yang* with hard tetany accompanied by cold dampness, however, is characterized by a pulse which comes and goes, advances and retreats, and is deep, slow, and fine. This differs from (the presentation of) febrile disease due to cold damage. To treat it, diaphoresis is not an appropriate therapy, and needling and moxaing is the best choice. If it is treated with medication, the *Ge Gen Tang* (Pueraria Decoction)[197] can be administered.[198]

For wind tetany characterized by arched-back rigidity, first take the blood vessel of the foot *tai yang* at the popliteal fossa[199] to let blood out. For tetany with cold in the center, take Three Li (*San Li*, St 36).[200]

For tetany, take the blood vessels at the yin motility vessel[201] and the three hair region[202] and bleed them.

(2)

For tetany, take Fontanelle Meeting (*Xin Hui*, GV 22) and Hundred Convergences (*Bai Hui*, GV 20), Celestial Pillar (*Tian Zhu*, Bl 10), Diaphragm Shu (*Ge Shu*, Bl 17), Upper Pass (*Shang Guan*, GB 3), and Bright Light (*Guang Ming*, GB 37) as the ruling points.

For tetany with inability to roll the eyes, needle Brain Door (*Nao Hu*, GV 17).

For tetany with arched-back rigidity, tugging and slackening, madness, and heavy headedness, Fifth Place (*Wu Chu*, Bl 5) is the ruling point.

For tetany with tugging (of the sinews) and susceptibility to fright, Celestial Surge (*Tian Chong*, GB 9) is the ruling point.[203]

For tetany with arched-back rigidity, heart pain, shortage of form and qi, distention and cold in the sacrococcygeal (region), and dribbling urinary block with yellowish urine, Long Strong (*Chang Qiang*, GV 1) is the ruling point.[204]

For tetany with spinal rigidity, tugging (of the sinews), aversion to wind, intermittent quivering with cold, throat *bi*, fullness of the great qi, dyspnea, oppression in the chest, generalized fever, dizziness, blurred vision, stiffness of the neck, cold and heat, collapse, inability to stand for any length of time, vexation, fullness and urgency in the abdomen, and inability to lie down quietly, Great Shuttle (*Da Zhu*, Bl 11) is the ruling point.[205]

For tetany with pain and stiffness and tugging of the sinews, Liver Shu (*Gan Shu*, Bl 18) is the ruling point.

For heat tetany, Spleen Shu (*Pi Shu*, Bl 20) and Kidney Shu (*Shen Shu*, Bl 23) are the ruling points.

For heat tetany with tugging (of the sinews), lack of perspiration, arched-back rigidity, pain inside the buttocks and pure heat wasting thirst *nue*, Urinary Bladder Shu (*Pang Guang Shu*, Bl 28) is the ruling point.[206]

For tetany with arched-back rigidity, tugging (of the sinews), abdominal distention, hypertonicity of the armpits, and a distressed sensation in the upper back sending a dragging pain to the lateral costal regions and inwardly to the heart region, Central Backbone Shu (*Zhong Lu Shu*, Bl 29) is the ruling point. Palpate each vertebrae from the nape of the neck down the spine and find the painful points in the paravertebral sinews. Needle three of these and this will afford instant relief.[207]

For tetany with tugging (of the sinews) and generalized fever, Burning Valley (*Ran Gu*, Ki 2) and Yi Xi (*Yi Xi*, Bl 45) are the ruling points.

For tetany with upturned eyes and abhorrence of wind, needle Silk Bamboo Hole (*Si Zhu Kong*, TH 23).[208]

For tetany with tugging (of the sinews) and stiff lips and corners of the mouth, Severe Mouth (*Li Dui*, St 45) is the ruling point.

For tetany with vexation and fullness, Gum Intersection (*Yin Jiao*, GV 28) is the ruling point.

For tetany with clenched jaw, tugging (of the sinews), dry mouth, and yellowish or dark reddish urine or intermittent incontinence of urination, Sauce Receptacle (*Cheng Jiang*, CV 24) is the ruling point.

For tetany with clenched jaw, Great Reception (*Da Ying*, St 5) is the ruling point.

For tetany with inability to speak, Wind Screen (*Yi Feng*, TH 17) is the ruling point.

For tetany, take first Great Ravine (*Tai Xi*, Ki 3) and then the source point of the great granary.[209, 210]

For tetany with spinal rigidity, abdominal urgency, and abdominal hypertonicity and pain, Water Divide (*Shui Fen*, CV 29) is the ruling point.

For tetany with spinal rigidity, inability to open the mouth, copious sputum, and difficult defecation, Stone Pass (*Shi Guan*, Ki 18) is the ruling point.

For tetany with arched-back rigidity, Capital Gate (*Jing Men*, GB 25) is the ruling point.

For tetany with an enlarged and hardened abdomen and inability to catch one's breath, Cycle Gate (*Qi Men*, Liv 14) is the ruling point.

For tetany with an ascension of qi, Fish's Margin (*Yu Ji*, Lu 10) is the ruling point.

For tetany with tugging (of the sinews), Wrist Bone (*Wan Gu*, SI 4) is the ruling point.

For febrile disease with lack of perspiration and frequent vomiting of bitter (fluid) and for tetany with arched-back rigidity, clenched jaw, frequent chattering of the jaws, lumbar pain with inability to look round or breaking pain in the lumbus arising on attempting to look round, and sentimentality, take (the points) both above and below [211] and bleed them. Relief will follow immediately upon the appearance of blood.[212]

For tetany with arched-back rigidity, clenched jaw, and throat *bi* with loss of voice, Three Li (*San Li*, St 36) is the ruling point.

For tetany with susceptibility to fright, tugging (of the sinews), feet which feel bound, and calves which feel as if they are about to split, Bundle

Bone (*Shu Gu*, Bl 65) is the ruling point.

For tetany with eyes upturned so that it is predominantly the whites which are visible, inhibited nose, sniveling of yellow nasal mucus, and blood in the stools ["which requires blood letting" in a variant version {later editor}], Capital Bone (*Jing Gu*, Bl 64) is the ruling point.

For tetany with rigid spine, spinning and ache of the head, feet which feel bound, and calves which feel as if they are about to split, Kun Lun Mountain (*Kun Lun*, Bl 60) is the ruling point.

For tetany with arched-back rigidity, Taking Flight (*Fei Yang*, Bl 58) is the ruling point.

Chapter Five

Mutual Suppression of Yin & Yang Producing Three Types of *Nue* [213]

(1)

The Yellow Emperor asked:

All types of *nue* are generated from wind. Some types attack once a day and at regular hours. How is this?[214]

Qi Bo answered:

Nue starts in the fine hair with (symptoms of) yawning and stretching. (This is followed by) quivering with cold, chattering of the jaws, and pain both in the lumbus and in the spine. After the disappearance of cold, heat both internally and externally ensues with splitting headache and thirst with desire for cold drinks.[215]

The Yellow Emperor asked:

What kind of qi causes (*nue*)?

Qi Bo answered:

Yin and yang contend above and below, vacuity

and repletion alternate, and yin and yang supersede one another (abnormally). If yang becomes incorporated into the yin, then the yin becomes replete and yang vacuous. If the *yang ming* is vacuous, there is quivering with cold and chattering of the jaws. If the *tai yang* is vacuous, there is pain in both the upper and lower back, the head, and the nape of the neck. When the three yang all become vacuous, yin qi ["the second yin" in a variant version {later editor}] prevails, and, with yin qi prevailing, there is cold and pain in the bones. Since cold is generated internally, it, therefore, presents itself both in the center as well as externally. If yang prevails, there is external heat. If yin prevails, there is internal heat. If there is both internal and external heat, this causes dyspnea and thirst which results in the desire for cold drinks.[216]

All this is contracted in summer as a result of damage done by summerheat. The heat qi, which is exuberant, is then hidden in the skin, outside the stomach and the intestines, (or more exactly,) in the dwelling place of the constructive qi. It causes people to perspire. This leaves a void behind and forces the interstices open. (Later, they) may contract autumn qi, be caught in wind while sweating, or contract water qi while taking a bath. (These evil qi then) lodge in the skin, residing in the defensive qi. Because the defensive qi moves in the yang during the day and in the yin during the night, the (evil) qi emerges during the yang (phase) and oppresses internally during the yin (phase). Because (the evil) oppresses (alternately) internally and externally, *nue*-like episodes occur once a day.[217]

The Yellow Emperor asked:

How is it that (some types of *nue*) attack every other day?

Qi Bo answered:

(In this case) the (evil) qi has settled deeply, oppressing yin internally, and the yang qi is left to act alone. With the yin evil lodging internally, yin, which is locked in a contention with yang, is unable to emerge (according to a daily law).

Thus, *nue* attacks every other day.[218]

The Yellow Emperor asked:

What kind of qi causes (*nue*-like episodes to occur) at an earlier and later hour than on each preceding day?

Qi Bo answered:

The evil qi invades the wind mansion and travels downward along the spinal column. The defensive qi has a grand meeting at the wind mansion once in a day and night, and, by the next day, the evil qi has moved to the next vertebra. Therefore, the attack is postponed. This presupposes the initial intrusion (of the evil) is located in the spine in the back. Each time (the defensive qi) arrives at the wind mansion, the interstices are open. The open interstices consequently provide the evil qi with an opportunity to penetrate. Each time the evil qi penetrates, a (*nue*-like) episode ensues. This (mechanism) explains the slight postponement of the attack. After leaving the wind mansion, the evil qi moves down one vertebra each day. On the twenty-first day, it has descended to the coccyx, and, on the twenty-second it submerges into the spine, pouring into the *tai chong* vessel.[219] [In the *Su Wen* twenty-fifth replaces the twenty-first, and twenty-sixth replaces the twenty-second; in addition, the deep-lying paravertebral sinews replace the *tai chong*. {later editor}] The evil qi then turns and travels upward for nine days, where it emerges at the basin-like depression. Because the (evil) qi is (lodged) a little higher each day, it is afforded an opportunity to attack earlier each day.[220]

(*Nue* that attacks) every other day is due to the internal oppression of the five viscera by evil qi and its transversely linking to the *mo yuan*.[221] Lodged here, its journey (to the surface) is distant, its penetration deep, and its action retarded. Because of this, (the evil qi) is unable to keep pace with the defensive qi and fails to emerge simultaneously with it. Therefore, (the evil qi) will only present itself every other day.[222]

The Yellow Emperor asked:

Each time the defensive qi arrives at the wind mansion, the interstices are effusive, and when they are effusive, the evil qi has an opportunity to penetrate. When the evil qi penetrates, this triggers a (nue) episode. Now, since the defensive qi responds one vertebra later each day, the attack of the (evil) qi should not occur (when the evil qi arrives at) the wind mansion. How is it still possible for the evil qi to attack once a day?[223]

Qi Bo answered:

[The following reply is preceded by eighty-eight characters in the *Su Wen* which are absent from the *Jia Yi Jing*. Therefore, they are not included here. {later editor}] Wind has no permanent mansion of its own. When the defensive qi is effusive, the interstices are surely open, and when the evil (wind) qi meets (the defensive qi), the disease presents itself ["makes its home there" in the *Su Wen*. {later editor}][224]

The Yellow Emperor asked:

Since wind and *nue* are of a kind and similar in nature, why is it that only wind appears persistently, while *nue* attacks intermittently?

Qi Bo answered:

Since wind qi typically becomes lodged in the place (where it invades), it appears persistently, while the *nue* qi, following the channels and network vessels to penetrate more deeply [the *Su Wen* adds "in order to lie deeply, and contend internally" {later editor}]. Therefore, (the *nue* qi) presents itself only when responding to the defensive qi.[225]

The Yellow Emperor asked:

Why is it that *nue*-like episodes first present as cold and then heat?

Qi Bo answered:

The damage done by the great summerheat in summer causes copious perspiration and opens the interstices. If one is assailed by a slight summer cool qi, (the evil cool qi) hides in the interstices and the skin. When wind damage is inflicted in the autumn, the illness then finally develops. Cold is a yin qi, while wind is a yang qi. Since cold damage precedes wind damage, cold is followed by heat. The disease attacks at fixed hours, and is called cold *nue*.[226]

The Yellow Emperor asked:

Why is it (that some *nue* episodes) first present with heat and then with cold?

Qi Bo answered:

First there is wind damage, and then there is cold damage. Thus heat comes first and then cold. (The *nue* episodes) occur at fixed hours as well. This is called warm *nue*.

Heat which is not followed by cold (in a *nue* episode) is the result of the prior expiry of the yin qi. When the yang qi alone is effusive, there is heat with diminished qi, vexation, hotness in the hands and feet, and desire to retch. This is known as pure heat wasting thirst *nue*.[227]

The Yellow Emperor asked:

The classic[228] explains that surplus requires drainage, while insufficiency requires supplementation. Now, heat is known as surplus and cold as insufficiency. (However,) the cold in *nue* cannot be warmed by boiling water or fire, and the heat in malaria cannot be cooled by iced water. If these two simply pertain to the classes of surplus and insufficiency, why then are even proficient practitioners unable to check them, finding themselves constrained to wait for the episode to abate of itself before they can preform needling?

Qi Bo answered:

The classic warns against needling to treat scalding heat, warns against needling in the case of a deranged pulse, and warns against needling cases of prodigious sweating. This is because, when the diseased (qi) counterflows, it is not yet opportune to treat it.[229]

At the outset of a *nue* episode, the yang qi is superseded by the yin. At this point, yang is vacuous and yin is exuberant, and qi is absent from the exterior. As a result, initially there is shivering with cold. Once the yin qi reaches its counterflow climax, it emerges and moves into a yang (phase) such that yang and yin are merged in the exterior. At this point, yin is vacuous and yang is replete, resulting first in heat and then thirst.[230]

Nue qi which is superseded by yang may lead to an overwhelming of yang, or when superseded by yin may lead to an overwhelming of yin. Overwhelming yin gives rise to cold while overwhelming yang to heat. As *nue* is a fulminant wind cold qi of capricious nature, the disease goes to its zenith and (some time) after, relapses. When it attacks, it is as hot as fire, and as irresistible as wind and rain. For this reason the classic states that (treatment) is doomed to failure if administered in the face of an exuberance (of evil) and yet may be a great success if administered when (the evil) is in decline. This is said (of *nue*).[231]

Prior to a *nue* episode, yin has not yet been superseded by yang nor has yang been superseded by yin. If (one) seizes the opportunity to regulate (yin and yang), the true qi will become quiet and the evil qi will escape. The practitioner, however, has no means of treating the disease in the midst of an episode because the (evil) qi is in a state of counterflow (at that moment).

At the onset of a *nue* episode, (that is,) when yin and yang are just about to supersede each other, (the episode) will invariably begin from the four extremities. When yang is damaged, yin tends towards it. Just before their qi have merged, (one may) anticipate (these pathological changes) and bind up the places to prevent the evil qi from entering and the yin qi from emerging. At the same time, one may take all the exuberant, hard, blood (filled) minute vessels found on examination. This is (a treatment) when (the evil qi) is about to enter but (yin and yang) have not yet superseded one another.[232]

The Yellow Emperor asked:

What happens when a *nue* episode is interrupted?

Qi Bo answered:

Nue is always (characterized by) alternating exuberance and vacuity. (A *nue* episode) is contingent upon the location of the (defensive) qi. When the diseased (qi) is in the yang, there is heat with an agitated pulse, whereas when it is in the yin, there is cold with a tranquil pulse. At the climax (of the attack), yin and yang are both exhausted, the defensive qi (and the evil qi) begin to separate from one another, and the episode ceases. The episode recurs, however, when (the evil qi) combines with the defensive qi once more.

The Yellow Emperor asked:

Some (types of *nue*) occur once every third day or at intervals of several days, some with and some without thirst. What is the reason for all these (differences)?

Qi Bo answered:

Intermittent episodes occur if the evil qi and the defensive qi become lodged in the six bowels and, (consequently,) cannot maintain synchronization. They may, on occasion, fail to meet with each other and, therefore, (the *nue*) remains dormant for several days before another episode.[233]

Yin and yang overwhelm one another. However, this will occur to a greater or lesser extent, and this accounts for thirst or an absence of thirst.

The Yellow Emperor asked:

(It is said that) summerheat damage inflicted in summer must develop into the disease of *nue* in autumn. Yet why are there cases which do not conform (to this axiom) today?

Qi Bo answered:

This (axiom is only seen in those illnesses) that are in accord with the seasonal disposition. A disease with an unusual form may manifest in a manner contrary to the seasonal disposition. A disease occurring in the autumn is characterized by severe cold. A disease occurring in the winter is characterized by slight cold. A disease occurring in the spring is characterized by aversion to wind. And a disease occurring in the summer is characterized by profuse sweating.[234]

The Yellow Emperor asked:

Where does (the evil qi of) warm *nue* and cold malaria lodge and in which viscus?

Qi Bo answered:

Warm *nue* is contracted during the winter and is due to wind cold stroke. The cold qi is hidden within the bone marrow, and, even when the yang qi begins to become effusive in the spring, the cold qi is unable to emerge. Only in cases of major (contractions of) summerheat, where the brain marrow becomes consumed, the muscles become emaciated, and the interstices are effusive and draining, or only upon exertion, will the evil qi emerge with perspiration. The disease has been lying hidden within the kidney, and the (evil) qi proceeds first from the internal toward the external. Thus, yin becomes vacuous and yang exuberant. When yang is exuberant, there is heat, and when it declines, the (evil) qi turns inward once more. Once it has turned inward, the yang becomes vacuous and this yang vacuity produces cold. For this reason, first there is heat and then there is cold. (Hence) the term warm *nue*.[235]

The Yellow Emperor asked:

What is pure heat wasting thirst *nue*?

Qi Bo answered:

Because heat has been present in the lung, there is an exuberance of qi within the body (as a whole. This exuberance of qi produces) an inversion of qi which counterflows upward. (Thus) the qi in the center becomes replete and fails to dissipate outward. As a result of exertion, the interstices may be open, allowing wind cold to reside in the skin and the border of the flesh where it becomes effusive. (When wind cold) becomes effusive, yang qi becomes exuberant. If yang qi remains exuberant without ever diminishing, this results in disease. Since this (yang) qi does not return to yin, there will only be heat which is followed by no cold. This (evil) qi is hidden internally within the heart and resides externally in the border of the flesh. It causes emaciation and shedding of flesh, (hence) the term pure heat wasting thirst *nue*.[236]

(2)

For *nue* with a pulse that is full, large, and urgent, prick the associated points on the back using a medium sized needle and/or each of the five axillary associated points beside them. (These points are) bled in an amount which is appropriate to the fatness or thinness (of the patient).[237]

For *nue* with a pulse that is small, replete, and urgent, moxa the lower legs on the (foot) *shao yin*[238] and needle the toe at the well point.[239]

For *nue* with a slow, large, and vacuous pulse, medication may be administered but needling is inappropriate.[240]

Whenever treating *nue*, (treatment) must be performed about the time it takes to eat a meal prior to an episode in order for the therapy to be successful. (If performed) later than this, the opportunity will be missed.

Item,[241] for *nue* with no thirst that occurs every other day, the *Jiu Juan* instructs that one take the foot *yang ming*, while the *Su Wen* instructs that one needle the foot *tai yang*. For *nue* with thirst that occurs every other day, the *Jiu Juan* instructs that one take the hand *shao yang*, while the *Su Wen* instructs that one needle the foot *shao yang*.[242]

Item, for warm *nue* with lack of perspiration, select from among the fifty-nine needling (points)[243] [that are indicated for febrile diseases {later editor}].

Item, foot *tai yang nue* causes people to suffer

from lumbar pain, heavy headedness, cold starting from the back, cold followed by heat and thirst, and once this thirst is quenched, then perspiration ensues. It is difficult to overcome [the phrase "cold followed by heat" is modified by the epithets "scalding and scorching" in the *Su Wen* {later editor}]. Episodes occur every other day, (requiring that one) prick (the vessel) at the popliteal fossa[244] to let out blood.[245]

Item, foot *shao yang nue* causes people to suffer from languor and lassitude, moderate cold, aversion to the sight of people, palpitation with apprehension. and abundant heat with profuse perspiration. (This condition requires that one) needle the foot *shao yang*.[246]

Item, foot *yang ming nue* causes people to first suffer from cold and shivering as if after having become soaked. The cold becomes severe and chronic and then is followed by heat. When the heat has departed, then perspiration emerges. (The patient) has a preference for the sight of sunlight, moonlight, and fire qi which can bring relief. (This condition requires that one) needle the foot *yang ming* at the instep, regulating the point Surging Yang (*Chong Yang, St 42*).[247]

Item, foot *tai yin nue* causes people to suffer from gloom and melancholy, a tendency to great sighs, a lack of desire for food, abundant cold and heat, and sweating. At the onset of an episode, there is a tendency to retch, and once this retching has occurred, there is some relief (of the *nue* symptoms. This condition requires that one) take the foot *tai yin*.[248]

Item, foot *shao yin nue* causes people to suffer from violent retching and vomiting, abundant cold with scant heat, and a preference for privacy with doors and windows shut. This disease is difficult to overcome. (This condition requires that one) take Great Ravine (*Tai Xi*, Ki 3).[249]

Item, foot *jue yin nue* causes people to suffer from lumbar pain, lower abdominal fullness, inhibited urination which resembles dribbling urinary block but is not in fact dribbling urinary block, frequent belching, susceptibility to fright, appre-

hension, insufficiency of qi, and discomfort in the abdomen. (This condition requires that one) needle the foot *jue yin*.[250]

Item, lung *nue* causes people to suffer from cold in the heart region and severe heat succeeding the cold. During the course of the heat, there is a susceptibility to fright with confused vision. (This condition requires that one) needle the hand *tai yin*[251] and *yang ming*.[252]

Item, heart *nue* causes people to suffer from severe vexation of the heart, desire for the sight of cold water, abundant cold ["despite abundant cold" in the *Su Wen*; "with abundant cold" in the *Tai Su* {later editor}], and moderate heat. (This condition requires that one) needle the hand *shao yin*, by which is meant Spirit Door (*Shen Men*, Ht 7).[253]

Item, liver *nue* causes people to suffer from a green-blue complexion ["sighing" is included in the *Su Wen* {later editor}] and death-like appearance. (This condition requires that one) prick the foot *jue yin*[254] to let blood out.

Item, spleen *nue* causes people to suffer from illnesses of abdominal pain in the case of cold, and rumbling of the intestines occurring in the case of heat, with sweat emerging when the rumbling ceases. (This condition requires that one) needle the foot *tai yin*.[255]

Item, kidney *nue* causes people to suffer from shivering with cold ["shivering with cold as after a soaking" in the *Su Wen* {later editor}], pain in the lumbar spine, difficult defecation, visual dizziness, and cold hands and feet. (This condition requires that one) needle the foot *tai yang*[256] and *shao yin*.[257]

Item, stomach *nue* causes people to suffer from cold diseases of the gallbladder. They may easily become hungry and yet be unable to ingest, and there may be a propping fullness in the abdomen on ingestion of food. (This condition requires that one) needle the foot *yang ming*[258] and prick the transverse vessel of the foot *tai yin*[259] to let blood out.[260]

Item, *nue* which occurs in episodes of generalized heat (requires that one) needle the moving vessel at the instep.[261] (The needle) hole should be widened. With bloodletting a chill immediately ensues.[262]

Item, just as a *nue* episode is about to become cold (but there are as yet no chills, one should) needle the hand *yang ming*,[263] hand *tai yin*,[264] foot *yang ming*,[265] and foot *tai yin*.[266]

Item, in all types of *nue* in which a pulse is not evident, (one should) prick the fingers and toes[267] to let blood out. Relief is certain to follow bloodletting. (One should) first locate all the red bean-like papules on the body and remove them.[268]

Item, the twelve types of *nue*[269] each attack at different times. (One should) study their characteristics as a means of identifying which channel has become diseased. Needling should be performed about as long as it takes to eat a meal prior to the occurrence of an episode. The first needling diminishes (the evil qi). By the second, one may know (that the illness has abated). And the third puts an end to it. If this is not the case, (one may) prick the two vessels under the tongue to let blood out. If this is ineffective, (one may) prick the exuberant channel at the popliteal fossa to let out blood in combination with needling the paravertebral points below the nape of the neck.[270] Recuperation is then a certainty. The two vessels under the tongue are (the point) Ridge Spring (*Lian Quan*).[271]

Item, in needling *nue*, one must first determine where the episode begins and this aspect must be needled first. If headache and heavy headedness (appears first, one should) first prick the head,[272] both temples[273] and (the point) between the eyebrows[274] to let blood out. If pain appears first in the nape of the neck and the upper back, (one should) first needle the nape[275] and the upper back.[276] If pain appears first in the lumbar spine, (one should) first prick the popliteal fossae[277] to let blood out. If pain appears first in the hands and arms, (one should) first needle the hand *shao yin* and *yang ming* at the ten fingers.[278] If there is aching pain appearing first in the feet and the lower legs, (one should) first prick the foot *yang ming* at the ten toes[279] to let blood out.[280]

For wind *nue* characterized by perspiration and aversion to wind occurring (at the onset) of an episode, (one should) prick the (viscus-)associated back points of the three foot yang channels[281] to let blood out.[282]

Aching pain in the lower legs which cannot bear the lightest pressure is called shin bone marrow disease. Pricking the Severed Bone (*Jue Gu*, GB 38) with the arrowhead needle to let blood out affords an instant cure. In the case of a slight generalized (aching) pain, (one should) needle the well points of the various yin channels once every other day without letting them bleed.[283]

(3)

For quartan *nue* (*jie nue*, 痎 虐), Spirit Court (*Shen Ting*, GV 24) and Hundred Convergences (*Bai Hui*, GV 20) are the ruling points.[284]

For quartan *nue*, Upper Star (*Shang Xing*, GV 23) is the ruling point. It is necessary to take first Yi Xi (*Yi Xi*, Bl 45) and finally Celestial Window (*Tian You*, TH 16) and Wind Pool (*Feng Chi*, GB 20).[285]

For quartan *nue*, Completion Bone (*Wan Gu*, GB 12), Wind Pool (*Feng Chi*, GB 20), Great Shuttle (*Da Zhu*, Bl 11), Heart Shu (*Xin Shu*, Bl 15), Upper Bone Hole (*Shang Liao*, Bl 31), Yi Xi (*Yi Xi*, Bl 45), Yin Metropolis (*Yin Du*, Ki 19), Great Abyss (*Tai Yuan*, Lu 9), Third Space (*San Jian*, LI 3), Union Valley (*He Gu*, LI 4), Yang Pool (*Yang Chi*, TH 4), Lesser Marsh (*Shao Ze*, SI 1), Front Valley (*Qian Gu*, SI 2), Back Ravine (*Hou Xi*, SI 3), Wrist Bone (*Wan Gu*, SI 4), Yang Valley (*Yang Gu*, SI 5), Pinched Ravine (*Xia Xi*, GB 43), Reaching Yin (*Zhi Yin*, Bl 67), Open Valley (*Tong Gu*, Bl 66), and Capital Bone (*Jing Gu*, Bl 64) are all the ruling points.

For *nue* characterized by shivering with cold, intense fever, and raving, Celestial Pivot (*Tian Shu*, St 25) is the ruling point.[286]

For *nue* with exuberant heat, Broken Sequence

(*Lie Que*, Lu 7) is the ruling point.

For *nue* characterized by cold inversion, heat with vexation of the heart, frequent retching, heart fullness, and sweating, pricking Lesser Shang (*Shao Shang*, Lu 11) to let blood out affords an immediate cure.[287]

For heat *nue* with dry mouth, Shang Yang (*Shang Yang*, LI 1) is the ruling point.

For *nue* with intense cold ["inclination to retching of foamy fluid" added in the *Qian Jin* {later editor}], Yang Ravine (*Yang Xi*, LI 5) is the ruling point.

For wind *nue* with a lack of perspiration, Veering Passageway (*Pian Li*, LI 6) is the ruling point.

For *nue* with red facial complexion and facial swelling, Warm Dwelling (*Wen Liu*, LI 7) is the ruling point.

For quartan *nue* with distention, fullness and pain in the region below the heart, and qi ascension, moxa Arm Five (*Shou Wu Li*, LI 13). For the right side, (one should) take the left (point); for the left, (one should) take the right.

For *nue* with pain in the nape of the neck and sudden fulminating counterflow, Armpit Gate (*Ye Men*, TH 2) is the ruling point.[288]

For *nue* episodes occurring regardless of the season with a red facial complexion and blurred vision, Central Islet (*Zhong Zhu*, TH 3) is the ruling point.

For *nue* episodes that are triggered during meals, heart pain, gloom, and melancholy, Celestial Well (*Tian Jing*, TH 10) is the ruling point.

For wind *nue*, Branch to the Correct (*Zhi Zheng*, SI 7) is the ruling point.

For *nue* characterized by shivering with cold of the paravertebral sinews in the back, pain in the nape of the neck sending a dragging (discomfort) to the elbows and axillae, lumbar pain sending a dragging (discomfort) into the lower abdomen,

and inability to lift the four limbs, Small Sea (*Xiao Hai*, SI 8) is the ruling point.[289]

For *nue* characterized by discomfort of an unknown location, Great Metropolis (*Da Du*, Sp 2) is the ruling point.

For *nue* with abundant cold but scant heat, Large Goblet (*Da Zhong*, Ki 4) is the ruling point.

For *nue* with counterflow cough, oppression of the heart with inability to lie down, violent retching, abundant heat but scant cold, preference of privacy with doors and windows shut, and cold inversion with hot feet, Great Ravine (*Tai Xi*, Ki 3) is the ruling point.

For *nue* with heat, diminished qi, cold lower legs which cannot be kept warm by themselves, abdominal distention, and lancinating pain radiating to the heart, Recover Flow (*Fu Liu*, Ki 7) is the ruling point.

For *nue* with no desire for food, Severe Mouth (*Li Dui*, St 45) is the ruling point.

For *nue* with tugging and slackening, susceptibility to fright, heaviness of the thighs and the knees ["heaviness in turning the knees" in the *Qian Jin* {later editor}], cramps of the lower legs, and dizziness and pain in the head, Ravine Divide (*Jie Xi*, St 41) is the ruling point.

For *nue* episodes which begin when the sun is in the west (*i.e.*, in the afternoon), On the Verge of Tears (*Lin Qi*, GB 41) is the ruling point.

For *nue* characterized by shivering with cold and swelling of the armpits, Hill Ruins (*Qiu Xu*, GB 40) is the ruling point.

For *nue* episodes that (begin) in the lower legs, Bundle Bone (*Shu Gu*, Bl 65) is the ruling point.

For *nue* with copious sweating, pain in the lumbus with inability to bend either forward or backward, (pain in the) eyes as if they were about to burst from their sockets, (pain in the) nape of the neck as if it were being pulled up, Kun Lun

Mountain (*Kun Lun*, Bl 60) is the ruling point.

For *nue* characterized by repletion resulting in pain in the upper and lower back or characterized by vacuity resulting in runny snivel nosebleeding, Taking Flight (*Fei Yang*, Bl 58) is the ruling point.

For *nue* with heavy headedness, cold that (originates) in the back, cold preceding heat, unquenchable thirst, and lack of perspiration until (water is drunk), Bend Middle (*Wei Zhong*, Bl 40) is the ruling point.

For *nue* with an absence of thirst that attacks every other day, Taking Flight (*Fei Yang*, Bl 58) is the ruling point.[290]

Endnotes

[1]Part 1 is derived from Chap. 31, *Su Wen (Basic Questions)*; Part 2 from Chap. 32, *Su Wen*; Part 3 is a combination of parts of Chap. 3, 5, and 31, *Su Wen*; Part 4 from Chap. 75, Vol. 11, *Ling Shu (Spiritual Pivot)*; Part 5 from Chap. 34, *Su Wen*; and Part 6 from Chap. 29, *Su Wen*.

[2]The governing vessel is the sea of all the yang channels, while the yang linking vessel connects with all the yang channels. Both meet at Wind Mansion and are ascribed to the *tai yang*. Therefore, it is justifiably said to govern the qi on behalf of all the yang channels. Moreover, the *tai yang* channel travels along the entire posterior of the body, and this is another reason for the assertion that the *tai yang* is the sea of all the yang channels. If a febrile disease affects a yang channel only, it will **not** be fatal. However, when both a yang channel and a yin channel are simultaneously damaged by cold, this is considered a dual affliction of cold. Since yin and yang are both damaged, the condition is critical.

[3]One should note the order of this transmission. It is of great significance in determining the patterns of cold damage and in prescribing their proper therapy. Any type of cold damage may manifest with fever, but cold damage of the *yang ming* is characterized by an especially high fever. This accounts for the special mention of fever in the case of *yang ming* affliction. It is well known that the bones are governed by the kidney, but here the author ascribes the bones to the *shao yang* and gallbladder. In a note for the "*Re Lun* (Treatise on Heat)", Chap.

31, the *Su Wen*, Quan Yuan-qi explains that, because the *shao yang* is matched with the *jue yin*, *i.e.*, the liver, which governs the sinews and the sinews gather at the bones and are nourished by the qi of the *shao yang*, it is understandable that the bones are said to be ascribed to the foot *shao yang*. In addition, Ni Wa Yuan-jian, a well known Japanese TCM scholar living in the early nineteenth century who authored such texts as *Su Wen Shi (A Conceptual Understanding of the Basic Questions)* and *Jin Gui Yao Lue Ji Yi (Exposition on Perplexing Issues in the Golden Cabinet)*, explains that it is quite natural and only reasonable to declare that the *shao yang* governs the bones since these lie between the exterior and the interior, while the skin is ascribed to the *tai yang* and the muscles to the *yang ming*. According to him, the *shao yang's* governing the bones provides the necessary completion of the tripartite system of the gradual penetration of the three yang into the interior of the body.

[4]The abatement of cold damage must also make its course around the six channels and, therefore, appears on the seventh day after contraction. If the disease does not progress, then after twelve days, when two rounds of the six channels are completed, the great qi or the fulminating evil cold qi is no longer capable of doing harm and the disease is overcome.

[5]Here, freeing the channel does not mean drainage or attacking therapies as this term often suggests in TCM. It merely means ridding the affected channel of evil or cold damage by whatever method is appropriate, be it drainage or supplementation. Before cold damage has lasted three days, the evil is in the yang channels and the exterior. Therefore, it can be exteriorized by diaphoresis. This is called exterior resolution. Beyond that period, the evil will have penetrated to the interior and the yin channels. Thus, diaphoresis is no longer appropriate.

[6]Both during and while recovering from cold damage, one should not eat much in general, and, in particular meat, since it may produce heat. When the heat produced from food and the remaining heat of the febrile disease meet, these two combined can cause a relapse. The key point in the treatment of residual heat is the identification of vacuity and repletion, and then and only then should one perform supplementation and drainage accordingly. The Chinese terms *ni shun* here are synonymous with vacuity and repletion.

[7]In a dual affliction, the symptoms are a combination of yin pattern and yang pattern since both yin and yang channels are involved. On the first day, for

example, there is headache. This is ascribed to the *tai yang* because this channel flows up to the head. At the same time, there is a dry mouth and vexation. These are due to counterflow in the *shao yin*. This is fire causing dryness and other fire patterns. Why death comes on the sixth day is explained in the next section.

[8]Both the *tai yang* and the *yang ming* are said to be leaders, but it should be noted that the *tai yang* is only the commander of the yang channels while the *yang ming* is the leader of all the channels and network vessels because all of them rely on the qi of the stomach. As a result of this the stomach qi is generally a decisive factor in making a prognosis.

[9]The course of the liver channel provides an explanation for these symptoms. That it circles the genitals accounts for the yellowish urine. That it travels by the stomach accounts for the abdominal pain, somnolence, and high fever for which the stomach is directly responsible. That the liver channel homes to the liver and connects with the gallbladder accounts for the flank pain. That it emerges from the feet and links with the hand *jue yin* accounts for the fidgeting of the hands and feet. And because the liver is wind, its affliction by heat naturally gives rise to ravings and susceptibility to fright.

[10]Because *geng*(S7) and *xin*(S8) are days when metal, the restraining phase of wood, is effulgent, disease involving the liver becomes worse or, in the extreme, results in death. Because *jia*(S1) and *yi*(S2) are days when wood is effulgent, diseases involving the liver tends to get better or cure then. Qi counterflow, which here means disorder or chaos of the righteous qi, is always the climax of cold damage, very critical.

[11]Because the heart governs joy, when it is afflicted, a certain gloominess appears. Because the *shao yin* heart channel starts in the heart, passing the throat and linking the eyes, and its associated channel, the hand *tai yang*, connects the inner and outer canthi, symptoms include vexation and oppression, frequent vomiting, headache, etc.

[12]Because the *ren*(S9) and *gui*(S10) are days when water, the restraining phase of fire, is effulgent diseases involving the heart become worse or, in the extreme, result in death on those days. *Bing*(S3) and *ding*(S4), on the other hand, are days when fire is effulgent, and this accounts for the tendency of heart diseases to improve or be cured on those days.

[13]There is a note in the "*Wu Zhang Re Bing* (Heat Diseases of the Five Viscera)", of the *Tai Su* to the effect that the foot *yang ming* channel, which is a channel associated with the spleen, travels along the hairline to the forehead. This accounts for heavy headedness and ache in the forehead. The fact that the spleen channel pours into the heart accounts for vexation of the heart. The fact that the foot *yang ming* runs down the throat, penetrates the diaphragm, homes to the stomach, connects with the spleen, and governs the muscles accounts for vomiting, generalized fever, abdominal fullness, and diarrhea. Lumbago is typical of kidney disease, but, when heat overwhelms the spleen, the evils of the spleen, *i.e.*, earth evil conquer water or rather the kidney, thus also giving rise to lumbago. This explanation can also be found in a note in the "*Wu Zang Re Bing Ci Fa* (Needling Techniques for Heat Diseases of the Five Viscera)" from the *Lei Jing*.

[14]On *jia*(S1) and *yi*(S2) days, wood is effulgent and tends to overwhelm spleen earth. Therefore, diseases involving the spleen become worse or, in the extreme, result in death on those days. *Wu*(S5) and *ji*(S6) are days when earth is effulgent. Therefore, diseases involving the spleen tend to improve or be cured on those days.

[15]The character *bei* refers to the area of the body from the nape down to the hip. However, in common Chinese parlance it is used to denote the area of the back above the waist, while the character *yao* is used to denote the lumbar region.

[16]First, it should be noted that inversion used here simply means a feeling of cold. A note in the "*Wu Zang Re Bing Lun* (Treatise on Heat Diseases of the Five Organs)" in the *Tai Su* says that the lung governs the skin and hair, thus accounting for cold shivering with gooseflesh. When heat in the lung steams upward, the tongue produces a yellow coating. Because the lung governs the circulation of the qi of the whole body, generalized fever occurs when it is affected.

The note by Wang Bing in the "*Ci Re Lun* (Treatise on Needling Heat [Diseases])", of the *Su Wen* explains that the lung, located above the diaphragm, rules respiration and that the gathering or ancestral qi governs the breasts and the chest where qi is stored. Therefore, dyspnea and coughing with pain in the breast and upper back occur when the channel of the lung is affected. Because the pain in the chest is severe, the patient dare not breathe deeply.

[17]A note in the "*Wu Zang Re Bing Lun* (Treatise on Heat Diseases in the Five Organs)" of the *Tai Su*, explains "The *shao yin* kidney vessel ascends, submerging in the calves, emerging from the medial

aspects of the hollows of the knees, running through the spine, and homing to the kidney. It connects with the urinary bladder, moving upward and penetrating the liver and the diaphragm. From there, it enters the lung, passing the throat and moving bilaterally to the root of the tongue. This accounts in febrile disease for lumbago, aching of the lower legs, tormenting thirst, and frequent drinking. The foot *tai yang* vessel deviates from the root of the nape of the neck, branches in the back into four routes altogether, and descends to the hollows of the knees. It penetrates the calves, reaching the lateral aspect of the small toes. This accounts for generalized fever, stiffness and pain of the nape of the neck, and cold and aching of the shanks. The foot *shao yang* starts from the soles of the feet, and this accounts for heat in the soles. It emerges from the lung to connect with the heart, and this accounts for heat with disinclination to talk."

[18]According to the above passages, cold damage is classified into affliction of a single channel, dual affliction of a yin and yang channel, affliction of the viscera, and, finally, qi counterflow which means chaotic righteous qi. This is the last stage leading to death. Prognosis is related to the five phases which are associated with days numbered by the heavenly stems. For exapmle, the restraining days of the lungs which are metal, are the days associated with fire, i.e., the *bing*(S3) and *ding*(S4). On these days, lung diseases may become worse. The restraining days for other viscera can be inferred this way in accordance with the five phases. On the contrary, i.e., days of the phase allotted to the particular viscus, the patient will recover easily. For example, the lung qi is at high tide on *geng*(S7) and *xin*(S8) days producing massive perspiration and resulting in a cure.

[19]*Zhi wei bing* literally means "treat not yet disease", i.e., treat a disease before it arises.

[20]The meaning of the term cycle is ambiguous. A note by Wang Bing, in the "*Ci Re Lun*" of the *Su Wen* says that three cycles means regulating the three yin and three yang vessels three times. Zhang Jing–yue explains in the *Lei Jing* that the sentence means that recuperation happens after three restrained days of the affected viscus have passed. In other words, recovery comes after the disease completes three circuits round the six channels. Gao Shi–shi (1637-?), in his *Su Wen Zhi Jie*, regards three cycles as referring simply to three days.

[21]For regions of the face associated with the various viscera and bowels, see "The Five (Facial) Colors", Chap. 15, Book 1, of this work. Roughly speaking, a disease involving a certain viscus displays a color at its associated region on the face is a favorable sign. Therefore, it is easy to treat and usually heals in due time, i.e., on the days associated with the phase of the affected viscus, *bing*(S3) and *ding*(S4) for the heart for instance. If there is nonconformity between the location of the pathological complexion and the affected viscus, this portends a difficult recuperation or even a fatal end.

Needling therapies should be preformed in accordance with vacuity and repletion. Evacuating a vacuity condition and replenishing a repletion condition delays recuperation. If such inappropriate treatment is done twice, the result may be fatal.

[22]See the next chapter in this book for an explanation of these points.

[23]The last two sentences are absent from the *Su Wen* and the *Tai Su*.

Drinking cold water before needling forces heat evils from the interior toward the exterior thus facilitating the effect of needling. Wearing thin clothes and living in cold a environment helps eliminate heat evils. When the body turns cold, this is the sign that heat evils have left the body.

[24]Because the *shao yang* travels laterally, thoracic and flank pain and fullness indicate a disease of the *shao yang*. This requires draining of the foot *shao yang*, usually through needling point Hill Ruins (*Qiu Xu*, GB 40) since febrile disease is usually due to an exuberance of yang. The foot *shao yang* is wood which restrains earth. Therefore, to treat the problem and to prevent transmission to the spleen earth, it is necessary to supplement the foot *tai yin*, usually at its well and brook points. However, this prescription of the foot *tai yin* is still open to discussion. Yang Shang–shan of the Tang dynasty argues in a note in an edition of the *Su Wen* that, although the earliest edition of that text gives the foot *tai yin*, this is, in fact, a literary convention. Huang–fu Mi was in the habit of capping a couplet of channels with the word foot and not specifying hand or foot in the second channel in the couplet if the two are both foot channels. Since the word foot is repeated in this passage, one must be mistaken. He felt "foot *tai yin*" was a mistake that should read hand *tai yin*, and many later scholars have agreed with him.

[25]Because the kidneys govern the bones and open into the ears, there are symptoms of generalized heaviness and deafness. Moreover, because the true yin, which is contained in the kidney, is damaged, the spirit and orientation become clouded, and this manifests as drowsiness. The points that should be chosen are also the well and brook points.

[26]This is evidently a complicated disease of the *shao yin* and *shao yang*. In this case, the *shao yin* is responsible for dizziness and fever, and the *shao yang* is responsible for thoracic and flank fullness.

[27]In our source edition of the *Jia Yi Jing*, the grammatical structure of the second sentence is broken and should read as follows: "Not yet perished brilliance tells that it will heal..."

The brilliant complexion referred to above is a red color and perished describes a dull, ghostly color. If a green–blue complexion, representing the liver or the *jue yin*, appears in the zygomatic region instead of a red complexion, this indicates that the *jue yin* vessel is vying for control of the situation. In this case, wood is insulting water which, in terms of channels, is the *tai yang* and *shao yin*. Since the kidney, *i.e.*, the *shao yin*, where the true yin is stored, is damaged, the condition is critical. A note in the *Wu Zang Re Bing* in the *Su Wen* explains, "The foot *tai yang* is water, while the foot *jue yin* is wood. Water engenders wood. If wood becomes exuberant while water is diminished, the color associated with water is replaced by that of wood. This is indicative of the demise of water. When heat links with the kidney in the interior, the kidney becomes damaged. This accounts for death in three days."

[28]According to the *Su Wen*, this section originally ended with the sentence "Death comes in three days."

Shao yin water is the mother of *shao yang* wood. When the mother restrains the child, the condition is decidedly fatal.

[29]This refers to the thoracic vertebra both here and hereafter.

[30]In our source edition, "ruling (point for) heat in the diaphragm" reads "...in the stomach". This has been corrected according to the *Su Wen* and *Tai Su*. The sentence "In the case...in the nape of the neck" is incomprehensible. A misprint is likely.

The points located in the spinal articulations are very important for treating febrile disease because the governing vessel is the sea of the yang vessels. Many proven therapies, not merely acupuncture, include these points. These include massage and scraping therapy (*gua sha*).

"Major conglomeration" is a reference to what is called major conglomeration diarrhea. This is characterized by abdominal urgency and rectal heaviness, difficult evacuation, and pain in the penis.

[31]This is an ancient acupuncture classic, now long lost. The *Ling Shu* contains a chapter (Chap. 75) with the same title.

[32]Disrobing is a poetic term describing an effect which is achieved as quickly as it takes to remove one's clothes.

[33]The "*Ci Jie Zhen Xie* (Needling Strategies and the True Evil)" states, "taking in whatever food and drink, good or bad" in place of "desire for drinks", Chap. 75, Vol. 11, of the *Ling Shu*. The "*Wu Jie Ci* (Five Needling Strategies)" of the *Tai Su* states "desire for whatever drinks good or bad" rather than "desire for drinks."

[34]This point is commonly known as *Zhong Lu Shu*.

[35]Literally, the passage reads, "supplementation of the hand–foot *tai yin* means that one checks sweating." All the reference materials available to the translators brought out in recent years, however, give an explanation similar to that in the text above.

It seems contradictory that the *tai yin*, for example, is prescribed for treatment, since the Yellow Emperor just asked about the reason for selecting the curious points, *i.e.*, the *ashi* points, of the yang channels. One plausible explanation is that the *tai yin* requires needling as well as the curious points of the yang vessels. Another point worth noting is the needling of Celestial Storehouse and Great Shuttle thrice. One plausible explanation is that one needles three *ashi* points around each of them. Another possibility is that thrice simply indicates that Celestial Storehouse is to be needled once bilaterally.

[36]This cite is from the Fifty-Eighth Difficult Issue. Yang vacuity with yin exuberance may mean that the defensive yang is in a state of vacuity, while the interior yin is in a state of exuberance of evil qi. This is a plausible understanding in many situations, and the later unknown editor would, in that case, be right commenting that the assertions in this passage are groundless.

On the other hand, vacuity in this context may mean subjection to evils or disease, and exuberance may sometimes be understood as freedom from evils or disease. It follows then that the phrase, "yang vacuity with yin exuberance," may be interpreted as a condition where the exterior is diseased, while the interior remains healthy. Such a condition, of course, requires diaphoresis. In this case, precipitation, should it be adopted, will impair the interior qi without doing anything to the disease in the yang or exterior. A similar explanation is applicable to yang exuberance with yin vacuity.

[37] According to the *Su Wen* edited by Quan Yuan–qi, "like a fire" should be omitted. In the *Tai Su*, it is "as burnt by moxaing."

[38] Wind is yang, while the limbs are also yang. These are the two yang to which the author refers. If the patient has been in the past subject to yin vacuity and yang exuberance (one should note that the definition of yin and yang is different from that in the previous section), the conspiracy of these two yang is sure to make the yin qi more meager. Overriding predominance of yang over yin makes engenderment or growth impossible. This accounts for fire–like heat in the limbs on exposure to wind.

The above is the classic interpretation of this text, and the English translation is based on this interpretation. The translators are of another opinion, however, which is stated below. Heat in the limbs is due to vacuity of yin qi and an exuberance of yang qi in the patient. This is a yang pattern. Because the patient already expresses an exuberance of yang qi, when wind intrudes, it also being yang in nature, these two yang are too much for the already scant yin qi to match. Therefore, they stir an effulgent fire, and this fire finds it easy to travel to the yang regions of the body, i.e., the limbs.

[39] The condition in discussion is different from the common febrile disease that is due to cold damage. It is caused by some internal factors rather than external affection. Yin qi here refers to the visceral qi and the constructive, while yang qi refers to the defensive.

[40] Zhang Jing–yue gives a detailed explanation of this passage in a note on the differences between the *tai yin* and *yang ming* in his *Lei Jing*. The following is an adopted translation of that note.

"The spleen is a viscus which is yin, while the stomach is a bowel which is yang. Yang governs the exterior, while yin governs the interior. Whereas yang governs above, while yin governs below. This is what is meant by a difference in location. When yin is in vacuity, yang is replete. This is what is meant by the difference in phase of vacuity and repletion.

"That which is diseased is in counterflow, and that which keeps fit is in conformity. This is what is meant by different counterflow and conformity. Yin qi travels first upward from the feet to the head and then turns downward to the tips of the fingers along the arms, whereas yang qi travels first upward from the hands to the head and then turns downward to the feet. This is a normal or conforming flow. Yang disease tends to turn downward after it reaches the upper extreme, whereas yin disease tends to turn upward after it reaches the lower extreme. This is counterflow.

"When a thieving wind and a vacuity evil attack, yang suffers, and they invade the bowels. While (in presence of) dietary irregularities and irregular lifestyle, from which yin suffers, (these evils) invade the viscera. This is what is meant by different tracks of invasion."

[41] Yang, in assimilating the heavenly qi, is responsible for protecting the exterior of the body, while yin, assimilating the earthly qi, is responsible for nourishing the interior. The yang track can be interpreted, in this context, simply as the yang. It is subject to external evil which often manifests itself as repletion evil. On the contrary, yin is subject to internal injury which is often caused by vacuity evils. Thieving wind, in this context, is synonymous with vacuity evil. It is an unseasonal wind which affects yang and intrudes upon the bowels. Overeating, going hungry, eating meals at irregular hours, and failing to keep regular hours in daily life more often than not damage the interior, i.e., the yin.

[42] Although the standard rendering for this word is "pharynx" the context in which it is used here explicitly defines it as the upper end of the esophagus.

[43] The larynx is an organ which controls the breath, i.e., the heavenly qi, while the upper end of the esophagus is a digestive organ which controls the earthly or grain qi. They pertain to yang and yin respectively and are the reason why yang, (i.e., the upper part of the body) is subject to wind qi, a species of yang, and yin, (i.e., the lower part of the body), is subject to damp qi, a species of yin.

[44] Part 1 is derived from Chap. 40, *Su Wen*; Part 2 from Chap. 33, *Su Wen*; Part 3 from Chap. 55, *Su Wen*; Part 4 from Chap. 28, *Su Wen*; Part 5 from Chap. 21, Vol. 5, *Ling Shu*; Part 6, a combination of parts of Chap. 23, Vol. 5, *Ling Shu* and Chap. 61, *Su Wen*; and Part 7 from the *Zhen Jiu Ming Tang Zhi Yao*.

[45] The first sentence can be interpreted in another manner, and this changes the rendering: "Febrile disease is reflected by a yang pulse with three yang vessels exuberant." There is yet another understanding, according to which the sentence should read, "Febrile disease..., with three types of exuberant yang pulse." In this context, a yang pulse means an exuberant or energetically pulsating pulse. Besides, both the *Su Wen* and the *Tai Su* sub-

stitute the word beating for the word exuberant, and this provides a sound reason for the latter interpretation.

The *ren ying* is the yang pulse because it is located in the neck, above the *cun kou* and along the route of the *yang ming*. It is, therefore, an indicator for yang disease. It should be noted that there seems to be a missing link in the above translation since it is implied in the original text that febrile disease is always accompanied by ache or, rather, headache, and that when it has been transmitted into the yin interior, it gives rise to abdominal distention in addition.

[46]When wind invades, the interstices are forced open and there is perspiration. When the *tai yang* is affected, it may bring the *shao yin* upward with it. Inversion here means just this kind of counterflow of the qi along the *shao yin*. Because the yin must be in a state of insufficiency when the yang evil is exuberant, the treatment should be to supplement the *shao yin* channel, *i.e.*, the interior, while draining the *tai yang* channel, *i.e.*, the exterior.

[47]This is a case of a simultaneous surplus of yang evil and an exhaustion of yin. Sweat is transformed from essence, a product of the grain qi. Sweating is loss of yin essence, and a failure of perspiration to resolve heat means that yang evils are overwhelming yin essence. In ordinary cases, sweating should be followed by a tranquilized pulse, but now, on the contrary, the pulse becomes even more agitated and racing after perspiration. This implies that the visceral qi is vanquished. What is worse, an inability to take in food develops. All the viscera and bowels rely upon the grain qi and, once deprived of it, none of them can hope to survive. The three signs for death are generalized fever with inability to ingest food, an agitated and exuberant pulse, and raving.

[48]Zhang Jing–yue explains in his *Lei Jing* that the influence of evil may be minimal or intense. When it is intense enough to predominate, repletion is seen. The righteous qi may be weak or strong. When it is debilitated, the condition is one of vacuity.

As for a great heat disease, Yao Zhi–an of the Qing dynasty, explains in his *Su Wen Jing Zhu Jie Jie (Annotations & Explanations of the Classic of the Basic Questions)* that this refers to repletion heat of the three yang patterns of cold damage, phlegm fire, and accumulated food in miscellaneous diseases. In these cases, there are repletion evils with true fire in the interior, and therefore great heat qi is observed externally with exuberant pulses. Because there is repletion both in the interior and exterior, it is called dual repletion. It should be

noted that in cross-referencing other sources, such as the *Su Wen*, it is clear that the word internal in the term internal great heat is a redundancy.

[49]In the *Su Wen Shi (Conceptual Knowledge About the Basic Questions)*, the Japanese TCM scholar Ni Wa Yuan–jian explains that the *mai kou* is for the examination of the channels, while the cubit skin is for the examination of the network vessels. The channels are interior or yin as are the route of the vessels, whereas the network vessels are yang, floating, and shallow.

A slippery pulse indicates exuberant yang. This is not fatal. If the pulse is choppy, yin evils are overwhelming and this is an unfavorable sign.

When speaking of vacuity or repletion, the main concern is with the vacuity or repletion of the materials. These are understood to be the viscera, bones, and flesh. Treatment should be designed in accordance with the vacuity or repletion of the materials. Although slippery, uninhibited viscera, etc. are invisible, they can be determined through examination of the *cun kou* pulse and cubit skin.

There are different interpretations for the last two sentences. One says that vacuity and repletion always begin in the materials. Therefore, when they are slippery, *i.e.*, uninhibited, a long life is maintained. This interpretation is apparently reinforced by the substitution of the word treat for the word initiated. Another interpretation asserts that humans are like all other living things in terms of vacuity and repletion. When things grow smoothly, they are in good form. When they are inhibited, they cease to grow. Similarly, when the five viscera, etc. are slippery or uninhibited, people enjoy a long life.

[50]In the case of abrupt ascension of cold qi which makes the pulse full and replete, a slippery quality signifies a triumph of yang qi, *i.e.*, the correct qi, which has not yet been conquered by cold qi. This is, therefore, a favorable sign. On the contrary, a choppy, astringent quality indicates a triumph of yin qi, *i.e.*, the cold qi. This is an ill sign. In the case of generalized fullness of the body, for example, with fullness in the chest and abdomen with rapid dyspneic breathing, the pulse should be large, hard, and urgent, and the cubit skin should be smooth and urgent. If the skin is otherwise, the condition is critical. Life and death are dependent upon the warmth of the extremities. It should be noted that cold extremities are said to be unfavorable. The word translated here as unfavorable (*ni*) also means counterflow. This meaning is implied in this context as well because counterflow is often responsible for cold hands and feet.

The second sentence may also be interpreted to mean that a replete, slippery, and smooth pulse indicates survival, while a pulse which is replete and counterflowing indicates death.

In the third sentence, our insertion of the words physical body is based on the corresponding passage in the *Su Wen* where those words appear.

[51]Erratic speech means broken speech with unpredictably long pauses. It is an obvious sign of extremely diminished ancestral qi which is ascribed to the lungs. Cubit muscles and skin reflect the muscles and flesh of the whole body. These are governed by the spleen, and the integrity of the gait is their indicator. The *cun kou* is the pulse of the *tai yin*, reflecting yin, *i.e.*, the internal viscera. A pulse not manifesting in accordance with its yin character means that the *cun kou* presents a quality of viscus vacuity. If, however, the pulse is slippery, even though it is vacuous, the qi is not yet exhausted, and there is, as yet, no threat to life.

[52]Vacuity of a visceral qi with qi counterflow, *i.e.*, cold hands and feet, is always critical, but the patient may survive when this occurs out of the season of the restrained phase of the affected viscus. The lung, for example, is metal, and summer fire which restrains metal is, therefore, the most unfavorable season for lung disease. If a lung disease happens in some season other than summer, there is hope of recovery. This prognosis can be inferred for the other viscera via five phase theory.

[53]A replete, full pulse with cold hands and feet, and heat in the head indicate separation of yin from yang. Zhang Jing–yue explains in the *Lei Jing*, "A replete and full pulse indicates superabundance of evils; cold hands and feet mean that yin counterflows below; and heat in the head indicates that yang evils exist above. With yin and yang separated and at odds, this is a disease of repletion above with vacuity below. Spring and autumn are seasons when yin and yang are in harmony and at peace, and (people) may take in the harmonious qi and, therefore, may survive. Winter and summer are seasons with yin and yang overwhelming each other. In summer, yang is intense, and in winter, yin is intense. This accounts for death (in these seasons). A replete, full pulse shows superabundance of evils; cold hands and feet are due to yin qi concentrating below; heat in the head is due to yang evil settling above. In a word this is a disease of repletion above and vacuity below. In spring and autumn, weather is mild when yin and yang in nature is in harmony. Thus such a case is not fatal. In summer or winter, however, the situation is quite different. In these seasons, yin or yang, *i.e.*, intense cold or hot weather, is prevailing one over the other. This overwhelming yin or yang in nature exacerbates the separation of yin from yang in the body and is, therefore, devastating."

[54]A floating pulse with generalized heat indicates a surplus of evils or overwhelming yang, while a choppy pulse is a sign of destitution of blood or meager yin. If both occur simultaneously, death is a certainty regardless of the season.

[55]A hot *mai kou* pulse means that it has a slippery quality. The cubit skin reflects the yang or the connecting vessel qi, while the *mai kou* is yin and reflects the channels. This is a case of an exuberance of yin and an insufficiency of yang. Yang vacuity cannot endure a season during which there is an exuberance of yin but benefits from a season of yang exuberance. In this case, that which is related to the disease includes not only vacuity and repletion, though, these are decisive in pathology and treatment, but also the seasonal dispositions which must be taken into account in treating the disease.

[56]Channel vacuity and fullness in the connecting vessel with hot, full cubit skin and a cold, choppy pulse (cold here just means choppy) are indicative of a disease of insufficient yin with superabundant yang.

In this context, when speaking of needling, drainage is implied, but when speaking of moxibustion, supplementation is implied. This is because, comparatively speaking, needling is particularly effective at drainage, while moxibustion is particularly effective at supplementation. The meanings of yin and yang may be interpreted in two possible ways. One holds that yin refers to a yin channel while yang refers to a yang channel. The other understanding asserts that yin refers to the channels, while yang refers to the network vessels. Because moxibustion is seldom applied to the network vessels, the former interpretation is more plausible.

[57]The author repeatedly instructs that different points should be chosen in accordance with the seasons. There is a detailed explanation of this in Chap. 1, Part 1, Book 5 of the present work.

In winter, qi is hidden deep, and extreme therapies should not be used which might stir the qi up. If so, the true yin may be exhausted.

[58]*I.e.*, Shang Yang (*Shang Yang*, LI 1) of the hand *yang ming* and Collection Hole (*Kong Zui*, Lu 6) of the hand *tai yin*

[59]*I.e.*, Celestial Pillar (*Tian Zhu*, Bl 10)

[60]*I.e.*, the transporting points of the channel

[61]*I.e.*, the hand *tai yin* channel's Fish Border (*Yu Ji*, Lu 10) and Great Abyss (*Tai Yuan*, Lu 9)

[62]Currently extant versions of the *Ling Shu* are identical to those of the *Jia Yi Jing* on this point.

[63]*I.e.*, Inner Court (*Nei Ting*, St 44) and Sunken Valley (*Xian Gu*, St 43)

[64]For diaphoresis, certain points of the hand *tai yin* lung channel and the hand and foot *yang ming* large intestine and stomach channels are particularly effective. Certain points of the hand *tai yin* and foot *yang ming* can be treated for the purpose either of inducing diaphoresis or checking perspiration. Diaphoresis is usually achieved by means of a draining manipulation, while supplementing manipulations are usually administered to check perspiration.

[65]The *qi kou* pulse is the yin pulse, while the *ren ying* is a yang pulse. A tranquil *qi kou* pulse suggests that the febrile disease remains lodged within the three yang channels and has not entered the yin phase. For a list of the fifty–nine points, see page 440–441 in the present chapter.

[66]Intense fever indicates a surplus of yang, but tranquil pulses at both the *cun kou* and the *ren ying* are an expression of a yin quality. Such an incongruity between the pattern and the pulse quality always prognoses a disastrous end. Further discussion of the various mortal signs and symptoms is given in the next paragraphs in the present chapter.

[67]*I.e.*, Lesser Shang (*Shao Shang*, Lu 11)

[68]While a stirring pulse is consistent with fever, it is a serious sign if accompanied by dyspnea and dizziness. This requires prompt treatment.

In the *Ling Shu*, the symptoms dyspnea and dizziness are replaced by the symptom of dyspnea with shortage (of qi).

[69]Hematuria and a dry mouth are signs that the yin has already been seriously damaged by heat. Moreover, a small and faint pulse in a febrile disease indicates that the yang qi has become substantially weakened.

[70]This is a case of overwhelming yang with an absence of yin.

[71]The pulse demonstrates that the evil is not advancing in a threatening manner, nor has it diminished. When perspiration occurs, the evil qi will be drained out and recovery achieved. If sweat refuses to come, this indicates an exhaustion of yin essence and death is a certainty.

[72]*I.e.*, the arrowhead needle

[73]Heat in the skin, etc. is due to evils lodging in the surface and is associated with the lung. Thus the lung should be treated by needling the skin. This means shallow insertion of the needle, not allowing it to go deeper than the skin, and at the points specifically effective for the skin which have been chosen from the fifty–nine points. If this fails, it is because there is a surplus of metal. In that case, fire, the restraining phase of metal, must be supplemented to restrain metal. That is to say, the heart channel should be needled with a supplementing manipulation. When heart fire is replenished, lung metal will be restored to normal.

[74]This syndrome is a disorder of the blood vessels. Therefore, points specific for the vessels are chosen. If the treatment fails, it is because fire has proven too exuberant. Since the vessels and heart pertain to fire, water, which is the restraining phase of fire, should be replenished. Therefore, the kidney channel should be needled with supplementing manipulation.

[75]*I.e.*, the round–sharp needle

[76]This is a syndrome where an evil has settled in the flesh. Thus it is a disease of the spleen channel. The needle should be inserted into the flesh at the points specific for the flesh. If this is ineffective, there is a surplus of evil in the spleen, and wood should be supplemented, since this is the restraining phase of earth.

[77]In the current versions of the *Ling Shu*, the symptom of pain in the brain is substituted for pain in the chest.

[78]*I.e.*, the sharp needle

[79]This syndrome is a type of sinew disease, *i.e.*, a liver disease, since the liver governs the sinews. Sinews usually start in the extremities, so one should needle the points between the sinews on the hands and feet. Unsteady steps and inability to walk due to sinew atony are known as sinew limpness, and, together with frequent lacrimation, this is still a sinew disease. Therefore, the same treatment should be performed. If this is ineffective, the evil there is a surplus of evil in liver wood, and lung metal should be supplemented.

[80]This is a blood disease due to blood heat toxin penetrating the heart. The *Lei Jing* explains,

"Susceptibility to fright in febrile disease is due to exuberance of heart evils. Tugging and slackening are due to heat intense enough to generate wind and cause damage to yin blood. And madness is due to extreme heat." Because madness is ascribed to extreme blood heat and hair is the surplus of blood, these two conditions occur together. One should prick the prominent blood network vessels to drain the heat toxin. Madness and loss of hair should be treated in the same way. If this fails, one should supplement kidney water.

The phrase "treat at the level of the vessels" may be a typographical error; it should be "treat at the level of the blood".

[81]This is apparently a bone disease, and the needle should penetrate deeply.

[82]Pain defying location is due to blood vacuity. Dry mouth, etc. are due to exhaustion of yin. Fever arising with yang, *i.e.*, during hot weather, and cold arising with yin, *i.e.*, during the night, are due to a complete imbalance of yin and yang. In other words, heat has penetrated the bones. In our original source edition, the first sentence begins with "Febrile disease without ability to locate the disease..." The present interpretation is made in accordance with the *Ling Shu* and the *Tai Su*.

[83]*I.e.*, the blunt needle

[84]This is a pattern due to an ascending counterflow of heat qi, otherwise known as inversion. Instead of tense vessels between the temples and eyes, the *Ling Shu* suggests the symptom of a sense of tugging in the eyes and pain in the vessel, while the *Tai Su* suggests tugging of the vessels around the eyes.

[85]*I.e.*, Supreme White (*Tai Bai*, Sp 3) and Sunken Valley (*Xian Gu*, St 43)

[86]*I.e.*, Severe Mouth (*Li Dui*, St 45), Inner Court (*Nei Ting*, St 44), etc.

[87]Heaviness is a manifestation of wasted or weakened muscles. These are governed by the spleen. Therefore, this is an illness affecting the spleen and stomach. Thus one should needle the rapids points of the stomach and spleen channels. The connecting vessel of the stomach mentioned in the text is point Bountiful Bulge (*Fei Long*, St 40). One should note that a point may be named after a vessel if it is the starting point of that vessel.

Zhang Jing–yue poses a plausible explanation for this passage in the *Lei Jing*, asserting, "The words cold and heat and piles read as if dangling and provoke suspicion of a typographical error."

[88]*I.e.*, Three Yin Intersection (*San Yin Jiao*, Sp 6)

[89]At first glance, the above two passages seem confusing but, in actuality there is no contradiction. They both describe a pattern of yang exuberance with yin exhaustion, and both are fatal illnesses. The first pattern, however, is characteristic of yang surplus leading to yin vacuity, while the second is typical of yin exhaustion contributing to a situation of solitary yang.

In the *Lei Jing*, Zhang Jing–yue gives an enlightening explanation of the above two passages. He asserts that an agitated and exuberant pulse is always an indication of overwhelming yang. Sweat is transformed from fluid. Diaphoresis relies on yang while its source lies in yin. A pulse which remains agitated and exuberant after sweating is because yang finds nowhere to home and is due to the advent of yin vacuity. A pulse which remains agitated and exuberant with lack of perspiration indicates that the yin is already exhausted in the interior. This is also ascribed to yin vacuity. Yin vacuity means absence of qi, and absence of qi means death. It follows that yin is the root of qi, and, without its root, qi collapses.

[90]*I.e.*, Great Ravine (*Tai Xi*, Ki 3)

[91]The translators find the source of the paragraph in Chapter 26 titled "Miscellaneous Diseases," Vol. 5 in the *Ling Shu* instead of the chapter of the *Su Wen* mentioned in the commentary remark.

[92]This is a syndrome of an upward counterflow of evil heat qi. Pricking the blood vessel in the hollow of the knee aims at draining this evil heat. If the great heat is so effulgent as to dry up fluid in the mouth, water should be replenished by needling the kidney channel with supplementing manipulation.

In the *Su Wen* and the *Tai Su*, there is no "which rules", and, without that phrase, the sentence is more coherent. In our source edition, the foot *shao yang* is prescribed instead of the foot *shao yin*. This is apparently a mistake, since the pattern involves the foot *tai yang* which is associated with the foot *shao yin*. There is nothing to do with the foot *shao yang*.

[93]In modern editions of the *Tai Su*, which are identical in respect to this paragraph, the statement is "lack of perspiration, reddening in the zygomatic region, and retching prognoses death."

[94]In the *Ling Shu* and the *Tai Su*, the first sentence reads "There are nine (types of) febrile disease that do

not allow of needling." In our source edition, the seventh pattern reads, "coughing with nose bleeding and sweating which does not reach the feet..." The rendering here is corrected in accordance with the *Ling Shu* and the *Tai Su*.

[95] These are Lesser Shang (*Shao Shang*, Lu 11), Central Hub (*Zhong Chong*, Per 9), and Lesser Thoroughfare (*Shao Chong*, Ht 9) on the radial aspect of the fingers and Lesser Marsh (*Shao Ze*, SI 1), Passage Hub (*Guan Chong*, TH 1), and Shang Yang (*Shang Yang*, LI 1) on the ulnar aspect. Counting these points bilaterally, there are twelve in all.

[96] These are Back Ravine (*Hou Xi*, SI 3), Central Islet (*Zhong Zhu*, TH 3), Third Space (*San Jian*, LI 3), and Lesser Mansion (*Shao Fu*, Ht 8). Counting these points bilaterally, there are eight in all.

[97] These are Bundle Bone (*Shu Gu*, Bl 65), Foot On the Verge of Tears (*Zu Lin Qi*, GB 41), Sunken Valley (*Xian Gu*, St 43), and Supreme White (*Tai Bai*, Sp 3). Counting bilaterally, there are eight in all.

[98] These are Fifth Place (*Wu Chu*, Bl 5), Light Guard (*Cheng Guang*, Bl 6), and Celestial Connection (*Tong Tian*, Bl 7), six in all bilaterally.

[99] These are Head On the Verge of Tears (*Tou Lin Qi*, GB 15), Eye Window (*Mu Chuang*, GB 16), Upright Nutrition (*Zheng Ying*, GB 17), Spirit Support (*Cheng Ling*, GB 18) and Brain Hollow (*Nao Kong*, GB 19), ten in all bilaterally.

[100] These are Auditory Convergence (*Ting Hui*, GB 2), Completion Bone (*Wan Gu*, GB 12), four in all bilaterally, Nectar Recepticle (*Cheng Jiang*, CV 24), and Mute's Gate (*Ya Men*, GV 15).

[101] These are Hundred Convergence (*Bai Hui*, GV 20), Fontanelle Meeting (*Xin Hui*, GV 22), Spirit Court (*Shen Ting*, GV 24), Wind Mansion (*Feng Fu*, GV 16), Ridge Spring (*Lian Quan*, CV 23), Wind Pool (*Feng Chi*, GB 20), and Celestial Pillar (*Tian Zhu*, Bl 10).

[102] The five lines refer to the five channels on the head, namely, the governing vessel, bilateral foot *tai yang* channel, and bilateral foot *shao yang* channel. The twenty–five points are Upper Star (*Shang Xing*, GV 23), Fontanelle Meeting (*Xin Hui*, GV 22), Before the Vertex (*Qian Ding*, GV 21), Hundred Convergence (*Bai Hui*, GV 20), Behind the Vertex (*Hou Ding*, GV 19), Fifth Place (*Wu Chu*, Bl 5), Light Guard (*Cheng Guang*, Bl 6), Celestial Connection (*Tong Tian*, Bl 7), Declining Connection (*Luo Que*, Bl 8), Jade Pillow (*Yu Zhen*, Bl 9), Head on the Verge of Tears (*Tou Lin Qi*, GB 15), Eye Window

(*Mu Chuang*, GB 16), Upright Nutrition (*Zheng Ying*, GB 17), Spirit Support (*Cheng Ling*, GB 18), and Brain Hollow (*Nao Kong*, GB 19).

[103] These eight points are Great Shuttle (*Da Zhu*, Bl 11), Central Treasury (*Zhong Fu*, Lu 1), Empty Basin (*Que Pen*, St 12), and Wind Gate (*Feng Men*, Bl 12) bilaterally. Note that the bosom point and the back point are Central Treasury and Wind Gate respectively.

[104] These eight points are Cloud Gate (*Yun Men*, Lu 2), Shoulder Bone (*Jian Yu*, LI 15), Bend Middle (*Wei Zhong*, Bl 40) and Horizontal Bone (*Heng Gu*, Ki 11) bilaterally. Note that the last point, the Marrow Hollow is believed to be Lumbar Shu (*Yao Shu*, GV 20) by many scholars. If they are right, there would be a problem with the text however, since Lumbar Shu is solitary. Thus the number of the points to drain the heat of the limbs would only be seven.

[105] These are bilaterally Po Door (*Po Hu*, Bl 42) beside Lung Shu (*Fei Shu*, Bl 13), Spirit Hall (*Shen Tang*, Bl 44) beside Heart Shu (*Xin Shu*, Bl 15), Hun Gate (*Hun Men*, Bl 47) beside Gallbladder Shu (*Gan Shu*, Bl 18), Reflection Abode (*Yi She*, Bl 49) beside Spleen Shu (*Pi Shu*, Bl 20), and Will Chamber (*Zhi Shi*, Bl 52) beside Kidney Shu (*Shen Shu*, Bl 23).

[106] The first list of the fifty-nine points is derived from Chap. 23, Vol. 5, the *Ling Shu* while the second from Chap. 61, the *Su Wen*.

[107] The last two passages contain two lists consisting of a total of one hundred points. The first list is derived from the *Ling Shu*, while the second from the *Su Wen*. The two sets have eighteen points in common, Hundred Convergence (*Bai Hui*, GV 20), Fontanelle Meeting (*Xin Hui*, GV 22), Fifth Place (*Wu Chu*, Bl 5), Light Guard (*Cheng Guang*, Bl 6), Celestial Connection (*Tong Tian*, Bl 7), On the Verge of Tears (*Lin Qi*, GB 15), Eye Window (*Mu Chuang*, GB 16), Upright Nutrition (*Zheng Ying*, GB 17), Spirit Support (*Cheng Ling*, GB 18), and Brain Hollow (*Nao Kong*, GB 19). According to Zhang Jie–bin, a.k.a. Zhang Jing–yue, the points in the first set are primarily located on the limbs and are used to drain root heat, while the points in the second set are used to drain heat in the local areas around the points themselves. This is seen as branch heat. In sum, the two sets are used for different purposes, and both are important. In addition, in the previous passages, the author has listed fourteen other points used specifically in the treatment of heat disease. They are Bountiful Bulge (*Feng Long*, St 40), *i.e.*, the connecting vessel of the stomach, Yin Mound Spring (*Yin Ling Quan*, Sp 9), Fish Border (*Yu Ji*, Lu 10), Great Abyss (*Tai*

Yuan, Lu 9), Great Metropolis (*Da Du*, Sp 2), and Three Yin Intersection (*San Yin Jiao*, Sp 6). All of these points belong to the hand and foot *yang ming* and *tai yin*.

[108]There is no "pain in the eyes" in our source edition. This insertion is made in accordance with the *Wai Tai Mi Yao (The Secret Medical Essentials of a Provincial Governor)* by Wang Tao.

[109]In this context, chilling inversion simply means shivering with cold.

[110]There is no such description in the current versions of the *Qian Jin*.

[111]The *Qian Jin* is practically identical to this work in relation to this section.

[112]Another name for *Ya Men*, GV 15

[113]Throat fistula implies a fistula in the neck. In the *Wai Tai Mi Yao*, it is throat *bi* with hunched back.

[114]"Inability to turn" is inserted in accordance with the *Wai Tai Mi Yao*.

[115]One source edition substitutes "perspiring" for "lack of perspiration." This correction is made in accordance with the *Qian Jin*.

[116]Repletion of qi here implies a surplus of wind cold. The *Wai Tai* states "cold damage with lack of perspiration" rather than "cold qi... despite the presence of fever."

[117]This syndrome results from an exposure to wind. In the *Wai Tai* it states, "For wind causing head dizziness, headache...." This reveals the causal relationship between the signs.

[118]Arm inversion is classified into four types according to cause. One is due to a diseased lung organ. One is due to a diseased lung channel. One is due to a diseased heart. And the last is due to a diseased heart channel. All share the symptoms of hypertonicity, cold, and debility of the fingers.

[119]In the current edition of the *Qian Jin*, Diaphragm Pass (*Ge Guan*, Bl 46) is given instead of Lumbar Yang Pass (*Yang Guan*, GV 3). One should note that many other reference materials such as the *Wai Tai* prescribe Diaphragm Pass as well. There is therefore, good reason to suspect a typographical error here in the *Jia Yi Jing*.

[120]The *Wai Tai* substitutes "wind causing headache" for "head wind headache", and "aversion to cold" for "cold and heat." Head wind headache, head wind for short, is a very severe headache, typically characterized by unexpected onset, which persists for a long period of time. It is due to wind fire, phlegm, and invasion of wind cold.

[121]Great qi is a fulminating evil qi. Qi clouding is blurred vision due to qi counterflow. Wind dizziness is a fitful kind of dizziness which attacks in an unpredictable way and is accompanied by counterflow retching. The symptom of nosebleed is somewhat problematic, since following it are disorders of the nose incompatible with it. The *Wai Tai* and the *Yi Xin Fang, (The Heart of Medicine Formulary)* may be right in replacing it with deep-source nasal congestion, a chronic disorder of the nose with constant running of foul turbid discharge.

[122]In our source edition, the sentence begins with "For head dizziness and disease of... " The correction here is made in accordance with an edition published in the Ming dynasty, and this agrees with its counterpart in the *Wai Tai* and the *Yi Xin Fang*.

[123]All these symptoms are due to lung qi vacuity. In our source edition, cough produces a dragging iscomfort in the coccyx rather than the testicles, and there is no "frothy eructation, and vomiting." These corrections are made in accordance with the *Wai Tai*.

[124]In our source edition, "manifested with" is followed simply by "the hands and feet at first"; eyes dropping is in place of upturned eyes; two *cun* in place of three *cun*; and lateral costal is in place of free rib. All these corrections are made in accordance with the *Wai Tai*.

[125]This entire chapter is derived from the *Zhen Jiu Ming Tang Zhi Yao*.

[126]One source substitutes tugging nosebleed for violent nosebleeding. Congestion implies nasal congestion.

[127]The *Qian Jin* is in error in prescribing *Tian Liao*.

[128]This is another name for Great Mound (*Da Ling*, Per 7).

[129]In our source edition, "incessant sweating" is substituted for "lack of perspiration." This correction is made in accordance with the *Qian Jin* and the *Wai Tai*. In the *Wai Tai*, "tormenting" replaces "melancholy."

[130]Loss of orientation is a state of partial loss of consciousness.

[131]The word agitated in the *Qian Jin* may be a typo-

graphical error for the character for spitting. In our source edition, sweating is said to be confined to the region above the shoulders rather than the eyebrows, and the characters are quite similar. This correction is made in accordance with the *Qian Jin* and the *Wai Tai*. In the above two references, the word "frigidity" replaces "green–blue cast to the forehead." It should be noted that native Chinese will often mistake *yan*, forehead, for face so that the symptom might be read as "facial frigidity."

[132]A seeping sore is a sore accompanied by fever. It is so named because it is capable of spreading. It itches and then breaks open, discharging a yellowish exudate.

Our source edition reads, "nose" in place of "shoulder bones", and "shoulder" in place of "upper back." These corrections are made in accordance with the *Wai Tai*.

[133]In our source edition, "Union Valley (*He Gu*, LI 4) is the ruling point" has been omitted and has been added here in accordance with the *Wai Tai*.

[134]Our source edition reads, "head" in place of "nape." This correction is made in accordance with the *Wai Tai*.

[135]In our source edition, "spinning and ache" is omitted and has been added here in accordance with the *Wai Tai*; and "inside" replaces "fullness." The syndrome ends with "inability to turn over the head", which, because it is redundant, has been deleted in accordance with the *Wai Tai*.

[136]Wind leakage is a pattern that occurs as a result of exposure to wind while sweating when the interstices are wide open. Aside from the above symptoms, it is characterized by dry mouth, generalized aching, and inability to exert oneself. It should be noted that the above passage actually includes two different patterns of wind leakage. In other words, wind leakage characterized by scarred scabies with itching is simply the initial stage of a broader pattern of wind leakage.

In our source edition, "reaching down to" is omitted; thus the passage may read "...perspiration, hypertonicity of the lower back and the nape with inability to exert oneself..." This correction is made in accordance with Chap. 2, Book 10 of the present work and the *Wai Tai*.

[137]Our source edition reads "heat" in place of "fever and chills"; "headache and pain in the nape" is in place of "spinning and ache of the head." These corrections are made in accordance with the *Wai Tai*.

[138]The *Wai Tai* replaces "heart pain with abdominal distention," with "inversion heart pain with abdominal distention and fullness." The *Ling Shu* gives "inversion heart pain with abdominal distention and chest fullness."

[139]This is a pattern involving the three channels of the liver, spleen, and stomach. Therefore, Three Li (*San Li*, St 36) should be needled first to remove heat evils from the *yang ming*. Then treat Supreme White (*Tai Bai*, Sp 3) and Camphorwood Gate (*Zhang Men*, Liv 13) to balance the qi of the *jue yin* and *tai yin*.

"Vexation and oppression" replaces "heart vexation" in our source edition and this correction was made in accordance with the *Su Wen*. "Chest fullness" replaces "abdominal fullness", and this correction was made in accordance with the *Su Wen* and the *Wai Tai*. "Frequent diarrhea" replaces "violent diarrhea", and this correction was made in accordance with the above two reference works. "Hunger" replaces "constant hungering", a correction also made in accordance with the above two works.

[140]In our source edition, the word "yang" follows "inversion", making the line read, "...inversion yang cold" and, according to the *Wai Tai*, this is an error.

[141]This is a pattern of the cold qi of the kidney counterflowing below. Therefore, one should first needle Burning Valley, (*Ran Gu*, Ki 2) to boost kidney yang, and then needle Great Ravine (*Tai Xi*, Ki 3) and Supreme Surge (*Tai Chong*, Liv 3) to boost the qi of the liver and kidney. It is of note that the moving vessel referred to here is not a blood vessel but Supreme Surge (*Tai Chong*, Liv 3). This is because *chong* in Chinese means penetrating, beating, charging, etc.

[142]*I.e.*, Shining Sea (*Zhao Hai*, Ki 6)

[143]*I.e.*, Horizontal Bone (*Heng Gu*, Ki 11)

[144]Because the yin motility vessel starts at Shining Sea (*Zhao Hai*, Ki 6), the point is named after the vessel.

[145]When cold reaches as far up as the elbows and knees, which are the joints referred to in this passage, the yang qi has been utterly vanquished and the desertion of yang inevitably results in death.

[146]This describes the effect of needling to abate heat in case febrile disease. It does not describe the progress of cold inversion.

[147]This section is omitted in our source edition. It has been added in accordance with the *Wai Tai* and the *Yi Xin Fang (Heart of Medicine Formulary)*.

[148]In our source edition, the words "frequent biting of cheeks, grinding of the teeth, and biting of lips" precede "febrile disease." This sentence has been deleted in accordance with the *Wai Tai*.

[149]There are several types of inversion headache. The above pattern is due to the upward counterflow of evils within the foot *yang ming*, and therefore, Bountiful Bulge (*Feng Long*, St 40), the connecting vessel of the *yang ming*, should be needled.

[150]Yang inversion is heat inversion. When heat has penetrated deeply and is oppressed in the interior, it can present a false picture of cold.

[151]In our source edition, "growing heat" replaces "gradual development of generalized heaviness"; "curled and dry tongue" replaces "curled tongue, dry mouth"; and the word "pain" in the phrase "pain in the inner aspect..." is omitted. This passage has been amended in accordance with the *Wai Tai*.

[152]The phrase "tearing on exposure to cold" may be interpreted in a different way. It may also mean counterflow of cold evil causing lacrimation.

[153]Inhibited nose means nasal congestion.

[154]It is commonly said that one must needle the *tai yang* in the case of sudden disease. Therefore, one should needle Bundle Bone (*Shu Gu*, Bl 65).

[155]In our source edition, "slackening" in the phrase "tugging and slackening" is omitted; and "...ache in the head" replaces "...ache in the vertex of the head." The text has been amended in accordance with the *Wai Tai*. Also, the *Wai Tai* gives "hunched back" for "generalized cold starting from the lower legs."

[156]In our source edition, "lumbar spine" replaces "pain in upper and lower back"; "hypertonicity of the heels of the feet" replaces "hypertonicity of the feet and pain in the heels"; and "spasms of the feet sending a dragging pain to the lower abdomen with sore throat" replaces "spasms of the feet, abdominal pain provoking sore throat." The text has been amended in accordance with the *Wai Tai*.

[157]Part 1 is a combination of parts of Chap. 30 and 49, *Su Wen*; Part 2 from Chap. 75, Vol. 11; and Part 3 from the *Zhen Jiu Ming Tang Zhi Yao*.

[158]The"*Yang Ming Mai Jie* (Explanation of the *Yang Ming* Vessels)", Chap. 31, *Su Wen*, instead of "prefers privacy ..." states, "remains composed when hearing bells and drums, but becomes frightened when hearing the sound of wood." Huang–fu Mi apparently altered this inquiry in order to achieve more consistency with the following explanation.

[159]I.e., Chap. 49, *Su Wen*

[160]Yin is by nature calm and tranquil, while yang is more dynamic in character. Therefore, when yin is victorious, the patient prefers solitude.

[161]In this case, dyspnea is caused by counterflow inversion which means upward counterflow of evil qi within the foot *yang ming*. If the counterflow evil qi enters the viscera, the interior becomes disordered. This is, therefore, fatal. If the counterflow evil affects only the channel, the disease does not lie deeply, and, therefore, the patient may survive.

[162]As a result of a contention between yin and yang, the limbs, which are understood as part of the exterior, may absorb yang, which is the heat evil of the foot *yang ming*. Thus these two yang merge. The yang evil in the exterior becomes superabundant so as to fill up the limbs. When the limbs are filled with repletion evil, they are capable of extraordinary things. Since the yang evil is exuberant, it produces chaos, giving rise to ravings, wild running, etc.

In the *Su Wen* and the *Tai Su*, "yang becomes exuberant" replaces "evil becomes exuberant"; "sing" is omitted.

[163]Before treatment can begin, it is necessary to determine whether the foot *yang ming* channel and its major connecting vessel, the apical vessel, are in a state of vacuity or repletion. If there is vacuity, one should needle with supplementing manipulation; if there is blood repletion, which may be reflected by prominent veins, for example, one should perform drainage. The author lists the appropriate points to be needled in the next paragraphs. It should be noted that when the author speaks of yang exuberance, he does not mean that it is an exuberance of the channel. In other words, channel vacuity may be accompanied by yang superabundance in the external. In addition, the dispersing technique by rubbing and rolling is effective against heat, and it can be applied along the spinal column and paravertebral regions.

In the *Ling Shu* and the *Tai Su*, "mania with" is in place of "manic speech, and"; and "pressing by either side of the pulsating vessels" in place of "pressing the pulsating vessels." These corrections are made in accordance with the *Tai Su*.

[164]Apprehension does not appear in the source edition but has been included here in accordance with the *Wai Tai*.

[165]Counterflow frigidity and inversion frigidity are different. The former is milder and usually confined to the hands and feet, while the latter is more severe and usually affects the forearms and lower legs. There are six types of both inversion frigidity and counterflow frigidity corresponding to the six channels, *i.e.*, the three yin and three yang channels. The patterns described in this passage are all *yang ming* type and, therefore, a *yang ming* point is chosen.

Our source edition reads, "inversion heat" in place of "counterflow frigidity." The text has been amended in accordance with the *Wai Tai*.

[166]Part 1 is derived from Chap. 45, *Su Wen*; Part 2 from Chap. 75, Vol. 11, *Ling Shu*; Part 3 a combination of parts of Chap. 9, Vol. 2, and Chap. 21, Vol. 5, *Ling Shu*; Part 4 from Chap. 26, Vol. 5, *Ling Shu*; Part 5 from Chap. 22, Vol. 5, *Ling Shu*; and Part 6 from the *Zhen Jiu Ming Tang Zhi Yao*.

[167]Zhang Jing–yue explains in a note in the *Lei Jing*, "Inversion is counterflow. When qi counterflows, there chaos results, thus giving rise to sudden spinning collapse, desertion, and expiry. Therefore, it is named inversion."

Wang Bing supplies a note to this paragraph in the *Su Wen*, saying, "Yang is known as the three foot yang vessels, while yin is known as the three foot yin vessels. Below implies the feet."

Ma Shi explains in his *Su Wen Zhu Zheng Fa Wei*, "When the channel qi of the three yang is debilitated below, yang qi becomes diminished and the yin qi exuberant. This is why the inversion is cold inversion. When the channel qi of the three yin is debilitated below, the yin qi becomes debilitated and yang qi exuberant. This is why the inversion is heat inversion."

[168]The pathways of all three foot yang channels traverse the dorsal surface of the feet including the toes, while the true yin, *i.e.*, the *shao yin* kidney channel, starts under the small toe and transversely travels across the soles. Heat inversion is caused when debilitated yin qi allows yang to become victorious, radiating a current of heat from the soles of the feet.

[169]Yin qi, the focus of this paragraph, should not be confused with the yin vessels which were the focus in the last paragraph. When yang qi becomes debilitated below, yin qi will become exuberant and then counterflow upward. This kind of inversion cold is generated within the body due to debilitation of yang qi.

[170]In this context, the *jue yin* refers to the genitals or the front yin which is surrounded by the foot *jue yin*, where all the sinew channels of the three foot yin, the foot *yang ming* and *shao yang*, the penetrating, conception, governing, and motility vessels gather. The author makes specific mention of the *yang ming* and *tai yin* because the stomach is the sea of water and grain, responsible for moistening the gathering sinews, and the Qi Thoroughfare (*Qi Chong*, St 30), a point on the stomach channel, is the meeting place of all the yin and yang sinews.

[171]In autumn and winter, the yang qi is diminished and sealed up, and people should take care to preserve it. If one defies the seasonal law, one may stir up the kidney qi, (*i.e.*, the lower qi) by engaging in sexual intercourse too frequently or by simply overworking. Hence the kidney qi will float upward to engage the qi of the upper burner in a struggle. The qi of the upper burner compels the essence qi to spill downward and becomes impaired. Now the yin qi is exuberant while the yang qi is overwhelmed. As a result, yin evil qi ascends and occupies the center, which is the spleen and stomach, and this further debilitates yang qi. Thus the yang qi is no longer able to nourish and operate the channels and network vessels. One should note that the term percolating and managing have specific meanings of their own. Percolating is understood as the infiltration of yang qi including the defensive qi from within the vessels. While managing is homonymous with the constructive, and includes the constructive and essence.

[172]Alcohol is an impetuous and hot yang qi derived from water and grain. When it enters the stomach, it does not flow within the channels but, following the defensive, runs into the skin to fill the network vessels. Therefore, after drinking, the network vessels become full and the channels empty. This kind of yang qi damages the spleen which works in the interest of the stomach. A damaged spleen means a vacuity of yin qi or spleen yin. In that case, the yang qi or hot qi takes advantage of this vacuity to enter the spleen and stomach. Consequently, the stomach comes into disharmony. The essence qi, all of which comes from the stomach, is now deprived of its source and is unable to nourish the limbs.

[173]Sexual intercourse consumes kidney essence or the true yin. The hot, impetuous alcoholic qi whittles the essence away as well as damages the spleen, while intoxication or overeating easily hurt the

spleen. These factors combine to produce a surplus of yang qi, causing heat in the hands and feet.

In the *Su Wen* and the *Tai Su*, "conflict with the grain qi" is followed by "heat becomes exuberant in the center."

[174]When it becomes exuberant above, yang qi must be inherently vacuous below. When yang is vacuous below, the transformation of qi is at a standstill, resulting in the abdomen becoming filled up by qi. The qi is then plunged into disorder below. This disorderly qi, naturally, ascends in a counterflow to join the yin qi above. One should note that evil qi here means abnormal qi or deranged qi as opposed to external wind or the like. This counterflow qi is bound to disorder the yang above, resulting in unconsciousness.

[175]In the *Su Wen* and the *Tai Su*, "retracted and swollen testicles" replaces "retracted testicles."

[176]The differences between these various types of inversion are primarily a function of the route and characteristics of the pertinent channels. Take the *shao yang* channel for example. It travels primarily in the lateral aspect of the body, and, therefore, inversion of the *shao yang* is characterized by sudden deafness, swollen cheeks, flank pain, etc. Since the *yang ming* is characterized by an exuberance at both qi and blood, when it becomes diseased this usually results in a high fever. Because of this, inversion of the *yang ming* is characterized by mental disorders, reddened face, etc., all resulting from great heat. This is in addition to symptoms of abdominal fullness and others that are easily explainable given the pathways of the stomach and intestine channel. Again, the presentations of *jue yin* inversion are easy to explain in terms of the pathways of the *jue yin* channel.

Subsequent passages discuss the treatment of inversion in detail, and the author advances a general principle. In the case of a neutral condition (*i.e.*, one of neither repletion or vacuity), treatment may be focused on the affected channel without handling other channels as prescribed below.

[177]Just as prosperous growth is a result of ample supplies of water hidden beneath the ground, qi, though intangible and hidden inside the body, can be evaluated by examination of the form. This is decisive in prescribing a proper treatment for resolution of inversion.

[178]In the *Tai Su*, the word rain is omitted, but is retained in other reference materials, such as the *Ling Shu*. In accordance with the *Tai Su*, the pertinent sentence should read, "...moisture is located above, and therefore..."

In our source edition, "...are reduced" is in place of "...are exuberant." This correction made in accordance with the *Ling Shu* and *Tai Su*.

[179]Our source edition reads, "skilled in cutting through" in place of "skilled in drilling." This correction made in accordance with the *Ling Shu* and *Tai Su*.

[180]The palms, armpits, etc. are the meeting places of the ravines and valleys and the joints between the large bones. Warming them via ironing introduces fire into the vessels, thereby freeing the flow of qi and blood within them. If the pulse is slippery, this means that the defensive qi is floating, making it necessary to calm it down. If, however, the pulse is hard and tense, a repletion of qi is indicated, warranting needling techniques to drastically drain the qi.

In the *Ling Shu* and *Tai Su*, after "Only then" is followed by "can they succeed in freeing flow of water and drilling the ground"; and "fire qi" replaces "broad highways."

[181]The stomach is the source of earthly qi. The clear component of the qi is the constructive qi which runs inside the vessels, while the turbid component of the qi is the defensive qi which flows outside the vessels. The ancestral qi, also called the great qi, is collected in two seas, the lower one, *i.e.*, the cinnabar field two *cun* below the umbilicus, and the upper one, *i.e.*, the chest. Thus there are three kinds of qi in the body: the constructive, the defensive, and the ancestral. From the lower sea of qi, qi travels via the qi thoroughfare of the stomach channel down to the feet, while from the upper sea, qi goes along the respiratory tract as breath. If there is counterflow of qi in the feet, the ancestral qi is no longer able to flow down, and, as a result, the vessels become congealed and stagnated. To treat this, ironing techniques must be applied before needling.

[182]The last sentence can be rendered differently as follows: "...before the place where qi is found stirring" or "before a qi is found reacting to the feeling hand." Since the author mentions various manual examination techniques, the last part most likely suggests that the acupuncturist should try to find various unusual signs, for example, pathological pulses or percussive reactions, in order to determine vacuity and repletion and locate the disease. In other words, the qi or the nature of the affliction (as we have put it), may refer to external manifestations of an illness found in the examination.

[183]A grand channel is simply a channel, and a transverse vessel as described here is a prominent vein.

[184]In the case of cold above and heat below, needling the nape of the neck and ironing the nape and scapulae is performed for the purpose of helping the heat below to ascend by means of directing the hot qi in the iron to join it. This technique is called pushing to assist ascent. The conduction to promote descent technique is aimed at conducting yang qi or hot qi in the upper part of the body downward by means of needling the sunken vessels.

The passages above give an account of two kinds of inversion. One is due to cold qi congealing the vessels; the other is due to transverse exuberant vessels forming blockage within a channel. Both require resolution of bondage but are treated in different ways. In the first case, needling must precede ironing techniques, while ironing techniques do not figure prominently in the second case at all.

[185]In treating heat inversion, retention of the needle may drive heat out and hence normalize the situation, while in treating cold inversion, retention of the needle may drive out cold normalizing the situation as well.

[186]In the case of heat inversion, it is necessary to perform drainage twice at a yin channel and supplementation once at a yang channel because the treatment focuses on clearing heat. In the case of cold inversion, it is necessary to perform drainage once at a yin channel and supplementation twice at a yang channel because the treatment aims at clearing cold. The meaning of the words once or twice in the original Chinese edition is ambiguous. They may be understood either as the selection of one or two points or that a single point is needled once or twice.

In the *Ling Shu* and *Tai Su*, "That which is referred to as one yang means that the yang is needled once" replaces "That which is referred to as two yang means that the yang is needled twice."

[187]All of the vessels indicated are needled at points on the feet.

[188]*I.e.*, swollen and distended lips

[189]In our source edition, "slight fullness" follows "cold hands and feet."

[190]Gusing Spring (*Yong Quan*, Ki 1) and Burning Valley (*Ran Gu*, Ki 2) of the foot *shao yin* and Severe Mouth (*Li Dui*, St 45), Inner Court (*Nei Ting*, St 44), Ravine Divide (*Jie Xi*, St 41), and Bountiful Bulge (*Feng Long*, St 40) of the foot *yang ming* are all points effective for counterflow inversion. In the *Ling Shu* and *Tai Su*, "vexation" replaces "distention." In our source edition, "choppy, large pulses" replaces "choppy pulses be they large or small"; and "(the trunk) is slack" replaces "(the trunk) is warm."

[191]It is common to experience a discomfort around the points, Camphorwood Gate (*Zhang Men*, Liv 13), Cycle Gate (*Qi Men*, Liv 14), etc. located in the lower lateral chest while coughing. The points Lung Shu (*Fei Shu*, Bl 13), Diaphragm Shu (*Ge Shu*, Bl 17), etc. on the back will often give relief to chest fullness when pressed, for example. These are the points implied by the author.

Our source edition reads, "three regions" instead of "two regions." This correction made in accordance with the *Ling Shu* and *Tai Su*.

[192]Part 1 is a combination of parts of Chap. 23, Vol. 5, *Ling Shu* and *Jin Gui Yao Lue (Prescriptions from the Golden Cabinet)* by Zhang Zhong–jing; and Part 2 is derived from the *Zhen Jiu Ming Tang Zhi Yao*.

[193]The following section with the exception of the first sentence consists of quotations from "*Zhi Shi Ye Bing Mai Zheng* (The Pulses and Symptoms of the Disease of Tetany, Dampness, and Summerheat Stroke)", Chap. 2, of the *Jin Gui Yao Lue*. Since the *Jin Gui* deals mainly with herbal medicine, there is some suspicion that this section was not authored by Huang–fu Mi but by some later known editor(s).

[194]In the *Ling Shu* and *Tai Su*, "(ending in) death" follows "Tetany due to heat."

[195]See Huang–fu Mi's Preface for more information on Zhang Zhong–jing.

[196]In the *Jin Gui Yao Lue*, there is no "hard" in the sentence "Hard tetany...", and the words "the patient" in the sentence "The patient must..." are absent in our source edition. "The *tai yang*" in the sentence "*Tai yang* disease with fever...is diagnosed as...tetany" is also absent.

[197]It is composed of Radix Puerariae (*Ge Gen*), 4 liang; Herba Ephedrae (*Ma Huang*), and raw Rhizoma Zingiberis (*Sheng Jiang*), each 3 liang; Ramulus Cinnamomi (*Gui Zhi*), mix–fried Radix Glycyrrhizae (*Gan Cao*), and Radix Paoniae Lactiflorae (*Shao Yao*), 2 *liang* for each of the above; plus Fructus Ziziphi Jujubae (*Da Zao*) 12 pieces.

[198]In the *Jin Gui*, "scant urine in spite of absence of perspiration" replaces "lack of perspiration, scant urine..."

[199]I.e., Bend Middle (*Wei Zhong*, Bl 40)

[200]Wind tetany is due to wind cold and dampness. It presents with sudden loss of consciousness and clenched jaw in addition to the symptoms mentioned in the text. For all practical purposes, it is tetany due to an affliction of dampness in wind stroke of the *tai yang* explained above.

In our source edition, "foot" is omitted in the term foot *tai yang* and has been supplemented in accordance with the *Wai Tai*. In the *Tai Su* and the *Ling Shu*, "For dribbling urinary block" replaces "For tetany."

[201]I.e., Shining Sea (*Zhao Hai*, Ki 6)

[202]I.e., Large Pile (*Da Dun*, Liv 1)

[203]In our source edition, "Supreme Surge (*Tai Chong*, Liv 3)" replaces "Celestial Surge (*Tian Chong*, GB 9)", and this correction is made in accordance with the *Wai Tai Mi Yao*.

[204]In the *Wai Tai*, "shortage of qi" replaces the passage "shortage...sacrococcygeal."

[205]Our source edition reads, "qi heat" in place of "generalized fever" and "dizziness, blurred vision" are omitted. "Great Hammer (*Da Zhui*, GV 14)" replaces "Great Shuttle (*Da Zhu*, Bl 11)." These corrections have been made in accordance with the *Wai Tai*.

[206]Our source edition reads, "sacrococcyx and arms" in place of "buttocks" and "*bi*" in place of "malaria." These corrections have been made in accordance with the *Wai Tai*.

[207]Our source edition reads "Lung Shu (*Fei Shu*, Bl 13) inside the paravertebral sinews" in place of "Central Backbone Shu (*Zhong Lu Shu*, Bl 29)"; "...the ruling point" is followed by "and needle the *yang ming*"; and the point Cubit Marsh (*Chi Ze*, Lu 5) is between "Needle" and "three of these." These corrections are made in accordance with the *Wai Tai*.

[208]In our source edition, the sentence ends with "which is the ruling point", an apparent error in transcription when compared to the treatment of similar conditions.

[209]I.e., Thoroughfare Yang (*Chong Yang*, St 42)

[210]In our source edition, the sentence ends with "which are the ruling points." This is an apparent redundancy.

[211]Above refers to points on the upper body which are effective for the treatment of tetany, such as Great Hammer (*Da Zhui*, GV 14). Below refers to points on the lower body effective for tetany, such as Bend Middle (*Wei Zhong*, Bl 40).

[212]One should note that bleeding a point implies the pricking of a prominent vein located nearby a standard point rather than piercing the point itself if no vein is prominently visible at that point.

[213]Part 1 is derived from Chap. 35, *Su Wen*; Part 2 from Chap. 36, *Su Wen*; and Part 3 from the *Zhen Jiu Ming Tang Zhi Yao*. As was stated in note 15, Chapter 1, Book 2, we have chosen not to translate *nue* as "malaria". *Nue* may include any syndrome characterized by alternating fever and chills.

[214]For the second sentence, the *Su Wen* and *Tai Su* read, "It is dormant and attacks at regular intervals."

[215]In our source edition, "desire to drink water" replaces "with desire for cold drinks" and has been corrected in accordance with the *Su Wen*. The *Tai Su* and the *Zhu Bing Yuan Hou Lun (Treatise on the Origins & Symptoms of Various Diseases)* are identical to the *Jia Yi Jing* in this aspect.

[216]Wang Bing notes in a commentary in the *Su Wen*, "The yang qi turns downward after travelling up to the summit, while the yin qi turns downward after travelling down to the nadir. This is what is meant by yin and yang contending above and below." This dynamic resembles the convection of cold and heat currents. It is of note that yin and yang qi here mean yin evils and yang evils respectively. The supersession of yang to yin can be understood as a subordination of yang to yin or yielding of yang to yin. When yang qi is merged in yin, then yang becomes vacuous and yin replete. Yang vacuity leads to external cold, while yin exuberance results in internal cold. Thus both the internal and the external are cold. If yin is merged in yang, then yin becomes vacuous while yang replete. Yin vacuity results in internal heat, whereas yang repletion gives rise to external heat. Thus heat occurs both externally and internally.

Because it enters the lower teeth, the foot *yang ming* channel gives rise to chattering of the jaws when vacuous. And because the foot *tai yang* travels along the back of the body and reaches the top of the head it causes pain along the route when vacuous. Overwhelming heat consumes fluid and humor, and this accounts for thirst and preference of cold drink to quench the heat fulminating in both the interior and exterior.

In our source edition, "yang becomes replete and yin vacuous" replaces "yin becomes replete and yang vacuous", and has been corrected in accordance with the *Su Wen* and *Wai Tai*. In the above two reference works, "lumbar spine" replaces "upper and lower back."

[217]The root of malaria is summerheat damage. The heat qi is hidden in the vessels where the constructive qi dwells. It forces the interstices open, producing perspiration and keeping sweat pores empty, and, as a result, when autumn comes, the clear depurating autumn qi or other evils are provided a chance to intrude. These yin cold qi lodge within the skin and circulate with the defensive qi. Since the defensive qi circulates according to a daily cycle (see Chap. 9, Book 1, present work), the evil malarial qi attacks once a day.

In our source edition, "oppresses externally" replaces "oppresses internally." This correction has been made in accordance with the *Su Wen* and *Tai Su*.

[218]As yin is retarded and unable to go with yang, the alternating yin (cold) and yang (heat) has to appear at longer intervals than one day. Also, refer to the immediate next question and answer between the Yellow Emperor and Qi Bo for further clarification.

[219]Collective name for the foot *shao yin* and the penetrating vessel

[220]The movement of evil qi up and down the spine has been verified by some clinicians who have found that there are tender points located along the back of malaria patients. Wind mansion here refers to the point Wind Mansion (*Feng Fu*, GV 16), but it should not invariably be understood as such in this chapter. It may sometimes also refer to the place where the wind evil or the malarial qi dwells. *Que Pen*, whose literal meaning is a basin-like depression, it is not the point Empty Basin (*Que Pen*, St 12) or the supraclavicular fossa. It is Celestial Chimney (*Tian Tu*, CV 22,) at the tip of the sternum. In understanding this and the following several paragraphs, the sentence, "This presupposes the initial intrusion (of the evil is) located in the spine in the back" is very important. It implies that, in other types of malaria, the evil qi may not affect the spine first but somewhere else.

The evil qi first intrudes at the wind mansion, and it moves down the spinal column at a rate of one vertebra per day. It launches an attack whenever the defensive qi comes into contact with the evil qi. This takes place once a day. Therefore, on the second day, when (the evil qi) is one vertebra lower, it takes a little longer to launch an attack. After the evil qi reaches the end of the spine, it

turns inward and upward, thus accounting for the gradual shortening of the time between attacks. The preceding section explained that the evil travels together with the defensive qi which moves twenty–five cycles within each yin and yang phase per day. This raises the question as to why Huang–fu Mi proceeds with an account of the evil qi moving one vertebra lower daily? The answer may be that the malaria qi simultaneously works somewhere in the interior, such as in the five viscera and circulates with the defensive qi but not at the same pace. After the evil qi reaches the end of the spine, it begins to travel upward. It takes nine days for the evil qi to complete its upward journey. This is a shorter duration than its descent because the evil qi now travels along the ventral aspect and is unimpeded by the vertebrae in its ascent.

In our source edition, "All this intrudes..." replaces "This presupposes the initial intrusion..." and has been corrected in accordance with the *Su Wen* and *Tai Su*.

[221]Membranes in the areas between the pleura and the diaphragm.

[222]Our source edition reads, "...keep pace with the constructive qi" in place of "...keep pace with the defensive qi" and has been corrected in accordance with the *Su Wen* and *Tai Su*.

[223]Our source edition reads, "...moves one vertebra down each day" in place of "...responds one vertebra later each day", and has been corrected in accordance with the *Ling Shu* and *Zhu Bing Yuan Hou*.

[224]The missing words are provided below for reference. They can be found in the "*Nue Lun Pian* (Treatise on Malaria)", Chap. 35, the *Su Wen*. This is because the evil qi intrudes the head and the nape of the neck and travels downward along the spine. Vacuity (evil) differs from repletion (evil), and, therefore, they may strike different places and it may happen that they fail to fall upon the wind mansion. If the evil happens to strike the head and the nape, a episode begins when the (defensive) qi arrives at the head and the nape. If it happens to strike the upper back, an episode begins when the (defensive) qi arrives at the upper back. If it happens to strike the lumbar spine, an episode begins when the (defensive) qi arrives at the lumbar spine. If it happens to strike the hands and feet, an episode begins when the (defensive) qi) arrives at the hands and feet. An episode begins wherever the (defensive) qi meet the evil qi."

In the *Su Wen* the last sentence is: "Wherever the

evil qi meets (with the defensive qi) is its mansion."

225Wind has no constant mansion. From this, it can be seen that the wind mansion mentioned in the text is not necessarily the point Wind Mansion (*Feng Fu*, GV 16). It is necessary to distinguish a wind disease, for example, wind stroke or hemilateral paraplegia from malaria, which may also be caused by an evil qi. A wind disease manifests constantly while malarial episodes are intermittent.

226Our source edition reads, "water" instead of "slight" and has been corrected in accordance with the *Su Wen*.

227According to the *Su Wen Jing Zhu Jie Jie (Annotations & Explanations of the Classic of the Basic Questions)*, expiry of yin should be understood as vanquished yin qi. This is not a true expiry of yin. A true case of yin expiry is a mortal illness, and malaria is not. Yin vacuity leads to internal heat, while yang exuberance results in external heat. The above is a case of prevailing yang with diminished yin. It is of note that although alternating cold and heat are not present, this illness is considered malarial because the fever arises at fixed hours.

228It is notable that the quotes here are from the *Su Wen*, but refer to the *Ling Shu*, Chap. 55.

229Counterflow here implies that the evil qi progresses with momentum.

230At the incipient stage, the yang defensive qi is subordinated to the yin, locked in the yin phase at the interior. As a consequence, the exterior is left devoid of yang qi, cold arises, and the patient shivers. An absence of qi in the exterior implies an external vacuity resulting from the merger of the defensive qi into the yin. Waxing and waning always follow each other. When yin passes its zenith, it becomes its opposite. Now the yin qi is subordinated to the yang qi, producing repletion of yang at the exterior, and, therefore, heat is generated with thirst.

231Our source edition reads, "malaria" instead of "malarial qi" and has been corrected in accordance with the *Su Wen* and *Tai Su*. In place of the clause "As malaria...nature" is given "As malaria, a wind cold qi, is irregular." This correction is made in accordance with the *Tai Su*.

232Before malaria attacks, yang at the exterior submerges into the interior, while yin struggles outward to the exterior. Then yang may be subordinated to yin, or yin to yang, giving rise to cold or

heat. The well points are located on the fingers and toes and it is from here that the yang turns inward. For this reason, malarial episodes are first experienced in the extremities. If one binds the extremities, usually at the fingers and toes just prior to an attack, then pathway of the yang's submergence and yin's emergence is occluded, and, by pricking the prominent blood vessels, the evil qi may be drained off.

The last sentence reads in the *Su Wen* "...when the true (qi) is about to leave but has not yet been superseded by the evil qi" and in the *Tai Su* reads, "This is (a treatment) to directly take what has not yet merged."

233There is a logical inconsistency in the first sentence. It should read, "(Malaria which is) intermittently episodic occurs when the evil qi become lodged in the six bowels and fails to maintain synchronization with the defensive qi. Thus it may, on some occasions, fail to meet with the defensive qi and so must remain dormant for several days before another episode."

234It is a general rule that summerheat damage breeds malaria in the autumn. Some cases, however, fail to conform with this axiom and do not develop in an ordinary manner. They may happen any time in the four seasons with distinctive manifestations. Since environmental cold is just accumulating in the autumn, illnesses occurring then are characterized by severe chills. Since the yang lies deeply during the winter, chills occurring at this time will be relatively mild. Since the interstices are open in the spring, there will be an aversion to wind at this time. And during the summer, summerheat fevers cause copious perspiration.

235The evil qi of warm malaria is hidden deep in the kidneys. Because it first emerges from the interior to the exterior at the beginning, the internal becomes vacuous and the yang exuberant. This results in heat. When yang has reached its extreme, it declines and begins to enter the interior. Thus, yang becomes vacuous and cold is generated.

In the *Su Wen* and *Tai Su*, "due to wind" is "due to wind cold"; and in our source edition, "heat declines" replaces "there is heat." These have been corrected in accordance with the *Su Wen*.

236At some point in the past, heat has become hidden in the heart and lung. The word "center" mentioned in the text refers specifically to the heart in this context. When this repletion heat conspires with external wind cold that has become lodged in the skin and border of flesh at the exterior, then there is a surplus of hot yang qi, wasting the flesh and causing intense fever. In this pattern, the yang qi does not turn inward. Therefore, there is only heat and cold is not present.

[237]A large, full, and urgent pulse reflects exuberant repletion heat and, therefore, requires draining. The five (viscus-)associated back points are Heart Shu (*Xin Shu*, Bl 15), Lung Shu (*Fei Shu*, Bl 13), Liver Shu (*Gan Shu*, Bl 18), Spleen Shu (*Pi Shu*, Bl 20), and Kidney Shu (*Shen Shu*, Bl 23), and the five points beside them, Po Door (*Po Hu*, Bl 42), Spirit Hall (*Shen Tang*, Bl 44), Hun Gate (*Hun Men*, Bl 47), Reflection Abode (*Yi She*, Bl 49), and Will Chamber (*Zhi Shi*, Bl 52) all of which are located near the axilla. These are, therefore, referred to as the auxiliary points. Note that this sentence may be interpreted in a number of ways: 1) "one of the axillary points is selected"; 2) "one of the axillary and one of the viscus–associated back points is selected"; 3) "the five axillary are chosen"; and 4) "the five axillary and the five viscus-associated back points are all chosen." The translator stands for the third interpretation.

[238]*I.e.*, Recover Flow (*Fu Liu*, Ki 7)

[239]*I.e.*, the well point of the foot *tai yang* at the small toe, Reaching Yin (*Zhi Yin*, Bl 67)

[240]These pulse qualities point to a vacuity condition. Although needling can be used for supplementation, it is prohibited in the case of serious vacuity.

[241]We have replaced the word "one" in this paragraph and the succeeding ones with the word "item." One would be a meaningless redundancy in English. In Chinese, it is used here to begin each section in a series of sections. In classical Chinese where there was no punctuation, this word is sometimes used to set off one item from the next.

[242]In our source edition, "foot *tai yin*" replaces "foot *tai yang*", and this has been corrected in accordance with the *Su Wen* and *Tai Su*. In the *Ling Shu* and the *Tai Su*, "hand *yang ming*" replaces "hand *shao yang*."

[243]See the preceding chapter for an explanation of the fifty–nine needling points.

[244]*I.e.*, Bend Middle (*Wei Zhong*, Bl 40)

[245]The presentation of this type of malaria is ascribed to the route of the foot *tai yang* channel which runs primarily along the back of the body. This explanation is applicable in the following sections as well.

[246]*I.e.*, Pinched Ravine (*Xia Xi*, GB 43)

[247]Since the *yang ming* is abundant in both qi and blood, when it becomes diseased, symptoms such as aversion to the sight of people and fire or even madness and wild running usually occur in this case. However, *yang ming* malaria makes the patient like fire and the sun. This is because of the presence of great cold in the interior, and this yin evil has overwhelmed the *yang ming*. This also accounts for the fact that, in this *yang ming* malaria, cold precedes heat.

[248]*I.e.*, Yin White (*Yin Bai*, Sp 1) and Offspring of Duke (*Gong Sun*, Sp 4)

Our source edition reads, "abundant cold but scant heat" instead of "abundant cold and heat", and this has been corrected in accordance with the *Su Wen* and *Tai Su*. The last sentence has probably been inserted by some later unknown editor(s) since it cannot be found in either the *Su Wen* or *Tai Su*.

[249]In the *Lei Jing*, Zhang Jing–yue explains, "If the disease is in the yin, there will be a preference for privacy with doors and windows shut. Because the kidney is a viscus of consummate yin, when evils become lodged within it, the disease is difficult to treat."

In the *Su Wen* and *Tai Su*, "abundant cold and heat with the heat being more and the cold less" replaces "abundant cold with scant heat." The last sentence is not found in the *Su Wen*, the *Tai Su*, or the *Zhu Bing Yuan Hou*.

[250]*I.e.*, Supreme Surge (*Tai Chong*, Liv 3)

Our source edition reads, "frequent voiding of stools" instead of "frequent belching." This correction has been made in accordance with a note in the *Jia Yi Jing* by an unknown editor and the *Su Wen*.

[251]*I.e.*, Broken Sequence (*Lie Que*, Lu 7)

[252]*I.e.*, Union Valley (*He Gu*, LI 4)

In our source edition, "succeeding the cold" is omitted. This correction is made in accordance with the *Su Wen* and *Tai Su*.

[253]"By which is meant Spirit Door (*Shen Men*, Ht 7)" is not found in the *Su Wen* or the *Tai Su*.

[254]*I.e.*, Mound Center (*Zhong Feng*, Liv 4)

[255]*I.e.*, Shang Hill (*Shang Qiu*, Sp 5)

256*I.e.*, Capital Bone (*Jing Gu*, Bl 64)

257*I.e.*, Guest House (*Zhu Bin*, Ki 9)

258*I.e.*, Severe Mouth (*Li Dui*, St 45), Ravine Divide (*Jie Xi*, St 41), and Foot Three Li (*Zu San Li*, St 36)

259*I.e.*, Shang Hill (*Shang Qiu*, Sp 5)

260In our source edition, the *Su Wen*, the *Wai Tai*, and the *Zhu Bing Yuan Hou Lun*, "a disease" replaces "cold diseases of the gallbladder." This correction has been made in accordance with the *Tai Su*. In this phrase there is a functional word which we fail to represent meaning "moreover." This ideogram is easily confused with the ideogram for gallbladder. This causes the confusion.

261The moving vessel here does not mean a beating or pulsating vessel, or the arterial vessel, needling of which is prohibited. It refers to the point Surging Yang (*Chong Yang*, St 42). Moving is a synonym for penetrating, and the moving vessel, *i.e.*, *dong mai* refers to the penetrating vessel.

262Bloodletting causes the fever to abate, leaving the body chilled.

263*I.e.*, Shang Yang (*Shang Yang*, LI 1)

264*I.e.*, Lesser Shang (*Shao Shang*, Lu 11)

265*I.e.*, Severe Mouth (*Li Dui*, St 45)

266*I.e.*, Yin White (*Yin Bai*, Sp 1)

267*I.e.*, the ten well points

268Red bean-like papules mean petechiae on the skin. According to Zhang Zhi–cong in his *Su Wen Ji Zhu (Condensed Annotations on the Basic Questions)* these occur when evils have penetrated the skin damaging the qi aspect.

269The twelve types of malaria are malaria of the six channels, the five viscera, and the stomach.

270*I.e.*, points of the foot *tai yang* such as Great Shuttle (*Da Zhu*, Bl 11), Wing Gate (*Feng Men*, Bl 12), and Lung Shu (*Fei Shu*, Bl 13)

271Ridge Spring (*Lian Quan*) is not the point Ridge Spring (*Lian Quan*, CV 23), since this is a single point belonging to the conception vessel, while the author declares that the point in question is two vessels and that it is a bilateral point. Wang Bing explains in a note in the *Su Wen*, "The bilateral point of the foot *shao yin* under the tongue is located in a depression anterior to a pulsating vessel before Man's Prognosis (*Ren Ying*, St 9). It is named the Root of the Tongue (*She Ben*), a bilateral point. This point may be a point located between the point Man's Prognosis and Ridge Spring."

272*I.e.*, Upper Star (*Shang Xing*, GV 23) and Hundred Convergence (*Bai Hui*, GV 20)

273*I.e.*, Suspended Skull (*Xuan Lu*, GB 5)

274*I.e.*, Bamboo Gathering (*Zan Zhu*, Bl 2)

275*I.e.*, Wind Pool (*Feng Chi*, GB 20) and Wind Mansion (*Feng Fu*, GB 16)

276*I.e.*, Great Shuttle (*Da Zhu*, Bl 11) and Spirit Path (*Shen Dao*, GV 11)

277*I.e.*, prominent veins around Bend Middle (*Wei Zhong*, Bl 40)

278*I.e.*, Lesser Surge (*Shao Chong*, Ht 9) and Shang Yang (*Shang Yang*, LI 1)

279*I.e.*, Severe Mouth (*Li Dui*, St 45)

280The points on the fingers of the hand *shao yin* and *yang ming* are prescribed as an example. If the pain in the hands and arms involves other channels than the hand *shao yang* or *yang ming*, points selected should be pertinent to the affected channels. This is also the case with the prescription of the foot *yang ming* to treat pain in the feet and lower legs.

In our source edition, "between the shoulders" replaces "between the eyebrows", and this correction has been made in accordance with the *Su Wen* and *Tai Su*.

281*I.e.*, Urinary Bladder Shu (*Pang Guang Shu*, Bl 28), Stomach Shu (*Wei Shu*, Bl 21), and Gallbladder Shu (*Dan Shu*, Bl 19)

282In the *Su Wen* and *Tai Su*, "three yang channels" replaces "the three foot yang channels."

283In our source edition, "elbows" replace "the lower legs", and this correction has been made in accordance with the *Su Wen* and *Tai Su*.

284*Jie nue* has three meanings. One is quartan malaria which attacks every seventy–two hours. The second is used as a collective term for all kinds of malaria. The last refers to malaria whose episodes occur at night (*jie*) and malaria launching attacks during the day. Because this section is intended to deal with various kinds of malaria, *jie nue* should be used in a narrow sense, and, therefore, it is rendered as quartan malaria. It is of note that, in the majority of the modern versions of the *Jia Yi Jing*, it is usually interpreted in a wide sense.

[285]In our source edition, the point Great Shuttle (*Da Zhu*, Bl 11) is also prescribed. However, it is omitted here in accordance with the *Wai Tai* and the *Qian Jin*.

[286]This is evil in the *tai yang* infecting the *yang ming*. Thus a point on the *yang ming* channel is indicated.

[287]In our source edition, "heat inversion" replaces "heat with", and this correction has been made in accordance with the *Wai Tai*.

[288]In the *Wai Tai*, "headache, dry eyes, and attack triggered by sudden counterflow (of qi)", replaces "sudden fulminating counterflow."

[289]In our source edition, "to the lower abdomen" replaces "into the lower abdomen", and "Lesser Sea (*Shao Hai*, Ht 3)" replaces "Small Sea (*Xiao Hai*, SI 8)." These have been corrected in accordance with the *Wai Tai* and the *Yi Xin Fang (The Heart of Medicine Formulary)*.

[290]In our source edition, Kun Lun Mountain (*Kun Lun*, Bl 60) replaces Taking Flight (*Fei Yang*, Bl 58).

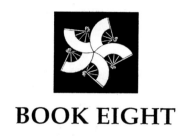

BOOK EIGHT

Chapter One

On the Transmission of Disease Among the Five Viscera Producing Cold & Heat (Part 1)[1]

(1)

The Yellow Emperor said:

The five viscera communicate with one another, and (disease) is passed (among them) in a sequential manner. Among the five viscera, disease is transmitted to the restrained (viscera). If left untreated, (the patient will survive only) three to six months or three to six days. Once (the illness) has been transmitted among all of the five viscera, death should occur. [The *Su Wen* describes the sequence of transmission in accordance with the restraining cycle of the five phases. {later editor}][2]

Therefore, it is said that identification of yang leads to an understanding of the origination of a disease, and identification of yin leads to an understanding of the date of death. This implies that death comes about at the subjugated (phase of the involved viscus).[3]

Wind is the leader of the hundred diseases. When wind cold intrudes, it causes a person's fine hair to stand on end. The skin closes (the interstices), thus generating heat. At this point, (the evil) may be effused through diaphoresis. (The evil may cause) numbness, insensitivity and painful swelling. At this point, drug ironing is indicated.

(This pathology) may also be removed by moxibustion ["moxibustion on the feet" in a variant version {later editor}] and needling.[4]

If left untreated, the disease enters and lodges in the lung. This is known as the lung *bi*, and produces coughing and an ascension of qi.[5]

If left untreated, the lung transmits (the evil) on to the liver. This disease is known as the liver *bi*. It is also known as inversion, (and is characterized by) pain in the lateral costal region and vomiting of food (upon ingestion). At this juncture, massage and acupuncture are indicated.[6]

If left untreated, the liver transmits (the evil) on to the spleen. This disease is known as spleen wind and produces jaundice with heat in the abdomen, vexation of the heart, sweating, and yellowing of the body [the word "sweating" is absent from the *Su Wen* {later editor}]. At this point massage, medication, and fire-branding ["bathing" in a variant version {later editor}] are indicated.[7]

If left untreated, the spleen transmits (the evil) on to the kidney. This disease is known as *shan* conglomeration. It is characterized by the symptoms of vexation, oppression, pain in the lower abdomen, and sweating ["discharge of white turbidity" in the *Su Wen*. {later editor}] It is also known as drum-distention (*gu*, 蛊). At this point, massage and medication are indicated.[8]

If left untreated, the kidney transmits (the evil) on to the heart. This disease is characterized by contraction and hypertonicity of the sinews and vessels and is known as tugging. At this point, moxibustion and medication are indicated.[9]

If this condition is left untreated, death should occur in ten days. Once the kidney has transmitted (the disease) to the heart, the heart transmits it once again to the lung, producing cold and heat. (In this case,) death should occur in three years.[10]

This is the sequence (of the transmission of) disease. There are some sudden (illnesses), however, that should not necessarily be treated based on this sequence. Transmission and transmutation that does not take place in (the above mentioned) sequence is due to worry, fright, sorrow, joy, and anger. Since (these factors) may cause (an illness to be transmitted) out of the expected sequence, people may suffer from major illnesses.[11]

As a consequence of joy, a great vacuity may be produced, and, therefore, the kidney qi overwhelms (the heart. Likewise,) anger causes the liver qi to overwhelm (the spleen). Sorrow causes the lung qi to overwhelm (the liver). Fright causes the spleen qi to overwhelm (the kidney). Worry causes the heart qi to overwhelm (the lung). This is a basic principle. It follows that these five types of disease, with five times five, i.e., twenty-five variations in (the manner in which diseases may be) transmitted and transmutated. Transmission is a term for overwhelming.[12]

(The presence of) desiccation and withering in the major bones, wasting and sinking of the major muscles, fullness of qi in the chest, and dyspnea and labored breathing causing the body to move place the time of death in six months. If the true visceral pulse appears, one's days are numbered.[13]

(The presence of) desiccation and withering of the major bones, wasting and sinking of the major muscles, fullness of qi in the chest, dyspnea and labored breathing, and internal pain radiating to the shoulders and the nape of the neck, place the time of death in one month. If the true visceral pulse appears, one's days are numbered.[14]

(The presence of) desiccation and withering of the major bones, wasting and sinking of the major muscles, fullness of qi in the chest, dyspnea and labored breathing, internal pain radiating to the shoulders and the nape of the neck, generalized fever, shedding of flesh and cleaving of major muscular masses, and the appearance of the true visceral pulse, place the time of death in ten days.[15]

(The presence of) desiccation and withering of the major bones, wasting and sinking of the major muscles, internal consumption of the marrow of the shoulders, and increasing decrepitude in the absence of the true visceral pulse, place the time of death in one year. If the true visceral pulse appears, ones days are numbered.[16]

(The presence of) desiccation and withering of the major bones, wasting and sinking of the major muscles, fullness of qi in the chest, abdominal pain, discomfort in the heart, heat in the shoulder and the nape, generalized heat, shedding of flesh and cleaving of major muscular masses, sunken eyes, the appearance of the true visceral pulse, and loss of eyesight mean impending death. If the sight is preserved, death will occur when (the evil) reaches its restrained phase.[17]

When vacuity abruptly strikes the body resulting in the sudden arousal (of evils), the five viscera become blocked and expiring, the passages of the vessels become congested, and the qi cannot come and go. This (condition) can be compared to that of those who are drowning or who have been fatally wounded in a fall. The exact time of their death is indeterminate. If the pulse is expiring, is not present, or beats five or six times during a single exhalation, death is also certain even though there is as yet no shedding of the fleshy form and even though the true visceral pulse is not yet present.[18]

The true liver pulse may be urgent both interiorly and exteriorly, like touching the sharp edge of a knife or like pressing the string of a musical instrument. (In this case,) when the complexion becomes a lusterless whitish green-blue and the hair becomes brittle, death ensues.

The true heart pulse may be hard and forceful,

like touching a string of hard Job's tears seeds. (In this case,) when the complexion becomes a lusterless reddish black and the hair becomes brittle, death ensues.[19]

The true lung pulse may be large and vacuous, like a feather touching the skin. (In this case,) when the complexion becomes a lusterless reddish white and the hair becomes brittle, death ensues.

The true spleen pulse may be weak, varying in rhythm and pace. (In this case,) when the complexion becomes a lusterless yellowish green-blue and the hair becomes brittle, death ensues.

The true kidney pulse may be forceful with expiry (of the stomach qi) like stone pellets hitting the fingers. (In this case,) when the complexion becomes a lusterless yellowish black and the hair becomes brittle, death ensues.

If any one of these true visceral pulses appears, death is a certainty (and the condition) cannot be treated.

(2)

The Yellow Emperor asked:

What kind of qi generates scrofula in the neck and axilla with cold and heat?

Qi Bo answered:

They are known as rats' tunnels (*shu lou*, 鼠瘘). They are the toxic qi of cold and heat that is trapped and persists in the vessels. The root of rats' tunnel is invariably found in the viscus, while its end exits upward into the neck or the axilla. If (the toxic qi) floats in the vessels and has not yet become fixed in the muscle, thus producing pus and blood externally, it is easily removed[20]

The Yellow Emperor asked:

How (are these lesions) removed?

Qi Bo answered:

One must track down the root and conduct the end in order to diminish and remove (the toxic qi) and succeed in exterminating cold and heat. (One should) examine and palpate the passageways and (needle) in accordance with them. Slow insertion and slow extraction (of the needle) should be performed in order to remove it. For (scrofula that is as) small as a wheat (grain), one needling will show (a result), and three needlings will eliminate it. A determination of life or death (is made possible through) examination of the eyes (with the eyelids) turned inside out. If the pupils appear to be suffused by red vessels from above to below, one such vessel predicts death in one year; one and a half such vessels, death in one and a half years; two such vessels, death in two years; two and a half such vessels, death in two and a half years; and three such vessels, death in three years. If the vessel (or vessels) have not penetrated down through the pupils, (the scrofula) is curable.[21]

(3)

The Yellow Emperor asked:

What signs help to identify those who have a tendency toward illnesses of cold and heat?

Qi Bo answered:

Those with small bones and weak muscles are subject to cold and heat. Because the cheekbones are the root of the bones, large cheekbones mean large bones, while small cheekbones mean small bones. Thin skin, weak flesh without prominent masses, flaccid arms, and a sooty complexion at the earth (region), which looks grimy and unusual, differing from that at the heaven (region), are all indications (of those subject to cold and heat). In those with thin arms, the marrow does not fill (the bones), and (these people), therefore, have a tendency toward cold and heat.[22]

(4)

An affliction by wind results in cold and heat. Cutaneous cold and heat (is characterized by) an unwillingness to touch one's skin to the mat, parched hair, a desiccated nose like dry, seasoned meat, and a lack of perspiration. (One should) take the connecting vessel of the third yang and supplement the hand *tai yin*.[23]

Muscular cold and heat is a disease characterized by pain in the muscles, parched hair, desiccated lips like dry, seasoned meat, and lack of perspiration. (One should) take the third yang below and let out blood and supplement the *tai yin* to induce perspiration.[24]

Bone cold and heat is characterized by pain that allows no peace and incessant perspiration. If the teeth are not yet desiccated, (one should) take the connecting vessel of the (foot) *shao yin* on the medial aspect of the thigh. If the teeth are already desiccated, the disease is fatal and cannot be remedied. This is also the case with bone inversion.[25]

(5)

For *gu*[26] disorder in males and morning sickness-like disorder in females with the body and the lumbar spine (in particular, flaccid) as if disintegrated, and no desire for food, first take Gushing Spring (*Yong Quan*, Ki 1) until blood appears, and then (prick) all the exuberant vessels found at the instep to let blood out.[27]

(6)

Moxa techniques for cold and heat involve moxibustion first at the nape at Great Hammer (*Da Zhui*, GV 14) using the same number of the cones as that of the patient's age. Then moxa the coccyx bone,[28] using the same number of the cones as that of the patient's age. Moxa the (viscus-)associated back points that have been found to be depressed[29] Moxa the point in a depression appearing in the shoulder when the arm is raised.[30] Moxa the point between the two (lowest) free ribs.[31] Moxa the end of the Severed Bone above the lateral malleolus.[32] Moxa the point between the small and the fourth toe.[33] Moxa the vessel in a depression under the calf.[34] Moxa the point posterior to the lateral malleolus.[35] Moxa

the place that feels hard like sinew above the clavicle bone.[36] Moxa the point in a depression at the middle of the breast bone.[37] Moxa the point on the palmar aspect below the bundle bone.[38] Moxa Origin Pass (*Guan Yuan*, CV 4) located three *cun* below the navel. Moxa the moving vessel in the region of the pubic hair.[39] Moxa the point between the two sinews three *cun* under the knee.[40] Moxa the foot *yang ming*, i.e., moxa the moving vessel at the instep.[41] Moxa the single point at the vertex.[42] And select and moxa the place bitten by the dog. (The bite) should be moxaed, three cones, as instructed in the Protocol for Dog's Injury. There are altogether twenty-nine places for moxibustion.[43, 44]

(7)

For cold and heat with headache, asthmatic wheezing and loss of eye-sight, Spirit Court (*Shen Ting*, GV 24) is the ruling point.

For (cold and heat with) tearing and absence of headache, Fontanelle Meeting (*Xin Hui*, GV 22) is the ruling point.[45]

For cold and heat with splitting headache, painful eyes that feel as if they are about to burst from their sockets, counterflow dyspnea with vexation and fullness, retching and vomiting, flowing perspiration and labored speech, Head Corner (*Tou Wei*, St 8) is the ruling point.

For cold and heat, needle Brain Door (*Nao Hu*, GV 17).

Chapter One

On the Transmission of Disease Among the Five Viscera Producing Cold & Heat (Part 2)[46]

For cold and heat, take Fifth Place (*Wu Chu*, Bl 5), and, Celestial Pool (*Tian Chi*, Per 1), Wind Pool (*Feng Chi*, GB 20), Lumbar Shu (*Yao Shu*, GV 2),

Long Strong (*Chang Qiang*, GV 1), Great Shuttle (*Da Zhu*, GV 14), Central Backbone Inner Shu (*Zhong Lu Nei Shu*, Bl 29), Upper Bone Hole (*Shang Liao*, Bl 31), Gum Intersection (*Yin Jiao*, CV 7), Upper Pass (*Shang Guan*, GB 3), Origin Pass (*Guan Yuan*, CV 4), Celestial Window (*Tian You*, TH 16), Celestial Countenance (*Tian Rong*, SI 17), Union Valley (*He Gu*, LI 4), Yang Ravine (*Yang Xi*, LI 5), Passage Hub (*Guan Chong*, TH 1), Central Islet (*Zhong Zhu*, TH 3), Yang Pool (*Yang Chi*, TH 4), Dispersing Riverbed (*Xiao Luo*, TH 12), Lesser Marsh (*Shao Ze*, SI 1), Front Valley (*Qian Gu*, SI 2), Wrist Bone (*Wan Gu*, SI 4), Yang Union (*Yang Gu*, SI 5), Lesser Sea (*Xiao Hai*, SI 8), Blazing Valley (*Ran Gu*, Ki 2), Reaching Yin (*Zhi Yin*, Bl 67), and Kun Lun Mountain (*Kun Lun*, Bl 60) are all the ruling points.

For cold and heat with pain in the bone, Jade Pillow (*Yu Zhen*, Bl 9) is the ruling point.

For cold and heat with languor and lassitude, aching and weakness in the lower legs, heaviness and pain in the four limbs and diminished qi with labored speech, Reaching Yang (*Zhi Yang*, GV 9) is the ruling point.[47]

For lung cold and heat with (inhibited) respiration causing inability to lie down, coughing due to ascension of qi, retching of foam, panting which comes in quick successive gasps, fullness in the chest, hypertonicity of the upper back and bosom, difficulty in breathing, quivering with cold, drum pulse, qi obstruction, heat existing in the chest with propping fullness and no desire for food, lack of perspiration, and pain in the lumbar spine, Lung Shu (*Fei Shu*, Bl 13) is the ruling point.[48]

For cold and heat with heart pain sending a dull and steady dragging pain to the upper back, oppression in the chest with inability to catch the breath, coughing and spitting of blood, copious drooling, vexation of the center, tendency to esophageal constriction, inability to ingest food, counterflow retching, lack of perspiration, *nue*-like (condition), blurred vision, and tearing sorrow and lamentation, Heart Shu (*Xin Shu*, Bl 15) is the ruling point.[49]

For coughing with retching, cold in the dia-

phragm, inability to ingest food, fever and chills, pain in the skin, flesh and bone, diminished qi with inability to lie down, fullness in the chest propping against the lateral costal regions, agitated diaphragm, pain in the lateral costal regions with abdominal distention, acute pain in the venter, qi ascension, cold and pain in the shoulders and upper back, lack of perspiration, throat *bi*, pain in the abdomen with masses and accumulations, taciturnity and somnolence, languor and lassitude with disinclination to move, a continuously damp body, heart pain, and inability to go about, Diaphragm Shu (*Ge Shu*, Bl 17) is the ruling point.[50]

For coughing with fullness and hypertonicity in the lateral costal regions, inability to catch the breath, inability to turn over, dragging (discomfort) between the axillae, the costal regions, and the navel, hypertonicity and pain of the sinews, arched-back rigidity, upturned eyes, dizziness, rolling of the eyes, pain in the eyebrows, fright mania, nosebleeding, lower abdominal fullness, blurred vision, white screen growing in the eye, cough initiating pain in the chest, sinewy cold and heat, spitting of blood, qi shortage, and sourness in the nose, Liver Shu (*Gan Shu*, Bl 18) is the ruling point.[51]

For cold and heat, marked emaciation in spite of a large food intake, dragging pain between the two lateral costal regions, surging pain below the heart, suspended sensation of the heart sending a dragging (discomfort) to the umbilicus, acute pain in the lower abdomen, fever, black facial complexion, blurred vision, dyspnea and cough, diminished qi, and turbid, dark colored urine, Kidney Shu (*Shen Shu*, Bl 23) is the ruling point.[52]

For bone cold and heat with difficult urination, Kidney Shu (*Shen Shu*, Bl 23) is the ruling point.

For cold and heat with headache, Water Trough (*Shui Gou*, GV 26) is the ruling point.

For cold and heat with scrofula in the neck, Great Reception (*Da Ying*, St 5) is the ruling point.

For pain in the shoulders affecting the nape of the neck, cold and heat, pain in the supraclavicular fossa, lack of perspiration, and heat and fullness in the chest, Celestial Bone Hole (*Tian Liao*, TH 15) is the ruling point.[53]

For cold and heat with swelling in the shoulders initiating pain in the scapulae and aching in the shoulders and arms, Upper Arm Shu (*Nao Shu*, SI 10) is the ruling point.

For cold and heat cervical scrofula with ringing in the ears and impaired hearing initiating heat and pain in the supraclavicular fossa and shoulder, and palsy of the arm with inability to lift it [palsy is absent from a variant version {later editor}], True Shoulder (*Jian Zhen*, SI 9) is the ruling point.[54]

For cold and heat scrofula with dim vision, coughing due to an ascent of qi, and spitting of blood, Mid Shoulder Shu (*Jian Zhong Shu*, SI 15) is the ruling point.

Cold and heat scrofula where the chest is full of great qi and there is pain in the supraclavicular fossae is fatal. However, if (the scrofulous masses) suppurate, the condition is not fatal. For shoulder pain affecting the nape of the neck, inability to lift the arm, pain in the supraclavicular fossa, lack of perspiration, throat *bi*, and coughing of blood, Empty Basin (*Que Pen*, St 12) is the ruling point.[55]

For coughing with ascension of qi, dyspnea, sudden loss of voice, green-blue veins in the fold beneath the tongue, great qi in the neck, throat *bi*, dry throat, distressed rapid dyspneic breathing, rale in the throat, mild cold and heat, swelling in the neck with pain in the shoulders, fullness in the chest, heat in the skin of the abdomen, nosebleeding, qi choking with heart pain, dormant papules, headache, hotness in the face with red complexion, and insensitivity of the muscles all over the body, Celestial Chimney (*Tian Tu*, CV 22) is the ruling point.[56]

For tension in the lung ligation, pain in the chest, aversion to cold, distressed fullness in the chest, frequent retching of bile, heat in the chest, dyspnea with qi counterflow, panting which comes in quick successive gasps, copious turbid phlegm, inability to catch the breath, aversion of the shoulders and upper back to wind, (spontaneous) sweating, swelling of the face and abdomen, esophageal constriction at the diaphragm, inability to ingest food, throat *bi*, shrugging the shoulders to facilitate breathing with the lung dilated, pain in the skin and the bone, and cold and heat with vexation and fullness, Central Treasury (*Zhong Fu*, Lu 1) is the ruling point.[57]

For cold and heat with fullness in the chest, pain in the neck, inability to lift the four limbs, swelling of the armpit, qi ascension, noise in the chest, and rale in the throat, Celestial Pool (*Tian Chi*, Per 1) is the ruling point.[58]

For coughing, gatherings and accumulations in the free rib regions, counterflow dyspnea, restless sleep, and occasional cold and heat, Cycle Gate (*Qi Men*, Liv 14) is the ruling point.

For cold and heat with abdominal distention and fullness, melancholy and inhibited respiration, Capital Gate (*Jing Men*, GB 25) is the ruling point.

For shivering as after bathing in cold water, heart vexation, insensitivity of the hands and the arms, foamy sputum, dry lips with copious drinking, cramp of the wrists, pain in the finger joints, distention of the lung, qi ascension, noise like wind blowing in the ears, coughing and counterflow dyspnea, finger *bi*, pain in the arms, retching and vomiting, inability to ingest food or drink, and bloating (of the abdomen), Lesser Shang (*Shao Shang*, Lu 11) is the ruling point.[59]

For spitting blood and intermittent alternating cold and heat, drain at Fish Border (*Yu Ji*, Lu 10) and supplement at Cubit Marsh (*Chi Ze*, Lu 5).

For arm inversion (characterized by) pain in the shoulder, bosom, and chest, growth of white screen in the eye, green-blue coloring of the eye, cramps (of sinews), hotness in the palm, alternating cold and heat, dragging pain in the supraclavicular fossae, frequent yawning, dyspnea with inability to catch the breath, pain in the inner side of the arm, vomiting from above the diaphragm, and vexation and fullness arising on drinking, Great Abyss (*Tai Yuan*, Lu 9) is the ruling point.[60]

For cold and heat with hypertonicity of the chest and upper back, throat *bi*, coughing, qi ascension dyspnea, heat in the palm, frequent yawning and stretching, and (spontaneous) sweating, needle Channel Ditch (*Jing Qu*, Lu 8).[61]

For poor memory, inversion frigidity of the four limbs, incessant laughing, and whitish urine, Broken Sequence (*Lie Que*, Lu 7) is the ruling point.

For bloated chest, and, in serious cases, visual distortion with arms crossed before the chest, sudden *bi*, and counterflow dyspnea, needle Channel Ditch (*Jing Qu*, Lu 8) and Celestial Storehouse (*Tian Fu*, Lu 3), the latter of which is called a grand point.[62]

For cold and heat, coughing, retching of foam, heat in the palm, and, in the case of vacuity, shivering of the shoulders and upper back with cold, diminished qi which is insufficient for respiration, cold inversion, visual distortion with arms crossed before the chest and foaming at the mouth, or, in the case of repletion, heat and pain in the shoulders and upper back, (spontaneous) sweating, fulminant swelling of the four limbs, a dank body ["warm body" in a variant version {later editor}], fidgeting, occasional fever and chills, vexation on hunger, tendency to abnormal facial complexion when having overeaten, clenched jaw, and aversion to wind and tearing, Broken Sequence (*Lie Que*, Lu 7) is the ruling point.[63]

For vexation of the heart, coughing, cold and heat and frequent retching, Palace of Toil (*Lao Gong*, Per 8) is the ruling point.

For cold and heat, dry mouth and lips, generalized fever, panting, acute pain of the eyes, and susceptibility to fright, Third Space (*San Jian*, LI 3) is the ruling point.[64]

For fullness in the chest, pain (in the region) anterior to the auricles, toothache, red painful eyes, swelling in the neck, cold and heat, thirst, and sweating upon drinking but the skin turning dry and hot while not drinking, Pool at the Bend (*Qu Chi*, LI 11) is the ruling point.

For cold and heat cervical scrofula and cough and difficulty breathing, moxa Fifth Place (*Wu Li*, LI 13). For (afflictions) on the left side, treat the right, and for (afflictions) on the right side, treat the left.

For cold and heat cervical scrofula with pain in and inability to raise the shoulders, Upper Arm (*Bi Nao*, LI 14) is the ruling point.[65]

For cold and heat due to wind, Armpit Gate (*Ye Men*, TH 2) is the ruling point.

For cold and heat with swelling in the neck and the submandibular region, Back Ravine (*Hou Xi*, SI 3) is the ruling point.

For cold and heat with frequent retching, Shang Hill (*Shang Qiu*, Sp 5) is the ruling point.

For retching, inversion cold, mild fever from time to time, propping fullness in the free rib regions, sore throat, dry throat, pain in the lateral aspect of the knees, aching and weakness of the lower legs, swollen armpits, saber scrofula, swollen lips, and lesions and pain in the corners of the mouth, Supreme Surge (*Tai Chong*, Liv 3) is the ruling point.[66]

For a suspended sensation of the heart ["heart pain" in the *Qian Jin* {later editor}], yin inversion, hypertonicity of the posterior border of the calf, inability to move either forward or backward, blood *yong*, intestinal *pi* with blood and pus in stools, pain in the instep, curled tongue with inability to speak, frequent laughing, atonic feet such that one no longer fits into their shoes, and green-bluish, reddish, yellowish, or blackish urine, take the well in the case of green-bluish urine, the brook in the case of reddish urine, the rapids in the case of yellowish urine, the stream in the case of whitish urine, or the confluence in the case of blackish urine.[67]

For bloody hemorrhoid, diarrhea, pressure in the rectum, abdominal pain as in dribbling urinary blockage, mania and collapse making support necessary (all the time), great qi, drooling, pain in the nostrils, thunderous rumbling in the abdomen, cold and heat in the bone giving no moment of rest, and incessant sweating, Recover Flow (*Fu Liu*, Ki 7) is the ruling point.[68]

For drum-distention-like disorder in males, and morning sickness-like disorder in females with cold and heat and lower abdominal swelling at one side, Yin Valley (*Yin Gu*, Ki 10) is the ruling point.

For lower abdominal pain, swill diarrhea and chyme-like stool, heat in the small and ring fingers, sunken vessels, fever and chills with generalized pain, dry lips, lack of perspiration, parched hair, shedding of the flesh, diminished qi, heat existing in the interior, disinclination to stir, diarrhea of pus and blood, the lumbus initiating a dragging pain to the lower abdomen, sudden fright (*i.e.*, panic), and outrageous ravings, the Lower Ridge of the Great Hollow (*Ju Xu Xia Lian*, St 39) is the ruling point.[69]

For fullness in the chest, swollen armpit, saber scrofula, frequent biting of the tongue and the cheek, swelling at Celestial Window (*Tian You*, TH 16),[70] aching and weakness in the lower legs, spinning of the head, pain in the occipital bone, submandibular region, and cheek, dry eyes, generalized *bi*, shivering with cold as after a soaking, propping fullness in the free rib region, fever and chills, and pain in the chest, lateral costal region, lumbus, abdomen, and lateral aspect of the knee, Overlooking Tears (*Lin Qi*, GB 41) is the ruling point.[71]

For cold and heat with swelling in the neck, Hill Ruins (*Qiu Xu*, GB 40) is the ruling point.

For cold and heat with swollen neck and armpit, Extending Vessel (*Shen Mai*, GB 62) is the ruling point.

For cold and heat with (generalized) aching and weakness, inability to lift the four limbs, swollen armpit, saber scrofula, throat *bi*, and slackening of the thigh, knee, and lower leg with aching, numbness, and insensitivity, Yang Support (*Yang Fu*, GB 38) is the ruling point.[72]

For cold and heat with debility of the thigh and lower leg, Yang Intersection (*Yang Jiao*, GB 35) is the ruling point.[73]

For cold and heat with the lumbus painful as if about to break, Bundle Bone (*Shu Gu*, Bl 65) is the ruling point.

For cold and heat with blurred vision, frequent coughing, and counterflow dyspnea, Open Valley (*Tong Gu*, Bl 66) is the ruling point.

For cold and heat with frequent sighing, heavy headedness, cold feet, no desire for food, and cramp of the feet, Capital Bone (*Jing Gu*, Bl 64) is the ruling point.

For cold and heat with protrusion of the perineum, Mountain Support (*Cheng Shan*, Bl 57) is the ruling point.[74]

For cold and heat with protrusion of the perineum, tugging and slackening, aching heaviness of the feet and calves, trembling with inability to stand for long, hypertonicity and swelling of the feet, cramps of the sinews of the insteps and feet, lower abdominal pain sending a dragging (discomfort) to the throat, and difficult defecation, Sinew Support (*Cheng Jin*, Bl 56) is the ruling point.[75]

For inversion frigidity of the heels, hypertonicity of the knees, pain in the lumbar spine sending a dragging (discomfort) to the abdomen, heat in the perineum and inner aspect of the thighs, violent pain in the perineum and genitals, fever and chills, and aching heaviness of the knees, Yang Union (*He Yang*, Bl 55) is the ruling point.

Chapter Two

Contraction of Disease Within the
Channels & Network Vessels Entering
the Intestines & Stomach Resulting in
Accumulations in the Five Viscera
Which in Turn Produce Deep-Lying
Beam, Inverted Cup Surging, Fat Qi,
Glomus Qi & Running Piglet[76]

(1)

The Yellow Emperor asked:

At the onset of the hundreds of diseases, the qi of
the three regions may each become damaged in
different ways. Please tell me the (principles
involved).

Qi Bo answered:

Joy or anger that is not in its proper measure
causes damage to the viscera, and when the viscera become damaged, disease arises in the yin. If
cool and dampness make an assault in a vacuity
condition, disease arises below. If wind and rain
make an assault in a vacuity condition, disease
arises above. These are the so-called three
regions. As for (the mechanisms of) sapping and
spreading, there are countless (categories of) disease.[77]

Wind and rain, cold and heat in the absence of a
vacuity evil can do no harm to people. Even after
being unexpectedly caught in furious wind and
crushing rain, some may remain (unhurt and) not
diseased. This is because no harm can be done to
people in absence of vacuity evil. A vacuity evil
wind in conjunction with a constitutional (vacuity) is required; these two kinds of vacuity work
together to intrude on the consitution. (On the
other hand,) when two types of repletion meet,
the muscles of the majority of people are simply
strengthened.[78]

The penetration of vacuity evils depend on the
seasonal disposition and the state of one's consti-

tution, and only from combined vacuity and
repletion does grave disease develop.[79]

(All) qi have fixed dwelling places and are named
for the regions in which they dwell. Accordingly,
(the body) is divided into three cardinal (regions):
above, below, the internal and external.[80]

It follows then that when a vacuity evil strikes an
individual, it begins with the skin. When the skin
becomes slack, the interstices are opened, and
when the interstices are opened, the evil intrudes
via the hair. After the intrusion, it will penetrate a
little deeper. When it is a little deeper, it makes
the hair stand on end, causing shivering and pain
in the skin. If it (is allowed to) become lodged
here and is not expelled, it will be transmitted to
and take up residence in the network vessels.
While (the vacuity evil) is in the network vessels,
there is pain in the muscles. Intermittent pain is
characteristic of this disease. Next the major
channels fall victum. If (allowed to) become
lodged here and not expelled, (the vacuity evil)
will be transmitted to and take up residence in
the channels. While it is in the channel, there will
be shivering as if one had become soaked and
susceptibility to fright. If it (is allowed to) become
lodged here and is not expelled, (the vacuity evil)
will then be transmitted to and take up residence
in the transport (vessel). While it is in the transport (vessel), the six channels are blocked with
pain in the joints of the four limbs and rigidity of
the lumbar spine. If it is (allowed to) become
lodged here and is not expelled, (the vacuity evil)
will then be transmitted to and take up residence
in the deep-lying penetrating vessel. While in the
deep-lying penetrating vessel, the body becomes
heavy and painful. If it (is allowed to) become
lodged here and is not expelled, (the vacuity evil)
will be transmitted to and take up residence in
the stomach and intestines. While it is in the
stomach and intestines, there will be abdominal
distention with thunderous sound. In the case of
abundant cold, there will be intestinal rumbling
and swill diarrhea with untransformed food, and
in the case of abundant heat, there will be diarrhea with chyme-like stools. If it (is allowed to)
become lodged and is not expelled, (the vacuity
evil) will be transmitted to and take up residence

301

in between membranes outside the stomach and the intestines. (At this point, the vacuity evil) becomes lodged in the vessels and if it becomes lodged here and is not expelled, it will stay and become an accumulation.[81]

(Accumulations) may settle in (many locations, including) the minute network vessels, the network vessels, the channels, the transport vessel, the deep-lying penetrating vessel, the paravertebral sinews, or the membranes of the stomach and intestines, which link with the slack sinew above. Thus, the evil qi may sap and spread in countless ways.[82]

When (evil) lodges in the minute network vessels and produces accumulations, (these accumulations) travel up and down. The arms and hands are the residence of the minute network vessels. Since (the minute vessels) are superficial and sluggish, they are unable to confine and arrest the movement of the accumulation. Therefore, the accumulation travels to and fro, causing the water inside the intestines to converge, percolate, pour, and irrigate. This produces a gurgling sound. (In addition,) if there is cold, this causes abdominal distention and thundering fullness. (All these factors) account for occasional lancinating pain.[83]

(Accumulations) lodging in the (foot) yang ming channel remain bilateral to the umbilicus, enlarging in satiety and lessening in hunger.[84]

Those that lodge in the slack sinews resemble the yang ming accumulations. They become painful in satiety but calm in hunger.

(Accumulations) lodging in the membranes of the stomach and intestines connect to the slack sinew externally when painful. They become quiet in satiety but painful in hunger.[85]

(Accumulations) lodging in the deep-lying penetrating vessel pulsate under the hand with pressure, but when one takes one's hands away, hot qi radiates down both thighs which then feel as if they are immersed in hot water. (Accumulations) lodging in the paravertebral

sinews lie behind the intestines. When hungry, these manifest themselves but when satiated, they disappear and are no longer palpable. (Accumulation) lodging in the transport vessel causes obstruction and blockage, arresting the descent of fluid and humor and drying the hollow portals. This is the course of the invasion of evil qi from the exterior to the interior and from above to below.[86]

The Yellow Emperor asked:

What happens at the initial stage of accumulation before it has matured?

Qi Bo answered:

At its genesis, the affliction of cold generates (accumulation), and it is the ascending (counterflow) of inversion (qi) that produces its shape.[87]

The Yellow Emperor asked:

How does it develop?

Qi Bo answered:

Inversion qi produces spillage in the feet ["distressed sensation in the feet" in the Ling Shu {later editor}], and spillage in the feet (in turn) produces cold in the lower legs. Cold in the lower legs congeals the blood in the vessels there. (Subsequently,) the cold qi ascends, entering the stomach and intestines. Once it has entered the stomach and intestines, there will be distention and fullness. This distention and fullness oppresses and gathers the sap and foam outside the intestines which are unable to dissipate. Thus the accumulation takes shape day by day.[88]

If one suddenly eats and drinks too much at a meal, this fills up the vessels, while an irregular lifestyle and overexertion damage the network vessels. If the yang network vessels are damaged, blood spills outward, resulting in nosebleeding. If the yin network vessels are damaged, blood spills inward, resulting in blood in the stools. When the network vessels outside the intestines are damaged, blood spills outside the intestines. If there is cold outside the intestines, the sap and foam and the blood will wrestle with one another, causing them to mingle, congeal, and coalesce together. Left with no way to dissipate, they develop into accumulation.[89]

As a result of a sudden external stroke of cold and internal damage due to worry and anger, the qi may counterflow upward. When qi counterflows upward, the six transport (channels) become blocked, so that the warm qi cannot circulate. (Hence) the blood congeals, massing up and becoming entangled without dispersing. Fluid and humor congeal and stagnate, becoming lodged and unable to leave. >From this, the various kinds of accumulations develop.[90]

The Yellow Emperor asked:

How is (accumulation) generated in the yin?

Qi Bo answered:

Worry and thought injure the heart. Dual cold injures the lung. Indignation and anger injure the liver. Sexual intercourse while intoxicated or when having overeaten and being exposed to a draft with sweating injure the spleen. Overexertion and sweating during or after taking a bath immediately after sexual intercourse injure the kidney[91]

This is how the disease is generated internally and externally in the three regions of the body. (One should) first examine (the nature of) the pain to determine (the nature of the imbalance) that it reflects. As for surplus and insufficiency, that which requires supplementation must be supplemented, while that which requires drainage must be drained. By never acting counter to the seasonal disposition, an immaculate treatment may be performed.[92]

(2)

The Yellow Emperor asked:

What are the indicators for those who tend toward gatherings and accumulations in the intestines?

Qi Bo answered:

(Those at risk have) thin and lusterless skin with weak and moist muscles. This being the case, the stomach and intestines are in bad condition. With them in bad condition, the evil qi becomes lodged and rests (inside them), giving rise to gatherings and accumulations in the stomach and intestines. (Furthermore, in the case of immoderate consumption of) cold and warm (food or drink), the evil qi ["a small amount of evil qi" in a variant version {later editor}] may reach (more deeply), where it accumulates and settles, building up. Thus great gatherings come into being.[93]

(3)

The Yellow Emperor asked:

What sort of disease is characterized by swelling all over the lumbus, the hips, the thighs, and the lower legs with pain around the umbilicus?

Qi Bo answered:

It is called the deep-lying beam. This is rooted in wind, and cannot be stirred; once stirred, it will give rise to water (stagnation), an illness characterized by rough urination[94]

A disease characterized by fullness in the lower abdomen with roots right and left, above and below, is called the deep-lying beam. Since there is a great amount of pus and blood wrapped within it, which is located outside the stomach and intestines, it cannot be treated. Pressing and palpating (for the purpose of examination often) results in death. When it moves down, it will depress the genitals, giving rise to pus and blood in the urine and stools. When it moves upward, it will press against the venter and may protrude through the diaphragmatic pass ["border" in variant version {later editor}] to cause internal *yong* around ["adjacent to" in a variant version {later editor}] the venter. It is a protracted disorder that is difficult to treat. (The prognosis is) unforvorable if located above the umbilicus, but favorable if located below the umbilicus. Efforts to snatch it by force are prohibited. Because its qi spills ["drains" in the *Su Wen* {later editor}] into the large intestine, and it fixes to the mesentery whose origination is found below the umbilicus, there is pain around the umbilicus.[95]

(4)

The *Nan Jing (Classic of Difficult Issues)* states[96] that accumulation of the heart is called deep-lying beam. It spreads upward from above the umbilicus to below the heart and is as big as the forearm. It can be a protracted (illness) and, (if left untreated), may present with vexation of the heart and heart pain. It is contracted on *geng* and *xin* days[97] during the autumn. Once a kidney illness has been transmitted to the heart, the heart should transmit it to the lung. However, since the lung presides over the autumn and cannot contract evils during this season, the disease must lodge and bind (in the heart) where it develops into accumulation.[98]

The *Nan Jing* states that accumulation of the lung is called inverted cup surging. It is located in the right lateral costal region and looks like a large, upside down cup. It can be a protracted illness and, if left untreated, may present with shivering and aversion to cold and qi counterflow dyspnea and coughing leading to lung *yong*. It is contracted on *jia* and *yi* days in spring. Once the heart has transmitted the disease to the lung, the lung should transmit it to the liver. However, since the liver presides over the spring and cannot contract evils in this season, the disease must lodge and bind (in the lung) where it develops into accumulation.[99]

(5)

The Yellow Emperor asked:

What sort of disease is characterized by fullness in the lateral costal region and qi counterflow, and which can last for two or three years?

Qi Bo answered:

This illness is called inverted cup surging (*xi ben*, 息贲). It does not affect food intake, nor may it

(be treated with) moxibustion or needling. (To treat it, one should) combine cultivation of qi with medication. Medication alone will not cure it.[100]

(6)

The *Nan Jing* states that accumulation of the liver is called fat qi. It is located in the left lateral costal region and looks like an inverted cup with a head and feet so that it resembles a turtle. It can be a protracted illness and, (if left untreated), is characterized by counterflow cough and *nue* which are perennial. It is contracted on *wu* and *ji* days in late summer. Once the lung has transmitted the disease to the liver, the liver should transmit it to the spleen. However, since the spleen presides over late summer and cannot contract evils in this season, the disease must lodge and bind (in the liver) where it develops into accumulation. This is similar to inverted cup surging.[101]

The *Nan Jing* states that accumulation of the spleen is called glomus qi. It is located in the venter and looks like a large inverted plate. It can be a protracted illness and, (if left untreated,) is characterized by debility of the four limbs, jaundice, and failure of food and drink to nourish the skin and muscles. It is contracted on *ren* and *gui* days in winter. Once the liver has transmitted the disease to the spleen, the spleen ought to transmit it to the kidney. However, since the kidney presides over winter and cannot contract evils in this season, the disease must lodge and bind (in the spleen) where it develops into accumulation.[102]

The *Nan Jing* states that accumulation of the kidney is called running piglet. It arises from the lower abdomen and reaches up to (the region) under the heart. When present, it moves up and down in an unpredictable manner. It can be a protracted illness causing people to suffer from counterflow dyspnea, atony of the bone, and diminished qi. It is contracted on *bing* and *ding* days in summer. Once the spleen has transmitted the disease to the kidney, the kidney should then transmit it to the heart. However, since the heart presides over summer and cannot contract evils in this season, the disease must lodge and bind (in the kidney) where it develops into accumulation.

(7)

For spitting of blood during an episode of inverted cup surging, Great Tower Gate (*Ju Que*, CV 14) is the ruling point.

For accumulation in the abdomen circulating up and down, Suspended Pivot (*Xuan Shu*, GV 5) is the ruling point.

For *shan* accumulation with pain in the chest and inability to catch the breath, Celestial Countenence (*Tian Rong*, SI 17) is the ruling point.[103]

For sudden heart and abdominal pain and (qi) surging up into the heart during frequent episodes of *shan* accumulation, Cloud Gate (*Yun Men*, Lu 2) is the ruling point.

For enlargement and hardening below the heart, Huang Shu (*Huang Shu*, Ki 16), Cycle Gate (*Qi Men*, Liv 14), and Central Venter (*Zhong Wan*, CV 12) are the ruling points.

For umbilical *shan*, periumbilical pain, and (qi) surging up into the chest with inability to catch the breath, moxa Qi Center (*Qi Zhong*, M-CA-10)[104]

For running piglet and qi ascension, abdominal distention and hardness with pain radiating to the genitals, inability to urinate, and retracted testicles, Yin Intersection (*Yin Jiao*, CV 7) is the ruling point.

For umbilical *shan* with periumbilical pain, Stone Gate (*Shi Men*, CV 5) is the ruling point.

For running piglet with qi ascension, distention and pain in the abdomen, rigidity of the mouth with loss of the ability to speak, penile swelling initially producing a dragging (discomfort) in the lumbus and later in the lower abdomen, hardness and pain in the lumbus, hips, and lower abdomen producing a dragging (discomfort) in the genitals, inability to urinate, and retracted testicles, Stone Gate (*Shi Men*, CV 5) is the ruling point.

For running piglet with cold qi penetrating the lower abdomen, occasional desire to retch, urination of blood due to internal damage, frequent urination, pain in the upper and lower back and the umbilicus producing a dragging (discomfort) in the genitals, hypertonicity of the abdomen which feels as if it were being drawn together, and incessant diarrhea, Origin Pass (*Guan Yuan*, CV 4) is the ruling point.

For running piglet with (qi) surging up into the heart and, in extreme cases, symptoms of inability to catch one's breath, an empty sensation in the heart with diminished qi, deathlike inversion, heart vexation and pain, hunger but inability to ingest food, frequent cold in the center with abdominal distention sending a dragging pain to the lateral costal region, sudden dragging pain between the lower abdomen and the spine, and occasional pressure in the rectum, Central Pole (*Zhong Ji*, CV 3) is the ruling point.

For gatherings and accumulations in the abdomen with occasional lancinating pain, Shang Bend (*Shang Qu*, Ki 17) is the ruling point.

For gatherings and accumulations with *shan* conglomeration and blood (stasis) in the uterus, Fourfold Fullness (*Si Man*, Ki 14) is the ruling point.

For umbilical *shan* with periumbilical pain and occasional (qi) surging upward into the heart, Celestail Pivot (*Tian Shu*, St 25) is the ruling point.

For qi *shan* with distressed retching, swollen face, and running piglet, Celestial Pivot (*Tian Shu*, St 25) is the ruling point.[105]

For running piglet with the testicles retracted into the abdomen initiating a dragging pain in the penis, Return (*Gui Lai*, St 28) is the ruling point.

For running piglet with (qi) moving up and down, Cycle Gate (*Qi Men*, Liv 14) is the ruling point.

For *shan* conglomeration with hypertonicity and pain in the upper thighs, (qi) surging up and down along the lateral costal regions and into the heart, and fullness in the abdomen with gathering and accumulations, Bowel Abode (*Fu She*, Sp 13) is the ruling point.

For running piglet with abdominal swelling, Camphorwood Gate (*Zhang Men*, Liv 13) is the ruling point.

For gatherings and accumulations in the lower abdomen, Palace of Toil (*Lao Gong*, Per 8) is the ruling point.

For periumbilical pain, penile contraction, testicular retraction, hardness and pain in the abdomen, and inability to lie down, Supreme Surge (*Tai Chong*, Liv 3) is the ruling point.

For cold *shan* extending into the abdominal striae and knees and lumbar region which are painful like cold water; (for) various *shan* in the upper abdomen ["the lower abdomen" in a variant version {later editor}] with cold extending down to the Crouching Rabbit (*Fu Tu*, St 32) when (the *shan* is) pressed; and (for) painful *shan* with abdominal distention and fullness, atonic inversion, and diminished qi, Yin Market (*Yin Shi*, St 33) is the ruling point.[106]

For large *shan* with hardness in the abdomen, Hill Ruins (*Qiu Xu*, GB 40) is the ruling point.

Chapter Three

Distentions of the Five Viscera & Six Bowels[107]

(1)

The Yellow Emperor asked:

How is distension reflected at the *cun kou* pulse?

Qi Bo answered:

A pulse that arrives large, hard, and straight as well as rough indicates distention.[108]

The Yellow Emperor asked:

How may visceral and bowel distention (respectively) be identified in the pulse?

Qi Bo answered:

The yin points to visceral (distension), while the yang to bowel (distension).[109]

The Yellow Emperor asked:

It is qi that causes people to suffer from distention. Does it lie in the blood vessels or within the viscera and the bowels?

Qi Bo answered:

It lies within both of them, but neither of them is the dwelling place of distention.[110]

The Yellow Emperor asked:

Please tell me the dwelling place of distention.

Qi Bo answered:

Distension of any kind lies outside the viscera and bowels. It presses on the viscera and the bowels and dilates the chest and lateral costal regions, distending the skin. (For) these reasons, it is called distention.

The Yellow Emperor asked:

Just as holy articles are kept in a box or cabinet, so the viscera and the bowels lie within the body. They reside in their proper sequence and carry different names although they are accommodated in the same place. While they dwell in the same region, their (respective) qi differ from one another. Please tell me about the reasons.

Qi Bo answered:

The chest and abdomen are the city precincts of the viscera and the bowels. The center of the chest is the central palace of the heart. The stomach is the great granary. The pharynx and larynx and the small intestine are the transport roads. The five openings of the stomach are the gates of the alley and neighborhood. And Ridge Spring (*Lian Quan*, CV 23) and Jade Beauty (*Yu Ying*, CV 18) are the roadways for fluid and humor. Thus, the five viscera and the six bowels each have their own boundaries and, when they are diseased, they each have a distinct presentation.[111]

If the constructive qi flows along inside the vessel but the defensive qi counterflows, then vascular distention ensues. If the defensive qi merges with the blood vessel and runs along the borders of the flesh, this produces cutaneous distention. [The *Ling Shu* states that, "If the defensive qi runs along the vessel, vascular distention ensues. If the constructive qi becomes subsumed within the vessel and runs in the borders of flesh, cutaneous distention ensues." {later editor}] (Distention requires that one) drain Three Li (*San Li*, St 36). For a recent case, one treatment ["one *fen* deep" in a variant version; the same hereafter {later editor}] is enough, and for a chronic case, three treatments are sufficient. Regardless of whether this is a case of vacuity or repletion, the task is one of prompt drainage.[112]

The Yellow Emperor asked:

Tell me how distension presents itself.

Qi Bo answered:

Heart distention is characterized by vexation of the heart, shortage of breath, and disturbed sleep. Lung distention is characterized by vacuity fullness, dyspnea, and cough. Liver distention presents with fullness in the region of the free ribs with pain radiating to the lateral lower abdomen. Spleen distention presents with tormenting retching, vexation and oppression of the four limbs, and generalized heaviness with inability (even) to dress oneself. Kidney distention is characterized by abdominal fullness sending a dragging (discomfort) to the back and vexing pain in the lumbus and upper thighs. Stomach distention is characterized by abdominal fullness, pain in the venter, a foul burning smell in the nose impairing the appetite, and difficult defecation. Large intes-

tine distention presents with rumbling and pain in the intestine and, in the case of cold, diarrhea containing untransformed food. Small intestine distention is characterized by lateral lower abdominal distention and fullness producing a dragging pain in the lumbus. Urinary bladder distention presents with fullness in the lower abdomen and dribbling urinary qi block. Triple burner distention is characterized by fullness of qi in the skin which seems taut but not solid. Gallbladder distension is manifested by pain and distention in the region of the free ribs, bitter taste in the mouth, and frequent sighing.[113]

(In the treatment of) the various types of distention, there is a unifying principle. A clear awareness of normal flow and counterflow will preclude any failure in the administration of acupuncture. If vacuity is drained and repletion is supplemented, the spirit will take leave of its office. This is inviting the evil and losing the correct so that the true (qi) is incapable of maintaining stability. The blunder of the inferior practitioner is tantamount to the taking of life. (Those who) treat vacuity by supplementation and repletion by drainage to send the spirit back to its office and fill the void for some time are considered superior practitioners.[114]

The Yellow Emperor asked:

How is distention generated and why is it so named?

Qi Bo answered:

The defensive qi usually travels in the body side by side with the vessels and runs along the borders of flesh. It flows up and down (in a regular way). When yin and yang flow with one another, heavenly harmony is maintained, the five viscera are all ruled in good order, the seasonal despositions are always conformed to, and the five grains are transformed. When there is inversion qi below, however, the constructive and defensive cease to flow, cold qi counterflows upward and the true and evil qi attack one another. The two qi are locked in a conflict and comingle, resulting in distention.[115]

The Yellow Emperor asked:

How is this confusion resolved?

Qi Bo answered:

It is entangled with the true, and three entanglements suffice.[116]

The Yellow Emperor asked:

(It is said that,) regardless of (whether the condition is one of) of vacuity or repletion, the task (of the practitioner consists of) prompt drainage. For a recent case, one treatment is enough, while for a chronic case, three treatments are sifficient. (If) three treatments fail to downbear (the evil qi), what accounts for this failure?

Qi Bo answered:

This statement presupposes that one has penetrated the interstices in the flesh to hit the qi point. If one fails to strike the point of qi, then the qi remains blocked and confined. If one fails to penetrate the interstices of the flesh, then the qi is unable to circulate. Failure to reach the intermediate flesh causes the defensive qi to become deranged, resulting in counterflow of yin and yang.[117]

When distended, it should be treated by drainage, and, if it is not drained, the (evil) qi will not descend. If three treatments (performed in a proper way) fail to downbear (the qi), one must change one's approach until the qi has descended. In one fails once more, try again. (This) ensures complete success, and there will not be a single case of failure.

(The treatment of) distention requires careful examination. That which requires drainage must be treated with drainage; that which requires supplementation must be treated with supplementation. As the drum responds to the beating of the stick, so this will downbear (the evil qi).[118]

(2)

For heart distention, Heart Shu (*Xin Shu*, Bl 15) is the ruling point, and Broken Sequence (*Lie Que*, Lu 7) may also be taken.

For lung distention, Lung Shu (*Fei Shu*, Bl 13) is the ruling point, and Supreme Abyss (*Tai Yuan*, Lu 9) may also be taken.

For liver distention, Liver Shu (*Gan Shu*, Bl 18) is the ruling point, and Supreme Surge (*Tai Chong*, Liv 3) may also be taken.

For spleen distention, Spleen Shu (*Pi Shu*, Bl 20) is the ruling point, and Supreme White (*Tai Bai*, Sp 3) may also be taken.

For kidney distention, Kidney Shu (*Shen Shu*, Bl 23) is the ruling point, and Great Ravine (*Tai Xi*, Ki 3) may also be taken.

For stomach distention, Central Venter (*Zhong Wan*, CV 12) is the ruling point, and Camphorwood Gate (*Zhang Men*, Liv 13) may also be taken.

For large intestine distention, Celestial Pivot (*Tian Shu*, St 25) is the ruling point.

For small intestine distention, Central Bone Hole (*Zhong Liao*, Bl 33) is the ruling point.

For urinary bladder distention, Crooked Bone (*Qu Gu*, CV 2) is the ruling point.

For triple burner distention, Stone Door (*Shi Men*, CV 5) is the ruling point.

For gallbladder distention, Yang Mound Spring (*Yang Ling Quan*, GB 34) is the ruling point.

For any of the distentions of the five viscera and the six bowels, (one should) take Three Li (*San Li*, St 36). Three Li is the most important point for distention.

Chapter Four

Water (Swelling), Skin Distention, Drum Distention, Intestinal Mushroom & Stone Conglomeration[119]

(1)

The Yellow Emperor asked:

How may water (swelling), skin distention, drum distention, intestinal mushroom (*chang tan*,肠覃), and stone conglomeration be distinguished?

Qi Bo answered:

At the onset of water (swelling), the eyelids are slightly swollen, looking as if one has just arisen from sleep. (When) the vessel in the neck beats (tangibly) and there is occasional cough, cold in the medial aspect of the thighs, swelling of the feet and lower legs, and abdominal enlargement, the water (swelling) is (fully) developed. Try pressing the abdomen with one's hand. If the dent fills up as if (the abdomen) were enveloped in water as soon as the hand is removed, this is an indicator (of water swelling).[120]

Skin distention is caused by the intrusion of cold qi into the skin which becomes taut but not solid with enlargement of the abdomen. There is swelling all over the body and thickening of the skin. If (one) presses the abdomen and the dent remains unchanged (after removal of the pressure) and the abdominal color remains normal, these are indicators (of skin distention).[121]

Drum distention is characterized by abdominal distention and generalized swelling, as in the case of skin distention. The color (of the abdominal skin) which is somber yellow and prominent abdominal sinews ["vessels" in a variant version {later editor}] are indicators (of drum distention).

Intestinal mushroom is caused by the intrusion of cold qi outside the intestines. The cold qi contends with the defensive qi, and, as a result, the righteous qi is unable to operate (in a normal way). This allows the (evil qi) to gain a footing and become glomus, which settles internally. (Then) the foul qi erupts, and a polyp is generated. At the beginning, the polyp is as large as a hen's egg, but it gradually grows bigger and bigger. When it is mature, it looks as large as a baby during pregnancy. A long-standing (lump) may last over a year. When pressed, it is hard. When pushed, it is movable. And menstruation comes in due time. These are indicators (of intestinal mushroom).[122]

Stone conglomeration grows within the uterus. When cold qi intrudes, the infant's gate shuts and becomes blocked, qi does not flow freely, and the foul blood cannot be discharged when it ought. (Thus) coagulated blood settles down and grows bigger and bigger until it looks like a child in pregnancy, and menstruation fails to come in due time. It grows in females only and can be treated by abducting precipitation.

The Yellow Emperor asked:

Can either skin or drum distention be treated by needling?

Qi Bo answered:

First prick the blood vessels in the abdomen, and then regulate the (pertinent) channel. In addition, (one) may remove the blood vessels (of the channel) by means of needling.

(2)

The Yellow Emperor asked:

What kind of disease is heart and abdominal fullness with inability to eat in the evening if breakfast is taken in the morning?

Qi Bo answered:

This is called drum distention. It can be treated with the Chicken Droppings Tincture (*Ji Shi Li*,鸡矢醴).[123] One dose will be able to show (improvement) and, with another, (the patient) will be cured.

309

The Yellow Emperor asked:

What causes relapse in some cases?

Qi Bo answered:

This is due to dietary irregularity which causes the disease to recur from time to time. Although the disease is very nearly resolved, (these dietary irregularities) are bound to cause the diseased qi to accumulate in the abdomen.

(3)

Wind water skin distention calls for the fifty-seven needling (points).[124] (One should) take the blood (vessels found) in the skin, leaving none unpricked. In the presence of water alone, (one should) first take the point three *cun* below the circling valley with a sword needle (*pei zhen*, 排针). Inserted deep, the needle should be (repeatedly) withdrawn and pushed in, extracted and inserted to drain out the water. (After that, the waist) should be bound up tightly. Binding of the waist loosely only produces vexation and oppression, while binding tightly quiets (the patient). Needling should be administered once every other day till the water has been drained off. (The patient) should drink blocking medicinals. Drink the medicinals just prior to needling, eating nothing else soon after or shortly before. In addition, a diet should be kept for one hundred and thirty-five days.[125]

(4)

Water swelling with a brimming philtrum and outturned lips ends in death. (For it,) Water Trough (*Shui Gou*, GV 26) is the ruling point.[126]

For water swelling with protuberant navel, moxa Center of the Navel (*Qi Zhong*, a.k.a. *Shen Que*, CV 8). Disappearance of skin texture on the abdomen means (the condition) is incurable.[127]

For water distention characterized by water qi moving within the skin, Yin Intersection (*Yin Jiao*, GV 28) is the ruling point.[128]

For water swelling characterized by an enlarged abdomen, water distention, and water qi moving within the skin, Stone Gate (*Shi Men*, CV 5) is the ruling point.

For stone water with pain initiating distention in the free rib regions, spinning and ache of the head, and generalized fever, Origin Pass (*Guan Yuan*, CV 4) is the ruling point.[129]

For stone water characterized by shivering with cold and an enlarged abdomen, Fourfold Fullness (*Si Man*, Ki 14) is the ruling point.

For stone water, needle Qi Surge (*Qi Chong*, St 30).

For stone water, Camphorwood Gate (*Zhang Men*, Liv 13) and Burning Valley (*Ran Gu*, Ki 2) are the ruling points.

For stone water, Celestial Spring (*Tian Quan*, Per 2) is the ruling point.

For exuberance of (cold) qi in the abdomen, abdominal distention, and counterflow dyspnea ["water distention and counterflow" in the *Qian Jin* {later editor}] with inability to lie down, Yin Mound Spring (*Yin Ling Quan*, Sp 9) is the ruling point.

For water swelling with retained rheum and propping fullness in the chest and lateral costal regions, prick Sunken Valley (*Xian Gu*, St 43). When the blood emerges, (the patient) will be cured on the spot.

For abdominal water distention with swollen skin, Three Li (*San Li*, St 36) is the ruling point.

For large *shan* conglomeration, gathering and accumulation in the uterus with a dragging pain in the external genitals, and tormenting vomiting above and diarrhea below, apply supplementation at Cubit Marsh (*Chi Ze*, Lu 5), Great Ravine (*Tai Xi*, Ki 3) and the hand *yang ming*[130] and the *cun kou*.[131, 132]

Chapter Five

Kidney Wind Producing Wind Water Puffy Facial Swelling[133]

(1)

The Yellow Emperor asked:

Why does the *shao yin* govern the kidney and why does the kidney govern water?

Qi Bo answered:

The kidney is the consummate yin, and the consummate yin is exuberant water. The lung is the great yin. Because the *shao yin*, a channel of winter, has its root in the kidney and its end in the lung, the kidney and the lung are both responsible for accumulation of water.[134]

The Yellow Emperor asked:

How is it that the kidney may gather water to generate disease?

Qi Bo answered:

The kidney is the pass of the stomach. When the pass gates are shut and inhibited, water will gather and appeal to that which is of its kind, spilling into the skin above and below. This results in puffy swelling. Puffy swelling is a disease generated from an accumulation of water.[135]

The Yellow Emperor asked:

Are all types of water governed by the kidney?

Qi Bo answered:

The kidney is a feminine viscus. The earthly qi which ascends is ascribed to and turned into water fluid by the kidney. For this reason, it is called the consummate yin.[136]

(Unscrupulously) striving to parade strength by overtaxation forces the kidney sweat to emerge. (If accidentally) exposed to wind, the emerging kidney sweat will find no way to enter the bowels and viscera internally or to effuse through the skin externally. Thus, it intrudes on the dark mansion and circulates within the skin to develop into puffy swelling. The disease is rooted in the kidney and is called wind water.[137]

(2)

The Yellow Emperor asked:

In kidney wind diseases, the face may become hideously puffy and swollen to the extent that it hampers speech. Can this condition be needled?

Qi Bo answered:

Vacuity (conditions of this nature) should not be needled. If needling is applied in defiance of this prohibition, after five days, the (evil) qi is sure to come.[138]

The Yellow Emperor asked:

What happens when the (evil) qi arrives?

Qi Bo answered:

When it arrives, the qi is invariably diminished. There is intermittent heat spreading from the chest and upper back up to the head with sweating, heat in the hands, dry mouth with a bitter taste (*ku*) and thirst, yellowish urine, swollen lower eyelids, rumbling in the abdomen, generalized heaviness with difficulty in walking, amenorrhea, vexation with inability to ingest food, and inability to lie supine or serious coughing when lying in a supine position. This disease is called wind water.[139]

The Yellow Emperor asked:

Please tell me the cause (of this illness).

Qi Bo answered:

Where the evil is drawn, the qi there must be vacuous, and where there is yin vacuity, yang must be drawn towards it. It follows that qi becomes diminished with intermittent heat, sweating, and yellowish urine. Yellowish urine is due to the existence of heat in the lower abdomen. Inability to lie supine is due to disharmony of the stomach. Severe coughing when lying in a supine position posture is due to upward oppression of the lung. In all types of water qi, slight swelling first appears in the lower eyelids.[140]

The Yellow Emperor asked:

What reasons do you have for saying this?

Qi Bo answered:

Water is yin and the lower eyelids are also yin. (Furthermore,) the abdomen is the abode where consummate yin dwells. Therefore, when water exists in the abdomen, it never fails to result in swelling in the lower eyelids. Since the true qi counterflows upward (in this case), this results in a bitter taste in the mouth, dry tongue, and inability to lie supine or severe coughing when lying supine with the emission of clear water. In any type of water disease, there arises inability to lie down. Lying down provokes fright, and fright causes serious coughing. Rumbling in the abdomen is because the disease has its root in the stomach. Since the spleen is oppressed, there is vexation and inability to ingest food. This inability of food to descend is due to obstruction in the venter. Generalized heaviness with difficulty in walking is because the channel of the stomach runs in the feet. Amenorrhea is due to blockage of the uterine vessel, a vessel belonging to the heart and connecting with the uterus. Now that the qi goes up to oppress the lung, the heart qi is no longer able to flow down, thus giving rise to amenorrhea.[141]

(3)

The Yellow Emperor asked:

There is a disease characterized by hideous water qi-like swelling with a pulse which feels large and tight, an absence of pain in the body, and no emaciation of the form in spite of inability to ingest food or a diminished food intake. What is the name of this disease?

Qi Bo answered:

This disease is governed by ["generated in" in the *Su Wen* {later editor}] the kidney and is called kidney wind. It (is characterized by) inability to ingest food and susceptibility to fright. {later editor}] If the heart qi wilts, it may be fatal.[142]

(4)

For wind water swelling of the face, the Upper Ridge of the Great Hollow (*Ju Xu Shang Liang*, a.k.a. *Shang Ju Xu*, St 37) is the ruling point.

For puffy swelling of the face, Upper Star (*Shang Xing*, GV 23) is the ruling point. It is necessary first to take Yi Xi (*Yi Xi*, BL 45) and finally Celestial Window (*Tian You*, TH 19) and Wind Pool (*Feng Chi*, GB 20).

For wind water puffy swelling of the face ["floating" instead of "swelling" in a variant version {later editor}], Surging Yang (*Chong Yang*, St 42) is the ruling point.

For wind water swelling of the face with a black complexion in the forehead, Ravine Divide (*Jie Xi*, St 41) is the ruling point.

Endnotes

[1]Part 1 is derived from Chap. 19, *Su Wen*; Part 2 from Chap. 70, Vol. 10, *Ling Shu*; Part 3 from Chap. 46, Vol. 7, *Ling Shu*; Part 4 from Chap. 21, Vol. 5, *Ling Shu*; Part 5 from Chap. 23, Vol. 5, *Ling Shu*; Part 6 from Chap. 60, *Su Wen*; and Part 7 from *Zhen Jiu Ming Tang Zhi Yao*.

[2]Disease is transmitted along the restraint cycle. For instance lung metal transmits to liver wood transmits to spleen earth transmits to kidney water transmits to heart fire. If a disease is transmitted at a pace of one viscus per night and one viscus per day, it takes it three days to return to the viscus of origin. If it is transmitted at a rate of one viscus per day, it takes six days to complete the circuit. If it is

transmitted at a tempo of one viscus every fort-night, it takes three months to do so. If disease is transmitted at a rate of one viscus per one month, it takes six months to complete a cycle. When the disease returns to the viscus of origin, death ensues.

3Yang pertains to the exterior and external manifesta-tions, while yin pertains to the interior and the condition of the internal viscera, the visceral qi. One can determine which channel is involved by examining the external signs. Thereby the origins of a disease may be understood. Determining a prognosis may be made based on an understand-ing of the visceral qi. Death comes when, for example, a disease involving the lung progresses to the phase restraining the lung, i.e., the phase of fire heart.

4All diseases are generated by wind. In other words, wind is responsible for an innumerable variety of illnesses since it is regarded as the leader of all dis-eases. The nature of wind cold evil is toward con-traction. Therefore, when it penetrates the body, it forces the interstices shut. Consequently, the defensive or yang qi can no longer effuse into the exterior and becomes depressed. This depression of the exterior invariably generates heat. If exter-nal wind cold enters the body and is not exterior-ized in a timely fashion, it will become lodged in the channels obstructing the qi and blood, and thus giving rise to numbness, etc. There is a com-plete description of drug ironing in Chapter 1, Book 10.

5The lung governs the skin and hair. If evils become lodged in the skin and hair and are not removed, they tend to intrude first upon the lung. Lung bi is caused by obstruction of the lung qi. Its symptoms are qi counterflow coughing and, in the extreme, counterflow retching.

6This is a case of lung metal restraining liver wood. If not cured, a lung disease will become a liver dis-ease. Because the liver qi tends to be undisciplined and to ascend, it easily develops into inversion. This implies chaotic movement or counterflow. When the liver qi counterflows, water and grain cannot descend but are brought up by the coun-terflow. As a result, one vomits immediately fol-lowing ingestion of food.

7When wind cold penetrates the spleen, it transforms into heat and combines with dampness to produce jaundice.

Our source edition reads, "diaphoresis" instead of "massage", and this is corrected in accordance with the Su Wen. Fire-branding means moxibus-tion and, in the Su Wen, it is replaced by "bathing."

8Gu was believed to be a kind of worm which could squeeze into the abdomen, sucking blood and causing an enlarged belly. There are two types of shan conglomeration. One is characterized by heat and pain in the lower abdomen with whitish urine, i.e., white turbidity. The other is character-ized by swollen masses in the lower abdomen with intermittent pain and an upsurge of qi. This latter type is referred to as shan in males and is called conglomeration in females.

9The blood vessels are governed by the heart and, therefore, they tend to be affected when the heart is diseased.

10If the transmission of disease is discontinued, death comes in ten days. If it is transmitted further through a second cycle, it will result in secondary damage to the five viscera. The five viscera cannot bear this new damage, and, as a result, death is hastened. Zhang Jing-yue explains in his Lei Jing (The Classified Classic), "The reason for death three years later is that when wind evils have passed round the five viscera, death should ensue imme-diately. If it does not, this means that the original qi has not yet been vanquished and the disease will progress at a slow speed. Once the lung has suffered from evils a second time, the lung will shift (the illness) on to the liver the next year. A year later, the liver will shift it on to the spleen, and in one more year, the spleen will shift the ill-ness on to the kidney. When the three yin have all been vanquished, death should come."

This explanation, however, is less plausible than that of Hua Shou who states in his Su Wen Chao (Transcribed Copy of the Basic Questions), "Three years should read three days." He explains that two rounds of the five viscera should end in death, and this process takes ten days. Because seven days has passed since the lung first transmitted the disease to its restrained viscus, it will take the disease three days to run through the rest of the viscera, i.e., the liver, spleen, and kidney from the heart and lung, and death is sure to come by then. When the kidney transmits the disease to the lung, fire and metal are locked in a conflict. In this case, cold arises if metal prevails or heat arises if fire prevails. Thus there may be symptoms of alternat-ing cold and heat.

11External contractions abide by the laws of transmis-sion of illnesses, while the seven affects do not. Therefore, they may have a devastating effect on the five viscera.

12Joy makes the heart vacuous. Since the heart is fire

and is restrained by water, the kidney qi may overwhelm it when it is weakened by joy. Anger makes the liver qi hyperactive and sorrow produces tension in the lung qi. This accounts for an overwhelming of the spleen and lung qi. Fright injures the kidney which is water, and, therefore, spleen earth overwhelms it. There are five kinds of diseases each of which involves one of the five viscera, and these illnesses may be transmitted in five ways. Thus there are twenty–five variant diseases. It is of note that these twenty–five variations should be considered only in the context of the normal transmission of illness. Since evils may be transmitted among the viscera in virtually any abnormal order, there are, in fact, a countless number of diseases. In TCM terms, overwhelming is defined specifically as one phase overwhelming the phase that it restrains. For example, lung metal restrains and may overwhelm liver wood.

13Withered bones indicate exhausted kidney qi. Wasted muscles reveal exhaustion of the spleen. Qi fullness with severe dyspnea such that the patient has to shrug his shoulders and keeps his mouth open is due to chaotic counterflow of the lung qi. Since three viscera border on expiry, death is inevitable. However, since the stomach qi is intact, the patient will survive six months. If the true visceral pulse, a pulse devoid of stomach qi, appears, then the patient is done for, and death will occur shortly after. The stomach or stomach qi referred to in the pulse refers to a quality of moderation.

14Internal pain in this context refers to true heart pain and is a more serious condition than the above. Death, therefore, arrives more quickly.

15Shedding of the flesh describes musculature which has become severely wasted. Cleaving of muscles describes a condition of emaciation where the bones are unusually exposed. They are apparently the result of being bedridden for a long period of time. In this case, the qi of the five viscera have certainly expired.

In our source edition, "generalized fever and pain" replaces "generalized fever", and this has been corrected in accordance with the *Su Wen*.

16Internal consumption of the shoulder marrow is characterized by scrawny, drooping shoulders together with clumsy movement. This suggests that the qi and essence have become irretrievably damaged.

This passage begins with "Internal consumption" in our source text. The first line has been added in accordance with the *Su Wen*.

17All essence qi pours into the eyes. When the eyes are deprived of sight, the essence and spirit must be utterly exhausted, and death will come any moment. Because the case is extremely critical, death is inevitable even if the eyes can see, although the patient may survive a little longer.

There is likely a lacuna in the line "the shoulder and the nape."

18Vacuity in this context means a vacuity of the correct qi. A sudden vacuity of the correct qi allows evils to intrude upon the body in a sudden and fulminating way. That the viscera are blocked and expiring implies that the nine portals are blocked and the qi of the five viscera has dissipated.

The order of the ideograms in the beginning of this passage is somewhat different in our source edition, thus changing its meaning. Our source edition reads, "When vacuity abruptly appears inside the body. . ." and "one breath" replaces "one exhalation". The above corrections have been made in accordance with the *Su Wen*.

19Our source edition reads, "tight" in place of "hard" and has been corrected in accordance with the *Su Wen* and the *Mai Jing*.

20If the scrofula has not yet become adhered to the surrounding tissues, its toxic qi is located just inside the vessels and hence is easy to treat.

The Chinese term for scrofula is composed of two characters *luo li*, both of which contain the disease radical. Their pronunciation suggests strings and may be better rendered as stringed lesions. Zhang Jing–yue explains in the *Lei Jing*, "*Luo li*, shaped in strings, linked together up and down, can present itself in both the neck and the axilla. It looks like the rat's hole. When this hole is blocked, another appears elsewhere. For this reason, it is referred to as the rat's tunnel." He goes on to say, "Nodes chained together are called *luo li*, while those long and shaped like clam shells are called saber. In addition, those growing in the lateral costal regions are said to be sabers."

21The treatment of this condition must aim at the root, *i.e.*, the involved viscus. The end can be regarded as the acupoint. When manipulating the needle at an acupoint point, one should have a definite view of the internal viscera. Prior to treatment the physician should determine which channel is involved and identify states of vacuity and repletion in the affected viscus. In case of vacuity, a supplementing manipulation should be performed with the needle inserted slowly but extracted quickly. In the case of repletion, a draining manipulation should be performed with the needle inserted quickly but extracted slowly. The red vessel(s) in the eyeballs are signs of the toxic evil penetrating the yin viscus. When the viscera are damaged, death is inevitable. The question of why more red vessels promise a longer life is a mystery.

22The bones are associated with the kidney, while the muscle is governed by the spleen. A small skeleton with weak muscles indicate an insufficiency of the kidney and spleen. These are the true yin. When the true yin is insufficient, yang evil easily afflicts the body, resulting in cold and heat. Here earth refers to the chin, while heaven refers to the forehead. An abnormal complexion in the earth region means that the true yin is in disorder.

Our source edition reads, "hollow of the knee" in place of "masses" and "heaven and earth" in place of "heaven". These have been corrected in accordance with the *Ling Shu (Spiritual Pivot)*.

23When wind intrudes the body, the skin is the first victim. Therefore, the skin becomes extremely hot and painful. Besides the skin and hair, the nose is also affected. This is because, when the skin is involved, the lung qi, which also governs the nose, must be affected, too. Since the third yang (*i.e.*, the foot *tai yang*) is the leader of all yang channels, it should be drained at Taking Flight (*Fei Yang*, Bl 58) which connects the foot *tai yang* with the foot *shao yin*, thus expelling the exuberant yang evil. At the same time, since the hand *tai yin* lung channel is involved, this should be supplemented at Broken Sequence (*Lie Que*, Lu 7).

Our source edition reads, "hand *tai yang*" in place of "hand *tai yin*", and has been corrected in accordance with the *Ling Shu* and the *Tai Su (Essentials)*.

24The muscles are governed by the spleen, and the efflorescence of the muscles finds its expression in the lips. Because of this relationship, the lips as well as the muscles are affected in this case. The prominent blood vessels of the foot *tai yang* should be pricked to drain the yang evil qi, and the hand and foot *tai yin* should be needled to induce perspiration. One should note that in Chap. 2, Book 7 or this work, the author has explained that the two *tai yin* channels are significant in both inducing and checking perspiration. The points used include Fish Border (*Yu Ji*, Lu 10), Great Abyss (*Tai Yuan*, Lu 9), Great Metropolis (*Da Du*, Sp 2), and Supreme White (*Tai Bai*, Sp 3).

Our source edition reads, "to check perspiration" instead of "to induce perspiration." We have cor-

rected this in accordance with the *Ling Shu* and *Tai Su*.

25The kidney governs the bones, and when the bones are diseased, the kidney must also be affected. The kidney is the consummate yin, and when it becomes vacuous, agitation must arise as is always the case with yin vacuity. Incessant sweating implies a collapse of yin essence. At this point Large Goblet (*Da Zhong*, Ki 4), the connecting vessel point of the foot *shao yin*, should be needled. One should note that the point is not actually located on the medial aspect of the thigh. The teeth are the ends of the bones and, when they become desiccated, the kidney as the governor of the bones, is surely exhausted. Thus death is inevitable. Bone inversion is due to an affliction of the foot *shao yin* channel. Its symptoms are hunger with inability to eat, coughing of blood, the heart suspended as in hunger, susceptibility to fright, blackish facial complexion, and dyspnea.

Our source edition reads, "If the roots of the teeth are desiccated and painful" instead of "If the teeth are not yet desiccated"; "If the teeth are tinged with a color of desiccation" instead of "If the teeth are already desiccated." We have corrected these in accordance with the *Ling Shu* and *Tai Su*.

26See note 8 above in this book for a discussion of the term *gu*. For a discussion of the demonological origins of this term, see *Medicine in China: A History of Ideas* by Paul U. Unschuld, University of California Press, 1985, Berkeley, pp 46–50.

27This pattern is characterized by an enlarged belly due to blood stasis in males and amenorrhea in females with obstructed visceral qi. .

28*I.e.*, Long Strong (*Chang Qiang*, GV 1)

29*I.e.*, points of the foot *tai yang* on the back

30*I.e.*, Shoulder Bone (*Jian Yu*, LI 15)

31*I.e.*, Capital Gate (*Jing Men*, GB 25)

32*I.e.*, Yang Assistance (*Yang Fu*, GB 38)

33*I.e.*, Pinched Ravine (*Xia Xi*, GB 43)

34*I.e.*, Mountain Support (*Cheng Shan*, Bl 57)

35*I.e.*, Kun Lun Mountain (*Kun Lun*, Bl 60)

36Here, no particular points are implied. Moxibustion may be performed at muscular nodes when found.

37*I.e.*, Celestial Chimney (*Tian Tu*, CV 22)

38*I.e.*, Great Mound (*Da Ling*, Per 7)

39*I.e.*, Surging Qi (*Qi Chong*, St 30)

40*I.e.*, Leg Three Li (*Zu San Li*, St 36)

41*I.e.*, Surging Yang (*Chong Yang*, St 42)

42*I.e.*, Hundred Convergences (*Bai Hui*, GV 20)

43One should note that the number of the points is counted bilaterally and that the dog bitten place is excluded.

44The author includes dog's bite because a bite from a rabid dog may cause cold and heat. The Protocol for Dog's Injury referred to by the author may be that described by Sun Si–miao in the *Qian Jin Yi Fang (Supplement to the Prescriptions Worth a Thousand Taels of Gold).* Suck the foul blood from the bite and then moxa a hundred cones immediately. Afterwards, moxa once daily for one hundred days.

Our source edition reads "above the calf" instead of "under the calf" and "three *cun* below the navel instead of "three *cun* under the knee." We have made these corrections in accordance with the *Su Wen.* In our source edition, the word "moxa" is dropped from "moxa the foot *yang ming*" and has been added in accordance with the *Su Wen* and *Tai Su.*

45Our source edition reads "Auditory Convergence (*Ting Hui*, GB 2)" instead of "Fontanelle Meeting (*Xin Hui*, GV 22)", and this is the case with the *Wai Tai* as well. This correction is made in accordance with the *Yi Xin Fang (The Heart of Medicine Formulary).*

46This entire chapter is derived from the *Zhen Jiu Ming Tang Zhi Yao.*

47Our source edition reads "putrefication" instead of "lassitude". It also contains a note inserted by some unknown editor(s), which states, "lassitude in a variant version." In a note in the *Zhen Jiu Ming Tang Zhi Yao (Acupuncture & Moxibustion Treatment Essentials of the Enlightening Hall)*, Yang Shang–shan explains, "When wind has brewed cold and heat, it produces sores which become putrefied."

48Our source edition reads "lung qi heat" instead of "lung cold and heat", "ascension of qi" instead of "coughing due to ascension of qi", and "lateral costal regions" in place of "upper back." These corrections have been made in accordance with the *Wai Tai* and the *Yi Xin Fang.*

49Our source edition reads "counterflow coughing" in place of "counterflow retching" and has been corrected in accordance with the *Wai Tai* and *Yi Xin Fang.*

50Our source edition reads "the skin and flesh" instead of "the skin, flesh and bone" and "constantly dank" instead of "a continuously damp body." These corrections have been made in accordance with the *Wai Tai (Secret [Medical] Essentials of a Provincial Governor).* "Chest and venter" instead of "venter", and this correction has been made in accordance with the *Wai Tai* and the *Qian Jin.* "Spleen Shu (*Pi Shu*, Bl 20)" replaces "Diaphragm Shu (*Ge Shu*, Bl 17)", and this correction is made in accordance with the *Wai Tai*, the *Yi Xin Fang*, and the *Qian Jin.*

51Since the liver governs the sinews, cold and heat of the sinew is simply an alternative expression for the liver cold and heat.

Our source edition reads "nape of the neck and the shoulders" instead of "eyebrows." The correction made in accordance with the *Wai Tai* and the *Yi Xin Fang.*

52Our source edition reads "tense face" instead of "black facial complexion" and "enduring dyspnea and cough" instead of "dyspnea and cough." These corrections have been made in accordance with the *Wai Tai.*

53In our source edition, the above section is divided into two parts as follows. "For pain in the shoulders affecting the nape of the neck, and cold and heat, Empty Basin (*Que Pen*) is the ruling point. For cold and heat (generalized fever in a variant version), lack of perspiration, and heat and pain in the chest, Celestial Bone Hole (*Tian Liao*) is the ruling point." The above rendering has been adopted with reference to the *Wai Tai* and the *Yi Xin Fang.*

54In our source edition, "ringing in the ears" is omitted. It is supplemented in accordance with the *Wai Tai* and *Qian Jin.*

55In this context, great qi may imply fulminating evil qi, severe distention/ fullness due to a surplus of qi, or both.

56Our source edition reads "swelling in the nape of the neck" instead of "swelling in the neck with pain in the shoulders." This correction is made in accordance with the *Wai Tai* and *Yi Xin Fang.* "Qi shortage and choking" appears instead of "qi choking." These corrections are made in accordance with the *Wai Tai* and Chapter 2, Book 12, the *Jia Yi Jing.*

57Our source edition reads "heat in the gallbladder with counterflow retching" instead of "frequent retching of bile", and "abdominal distention" instead of "swelling of the face and abdomen." These corrections are made in accordance with the *Wai Tai*.

58Our source edition reads "headache" instead of "pain in the neck." This correction is made in accordance with the *Wai Tai*.

59In the *Wai Tai*, "malaria, cold and heat" appear in place of "shivering...heart vexation." Besides, our source edition reads "vexation of the tongue" instead of "heart vexation." These corrections are made in accordance with the *Wai Tai*. Also in our source edition, "finger" is dropped from the phrase "finger *bi*."

60Our source edition reads "frequent coughing" instead of "frequent yawning" and "arm flesh aspect" instead of "inner side of the arm." These corrections are made in accordance with the *Wai Tai*.

61In some variant versions, this section and the following have been combined into one, and the author prescribes a single point, Broken Sequence (*Lie Que*, Lu 7). "Needle Channel Ditch (*Jing Qu*, Lu 8)" has been added in accordance with the *Wai Tai*.

62Celestial Storehouse (*Tian Fu*, Lu 3) is one of the so-called five grand points, or grand points of the five organs. These include Celestial Window (*Tian You*, TH 16), Protuberance Assistant (*Fu Tu*, LI 18), Celestial Pillar (*Tian Zhu*, Bl 10), and Man's Prognosis (*Ren Ying*, St 9) in addition to Celestial Storehouse.

63Our source edition reads, "shoulders and arms" instead of "shoulders and upper back."

64In our source edition, "generalized fever" does not appear. It has been added here in accordance with the *Qian Jin*, *Wai Tai*, and *Yi Xin Fang*.

65Our source edition reads, "inability to raise the shoulders and arms" instead of "pain in and inability to raise the shoulders." This correction has been made in accordance with the *Wai Tai*. In some variant versions, Upper Arm Shu (*Nao Shu*, SI 10) has been inserted by unknown editor(s).

66Our source edition reads, "swollen shoulder" instead of "swollen lips" and has been corrected in accordance with the *Wai Tai*.

67Yin inversion is cold inversion initiated by debilitated yang below. This manifests as cold throughout the body, in the upper, middle, and lower. Atonic feet that no longer fit ones shoes is a descriptive term. It evokes a picture of feet that have become so debilitated and atrophied that the shoes have become too large for them. As for the five colors of the urine and their significance to needling, the explanation is based on the inter-restraining relationship between the five phases. Spring is metal; brook is water; rapids is wood; stream is fire; confluence is earth. As green-blue for example, is associated with wood, which is restrained by metal, spring is chosen for the treatment of a disease with a green-blue complexion.

68Our source edition reads, "constant rumbling" instead of "thunderous rumbling." This correction is made in accordance with the *Wai Tai*.

69Our source edition reads, "diarrhea" instead of "swill diarrhea", and "thirsty, not dry lips, sweating" instead of "dry lips, lack of perspiration." These have been corrected in accordance with the *Wai Tai*.

70The region around point Celestial Window (*Tian You*, TH 16)

71Our source edition reads, "swelling in the occipital..." instead of "pain in the occipital...." This correction is made in accordance with the *Yi Xin Fang*. Also, "the chest" is dropped from "pain in the chest..." It is supplemented in accordance with the *Wai Tai*.

72Our source edition reads, "neck" instead of "lower leg." This correction is made in accordance with the *Wai Tai*.

73In our source edition, "*bi* and debility of the lower leg" is in place of "debility of the thigh and lower leg." This correction is made in accordance with the *Wai Tai*.

74Protrusion of the perineum implies the presence of a hemorrhoid.

75In our source edition, "cramps of the sinew insteps..." is in place of "cramps of the sinews..." This correction is made in accordance with the *Wai Tai*.

76Part 1 is derived from Chap. 66, Vol. 10, *Ling Shu*; Part 2 from Chap 46, Vol 7, *Ling Shu*; Part 3 from Chap 40, *Su Wen*; Part 4 from the 56th Difficulty, *Nan Jing*; Part 7 from the *Zhen Jiu Ming Tang Zhi Yao*.

77Inordinate joy and anger damage the internal viscera, and with the viscera damaged, the yin channels become diseased. This is internal damage. Cool dampness is a yin evil, and it easily capitalizes on a vacuity condition to intrude below, thus giving rise to disease in the lowe part of the body. Wind and rain are yang evils, and easily capitalize on a vacuity condition to intrude above, thus giving rise to disease in the upper part of the body. The interior, above, and below are the three regions that are vulnerable to an intrusion of evils.

[78]Wind in winter, however cold, is not a vacuity evil. Similarly, a fierce storm in summer is only a repletion wind rather than an evil vacuity wind. On the other hand, if in the spring, a cold rather than warm wind blows, this is considered a vacuity wind and is, as such, a vacuity evil. In terms of ones constitution or, more literally, ones formal body, repletion is understood to be ample righteous qi. People are able to adapt themselves to weather changes and remain fit unless they have developed an internal vacuity and have then contracted a wind evil of a vacuity nature.

[79]The author reiterates the importance of the combined action of weather changes and the condition of one's physique in contracting or keeping immune to disease. Vacuity here means the vacuity of the righteous qi within the body, while repletion is understood to be superabundant evil qi. Serious disease may develop only when repletion evils occur within the context of a constitutional vacuity.

[80]The qi referred to here is evil qi as is often the case in TCM terminology. According to a note in the *Tai Su*, the last sentence, which seems illogical, implies that, in terms of the location of evils, the body is divided into three regions, *i.e.*, the head and face above, the abdomen in the middle, and the region from the hips down to the feet below. Evils may strike either the external or internal aspects of the above three regions.

[81]While the evil is lodged in the surface, it causes people to shiver with cold. However, when it becomes lodged in the channels, which link the exterior to the interior, people may be cold, which is an external sign, as well as susceptible to fright, which is a sign of an internal disorder. The *shu* or transport vessel mentioned in this passage refers to the foot *tai yang* channel, along which the various points associated with viscera and bowels are located. If a vacuity evil becomes lodged in this channel, the channels of the viscera and bowels will most definitely become obstructed, and this accounts for pain in the articulations of the extremeties, etc. The penetrating vessel lies deeply and serves as a sea for all the channels and vessels, irrigating the whole body with essence and blood, including all the channels and network vessels and the five viscera and six bowels. When it is affected, the body loses its supply of

essence and blood, and, therefore, symptoms of heaviness and pain occur. When a vacuity evil becomes lodged in the stomach and intestines, gastrointestinal disorders develop. When it finally lodges outside the stomach and intestines, the vacuity evil settles into the curves and convulsions of the bowels which provide it with good hiding places. From there, the evil qi work inside the vessels, transforming qi and blood into accumulations.

[82]Another interpretation of the passage is that it is not the accumulations themselves but the evil qi from which accumulations develop that settles in the minute connecting vessel, etc. The following passages justify the rendering that appears in the primary text. One should note that the slack sinew refers to the part of the sinew channel of the foot *yang ming* that runs upward from the pubic bone bilateral to the navel through the abdomen. One should note that although there are quite a number of places where accumulations may settle, all of these locations are considered to be in close proximity to the stomach and intestines.

[83]The arms and hands are mentioned here only to point out the fact that the minute vessels everywhere are superficial and slack rather than to imply that the accumulation involves the hands and arms.

[84](Accumulations) lodging in the slack sinew, like that of the (foot) *yang ming*, produce pain when satiated but are calm when hungry.

[85]Because the *yang ming* is the channel of the stomach, accumulation in the foot *yang ming* enlarge when the stomach receives food and drink, but diminish in size when the stomach is empty. An accumulation of the slack sinew runs bilateral to the navel through the abdomen. It will produce pain and become enlarged when the stomach is full and calm down and diminish in size when the stomach is empty.

[86]The penetrating vessel pours into the major connecting vessel of the foot *shao yin*, emerging from the qi thoroughfare and travelling down the inner aspect of the thighs. When there is accumulation in the vessel, heat tends to be produced and the thighs are easily affected. Since the pravertebral sinew lies behind the stomach and intestines, accumulations in it become visible when the stomach and intestines are empty but are occluded they are full. The transport vessel, as explained above, is the foot *tai yang* channel which governs all the viscus-associated back points. It is ascribed to the urinary bladder and connects with the kidney.

Therefore, in the case of an accumulation within it, the passageways of water are obstructed, the stools dry up, and urination and defecation are inhibited. This is what is implied by dried up portals.

[87]When cold qi counterflows upward, it becomes lodged in between the stomach and intestines which is where the actual lump takes form.

[88]Spillage here does not mean spillage of water but spillage of cold qi. Inversion qi is a cold qi. When it counterflows below, the feet are affected first. These become distended and full due to congelation of blood and obstruction. This is what is meant by the term spillage. Since the lower part of the body is obstructed by inverted qi, the legs become cold. Thus the cold qi finds its way into the stomach and intestines. Next the fluid outside the intestines is congealed by the cold and compressed into a mass. This mass is the accumulation.

[89]It is of note that, in the *Ling Shu*, eating too much is said to fill up the intestines rather than the vessels. A yin vessel is a connecting vessel of a yin channel, whereas a yang vessel is a connecting vessel of a yang channel.

[90]Since the channels are responsible for conveyance and transportation of qi and blood, they are often refered to as *shu* (transporters), a homonym with the acupoint designation. Thus the six *shu* are the six channels. One should note that this passage gives an etiology for accumulations that differs from that in the preceding passage. There are a variety of different accumulations and their genesis differs as well.

[91]A cold body and eating cold substances are referred to as dual cold. See Chap. 1, Book 1, of the present work for the relationships of the viscera to the emotions.

[92]This is a summary of the preceding passages. Accumulations may be initiated by external intrusion of vacuity wind and internal injuries of a vacuity nature caused by, for example, inordinate emotional changes. Once developed, accumulations may lodge anywhere in the three regions of the body. To treat them, one may determine which viscus, bowel, channel, or connecting vessel is involved as well as its state of vacuity and repletion by examination of the painful area. Vacuity is treated by supplementation and repletion by drainage. Moreover, obeying the seasonal disposition is significant in achieving success. In TCM, the term seasonal disposition is laden with meaning. Each of the four seasons sees a particular, distinctive supersession between yin and yang, and the five viscera each correspond to the status of yin and yang in thier own ways. This should all be taken into account in treatment.

[93]Moist muscles may be a typographical error and should probably read dried up muscles, which is just the opposite condition. Thin, lusterless skin indicates a vacuity of qi and an inability to replenish the skin and hair, while weak, dried muscles indicate a lack of fluid and humor, apparently as a result of a failure of transformation and transportation within the spleen and stomach. This condition may be aggravated if one is not careful about the spiciness and coldness of the food one eats.

[94]The root cause of deep-lying beam is wind. Drastic measures such as precipitation are indicated to treat it. Otherwise, water will become stagnated, causing inhibited urination.

[95]There are various types of deep-lying beam disease mentioned in different sources, including the *Su Wen*, *Ling Shu*, and *Nan Jing*. Huang-fu Mi has gathered them here and treated them in a systematic manner. Snatching by force implies drastic or offensive therapies such as precipitation.

[96]The Fifty-Sixth Difficulty

[97]The disease affects the lung when the lung qi is prevailing, thus accounting for the lung being immune to the accumulation. The lung is metal, which is associated with autumn in the four seasons, and *geng* and *xin* in the celestial stems.

[98]In the preceding passages, the author describes three categories of deep-lying beam, each with a different pathogenesis and symptom pattern. Their common symptom is the presence of gathering and accumulations in the form of hardened masses in the abdomen. An accumulation in the heart, for instance, may be understood from the perspective of the five phases. The malady begins with the kidney on the lung-prevailing days, that is, *geng* and *xin* days, and in the lung-prevailing season, *i.e.*, autumn. The kidney is water and, therefore, it should transmit the illness to the fire viscus or heart via the restraining cycle. From there, the problem should be transmitted further to the fire-restraining phase which is lung metal. However, since the lung is strong enough in its own season to repel this disease, the heart is afflicted in its place.

[99]Lung *yong* is a disease characterized by coughing,

dyspnea, stinking sputum, and spitting of mixed pus and blood. *Jia* and *yi* days are days when wood prevails.

[100]In a note in the *Su Wen*, Wang Bing explains that inverted cup surging is invisible but quite recalcitrant. It is primarily characterized by difficult breathing. This is what the Chinese term *xi ben* actually means. From this point of view, the English term is less than precise. The term "gasping" or "panting" may make for a better translation. As such, the condition does not affect the stomach. Therefore, food intake remains normal. Moxibustion may lead to fulminating fire in the interior, while needling may drain the channels resulting in vacuity. The only choice is to conduct and normalize the qi little by little and to administer medicinals over an extended period to disperse internal qi stasis.

The term "breathing accumulation (*xi ji*)", is used instead of "inverted cup surging" in the *Su Wen* and *Tai Su*.

[101]In a comment on "The Fifty-Sixth Difficulty" of the *Nan Jing*, Yang Xuan-cao notes: "Fat qi means fatness and exuberance, and this means that fat qi gathers in the free rib regions to form a protruding inverted cup like mass, similar to fat exuberant flesh."

[102]A note in the *Hua Shi Ben Yi (Precise Meanings of Master Hua)* states that "Glomus qi is a lump-forming obstruction and blockage." The modern physician Qin BoBwei was of the opinion that the symptoms associated with fat qi in the *Nan Jing* are actually spleen related symptoms, while the symptoms associated with glomus qi are actually liver related symptoms. He asserts that the two terms should be reversed if they are to make any sense at all.

[103]*Shan* in this context implies abdominal pain.

[104]Our source edition reads, "Central Pole (*Zhong Ji*, CV 3) is the ruling point" instead of "moxa Qi Center (*Qi Zhong*)." This has been corrected in accordance with the *Wai Tai*.

[105]Running piglet here is not an independent illness but synonymous with qi surging up.

[106]Atonic inversion is a combined pattern of atony and inversion characterized by atonic weakness of the limbs with frigidity.

[107]Part 1 is derived from Chap. 35, Vol. 6, *Ling Shu*; Part 2 from *Zhen Jiu Ming Tang Zhi Yao*.

[108]Zhang Jing-yue has a note in the *Lei Jing* to the effect that a large pulse indicates an exuberance of evils, a hard pulse indicates repletion evils, and a choppy pulse is astringed due to qi and blood vacuity. Stomach qi reflected in the pulse should have a moderate quality. As a rule, a large, surging pulse invariably indicates an exhaustion of yin qi, while a hard and strong pulse demonstrates that the stomach qi must be damaged. Therefore, this pulse image reveals distention.

[109]Yin and yang here are qualities of the pulse. There are several different interpretations of a yin and yang pulse. One asserts that a floating, slippery, long, large, or stirring pulse is yang and that floating and rapid are the key indicators. A deep, rough, short, faint, weak, or wiry pulse is yin, with the deep and slow qualities being the key indicators. Based on this interpretation, a slow pulse is a yin pulse, and a rapid pulse is a yang pulse. Another interpretation defines the *chi* section of the *cun kou* pulse as yin and the *cun* section as yang, and a diseased pulse image occurring in these places is indicative of distention in the viscus or bowel respectively.

[110]The qi lies within the blood vessels as well as in the viscera and bowels.

[111]The stomach stores water and grain. Therefore, it is named the great granary responsible for supplies for all the five viscera and six bowels. The five openings, the throat, cardia, pylorus, anus, and ileocecal valve are considered doors of the stomach even though some of them pertain to the large and small intestines. It is of note that the entire length of the large and small intestine and the digestive tract in general is ascribed to the stomach. As the building blocks of the social structure in ancient China, five households comprised one alley (*lu*) and fifty households were organized into a neighborhood (*li*). In this context, these units refer to the intestines, etc. Ridge Spring (*Lian Quan*, CV 23) and Jade Beauty (*Yu Ying*) commonly known as Jade Hall (*Yu Tang*, CV 18). These are ascribed to the conception vessel and act as sluiceways for fluid and humor.

[112]In normal cases, the constructive qi runs inside the vessels, while the defensive travels outside the vessels, and they should do so along prescribed pathways. If the defensive qi counterflows outside the vessel or encroaches upon the vessel, this produces distention. To treat distention, Leg Three Li (*Zu San Li*, St 36) is the first choice. Since distention is always due to the counterflow of defensive qi, drainage is required regardless of the state of vacuity or repletion. A recent case

requires but one needling since the evil has not yet fulminated. However, an old case is not so easy to treat. One should note that generally, at this stage, distinction is fresh and has not yet caused substantial vacuity or repletion. Otherwise one should administer needling in accordance with vacuity and repletion.

[113]In Chinese medical terminology, in most cases, *shao fu* and *xiao fu* mean the same thing. They both refer to the lower abdomen. However, in the context of the relationship of the abdomen to liver and gallbladder disorders, they must sometimes be distinguished. Lateral lower abdominal pain relates to the liver, while lower abdominal pain often relates to the kidney. We have rendered *shao fu* as lateral lower abdomen and *xiao fu* as lower abdomen when this distinction must be made.

[114]All types of distention are caused by chaos or counterflow of the defensive qi and should be treated according to the same general principle. Successful treatment depends on a clear understanding of whether the constructive and defensive qi are in a state of normal flow or counterflow. Inappropriate needling may well promote the evil and play havoc with the orginal qi. The proper approach to needling is to supplement vacuity and drain repletion. Only in this way can the practitioner succeed in making the channels and network vessels, the viscera and bowels replenished with qi for long.

[115]The defensive qi runs outside and along the vessels. It travels sequentially from the yin phase to the yang phase and from the yang phase to the yin phase. The constructive qi is yin and the defensive qi is yang. These two flow side by side in harmony, visiting the five viscera one by one. In this way, the body can adapt to changes in weather throughout the year, and the spleen/stomach work well, transforming water and grain to provide supplies for the whole body. If there is inversion qi below, the constructive and defensive qi will become stagnated and obstructed, and this allows cold qi to ascend. The true qi, which in this case is the defensive qi, and the cold qi consequently become engaged in conflict. The entanglement of the two qi results in distention.

[116]Both the question and the answer are abstruse. There are diametrically opposing interpretations as to just what is being asked here. Two different interpretations are paraphrased below.

"The Yellow Emperor asks: I am still not clear as to the cause of distention. Would you explain further to resolve my confusion?" Or, "The Yellow Emperor asks: How is distension differentiated?" The answer can be paraphrased as follows. "Inversion qi arises below to contend with the true qi. The result is an entanglement of inversion qi and defensive qi or the true qi. This may happen in three places, i.e., the blood vessels, the five viscrea, and the six bowels."

[117]The author focuses on the importance of needling the point at the correct location and to the correct depth. Needling otherwise will not set free the blocked true qi or remove the evil qi. If one needles too shallowly, rather than achieving positive results, one will only aggravate the condition.

[118]Even three properly administered treatments may fail to eliminate the counterflow qi. In this case, other related points should be chosen. At the initial stages, distention should be treated by drainage, regardless of whether it is a recent case or a chronic one. While at later stages, when the viscera and bowels are involved, the problem of a mixed vacuity and repletion pattern arises, and drainage alone is not an appropriate therapy.

[119]Part 1 is derived from Chap. 57, Vol. 9, *Ling Shu*; Part 2 from Chap. 40, *Su Wen*; Part 3 from Chap. 19, Vol. 4, *Ling Shu*; and Part 4 from the *Zhen Jiu Ming Tang Zhi Yao*.

[120]In Chinese medical terminology, water is often referred to as water swelling, or water qi. Water swelling is due to exuberant water with earth no longer able to restrain it. Instead, water rebels against earth. Earth is the foot *yang ming* which travels via Man's Prognosis (*Ren Ying*, St 9), where a vessel can be observed pulsating, down through the interior of the abdomen. This accounts for violent beating of the cervical vessel and abdominal enlargements. Water is the child of metal. A disease of the child may affect the mother, i.e., the lungs. For this reason, a water problem often involves the stomach and the lungs as well and this accounts for coughing.

[121]When cold qi invades the skin, the yang qi becomes obstructed and its flow comes to a standstill. Since the disease is a disorder of the qi, the abdomen looks like a drum, taut but not solid. Because qi penetrates, every part of the body becomes swollen. Water swelling occurs at the specific location where water spills over, while qi distention is seen throughout the body. Water swelling usually produces a glossy tinge to the affected area because water is shiny, while qi distention does not change the color of the skin.

[122]According to another understanding, the passage

from "This allows" to "become glomus" can be rendered as "Because there is something for it to hold onto, pi." *Pi*, though the same word as in the commonly known term intestinal *pi*, refers to a mass or lump of blood and putrid substances before it takes shape, and we render it as glomus because the character *pi* may carry another implication. The term polyp in Chinese medicine often suggests a mass of putrid substances, a synonym with *pi* in the advanced stage. Because the mass feels like a mushroom, the illness is called intestinal mushroom.

[123]There are several ways of preparing this tincture. The common one is to collect one *sheng* (liter) of dry cock droppings. Grind, bake, and then boil these in about two liters of wine until half of the liquid is left. After filtering, the tincture is taken warm early in the morning.

[124]The fifty-seven needling points include Long Strong (*Chang Qiang*, GV 1), Lumbar Shu (*Yao Shu*, GV 2), Life Gate (*Ming Men*, GV 4), Suspended Pivot (*Xuan Shu*, GV 5), and Spinal Center (*Ji Zhong*, GV 6) which are needled unilaterally and White Ring Shu (*Bai Huan Shu*, Bl 30), Central Backbone Shu (*Zhong Lu Shu*, Bl 29), Bladder Shu (*Pang Guang Shu*, Bl 28), Small Intestine Shu (*Xiao Chang Shu*, Bl 27), Large Intestine Shu (*Da Chang Shu*, Bl 25), Sequential Limit (*Zhi Bian*, Bl 54), Bladder Huang (*Bao Huang*, Bl 53), Will Chamber (*Zhi Shi*, Bl 52), Huang Gate (*Huang Men*, Bl 51), Stomach Granary (*Wei Cang*, Bl 50), Horizontal Bone (*Heng Gu*, Ki 11), Great Manifestation (*Da He*, Ki 12), Qi Point (*Qi Xue*, Ki 13), Fourfold Fullness (*Si Man*, Ki 14), Central Flow (*Zhong Zhu*, Ki 15), Surging Qi (*Qi Chong*, St 30), Return (*Gui Lai*, St 29), Waterway (*Shui Dao*, St 28), Great Gigantic (*Da Ju*, St 27), Outer Mound (*Wai Ling*, St 26), Large Goblet (*Da Zhong*, Ki 4), Shining Sea (*Zhao Hai*, Ki 6), Intersection Reach (*Jiao Xin*, Ki 8), Guest House (*Zhu Bin*, Ki 9), and Yin Valley (*Yin Gu*, Ki 10) which are needled bilaterally.

[125]Wind water skin distention is caused by being exposed to wind while sweating and presents with fever, aversion to wind, swelling appearing initially in the face and subsequently generalized water swelling with pain in limb joints, and a floating pulse. After needling one or more of the fifty-seven points, the prominent veins in the skin should be pricked and bled. If there are no signs of wind, such as aversion to wind, Origin Pass (*Guan Yuan*, CV 4) should be needled. This is located three *cun* below the navel. This is the point inferred by the reference to circling valley. There is no concensus as to what type of needle should be used. One should note that although we cite the sword needle as a type of needle, the

author may refer to it here in quite a different manner, since the term *pai zhen* has multiple meanings. It may refer to a needling technique which is characterized by slowly pushing in the needle to a great depth. Following acupuncture, the patient should be bound at the waist to prevent a recurrence of this condition. At the same time, disinhibiting agents should be administered. One should note that in the Chinese medical terms, a therapy or medicinal for a disease may be named after the disease, and so blocking medicinals are medicinals that eliminate blockage. After the swelling is eliminated, the patient should be placed on a diet free of water-/dampness-assisting foods, or foods that may damage the spleen. Sweet, salty, and cold substances as well as meat are prohibited.

[126]A swollen philtrum as if it is brimming over and outturned lips are signs of expiry of spleen qi and are prognosticative of death.

[127]When swelling is so serious as to make the skin textures invisible, the situation is hopeless.

[128]Running water in the skin refers to migratory swelling of the skin.

[129]Stone water is swelling in the lower abdomen which feels as hard as rock. This is due to yin cold in the liver and kidney and congelation and concentration of water qi in the lower burner. It is of note, however, that there is another category of stone swelling that develops from gathering and accumulation or concretion and conglomeration. This latter type is characterized by a hard mass of enormous size in the abdomen. Huang-fu Mi refers to the former sometimes and the latter in other instances in the following sections.

[130]*I.e.*, Veering Passageway (*Pian Li*, LI 6)

[131]*I.e.*, Great Abyss (*Tai Yuan*, Lu 9)

[132]In our source edition, this paragraph ends with "All must be (needled) with a supplementing (technique)." This has been omitted here as it is a redundancy even in Chinese.

[133]Part 1 is derived from Chap. 61, *Su Wen*; Part 2 from Chap. 33, *Su Wen*; Part 3 from Chap. 47, *Su Wen*; and Part 4 from the *Zhen Jiu Ming Tang Zhi Yao*.

[134]A note in the *Su Wen* given by Wang Bing explains, 'Yin is said to be cold, and winter is a state of extreme cold. The kidney is matched and corresponds (with winter). For this reason, the kidney is said to be the consummate yin. Water rules it in

winter, and therefore, the consummate yin is said to be exuberant water.'

The western reader may ask why water is not said to be exuberant in summer since that season sees most ample rainfall? In summer, dampness and heat are most conspicuously characteristic and rain evaporates and is absorbed by earth quickly. On the contrary, in winter water becomes iced and it greets your eyes everywhere, and water exhibits in a most striking way its cold nature. Since the kidney is associated with winter, it is justified that the kidney is exuberant water.

Ma Shi explains this point from another angle by saying, 'The kidney is located in the lower burner, the yin within yin, and therefore said to be the consummate yin. Water is yin, so is the kidney. Now that the kidney is the consummate yin, water disease is exuberant water.'

Regarding the relationship between the kidney and the lung in water problems, Zhang Jing-yue explains, 'The channel of the lung is the hand *tai yin*, and the viscus is ascribed to metal. The channel of the kidney is the foot *shao yin*, and the viscus is ascribed to water. Because the *shao yin* starts from the kidney, upwards penetrating the liver and the diaphragm to enter the lung, when the evils of the kidney counterflows upwards, water intrudes the lung. On the account, in all the cases of water disease, the root is in the kidney while the end is in the lung. Besides, as metal engenders water, and the mother and the child have common qi, (the kidney and the lung) are both capable of water.'

The kidney governs water for the whole body, but the lung, the governor of qi, takes the responsibility of regulating, coursing, and freeing flow of water with qi. The kidney is located in the lower while the lung in the upper. For that reason the kidney is the root and the lung is the branch or upper end in connection of water. Pathologically, it proves that water disease certainly involves the kidney but often with some manifestations of qi problems. Therefore we see swelling not infrequently with dyspnea.

[135]A pass is a strategic place for entry and exit. The kidney governs the lower burner, opening into the anterior and posterior yin organs, *i.e.*, the genitals and anus. Water and grain should enter the stomach where they are transformed. After that, they become gradually wasted substances, the liquid part discharged from the anterior yin, while the solid is evacuated from the posterior yin. Therefore, the two yin are said to function as passes and they both pertain to the kidney.

When the kidney works well, the two yin are uninhibited. But when the kidney qi is vacuous, they are blocked. When the water passageways are obstructed, water has to gather. In these circumstances, qi becomes obstructed and stagnated. Then the stagnated qi, in turn, facilitates an accumulation of water. This vicious circle progresses to cause swelling. It is of note that water and qi are regarded as having the same nature. About this point of view, the reader may refer to Chap. 13, Book 1, present work. The above is what is suggested by water appealing to that which is of its kind.

[136]The kidney is located below and is associated with water. Since a lower position and water are both yin, the kidney is called feminine, a synomyn with yin. Food and drink, after undergoing transformation in the stomach, which is earth, transforms into qi ascending from the stomach into the lung. This ascending process relies entirely on the transformation of the kidney qi. In addition, this ascending earthly qi or qi from the stomach can be transformed later into water based entirely on the strength of the kidney qi as well. From this angle, the kidney is the spring situated below, and it is called the consummate yin, or yin within the yin for good reason.

[137]The consumption of hot water produces immediate perspiration. Sweat of this kind, coming from the exterior, is ascribed to hot qi which opens the interstices and allows fluid to exit. At a moderate ambient temperature, when one overworks, the sweat comes from the kidney in the interior which governs water. In the course of sweating, if one is caught in a draught, the dark mansion, *i.e.*, the sweat pores because sweat is tinged a dark shade, become blocked. The sweat, trapped in its mansion, is unable either to penetrate inward or effuse outward. It must, therefore, produce swelling.

[138]Zhang Jing-yue explains, "Vacuity should not be treated by needling. If swelling is mistaken for a case of repletion and drained by means of needling, vacuity of the true qi will be further exacerbated, and, as a consequence, the evil qi will surely arrive. Because it takes the diseased qi five days to cycle around the five viscera, it returns to the originally affected viscus after as many days."

[139]Zhang Zhi-cong explains in *Su Wen Ji Zhu*, "When wind evils damage the kidney, the essence qi must be vacuous, and, in the case of yin vacuity, yang takes advantage to assault. For this reason, heat arises from time to time. The kidney is the source of the vital qi. This accounts for dimin-

323

ished qi. When yang imposes on yin, sweat is exuded."

Since the Chinese word *ku* is sometimes misleading in this context, some Chinese may interpret "a bitter taste and thirst" as "tormenting thirst." In Chinese, *ku* means both bitterness as taste and bitterness as suffering.

[140]Because the true essence and qi is diminished, heat is generated. As the saying goes, yin vacuity always engenders internal heat. This accounts for heat in the hands, dry mouth with thirst, yellowish urine, etc. Because there is heat in the lower abdomen and disharmony of the stomach, the evil qi surges up to oppress the lung. As a result, while lying supine, the patient coughs severely.

[141]The commonplace saying in Chinese medicine, that like attracts like, underlies the explanation for water in the abdomen being accompanied by swelling in the lower eyelids. The true qi is the kidney qi which is water. When water ascends, heart fire is threatened and has to escape upward causing signs peculiar to heat, such as dry mouth for example. Because the water qi ascends to oppress the lung, the patient finds it difficult to lie supine and if one is forced to assume that posture, the resultant coughing may cause the expectoration of watery sputum. From the discussion in the preceding passages, it is clear that water problems are rooted in the kidney whose qi governs the conveyance and transformation of water, and that the lung is often involved because it is responsible for maintaining the free flow of water. Since water and grain must be processed in the spleen/stomach before they become earthly qi, the spleen/stomach are also usually involved in water problems.

[142]In the case of kidney wind, there is a vacuity of kidney qi which is water. If, in addition, the heart qi or fire becomes vacuous as well, then the true yin and true yang both become exhausted and death is inevitable.

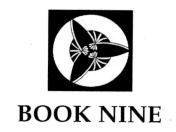

BOOK NINE

Chapter One

Great Cold Penetrating into the
Bone Marrow or Yang Counterflow
Producing Headache[1]
(with Appendices on Pain in the
Submandibular Region &
the Nape of the Neck)

(1)

The Yellow Emperor asked:

What kind of disease is characterized by headache which persists for years?

Qi Bo answered:

There must be affliction of great cold which has penetrated the bone marrow. Since the marrow of the bones is governed by the brain, when there is a counterflow in the brain, headache as well as toothache result.

(2)

For yang counterflow headache with fullness in the chest and inability to catch one's breath, take Man's Prognosis (*Ren Ying*, St 9).[1]

For inversion headache, take the foot *yang ming* and *tai yin* if it is accompanied by a swollen face and vexation of the heart.[3]

For inversion headache with pain in the vessels of the head, and sadness with frequent crying, locate the pulsating, prominent vessels in the head and prick them, letting blood out of them all, and then regulate the foot *jue yin*.[4]

For inversion headache which cannot be located by palpation with belching and poor memory, first take the pulsating vessels at the sides of the head and face and then the foot *tai yang* ["*tai yin*" in a variant version {later editor}].[5]

For inversion headache with swimming and pain of the head ["swimming of the head and heavy headedness" in the *Ling Shu* {later editor}], drain at the five points in the five columns each on the head. First take the hand *shao yin* and then take the foot *shao yin*.[6]

For inversion headache where the nape of the neck becomes painful first and then involves the lumbar spine, first take Celestial Pillar (*Tian Zhu*, Bl 10) and then take the foot *tai yang*.[7]

For inversion headache with severe pain and heat in ["surging of" in a variant version {later editor}] the vessels and bones both anterior and posterior to the auricles, drain first the blood (from the vessels) and then take the foot *tai yin* and *shao yin* ["*shao yang*" in a variant version {later editor}].[8]

For inversion headache with severe pain and surging of the vessels both anterior and posterior to the auricles which is due to heat, drain the blood (from the vessels) and then take the foot *shao yang*.

True headache with severe pain, pain throughout the brain, and cold in the hands and the feet which extends to the articulations (of the elbows and the knees) is fatal and cannot be treated.[9]

(Some) headaches may not be treated with transporting points. In the case of foul blood lodging internally, such as in an impact injury inflicted in wrestling or a fall, or in the case of pain due to an internal injury where the pain is persistent, these situations may be treated by needling local points but may not be needled with distant points.[10]

(Some) headaches may not (respond) to needling, such as those cases where great *bi* plays havoc and attacks on windy days. This can be relieved somewhat but cannot be eliminated.[11]

For hemilateral cold and pain in the head, first take the hand *shao yang* and *yang ming* and then the foot *shao yang* and *yang ming*.[12]

(3)

For pain in the submandibular region, needle the hand *yang ming*[13] and (prick) the exuberant vessels at the submandibular region to let out blood.

For pain in the nape of the neck with inability to bend (the body) either forward or backward, needle the foot *tai yang*. And for inability to look around, needle the hand *tai yang* ["hand *yang ming*" in a variant version {later editor}].[14]

For pain in the submandibular region, prick the pulsating vessel of the foot *yang ming* which may be observed at the curved surround (and the patient will be) cured on the spot. If this is not the case, press the channel and needle Man's Prognosis (*Ren Ying*, St 9, and the patient will be) cured on the spot.[15]

(4)

For headache, Eye Window (*Mu Chuang*, GB 16), Celestial Surge (*Tian Chong*, GB 9), and Wind Pool (*Feng Chi*, GB 20) are the ruling points.

For inversion headache, Collection Hole (*Kong Zui*, Lu 6) is the ruling point.

For inversion headache with a swollen face, Shang Hill (*Shang Qiu*, Sp 5) is the ruling point.

Chapter Two

Intrusion of Cold Qi into the Five Viscera & Six Bowels Producing Sudden Heart Pain, Chest Bi, Heart Shan, & Three Worms[16]

(1)

Inversion heart pain which radiates pain to the back with frequent tugging, a sensation (of the heart) being poked from the back, and hunched back is kidney heart pain. First take Capital Bone (*Jing Gu*, Bl 64) and Kun Lun Mountain (*Kun Lun*, Bl 60). (The patient) will be cured immediately upon (extraction) of the needles. If this is not the case, take Burning Valley (*Ran Gu*, Ki 2).[17]

Inversion heart pain characterized by sudden diarrhea and abdominal distention and fullness in addition to severe heart pain is stomach heart pain. Take Great Metropolis (*Da Du*, Sp 2) and Supreme White (*Tai Bai*, Sp 3).

Inversion heart pain which is characterized by a sensation of the heart being pricked by an awl in addition to the severity of the heart pain is spleen heart pain. Take Burning Valley (*Ran Gu*, Ki 2) and Supreme Ravine (*Tai Xi*, Ki 3).

Inversion heart pain characterized by a deathlike, somber, ashy complexion and inability to produce a sigh for a day is liver heart pain. Take Moving Between (*Xing Jian*, Liv 2) and Supreme Surge (*Tai Chong*, Liv 3).

Inversion heart pain which abates when lying down or when alone but increases with movement and is characterized by no change of complexion is lung heart pain. Take Fish Border (*Yu Ji*,

Lu 10) and Great Abyss (*Tai Yuan*, Lu 9).

True heart pain characterized by severity of the pain and frigidity in the hands and feet extending up to the elbows and knees causes death in the evening if it occurs in the morning or death in the morning if it occurs the previous evening.

(Some forms of) heart pain may not be needled, and, in the case of exuberant gatherings in the center, one cannot take the channel points (*shu*, 腧).[18]

(Heart pain due to) worm conglomerations in the intestines or the biting of roundworms may not be punctured with the small needle.

Heart and abdominal pain with swelling and gathering moving up and down in intermittent episodes of pain and with heat in the abdomen and frequent drooling is caused by the biting of roundworms. (One should) press the gathering and hold on lest it should move. Then thrust in a large needle, retaining it for an extended period of time. When the worm no longer moves, the needle may be withdrawn.

(2)

For heart pain radiating to the lumbar spine with desire to retch, needle at the foot *shao yin*.

For heart pain with abdominal distention and (qi stagnation) producing labored defecation, take the foot *tai yin*.

For heart pain radiating to the upper back such that one cannot catch one's breath, needle at the foot *shao yin*. If there is no result, take the hand *shao yin*.[19]

For heart pain which moves up and down without a fixed location and produces lower abdominal fullness and difficult urination and defecation, needle at the foot *jue yin*.

For heart pain characterized solely by diminished qi which is insufficient to allow one to catch one's breath, needle the hand *tai yin*.

(3)

For heart pain exacerbated by the slightest pressure and accompanied by vexation of the heart, Great Tower Gate (*Ju Que*, CV 14) is the ruling point.[20]

For heart pain due to three kinds of worms with copious drooling and inability to turn the body over, Upper Venter (*Shang Wan*, CV 13) is the ruling point.[21]

For heart pain with generalized cold, difficulty in bending (the body) either forward or backward, heart *shan*, qi surging dizziness, and utter loss of consciousness, Central Venter (*Zhong Wan*, CV 12) is the ruling point.[22]

For heart pain with qi surging up into the heart, no desire for food, and propping pain in the diaphragm, Interior Strengthening (*Jian Li*, CV 11) is the ruling point.

For sudden heart and abdominal pain with sweating, Stone Door (*Shi Men*, CV 5) is the ruling point.[23]

For a dragging pain between the chest, lateral costal regions, and upper back with a jumbling sensation below the heart, vomiting and retching, copious sputum, and inability to ingest food, Dark Gate (*You Men*, Ki 21) is the ruling point.

For chest *bi* with qi counterflow, cold inversion hypertonicity (of the four limbs), vexation of the heart, frequent spitting, retching, and belching, fullness in the chest, shouting, counterflow ascension of the stomach qi, and heart pain ["lung distention and counterflow of the stomach" in the *Qian Jin* {later editor}], Great Abyss (*Tai Yuan*, Lu 9) is the ruling point.

For distending heart pain ["vexation, oppression, and flusteredness" in the *Qian Jin* {later editor}] with diminished qi which is insufficient to allow one to catch one's breath, Cubit Marsh (*Chi Ze*, Lu 5) is the ruling point.

For heart pain with coughing, dry retching, vexa-

327

tion, and fullness, Guarding White (*Xia Bai*, Lu 4) is the ruling point.

For sudden heart pain with contraction between (the sinews), pain in the inner side of the elbow, and a burning and turning sensation in the heart region, Intermediary Courier (*Jian Shi*, Per 5) is the ruling point.

For heart pain with nosebleeding, retching of blood, susceptibility to fright and apprehension with fearing the presence of people, and insufficiency of spirit and qi, Cleft Gate (*Xi Men*, Per 4) is the ruling point.

For heart pain with sudden coughing with (qi) counterflow, Marsh at the Bend (*Qu Ze*, Per 3) is the ruling point.

For sudden heart pain with sweating, Large Pile (*Da Dun*, Liv 1) is the ruling point. When blood emerges, one is cured on the spot.

For chest *bi* sending a dragging (discomfort) to the upper back with intermittent cold, Intermediary Courier (*Jian Shi*, Per 5) is the ruling point.

For chest *bi* with heart pain and numbness and insensitivity in the flesh of the shoulders, Celestial Well (*Tian Jing*, TH 10) is the ruling point.

For chest *bi* with heart pain, inability to catch the breath and migratory pain ["inability to turn over" in the *Qian Jin* {later editor}], Overlooking Tears (*Lin Qi*, GB 41) is the ruling point.

For heart *shan* with sudden (heart) pain, take the foot *tai yin* and *jue yin*. Prick all the blood network vessels found.[24]

For throat *bi* with a curled tongue, dry mouth, vexation of the heart, heart pain, and pain in the surface of the arms ["pain in the medial region of the back" in the *Ling Shu* and *Tai Su* {later editor}] with inability to raise them to the head, take Passage Hub (*Guan Chong*, TH 1). This is located a leek leaf distant from the corner of the nail of the finger next to the small one. [The instruction

that the point on the right side is chosen for problems on the left, and the point of the left is chosen for problems of the right is added in a variant version. {later editor}]

Chapter Three

Evils in the Lung Causing Disease in the Five Viscera & Six Bowels Producing an Ascending Counterflow of Qi & Cough[25]

(1)

Evils in the lung result in pain in the skin, fever and chills, qi ascension dyspnea, sweating, and cough shaking the shoulders and upper back. Take the points on the lateral side of the bosom and the point by the side of the third vertebra.[26] Press the points swiftly and then needle those which yield a comfortable sensation upon the pressure. After that, take Empty Basin (*Que Pen*, St 12) to oust (the evil).[27]

(2)

The Yellow Emperor asked:

Why does the lung cause people to cough?

Qi Bo answered:

Each of the other viscera and the six bowels may cause people to cough; it is not the lung alone. The skin and hair are associated with the lung. The skin and hair are the first to be afflicted by evil qi, and then the evil qi is inclined to pursue its associated (viscera). If cold (evil) enters the stomach with food and drink, it will follow the channel of the lung up to the lung, giving rise to cold in the lung. When the lung becomes cold, both internal and external evils conspire to lodge in the lung, giving rise to lung cough.[28]

Each of the five viscera (is most likely to) contract disease in its prevalent season, and, in a season other than this, it receives a disease through transmission (from another viscus). As humans interact with heaven and earth, each of the five viscera may be affected by cold and hence suffer from a disease in its governing season, coughing in a slight case and diarrhea and pain in a serious case. In autumn, the lung is the first to suffer from evils. In spring, the liver is the first to suffer. In summer, the heart is the first to suffer. In the consummate yin, the spleen is the first to suffer. And in winter, the kidney is the first to suffer.[29]

The presentation of lung cough includes coughing, dyspneic rale, and, in serious cases, spitting of blood.

The presentation of heart cough includes heart pain arising with coughing, wheezing ["shrieking" in the *Su Wen* {later editor}] in the throat as if there were a lump in it and, in serious cases, swollen pharynx with throat *bi.*

The presentation of liver cough includes cough inducing pain in the subaxillary ["free rib" in the *Su Wen* {later editor}] regions and, in serious cases, inability to turn over (the body) or the free rib regions ["subaxillary regions" in the *Su Wen* {later editor}] becoming full on attempting to turn.

The presentation of spleen cough includes pain in the right subaxillary ["free rib" in the *Su Wen* {later editor}] regions, deep, dull, dragging pain between the shoulders and upper back and, in serious cases, inability to move (as in turning over), since movement exacerbates the cough.

The presentation of kidney cough includes a cough producing a dragging pain between the upper and lower back and, in serious cases, drooling when coughing.

Long-standing coughs related to the five viscera will be transmitted to the six bowels. If spleen cough persists, the stomach will contract (the evil). The presentation of stomach cough includes coughing, retching, and, when the retching is severe, the expulsion of round worms.

If liver cough persists, the gallbladder will con-

tract (the evil). The presentation of gallbladder cough includes coughing and retching of bile.

If lung cough persists, the large intestine will contract (the evil). The presentation of large intestine cough includes coughing and fecal incontinence.

If heart cough persists, the small intestine will contract (the evil). The presentation of small intestine cough includes coughing and passing fecal qi. The qi and coughing happen simultaneously.[30]

If kidney cough persists, the urinary bladder will contract (the evil). The presentation of bladder cough include coughing and fecal ["urinary" in the *Su Wen* {later editor}] incontinence.[31]

If the cough is long-standing and persistent, the triple burner will contract (the evil). The presentation of triple burner cough includes coughing and abdominal fullness with no desire for food.

All these types of cough are due to concentration (of evil qi) in the stomach and the involvement of the lung which result in copious snivel and sputum, puffy swelling of the face, and qi counterflow.[32]

To treat visceral (coughs), the rapids should be treated. To treat bowel (coughs), the confluence points should be treated. And for water swelling, the stream should be treated

.

Damage by dampness in autumn will lead to contraction of cough in winter.[33]

(3)

The Yellow Emperor asked:

Speaking of dusting, the *Jiu Juan (Ninefold Volume)* explains that needling at the external channels removes yang disease. I would like to learn about it in detail.[34]

Qi Bo answered:

When there is a major counterflow of yang qi, it

fills up the chest, dilating the chest. In this case, there is shrugging of the shoulders to facilitate breathing. When the great qi counterflows upward, there is dyspneic wheezing with forced sitting posture and body bent forward, esophageal constriction, and inability to catch the breath. (In this case,) take Celestial Countenance (*Tian Rong*, SI 17). If coughing is accompanied by qi ascension, bent body, and chest pain, take Ridge Spring (*Lian Quan*, CV 23). In taking Celestial Countenance (*Tian Rong*, SI 17), the needle should not be inserted over one *li* deep [the word *li* is probably an error {later editor}]. In taking Ridge Spring (*Lian Quan*, the operation) should not be stopped until the blood (of the patient) has changed (to normal).[35]

(4)

For counterflow cough ascension of qi, Po Door (*Po Hu*, Bl 42), Qi Abode (*Qi She*, St 11), and Yi Xi (*Yi Xi*, Bl 45) are the ruling points.

For counterflow cough ascension of qi and vacuity dyspnea, Yi Xi (*Yi Xi*, Bl 45) is the ruling point.[36]

For counterflow cough ascension of qi, rales in the throat, and dyspnea, Protuberance Assistant (*Fu Tu*, LI 18) is the ruling point.

For counterflow cough ascension of qi with spitting of foamy substance, Celestial Countenance (*Tian Rong*, SI 17) and Moving Between (*Xing Jian*, Liv 2) are the ruling points.

For counterflow cough ascension of qi, *yong* swelling in the throat, respiratory qi shortage, and dyspneic difficult breathing, Water Prominence (*Shui Tu*, St 10) ["Celestial Prominence (*Tian Tu*, CV 21)" in a variant version {later editor}] is the ruling point.[37]

For counterflow cough ascension of qi with coughing and dyspnea making it impossible to speak, Florid Canopy (*Hua Gai*, CV 20) is the ruling point.

For counterflow cough ascension of qi, (frequent) spitting, dyspnea, shortness of qi such that one cannot catch one's breath, and inability of the mouth to articulate, Chest Center (*Dan Zhong*, CV 17) is the ruling point.

For counterflow cough ascension of qi, dyspnea with inability to catch the breath, retching and vomiting, thoracic fullness and inability to ingest food and drink, Transport Mansion (*Shu Fu*, Ki 27) is the ruling point.

For counterflow cough ascension of qi, drooling, copious spitting, rapid dyspneic breathing with palpitation, and restlessness whether sitting or lying, Lively Center (*Yu Zhong*, Ki 26) is the ruling point.

For thoracic fullness, counterflow coughing, dyspnea with inability to catch the breath, retching and vomiting, vexation and fullness, and inability to ingest food and drink, Spirit Storehouse (*Shen Cang*, Ki 25) is the ruling point.

For stuffy fullness in the chest and lateral costal regions, counterflow cough ascension of qi, inhibited respiration, and frequent spitting of turbid foam, pus, and blood, Storeroom (*Ku Fang*, St 14) is the ruling point.

For coughing, dyspnea with inability to catch one's breath, forced sitting posture with inability to lie down, gasping for breath, inability to swallow, and heat in the chest, Cloud Gate (*Yun Men*, Lu 2) is the ruling point.

For stuffy fullness in the chest and lateral costal regions, inability to bend (the body) either forward or backward, suppurative *yong*, counterflow cough ascension of qi, and rale in the throat, Great Ravine (*Tai Xi*, Ki 3) is the ruling point.

For incessant counterflow coughing with water qi in the triple burner and inability to ingest food, Linking Path (*Wei Dao*, GB 28) is the ruling point.

For counterflow coughing, vexation and oppression with inability to lie down, fullness in the chest, dyspnea with inability to catch the breath, and backache, Great Abyss (*Tai Yuan*, Lu 9) is the ruling point.

For counterflow cough ascension of qi, dry tongue, pain in the lateral costal regions, heart vexation, cold shoulders, diminished qi such that one cannot catch one's breath, and abdominal distention with dyspnea, Cubit Marsh (*Chi Ze*, Lu 5) is the ruling point.

For coughing, dry retching, and vexation and fullness, Guarding White (*Xia Bai*, Lu 4) is the ruling point.

For coughing due to ascension of qi, dyspnea with inability to catch the breath, and sudden internal counterflow of pure heat and transmission (of the evil qi) between the liver and lung (with) oral and nasal bleeding, generalized distention, counterflow breathing, and inability to lie down, Celestial Storehouse (*Tian Fu*, Lu 3) is the ruling point.[38]

For shivering with cold, coughing, vomiting of blood, qi counterflow, susceptibility to fright, and heart pain, the cleft point of the hand *shao yin*[39] is the ruling point.

For coughing with thoracic fullness, Front Valley (*Qian Gu*, SI 2) is the ruling point.

For coughing with facial redness and heat, Branch Ditch (*Zhi Gou*, TH 6) is the ruling point.

For coughing, rale in the throat, and coughing and spitting of blood, Large Goblet (*Da Zhong*, Ki 4) is the ruling point.

Chapter Four

The Liver Contracts Disease and the Defensive Qi Lodges & Accumulates Producing Fullness & Pain in the Chest & the Lateral Costal Regions[40]

(1)

Evils in the liver result in illnesses characterized by pain in the lateral costal regions, cold in the center, foul blood in the interior, and tendency to swelling and tugging in the lower leg joints. (In this case,) take Moving Between (*Xing Jian*, Liv 2) to guide (the evils) away from the lateral costal regions, apply supplementation at Three Li (*San Li*, St 36) to warm the stomach, take the blood vessels to dissipate the foul blood, and take the green-blue vessels around the auricles to relieve tugging.[41]

(2)

The Yellow Emperor asked:

When lodged in the vessels ["the abdomen" in the *Tai Su* {later editor}], the defensive qi accumulates and stagnates. Since this accumulated stale qi cannot circulate (properly) and this accumulated stale qi has no constant dwelling place, this results in ["it causes people" in the *Ling Shu* {later editor}] stuffy fullness in the lateral costal regions, dyspneic wheezing, and counterflow breathing. How are (these disorders) removed?[42]

Bo Gao answered:

When the qi accumulates in the chest, take (the points) in the upper (part of the body). When (the qi accumulates) in the abdomen, take (the points) in the lower (part of the body). If both the upper and the lower (parts of the body) are filled up (with qi), take (the points) on the sides (in addition). For (accumulation) above, apply drainage at Man's Prognosis (*Ren Ying*, St 9), Celestial Prominence (*Tian Tu*, CV 22) and the throat center.[43] For accumulation below, apply drainage at Three Li (*San Li*, St 36) and Qi Thoroughfare (*Qi Chong*, St 30). If both the upper and the lower (aspects of the body) are filled up, take (the points) both above and below (in addition to the point) one *cun* below the free ribs,[44] and, for serious cases, take them with the chicken's claw needling.[45]

Those whose pulses are diagnosed as large, strong, and urgent, with expiring and impalpable pulses, or those whose abdominal skin is extremely taut may not be needled.

For counterflow qi ascension, needle the depression in the bosom and the pulsating vessel in the region of the free ribs.[46]

(3)

For thoracic fullness, unproductive retching, bitter taste in the mouth, dry tongue, and inability to ingest food and drink, Gallbladder Shu (*Dan Shu*, Bl 19) is the ruling point.

For thoracic fullness, asthmatic breathing, and the body bent with inability to catch one's breath, needle Man's Prognosis (*Ren Ying*, St 9) to a depth of four *fen*. Inappropriate needling may kill the patient.

For thoracic fullness and pain, Jade Pivot (*Xuan Ji*, CV 21) is the ruling point.

For stuffy fullness in the chest and lateral costal regions with pain radiating to the inside of the chest, Florid Canopy (*Hua Gai*, CV 20) is the ruling point.

For stuffy fullness in the chest and the lateral costal regions, *bi* pain, pain in the bones, inability to ingest food and drink, counterflow retching ["coughing" in the *Qian Jin* {later editor}], qi ascension, and vexation of the heart, Purple Palace (*Zi Gong*, CV 19) is the ruling point.

For fullness in the chest, inability to catch the breath, pain in the lateral costal regions, pain in the bones, counterflow qi ascension dyspnea, retching and vomiting, and vexation of the heart, Jade Hall (*Yu Tang*, CV 18) is the ruling point.

For stuffy fullness in the chest and lateral costal regions, diaphragmatic obstruction with inability of food to descend, and reflux retching and vomiting, Center Palace (*Zhong Ting*, CV 16) is the ruling point.[47]

For stuffy fullness in the chest and lateral costal regions with pain radiating to the bosom and inability to catch the breath, oppression, confusion, vexation, fullness, and inability to ingest food and drink, Spirit Homeland (*Ling Xu*, Ki 20) is the ruling point.

For stuffy fullness in the chest and the lateral costal regions, inability to catch the breath, counterflow cough, breast *yong*, shivering as if after a soaking, and aversion to cold, Spirit Seal (*Shen Feng*, Ki 23) is the ruling point.

For fullness in the chest and lateral costal regions, counterflow and obstruction of the diaphragmatic (qi), diminished qi impairing respiration, dyspneic breathing, and inability to lift the arms, Corridor Walk (*Bu Lang*, Ki 22) is the ruling point.

For stuffy fullness in the chest and lateral costal regions, counterflow qi ascension dyspnea, shrugging of the shoulders to facilitate breathing, and inability to taste food, Qi Door (*Qi Hu*, St 13) is the ruling point.

For throat *bi* and sudden counterflow in the chest, take first the penetrating vessel[48] and then Three Li (*San Li*, St 36) and Cloud Gate (*Yun Men*, Lu 2), all with the draining (manipulation).

For stuffy fullness in the chest and lateral costal regions initiating a dragging pain to the upper back and inability to turn over while lying, Chest Village (*Xiong Xiang*, Sp 19) is the ruling point.

For qi accumulation due to damage by worry, dejection, and thought, Central Venter (*Zhong Wan*, CV 12) is the ruling point.

For thoracic fullness, saber lumps, and inability to raise the arms, Armpit Abyss (*Yuan Ye*, GB 22) is the ruling point.

For great qi with inability to breathe (deeply) or pain in the chest and lateral costal regions arising with (deep) breathing and, in the case of repletion, cold all over the body, or in the case of vacuity, slackness of all the hundreds of joints, Great Bladder (*Da Bao*, Sp 21) is the ruling point.[49]

For sudden thoracic fullness, inability to lie down, and dyspnea, Sinew Seat (*Zhe Jin*, GB 23) is the ruling point.

For stuffing fullness in the chest and lateral costal regions, tugging and slackening initiating pain around the umbilicus and in the (lower) abdomen, qi shortage, vexation, and fullness, Great Tower Gate (*Ju Que*, CV 14) is the ruling point.

For accumulation of qi and binding pain in the abdomen, Beam Gate (*Liang Men*, St 21) is the ruling point.

For fullness in the lateral costal regions due to food damage, inability to turn over in bed, green-blue eyes, and retching, Cycle Gate (*Qi Men*, Liv 14) is the ruling point.

For stuffy fullness in the chest and lateral costal regions, Palace of Toil (*Lao Gong*, Per 8) is the ruling point.

For somnolence, frequent spitting, fullness in the chest, and rumbling in the intestines, Third Space (*San Jian*, LI 3) is the ruling point.

For fullness in the chest, inability to catch one's breath, and swelling in the neck and submandibular region, Yang Valley (*Yang Gu*, SI 5) is the ruling point.

For distention in the chest and lateral costal regions and rumbling of the intestines with lancinating pain ["stuffing fullness in the chest and the lateral costal regions, and lancinating pain in the abdomen" in a variant version {later editor}], Supreme White (*Tai Bai*, Sp 3) is the ruling point.

For sudden (abdominal) distention, stuffy fullness in the chest and lateral costal regions, cold feet, difficult defecation, white facial and labial complexion, and retching of blood from time to time, Supreme Surge (*Tai Chong*, Liv 3) is the ruling point.

For stuffy fullness in the chest and lateral costal regions, aversion to the voice of people and the sound of wood, the Upper Ridge of the Great Hollow (*Ju Xu Shang Liang*, St 37) is the ruling point.

For stuffy fullness in the chest and lateral costal regions and coldness in the body as if exposed to a draught, Pinched Ravine (*Xia Xi*, GB 43) is the

ruling point.

For pain in the chest and lateral costal regions, frequent sighing and inflating distention of the chest ["rigidity of the chest sinew" in the *Qian Jin* {later editor}], Hill Ruins (*Qiu Xu*, GB 40) is the ruling point.

For stuffy fullness in the chest and lateral costal regions, headache, and cold and heat in the nape of the neck, Outer Hill (*Wai Qiu*, GB 36) is the ruling point.

For stuffy fullness in the chest and subcostal regions and counterflow retching and vomiting, Yang Mound Spring (*Yang Ling Quan*, GB 34) is the ruling point.

Chapter Five

Evils in the Heart, Gallbladder, & Other Viscera & Bowels Producing Sorrow, Apprehension, Sighing, Bitter Taste in the Mouth, Melancholy, and Susceptibility to Fright[50]

(1)

The Yellow Emperor asked:

(It is said that) for bitter taste in the mouth, it is necessary to treat *Yang Ling Quan* (GB 34). What is the name of this disorder and how does it occur?

Qi Bo answered:

The disease is called biliary pure heat. The gallbladder is the bowel of the central essence. [The above nine characters are absent from the *Su Wen*, but instead are found "the liver holds office of the general in the center." {later editor}] The five viscera depend on it for decision. It has the pharynx at its disposal. Therefore, people (whose gallbladder is diseased) falter even after long consideration. When the biliary qi spills ["and is vacuous" in the *Su Wen* {later editor}] above, there is a bitter taste in the mouth. It is treated through the alarm point and the (back-associated) point of the gallbladder.[51] This is prescribed in the *Yin Yang Shi Er Guan Xiang Shi (The Inter-Potentiating of the Yin/Yang Twelve Organs).*[52]

(2)

For irritability, no desire for food, and ever growing silence, needle the foot *tai yin.*

For irascibility and loquaciousness, needle at the foot *shao yang.*

(3)

For qi shortage, heart *bi*, sorrow, irascibility, qi counterflow, and apprehension and mania, Fish Border (*Yu Ji*, Lu 10) is the ruling point.[53]

For heart pain, sentimentality, counterflow inversion, the sensation of a suspended heart as if hungering, faltering and stirring of the heart, susceptibility to fright, and apprehensiveness, Great Mound (*Da Ling*, Per 7) and Intermediary Courier (*Jian Shi*, Per 5) are the ruling points.

For faltering and stirring of the heart, susceptibility to fright, apprehension, and sorrow of the heart, Inner Pass (*Nei Guan*, Per 6) is the ruling point ["Marsh at the Bend (*Qu Ze*, Per 3)" in the *Qian Jin* {later editor}].

For susceptibility to fright, sorrow and melancholy, inversion, heat in the lower legs and soles of the feet, heat all over the face, and dry throat and thirst, Moving Between (*Xing Jian*, Liv 2) is the ruling point.

For spleen vacuity producing diseases of cold, melancholy, and frequent sighing in patients, Shang Hill (*Shang Qiu*, Sp 5) is the ruling point.

For somber green-blue complexion, sighing, death-like appearance, quivering with cold, whitish urine, and difficult defecation, Mound Center (*Zhong Feng*, Liv 4) is the ruling point.

For the sensation of a suspended heart, sorrow, confusion, irritability, swelling inside the throat, apprehensiveness and fearfulness as if afraid of arrest, profuse drooling, dyspnea, diminished qi, ebbing breath, and inability to catch the breath, Burning Valley (*Ran Gu*, Ki 2) is the ruling point.

For susceptibility to fright, sentimentality, melancholy, the sensation of falling from a height, lack of perspiration, a dusty, black facial complexion, and (constant) hungering yet with no desire for food, Shining Sea (*Zhao Hai*, Ki 6) is the ruling point.

For dizziness, cold inversion, pain in the arms and hands, susceptibility to fright of the gallbladder, ravings, a red facial complexion, and tearing, Armpit Gate (*Ye Men*, TH 2) is the ruling point.

For great fright with pain in the breast, Beam Hill (*Liang Qiu*, St 34) is the ruling point.

(4)

Evils in the heart result in diseases characterized by heart pain, sentimentality, and intermittent spinning collapse. (One should) determine surplus and insufficiency and then regulate the *shu.*[54]

Gallbladder disease is characterized by frequent sighing, bitter taste in the mouth, retching of stale water ["stale juice" in the *Ling Shu* {later editor}], faltering and stirring of the heart, apprehension as if fearing arrest, throat choked as if by a lump, and frequent spitting. Its signs are reflected in the foot *shao yang* from its origin to its endpoint. (One should) also moxa the sunken vessels found along the channel. For a case with cold and heat, take Yang Mound Spring (*Yang Ling Quan*, GB 34).[55]

Evils in the gallbladder result in counterflow in the stomach. When the bile spills, this results in a bitter taste in the mouth. Counterflow of stomach qi causes retching of bitter juice which is, therefore, called retching of gall. Take Three Li (*San Li*, St 36) to downbear stomach counterflow, prick the blood vessels of the foot *shao yang* to shut the gallbladder, and (finally) regulate vacuity and repletion to remove evil.

Chapter Six

Loss of Use of the Four Limbs Due to the Spleen Contracting Disease[56]

(1)

The Yellow Emperor asked:

Why is it that when the spleen becomes diseased this results in loss of use of the four limbs?

Qi Bo answered:

All four limbs depend on the stomach for their supply of qi, but the channels (in the limbs) have no (direct) access to (the fluid and humor of the stomach). They must rely on the spleen for their supplies. Once the spleen becomes diseased, it is no longer able to transport fluid and humor on behalf of the stomach, and, subsequently, the four limbs are not supplied with the qi from grain and water. As a result, qi diminishes day by day, the vessel passages become blocked, and the sinews, bones, and muscles can no longer function for lack of qi. In the end there is loss of use (of the four limbs).

The Yellow Emperor asked:

Why does the spleen rule no (particular) season?

Qi Bo answered:

The spleen is earth, and earth is located in the center. (Therefore,) it promotes the growth of the other four viscera in the four seasons, and they each spare eighteen days (of their reign for this. For this reason) it does not rule one entire season. The spleen, the viscus of earth, constantly stores the essence of stomach earth. Like the earth (in nature) which gives birth to the ten thousand things and in compliance to the laws of the heaven and the earth, (the spleen nourishes the entire body) from top to bottom, the head to the feet, and consequently cannot rule one (particular) season.[57]

The Yellow Emperor asked:

Since the spleen and stomach are linked by membranes, how is (the spleen) able to move fluid and humor (on behalf of the stomach)?

Qi Bo answered:

The foot *tai yin* is the third yin. Its vessel penetrates through the stomach, homes to the spleen, and connects with the throat. For this reason, the *tai yin* circulates qi to the three yin (on behalf of the stomach). The *yang ming* channel is the exterior (associate of the *tai yin*), and the sea of the five viscera and six bowels, and it circulates qi on behalf (of the *tai yin*) to the three yang. The viscera and bowels receive qi from the *yang ming* through the (*tai yin*) channel. That is how (the spleen) can circulate fluid and humor on behalf of the stomach. Because the limbs cannot receive supplies of water and grain qi, their qi is diminishing day by day, and the yin tracts are inhibited. Therefore, the sinews, bones, muscles, and flesh cannot sustain any longer and consequently lose their uses.[58]

(2)

For generalized heaviness and atony of the bones with insensitivity, Supreme White (*Tai Bai*, Sp 3) is the ruling point.

Chapter Seven

Contraction of Disease by the Spleen, Stomach, & Large Intestine Producing Abdominal Distention & Fullness, Rumbling of the Intestines, and Shortage of Qi[59]

(1)

Evils in the spleen and stomach result in illnesses characterized by pain in the muscles. If there is a surplus of yang qi while the yin qi is insufficient, this results in heat in the center with constant hunger. If the yang qi is insufficient while there is a surplus of yin, this results in cold in the center with rumbling of the intestines and pain in the abdomen. If both the yin and yang (qi) are in a state of either surplus or insufficiency, this results in cold and heat. For all of the above cases, regulate through Three Li (*San Li*, St 36).[60]

(2)

Inability of food and drink to descend with congestion of the diaphragm and throat is caused by evil in the stomach venter. If (the evil) exists in the upper venter, repress and downbear it. If it exists in the lower venter, disperse and remove it.[61]

For stomach disease characterized by abdominal distention and fullness, pain in the venter just opposite to the heart, propping fullness of the lateral costal regions, congestion of the diaphragm and throat, and inability of food and drink to descend, take Three Li.

Thunderous ["constant" in a variant version {later editor}] rumbling in the abdomen, qi surging up into the chest, dyspnea, and inability to stand for long are due to evil in the large intestine. Needle the membrane source,[62] the Upper Ridge of the Great Hollow (*Ju Xu Shang Lian*, St 37) and Three Li.

For anomalies in the abdomen, take Three Li. In the case of repletion, drain it, and in the case of vacuity, supplement it.[63]

For large intestine disease characterized by lancinating pain and gurgling of the intestine, and, in the case of dual cold in winter days, diarrhea, periumbilical pain, and inability to stand for long, the treatment is the same as with the stomach (disease), taking the Upper Ridge of the Great Hollow (*Ju Xu Shang Lian*, St 37).

(3)

For abdominal fullness, inhibited evacuation of stools, enlarged abdomen, (the water qi) surging up into the chest and throat [followed by the two words "dyspneic breathing" in the *Su Wen* {later editor}], and wheezing, take the foot *shao yin*.

For abdominal fullness, inability to transform food, rumbling (of the intestine), and inability to defecate, take the foot *tai yin*.

For abdominal pain, needle the pulsating vessels by either side of the umbilicus.[64] After extraction of the needle, press (the painful place) and the pain will be relieved on the spot. If not, then needle the Qi Thoroughfare (*Qi Chong*, St 30). After extraction of the needle, press (the painful place) and the pain will be relieved on the spot.

(4)

For sudden fullness in the abdomen such that (the abdomen) resists pressure, take the blood network vessels of the *tai yang* channels and relief will follow. In addition, needle the *shao yin* (associated back) point[65] ["the *shao yang* (associated back) point" in a variant version {later editor}], which is located one and a half *cun* bilateral to the spine, five times with a round-sharp needle. In about the time for a meal after the treatment, relief will be effected. This repeated needling, however, can be performed at the yang parts where the channel passes.[66]

(5)

For abdominal fullness with inability to ingest food, needle Spinal Center (*Ji Zhong*, GV 6).

Qi distention in the abdomen producing pain in the spine and emaciation in spite of large food intake are known as food withering. First take Spleen Shu (*Pi Shu*, Bl 20) and then take (the point at) the free rib region.[67]

For rolling of qi in the large intestine which when palpated feels like an inverted cup, with heat producing stomach pain, cold spleen qi, hypertonicity of and vexation in the four limbs, and no desire for food, Spleen Shu (*Pi Shu*, Bl 20) is the ruling point.

For cold and distention in the stomach, emaciation in spite of large food intake, fullness and rumbling in the abdomen, abdominal distention, wind inversion, stuffy fullness in the chest and lateral costal regions, retching and vomiting, hypertonicity of and pain in the spine, cramps of the sinews, and inability of food to descend, Stomach Shu (*Wei Shu*, Bl 21) is the ruling point.[68]

For headache, inability of water or food to descend, rumbling of the intestine, distention of the skin of the abdomen, desire to retch, and intermittent diarrhea, Triple Burner Shu (*San Jiao Shu*, Bl 22) is the ruling point.

For abdominal fullness with distention of the skin of the abdomen and thin-stool diarrhea, Reflection Abode (*Yi She*, Bl 44) is the ruling point.

For distention of the skin of the abdomen, water swelling, inability of food or water to descend, and abundant cold ["frequent aversion to cold" in the *Qian Jin* {later editor}], Stomach Granary (*Wei Cang*, Bl 45) is the ruling point.

Cold in the center and damage from gluttony with inability to transform food and drink, distention, stuffy fullness and distention in the heart, abdominal, thoracic, and lateral costal regions may generate hundreds of diseases if the pulse is vacuous. Upper Venter (*Shang Wan*, CV 13) is the ruling point.

For abdominal distention and blockage, cold in the center, damage from gluttony, and inability to transform food and drink, Central Venter (*Zhong Wan*, CV 12) is the ruling point.

For inability to transform food and drink and stomach reflux, Lower Venter (*Xia Wan*, CV 10) is the ruling point.

For frequent rumbling of the intestines and intermittent (qi) surging up into the heart, moxa the Center of the Navel (*Qi Zhong*, CV 8).

For heart fullness with qi counterflow, Yin Metropolis (*Yin Du*, Ki 19) is the ruling point.

For cold ["*shan*" in the *Qian Jin* {later editor}] in the large intestine with dry stool and lancinating pain in the abdomen, Huang Shu (*Huang Shu*, Ki 16) is the ruling point.

For pain over the entire abdomen, Outer Mound (*Wai Ling*, St 26) is the ruling point.

For rumbling of the intestines with qi chasing each other, and inability to lie on the side, Assuming Fullness (*Cheng Man*, St 20) is the ruling point.

For abdominal distention and a tendency to fullness with accumulation of qi, Pass Gate (*Guan Men*, St 22) is the ruling point.

For inability of food and drink to descend, thunderous rumbling in the abdomen, fecal incontinence, and yellowish or dark colored urine, Yang Headrope (*Yang Gang*, Bl 43) is the ruling point.

For abdominal distention, rumbling of the intestine, qi surging up into the chest, inability to stand for long, gurgling in the abdomen with pain, and, in the case of dual cold in winter days, resultant in diarrhea, periumbilical pain, qi wandering in the intestines with lancinating pain, inability to transform food, no desire for food, generalized swelling ["heaviness" in a variant version {later editor}] and hypertonicity around the umbilicus, Celestial Pivot (*Tian Shu*, St 25) is the ruling point.

For great heat in the abdomen, restlessness, great qi in the abdomen, sudden abdominal distention and fullness, dribbling urinary block, and (generalized) aching and weakness, Surging Qi (*Qi Chong*, St 30) is the ruling point.

Abdominal fullness and pain with inability to catch one's breath requires needling *Qi Chong* too, with the patient made to lie supine, one leg bent and the other stretched. Insert the needle three *cun* upward and perform drainage when the qi arrives.

For abdominal fullness of cold qi, urinary dribbling block, (generalized) aching and weakness, generalized fever, and gatherings and accumulations in the abdomen with pain, Surging Gate (*Chong Men*, Sp 12) is the ruling point.

For gurgling in the intestines inside the abdomen,

inability to transform food, pain in the lateral costal regions with inability to lie down, vexation, fever, dry mouth, no desire for food, stuffy fullness in the chest and lateral costal regions, dyspneic breathing with (qi) surging against the diaphragm, vomiting, heart pain, damage from gluttony, generalized jaundice, aching and weakness, and marked emaciation, Camphorwood Gate (*Zhang Men*, Liv 13) is the ruling point.

For intestinal rumbling and pain, Warm Dwelling (*Wen Liu*, LI 7) is the ruling point.

For abdominal distention with intermittent cold and lumbar pain with inability to lie down, Hand Three Li (*Shou San Li*, LI 10) is the ruling point.

For cold qi in the abdomen, Hidden White (*Yin Bai*, Sp 1) is the ruling point.

For fullness and gurgling in the abdomen, constipation, and cold and pain below the heart, Shang Hill (*Shang Qiu*, Sp 5) is the ruling point.

For either heat or cold in the abdomen, frequent rumbling of the intestines, yawning but with difficulty, intermittent pain in the internal, sorrow, qi counterflow, and abdominal fullness, Leaking Valley (*Lou Gu*, Sp 7) is the ruling point. If, after needling (the point) above the medial malleolus, qi (counterflow) is not checked, with abdominal distention and qi giving a pleasant relief to the elbows and the region of the free ribs, this point is also the ruling point.[69]

For abdominal qi distention with groaning,[70] no desire for food, and fullness in the region of the free ribs, Yin Mound Spring (*Yin Ling Quan*, Sp 9) is the ruling point.

For dyspnea, diminished qi which is insufficient to allow one to catch one's breath, abdominal fullness, difficult defecation, intermittent (qi) ascension, rale in the chest with distention and fullness, dry tongue and mouth, stirring (of the tongue) in the mouth, susceptibility to fright, sore throat with difficulty in swallowing food, irascibility, apprehension, and melancholy, Large Goblet (*Da Zhong*, Ki 4) is the ruling point.

For dry throat, tugging pain in the abdomen, blurred vision upon sitting up, irascibility, and talkativeness, Recover Flow (*Fu Liu*, Ki 7) is the ruling point.

For cold in the abdomen with distention and fullness, Severe Mouth (*Li Dui*, St 45) is the ruling point.

For abdominal enlargement with no desire for food, Surging Yang (*Chong Yang*, St 42) is the ruling point.

For ascending counterflow of inversion qi, Great Ravine (*Tai Xi*, Ki 3) is the ruling point.

For heat in the large intestine with rumbling of the intestine, abdominal fullness, periumbilical pain, inability to transform food, dyspnea, and inability to stand for long, the Upper Ridge of the Great Hollow (*Ju Xu Shang Lian*, St 37) is the ruling point.

For cold in the intestines with distention and fullness, frequent belching, aversion to the smell of food, insufficiency of the stomach qi, rumbling of the intestines, pain in the abdomen, diarrhea of untransformed food in stools, and distention (in the region) below the heart, Three Li (*San Li*, St 36) is the ruling point.

For abdominal fullness, heat in the stomach and no desire for food, Suspended Bell (*Xuan Zhong*, GB 39) is the ruling point.

For large intestine repletion resulting in pain in the upper and lower back, cold *bi*, cramps of the sinews, and spinning and ache of the head, or large intestine vacuity resulting in nosebleeding, madness, lumbar pain, a drenching sweat, and intensified desire for food and to walk about, Sinew Support (*Cheng Jin*, Bl 56) is the ruling point. Take the third fold of the foot and let blood out of the prominent transverse blood vessel.[71]

Chapter Eight

Contraction of Disease by the Kidney &
the Small Intestine Producing
Abdominal Distention & Lumbar Pain
Sending a Dragging (Discomfort) to the
Upper Back & Lower Abdomen and a
Dragging Pain to the Testicles[72]

(1)

Evils in the kidney result in bone pain and yin *bi*. For yin *bi* which cannot be located by palpation with abdominal distention, lumbar pain, difficult defecation, stiffness and pain of the shoulders, upper back, and neck, and intermittent dizziness, take Gushing Spring (*Yong Quan*, Ki 1) and Kun Lun Mountain (*Kun Lun*, Bl 60) and take all the blood vessels found.[73]

(2)

If the lower abdomen initiates a dragging pain in the testicles, which, (in turn,) produces a dragging (discomfort) in the lumbar spine with an ascending surgance (of qi) into the heart and the lung, then there is evil in the small intestine. (This is because) the small intestine links with the testicular ligation, homes to the spine, penetrates the liver and lung, and connects with the heart ligation. If its qi is exuberant, this will result in counterflow inversion, surging up into the stomach and intestines, stirring the liver and lung, dispersing into the mesentery, and binding in the umbilicus. Therefore, take the origin of the mesentery[74] to disperse (the binding), needle the *tai yin* to make up for (the lung vacuity), take the *jue yin* to precipitate (the repletion of the liver), take the Upper Ridge of the Great Hollow (*Ju Xu Shang Lian*, St 37) to remove (the evil qi from the small intestine), and regulate the channels visited (by the evil qi).[75]

(3)

When the small intestine is diseased, there is lower abdominal pain, a dragging sensation in the lumbar spine producing testicular pain with an occasional awkward feeling in the posterior,

either heat or intense cold (in the regions) anterior to the auricles, or a feeling of intense heat exclusively in the shoulders, and heat between the small and the ring finger or sunken vessels. These are the manifestations (of a disease of small intestine).[76]

(4)

The Yellow Emperor asked:

In inversion diseases, the pulse at the right side may be found to be deep and hard, while the pulse at the left is floating and slow. I wonder where the disease exists.

Qi Bo answered:

When examined in the winter, the right pulse should be deep and hard in correspondence with the season. If the left pulse is floating and slow, this is incongruent to the seasonal disposition. The left pulse should indicate disease. The examination of the left demonstrates (disease) in the kidney. There will be lung involvement as well, and there will be lumbar pain.[77]

The Yellow Emperor asked:

Why do you say this?

Qi Bo answered:

The *shao yin* vessel penetrates the kidney and connects with the lung. Now we have got the lung pulse, the kidney is diseased, and therefore there is lumbar pain.[78]

(5)

The foot *tai yang* vessel causes people to suffer from lower back pain which initiates a heaviness in the nape of the neck, spine, and sacrococcygeal areas as if one were bearing weights. Needle the cleft point. That is, let blood out at its primary channel. In spring, however, bleeding (therapy) is prohibited.[79]

The *shao yang* causes people to suffer from lower

back pain which feels like the skin is being pricked by needles, with restricted movement and inability to bend the body either forward or backward or to turn it round. Prick the (foot) *tai yang* at the end of the supporting bone (tibia) to let blood out. The (upper end of) the supporting bone is the outstanding prominence of the bone at the lateral border of the knee. In summer, however, bleeding (therapy) is prohibited.[80]

The *yang ming* causes people to suffer from lower back pain with inability to turn (the lumbus) round or confused vision when one attempts to turn round, and sentimentality. Prick the (foot) *yang ming* with three punctures anterior to the tibia to harmonize above and below by bloodletting. In autumn, however, bleeding (therapy) is prohibited.[81]

The foot *shao yin* causes people to suffer from lower back pain which radiates to the inside of the spine. Prick the foot *shao yin* (at the point) above the medial malleolus[82] twice. In spring, however, bleeding (therapy) is prohibited; copious bleeding leads to irretrievable vacuity.

The *jue yin* vessel causes people to suffer from pain in the lower back which is (tense) like the full drawn bow-string. Needle the *jue yin* vessel outside the fish belly between the calf and the heel, pricking (the place) that feels like a cluster of small balls on palpation. This disease makes the patient silent and lethargic. Prick three times.[83]

The unraveled vessel (*jie mai*, 解脉) causes people to suffer from lower back pain radiating to the shoulders with blurred vision and intermittent enuresis. Prick the unraveled vessel at the border of the flesh between the sinews below the knee, at the transverse vessel lateral border of the popliteal fossa. When the blood turns (to a normal color) stop pricking.[84]

The merging-into-yin vessel (*tong yin zhi mai*, 同阴之脉) causes people to suffer from lower back pain which is like being pierced by small awls, and is characterized by raging swelling. Prick the merging-into-yin vessel at the end of the severed bone at the lateral malleolus three times.[85]

The unraveled vessel causes people to suffer from splitting lower back pain ["as if dragged by a belt" in the *Su Wen* {later editor}] with irascibility. (The low back) is often bent. Needle the unraveled vessel in the popliteal fossa, pricking the binding connecting vessel there which is like a millet grain. Upon being pricked, the vessel will ejaculate black blood and, once the blood turns red, the treatment may be stopped. [Qian Yuanqi[86] says, "There are two unraveled vessels, each of which has a distinct pathogenicity." An error is suspected here but it remains to be confirmed. {later editor}][87]

The yang linking vessel causes people to suffer from lower back pain with raging swelling in the painful place. Prick the yang linking vessel at the place where the vessel meets the (foot) *tai yang* below the calf, one *chi* or so above the ground.[88]

The transverse connecting vessel (*heng luo zhi mai*, 衡络之脉) causes people to suffer from lower back pain with ability to bend forward but not backward for fear of falling. This is caused by damage to the lower back in lifting heavy weights. The transverse connecting vessel is ruptured and damaged, and foul blood has collected (there). Prick between the sinews at the yang (lateral) border of the popliteal fossa and the (vessel) lying transversely several *cun* above the popliteal fossa. Prick with two punctures to let blood out.[89]

The meeting-yin vessel causes people to suffer from lower back pain with soaking perspiration on attack of the pain, desire for drinks after the sweat is dried, and desire to walk after drinking. Prick the straight yang vessel with three punctures at the transversely lying vessel. This is located three *cun* above the (yang) motility vessel and (three *cun*) below the cleft. Let out blood from the vessel found to be exuberant. [In the *Su Wen*, "soaking" is replaced by "downpour" and "three *cun*" by "five *cun*." {later editor}][9000]

The soaring yang vessel (*fei yang zhi mai*, 飞阳之脉) causes people to suffer from lower back pain with raging (swelling) in the painful place, and, in serious cases, to experience sorrow and apprehension. Prick the soaring yang vessel at two *cun* ["five *cun*" in the *Su Wen* {later editor}] above the medial malleolus ["anterior to the foot *shao yin*" in the *Su Wen* {later editor}] where the soaring yang vessel meets with the yin linking vessel.[91]

The glorious yang vessel (*chang yang zhi mai*, 昌阳之脉) causes people to suffer from lower back pain radiating to the bosom with blurred vision, and, in serious cases, arched-back rigidity and curled tongue with inability to speak. Prick the inner sinew with two punctures, (or, more exactly, the point) which is above the medial malleolus anterior to the major sinew but posterior to the (foot) *tai yin*, two *cun* or so above the malleolus.[92]

The dispersing vessel causes people to suffer from lower back pain and heat, with intense heat producing vexation and a sensation of a wooden bar crossing inside the body below the lumbus. In severe cases, there is even enuresis. Prick the dispersing vessel anterior to the knee at the juncture between the flesh and the bone where the lateral aspect of the knee is connected by the binding sinew connecting with the lateral aspect of the knee. Make three punctures.[93]

The interior flesh vessel (*rou li zhi mai*) causes people to suffer from lower back pain such that one does not dare cough or suffers from hypertonicity when one does cough. Prick the interior flesh vessel with two punctures lateral to the (foot) *tai yang* at the end of the severed bone where the (foot) *shao yang* (passes).[94]

For lower back pain with paravertebral pain, rigidity extending up to the head, blurred vision, and a tendency to collapse, prick the foot *tai yang* at the popliteal fossa to let out blood.[95]

For lower back pain radiating to the lower abdomen and sending a dragging (discomfort) into the lateral abdomen with inability to bend (the body) either forward or backward, prick the meeting (point) at the lumbo-sacrococcygeal area (which is located) at the paravertebral muscle at the iliac crest. The number of the punctures is determined by the waxing and waning of the moon. With extraction of the needle one will be cured immediately. [The *Su Wen* adds, "For problems of the right, choose the point at the left and for problems of the left, choose the point on the right." {later editor}][96]

For lower back pain with cold in the upper (body), take the foot *tai yang* and *yang ming*. In the case of heat in the lower (body), take the foot *jue yin*. In the case of inability to bend (the body) either forward or backward, take the foot *shao yang*. In the case of heat in the center with dyspnea, take the foot *shao yin* or the blood vessel in the popliteal fossa.[97]

(6)

For lower back pain with cold in the painful place, and, in the case of repletion, hypertonicity, and rigidity of the spine, Long Strong (*Chang Qiang*, GV 1) is the ruling point.

For lower abdominal pain and heat sending a dragging pain to the testicles and a dragging (discomfort) to the lumbar spine, *shan* pain, an ascending surge of (qi) into the heart, rigidity of the lumbar spine, difficult voiding of yellowish or dark-colored urine, and dry mouth, Small Intestine Shu (*Xiao Chang Shu*, Bl 27) is the ruling point.

For pain in and rigidity of the lumbar spine sending a dragging (discomfort) to the upper back and lateral lower abdomen, difficulty in bending either forward or backward, inability to breathe in supine posture, atony and heaviness of the feet, inability to lift the sacrococcygeal region, reddish urine, frigidity and insensitivity from the lumbus down through the feet, and inability to sit up, Bladder Shu (*Pang Guang Shu*, Bl 28) is the ruling point.

For lower back pain with inability to bend either forward or backward, Central Backbone Inner Shu (*Zhong Lu Nei Shu*, Bl 29) is the ruling point.

For pain and frigidity in the lumbar spine with habitual stooping posture and testicular retraction, Upper Bone Hole (*Shang Liao*, Bl 31) is the ruling point.

For distressing lower back pain and inability to bend either forward or backward, insensitivity extending from the lumbar region down through the feet, and (cold) entering the spine with cold in the upper and lower back, Second Bone Hole (*Ci Liao*, Bl 32) is the ruling point. First take Empty Basin (*Que Pen*, St 12) and then the tail bone[98] and the eight bone holes.[99]

For lower back pain with difficult defecation, swill diarrhea, and cold in the lumbus and sacro-coccygeal (region), Central Bone Hole (*Zhong Liao*, Bl 33) is the ruling point.

For lower back pain with hypertonicity of the spine, fullness in the region of the free ribs, and hardness and hypertonicity of the lower abdomen, Will Chamber (*Zhi Shi*, Bl 47) is the ruling point.

For pain in the lumbar spine, aversion to cold, hardness and fullness of the lower abdomen, dribbling urinary block with a sensation of pressure in the bladder, and inability to void urine, Bladder Huang (*Bao Huang*, Bl 48) is the ruling point.

For lower back pain with cold in the sacrococcygeal (region), inhibition and difficulty in bending (the body) either forward or backward, pain in the genitals accompanied by a sensation of being weighted down, and inability to void urine, Sequential Limit (*Zhi Bian*, Bl 54) is the ruling point.

For lower back pain sending a dragging (discomfort) into the testicles, lower abdomen, and thighs with inability to bend (the body) backward once bent forward, needle Qi Thoroughfare (*Qi Jie*, St 30).

For lower back pain with inability to turn round, Camphorwood Gate (*Zhang Men*, Liv 13) is the ruling point.

For lower back pain with inability to stand for long or to bend either forward or backward, Capital Gate (*Jing Men*, GB 25) and Moving Between (*Xing Jian*, Liv 2) are the ruling points.

For lower back pain and lower abdominal pain, Lower Bone Hole (*Xia Liao*, Bl 34) is the ruling point.

For lower back pain with inability to bend either forward or backward, Yin Mound Spring (*Yin Ling Quan*, Sp 9) is the ruling point.

For lower back pain, fullness in the lower abdomen, urinary inhibition as if blocked, marked emaciation, apprehension and fearfulness, and insufficiency of qi and distressing discomfort in the abdomen, Supreme Surge (*Tai Chong*, Liv 3) is the ruling point.

For lower back pain and lower abdominal pain, Yin Bladder (*Yin Bao*, Liv 9) is the ruling point.

For lower back pain and difficult defecation ["a dragging {pain} in the lumbar spine as if disintegrating" in the *Qian Jin* {later editor}], Gushing Spring (*Yong Quan*, Ki 1) is the ruling point.

For dribbling urinary block, shivering (with cold), pain in the lumbar spine, rolling of the eyes, somnolence, and heat in the mouth in the case of repletion, or lower back pain, cold inversion, and vexation of the heart with oppression in the case of vacuity, Large Goblet (*Da Zhong*, Ki 4) is the ruling point.

For lower back pain radiating to the inner aspect of the spine, Recover Flow (*Fu Liu*, Ki 7) is the ruling point. In spring, bleeding is prohibited; copious bleeding leads to irretrievable vacuity [same as the previously discussed lower back pain of the foot *shao yin* {later editor}].

For lower back pain with inability to raise the feet or to sit even for a short time and a burning sensation in the lower legs as if having bumped them in getting off a cart, Extending Vessel (*Shen Mai*, Bl 62) is the ruling point.

For lower back pain which feels as if it were being pierced by small awls, raging swelling and pain, not daring to cough, or contraction and hypertonicity of the sinews upon coughing, pain in various joints with no fixed location, and cold and heat, Yang Assistance (*Yang Fu*, GB 38) is the ruling point.

For lower back pain with inability to lift (the lumbus), pain in the heels and the region posterior to the malleolus, and atony of the feet, Kneeling Visitor (*Pu Can*, Bl 61) is the ruling point.

For lower back pain with rigidity of the paravertebral regions extending to the head and blurred vision, Bend Middle (*Wei Zhong*, Bl 40) is the ruling point [same as the previously discussed lower back pain of the foot *tai yang* with bleeding therapy at the cleft point {later editor}].

For lower back pain which was contracted by lifting heavy weights and which causes foul blood to collect with ability to bend forward but not backward for fear of falling over, Gate of Abundance (*Yin Men*, Bl 51) is the ruling point [same as the previously discussed lower back pain of the transverse connecting vessel {later editor}].

For intense pain in the lumbar spine, sacrococcygeal (region), thighs, and buttocks due to yin cold, and, in the case of vacuity, stirring blood, or in the case of repletion, heat and pain, (and for) hemorrhoids, pain in the perineum, pain in the hips, and fecal incontinence, Support (*Cheng Fu*, Bl 50) is the ruling point.

Chapter Nine

Contraction of Disease by the Triple Heater & Urinary Bladder Producing Swelling in the Lower Abdomen & Difficult Urination[100]

(1)

Lower abdominal swelling and pain with difficult urination is due to evil in the triple burner. (It is this evil) which is the constrictor. (For this,) take the major connecting vessel of the foot *tai yang*[101] and the network vessels of the channel and locate the small network vessels of the (foot) *jue yin* which are bound with blood. If the swelling extends upward to the venter, take Three Li (*San Li*, St 36).[102]

(2)

Disease of the triple burner is characterized by abdominal distention and qi fullness with extreme hardness in the lower abdomen (upon palpation) and an inability to void urine accompanied by an awkward urgency. If (water) spills, this results in water (swelling). If (water) is retained, this results in distention. Indicators can be found in the major connecting vessel lateral to the foot *tai yang*, (more exactly,) between the foot *tai yang* and the foot *shao yang*,[103] where a redness can be observed in the vessels. Take Bend Yang (*Wei Yang*, Bl 53).[104]

Disease of the urinary bladder is characterized by swelling and pain throughout the lower abdomen, hand pressure (on the lower abdomen causing) a desire to urinate yet inability to do so, heat above the eyebrows ["in the shoulders" in a variant version {later editor}], and possibly, a sunken pulse with heat all along the lateral aspect of the small toe, lower legs, and the region posterior to the malleolus. For this, take Bend Middle (*Wei Zhong*, Bl 40).[105]

(3)

Diseases characterized by pain in the lower abdomen with inability to urinate and defecate is defined as *shan*. With affliction by cold, there is lower abdominal distention and cold in the medial aspect of the thighs. Needle (the points) between the lumbar region and iliac crest, choosing a sufficient number (of points). Once one has needled and the entire (lower abdomen) has become hot, the disease will be cured.

For lower abdominal fullness and enlargement, (qi counterflow) penetrating the stomach and extending to the heart, chilling, intermittent, generalized cold and heat, and inhibited urination, take the foot *jue yin*.

(4)

For fetal shifting (such that it presses on the urinary bladder) prohibiting urination, and lower abdominal fullness, Origin Pass (*Guan Yuan*, CV 4) is the ruling point.

For difficult urination, water distention and fullness, scanty urine, and fetal shifting (such that it presses on the urinary bladder) prohibiting urination, Curved Bone (*Qu Gu*, CV 2) is the ruling point.

Lower abdominal distention and hypertonicity, urinary inhibition, and inversion qi extending to the head, Leaking Valley (*Lou Gu*, Sp 7) is the ruling point.

For difficulty and pain on urination, white turbidity, sudden *shan*, lower abdominal swelling, counterflow coughing, retching and vomiting, sudden retraction of the testicles, lumbar pain with inability to bend either forward or backward, somber, black facial complexion, heat, abdominal distention and fullness, generalized fever, and inversion pain, Moving Between (*Xing Jian*, Liv 2) is the ruling point.

For lower abdominal fullness and heat blockage causing inability to urinate, the Foot Five Li (*Zu Wu Li*, Liv 10) is the ruling point.[106]

For lower abdominal fullness ["pain" in variant version {later editor}] with urinary inhibition, Gushing Spring (*Yong Quan*, Ki 1) is the ruling point.

For hypertonicity of the sinews and generalized fever, lower abdominal hardness and swelling with intermittent fullness, difficult urination, cold in the sacrococcygeal (region) and thighs, and pain in the hip joints radiating to the region of the free ribs and internally sending a dragging pain to the eight bone hole region, Bend Middle (*Wei Zhong*, Bl 40) is the ruling point.

For cold in the urinary bladder with urinary inhibition, Support (*Fu Cheng*, Bl 50)[107] is the ruling point.

Chapter Ten

Internal Blockage & Constriction of the Triple Heater, Causing Inability to Urinate or Defecate[108]

(1)

For inability to urinate due to internal blockage,

needle the foot *shao yin*, (the foot) *tai yang*[109] and the tail bone[110] with a long needle. For qi counterflow, take the (foot) *tai yin* and *yang ming*.[111] If the inversion is severe, treat the moving vessels of the (foot) *shao yin* and *yang ming*.[112]

(2)

For constriction of the triple burner producing an inability to urinate and defecate, Waterway (*Shui Dao*, St 28) is the ruling point.

For difficult defecation, Central Flow (*Zhong Zhu*, Ki 15) and Supreme White (*Tai Bai*, Sp 3) are the ruling points.

For difficult defecation, Large Goblet (*Da Zhong*, Ki 4) is the ruling point.

Chapter Eleven

Stirring in the Vessel of the *Jue Yin* and Constant Joy & Anger Causing *Tui Shan*, Enuresis, & Dribbling Urinary Blockage[113]

(1)

The Yellow Emperor asked:

The *Ci Jie (Needling Strategies)* explains that undressing (*qu yi*, 去衣) requires that one needle the branch connecting vessel at the joints. Please tell me about this in detail.[114]

Qi Bo answered:

The lumbar spine is composed of the key joints in humans. The upper and the lower legs are responsible for nimbleness in movement in humans. The penis and the testicles are the crucial mechanism in the body, reflecting (the state of) the yin essence and providing a passageway of fluid and humor. Either dietary irregularities or constant joy and anger may cause the inward flow of fluid and humor. They spill downward into the testicles, causing obstruction to the water passageway there. As a result, (the scrotum) becomes bigger day by day, (the body) bends with ever more difficulty, nimble movement becomes impossible, water accumulates gradually, and the (qi) can neither ascend nor descend. When a sword needle is used, the (water) form will find nowhere to hide and be divested of any cover. (This technique) is called undressing.[115]

(2)

The Yellow Emperor asked:

There is a species of dribbling urinary block with urinating many tens of times per day, and this is a manifestation of an insufficiency. There may be generalized fever as high as burning charcoal, repellence-like disorder in the neck and bosom, an agitated and exuberant *ren ying* pulse, and dyspneic breathing with counterflow qi ascension [in the *Su Wen* "prodigal exuberance of the yang qi in the exterior with insufficiency of the yin qi" is added {later editor}], and these are manifestations of surplus. The *tai yin* pulse may be faint and fine like a hair, and this is a manifestation of an insufficiency. Where does the disease lie?[116]

Qi Bo answered:

It lies in the *tai yin*, while the exuberance lies in the stomach and involves the lung to a large extent. The disease is called inversion. It ends in death and is without remedy. This is the result of a fivefold surplus and dual insufficiency.[117]

The Yellow Emperor asked:

What is (the nature of) this so-called fivefold surplus and dual insufficiency?

Qi Bo answered:

That which is referred to as five fold surplus is a surplus of diseased qi, and, in the case of dual insufficiency, the diseased qi is insufficient (in nature). Since there is a fivefold surplus externally and a dual insufficiency internally, this is neither simply an exterior nor an interior (problem).

It is evident that death is a certainty.[118]

(3)

For fox-like *shan* with susceptibility to fright, palpitation, and diminished qi, Great Tower Gate (*Ju Que*, CV 14) is the ruling point.

For yin *shan* sending a dragging pain to the testicles, Yin Intersection (*Yin Jiao*, CV 7) is the ruling point.[119]

For lower abdominal fullness, difficult urination, and slackened genitals, Pubic Bone (*Heng Gu*, Ki 11) is the ruling point.

For lower abdominal *shan* with susceptibility to fright while sleeping, Sea of Qi (*Qi Hai*, CV 6) is the ruling point.

For sudden *shan* pain with intense heat in the lower abdomen, Origin Pass (*Guan Yuan*, CV 4) is the ruling point.

For yin *shan* and qi *shan*, Celestial Pivot (*Tian Shu*, St 25) is the ruling point.[120]

For *tui shan*, Great Gigantic (*Da Ju*, St 27), Earth's Crux (*Di Ji*, Sp 8) and Central Cleft (*Zhong Xi*, GB 32) are the ruling points.

For yin *shan* with impotence, pain in the penis, bilateral testicular retraction and pain, and inability to lie supine, needle the Qi Thoroughfare (*Qi Jie*, St 30).

For yin *shan*, Surging Gate (*Chong Men*, Sp 12) is the ruling point.

For yin *shan* in males with intermittent retraction of the testicles and lower abdominal pain, Fifth Pivot (*Wu Shu*, GB 27) is the ruling point.

For pain in the medial aspect of the thigh, qi counterflow, fox-like *shan* moving up and down and initiating pain in the lower abdomen, and inability to bend (the body) either forward or backward, Shang Hill (*Shang Qiu*, Sp 5) is the ruling point.

For fox-like *shan*, Supreme Surge (*Tai Chong*, Liv 3) is the ruling point.

For testicular retraction, enuresis, urinary difficulty and pain, testicles withdrawn upward into the abdomen, cold *shan*, vaginal protrusion, enlargement and swelling of one testicle, periumbilical abdominal pain, and dull discomfort in the abdomen, Large Pile (*Da Dun*, Liv 1) is the ruling point.

For abdominal pain radiating (counterflow qi) up into the heart, fullness below the heart, dribbling urinary block, pain in the penis, glaring in anger with aversion to the sight of anything, tearing and frequent deep sighing, Moving Between (*Xing Jian*, Liv 2) is the ruling point.

For *tui shan* with sudden pain in the genitals, Mound Center (*Zhong Feng*, Liv 4) is the ruling point.

For *shan*, dribbling urinary block, a dragging pain between the umbilicus and the lateral lower abdomen, and lower back pain, Mound Center (*Zhong Feng*, Liv 4) is the ruling point.

For dribbling urinary qi blockage with yellowish urine, qi fullness, and, in the case of vacuity, intermittent generalized fever and chills, counterflow vomiting, difficult urination, and fullness in the abdomen, Stone Gate (*Shi Men*, CV 5) is the ruling point.[121]

For dribbling urinary qi blockage and *tui shan* with genital hypertonicity and pain in the medial aspect of the upper thigh and calf, Intersection Reach (*Jiao Xin*, Ki 8) is the ruling point.

For testicular retraction and lower back pain accompanied, in the case of repletion, by persistent (penile) erection, fever and chills, hypertonicity, sudden pain in the genitals, enuresis and enlargement of one testicle and, in the case of vacuity, fulminant itching (of the genitals), qi counterflow, swollen testicles, sudden *shan*, dribbling, block-like inhibited urination, frequent belching, apprehension, palpitation, insufficiency of qi, discomfort

in the abdomen, pain in the lower abdomen, heat in the throat producing a sensation of a fleshy polyp there (which nearly protrudes), and hypertonicity of the back with inability to bend either forward or backward, Woodworm Canal (*Li Gou*, Liv 5) is the ruling point.

For *tui shan* in males with testicular retraction causing pain to radiate into the perineum, inability to urinate, abdominal distention, stuffy fullness in the region of the free ribs, dribbling urinary block, impotence, intermittent mild diarrhea, debilitation of the four extremities, and, in the case of repletion, generalized fever and pain, headache, lack of perspiration, blurred vision, a raging impulse to commit murder, sudden pain (in the genitals) radiating to the lower joints in the lower back, intermittent heat qi, hypertonicity of the sinews, pain in the knees with inability to contract or stretch, disorder like newly contracted mania, nosebleeding, refusing to eat, dyspneic wheezing, lower abdominal pain sending a dragging (discomfort) to the throat and inversion pain in the feet, Spring at the Bend (*Qu Quan*, Liv 8) is the ruling point.

For dribbling urinary block with *shan*, Blazing Valley (*Ran Gu*, Ki 2) is the ruling point.

For sudden *shan* with lower abdominal pain, Shining Sea (*Zhao Hai*, Ki 6) is the ruling point. For problems on the left, choose the point on the right, and for problems on the right, choose the point on the left. (The patient) will be cured on the spot.

For sudden *shan* in the genitals with pain and weakness in the four limbs and heart oppression, Shining Sea (*Zhao Hai*, Ki 6) is the ruling point.

For *shan*, Reaching Yin (*Zhi Yin*, Bl 67) is the ruling point.

For enuresis, Pass Gate (*Guan Men*, St 22), Spirit Gate (*Shen Men*, Ht 7), and Bend Middle (*Wei Zhong*, Bl 40) are the ruling points.

For inflating fullness of the chest accompanied, in

the case of repletion, by dribbling urinary block and swelling and pain in the axillae, and, in the case of vacuity, by enuresis, hypertonicity and twitching of the feet, hypertonicity and pain of the sinews, inability to urinate or defecate, and lower back pain sending a dragging (discomfort) to the abdomen with inability to bend either forward or backward, Bend Yang (*Wei Yang*, Bl 53) is the ruling point.

For dribbling urinary qi blockage in males, Central Bone Hole (*Zhong Liao*, Bl 33) is the ruling point.

For dribbling urinary qi block with yellowish urine, Origin Pass (*Guan Yuan*, CV 4) and Yin Mound Spring (*Yin Ling Quan*, Sp 9) are the ruling points. ["For kidney disease with inability to bend the body either forward or backward due to heedlessness of cold and heat" in the *Qian Jin*. {later editor}]

For dribbling urinary qi blockage with yellowish urine, qi fullness, and, in the case of vacuity, enuresis, Stone Gate (*Shi Men*, CV 5) is effective.

For dribbling urinary blockage, enuresis, pain in the groin, and difficult urination of whitish urine, Cycle Gate (*Ji Men*, Sp 11) is the ruling point.

For urinary difficulty with heat in the portal accompanied, in the case of repletion, by pain in the abdominal skins or, in the case of vacuity, by itching, Meeting of Yin (*Hui Yin*, CV 1) is the ruling point.[122]

For heat in the small intestine with yellowish or dark colored urine, Central Venter (*Zhong Wan*, CV 12) is the ruling point.

For yellowish urine, Lower Ridge (*Xia Lian*, LI 8) is the ruling point.

For yellowish or dark colored urine, Completion Bone (*Wan Gu*, GB 12) is the ruling point.

For yellowish urine and peals of rumbling in the intestine, Upper Ridge (*Shang Lian*, St 37) is the ruling point.

For taxation pure heat wasting thirst and difficult voidings of dark colored urine, Front Valley (*Qian Gu*, SI 2) is the ruling point.

Chapter Twelve

Stirring in the Vessel of the Foot Tai Yang Causing Piles & Prolapse of the Rectum in the Lower (Part of the Body)[123]

For hemorrhoidal pain, Bamboo Gathering (*Zan Zhu*, GB 2) is the ruling point.

For hemorrhoids, Meeting of Yin (*Hui Yin*, CV 1) is the ruling point. In all cases, hemorrhoids with perforation into the genitals results in death. This is also the ruling point for any diseases involving the two yin with a dragging pain between the anterior and the posterior yin and inability to urinate or defecate.[124]

For hemorrhoids and bone erosion, Shang Hill (*Shang Qiu*, Sp 5) is the ruling point.[125]

For hemorrhoids with pain in the perineum, Flying Yang (*Fei Yang*, Bl 58), Bend Middle (*Wei Zhong*, Bl 40), and Support (*Fu Cheng*, Bl 50)[126] are the ruling points.

For hemorrhoids with pain in the perineum, Sinew Support (*Cheng Ji*, Bl 56) is the ruling point.

For prolapse of the rectum with diarrhea, the Qi Thoroughfare (*Qi Jie*, St 30) is the ruling point.

Endnotes

[1]Part 1 is derived from Chap. 47, *Su Wen (Basic Questions)*; Part 2 from Chap. 21 and 24, Vol. 24, *Ling Shu (Spiritual Pivot)*; Part 3 from Chap. 26, Vol. 5, *Ling Shu*; and Part 4 from the *Zhen Jiu Ming Tang Zhi Yao (Acupuncture & Moxibustion Treatment Essentials of the Enlightening Hall)*.

[2]When yang evils counterflow in the yang channels, qi becomes chaotic in the upper part of the body causing headache.

[3]If the evil counterflows in the channels and goes up to affect the head and brain, the headache is called inversion headache.

[4]Pain in the vessels of the head is not a headache that afflicts the brain. Rather it is an ache in the muscles, vessels, and skin on the head. Since the qi counterflows in the liver. This causes sadness, etc. This disorder should be treated by bloodletting to drain the evil and then by supplementation of the liver at, for example, Supreme Surge (*Tai Chong*, Liv 3), the source point of the *jue yin*.

[5]This pattern is due to counterflow of the foot *yang ming*, and, therefore, the superficially prominent vessels adjacent to the points of the *yang ming* on the head should be pricked.

[6]Regarding the points on the five columns on the head, see Chap. 1 (Part 2), page 418, Book 7, of the present work. Needling these points on the head drains evil qi. In order to exterminate the evil, the root should be assisted by draining fire and supplementing kidney water. For that purpose, Palace of Toil (*Lao Gong*, Per 8) of the hand *jue yin* and then Great Ravine (*Tai Xi*, Ki 3) on the foot *shao yin* may be needled. One should note that points of the hand *jue yin* are often used instead of points of the hand *shao yin* when only the channel is involved.

[7]*I.e.*, points of the channel in the lower of the body

[8]This section is quite similar to the next section and is absent from the *Ling Shu* and *Tai Su*.

[9]The "Sixtieth Difficulty" in the *Nan Jing (Classic of Difficult Issues)* explains, "When the three hand yang vessels are subject to wind cold, which, lying hidden, lingers on, the headache is called an inversion headache; but if wind cold penetrates the brain, it is called a true headache.

[10]Needling the transporting points below the knees and elbows treats headache due to counterflow in the channels. For other kinds of headache, this therapy is inappropriate.

[11]Great *bi* is understood as fulminating cold dampness. Once it penetrates the brain, the headache is quite difficult to treat.

[12]The hand-foot *shao yang* and *yang ming* all ascend to the head, but the foot *yang ming* alone travels contralaterally after reaching the face. Therefore, if there is pain on the left side of the head, we should first needle the hand *shao yang* and *yang ming* on the left side and then needle the foot *shao yang* and *yang ming* on the right side. The treatment is reversed if the right side is involved.

[13]*I.e.*, Shang Yang (*Shang Yang*, LI 1)

[14]Inability to bend the body involves the foot *tai yang* which runs through the entire posterior aspect of the body, while inability to turn the neck relates specifically to the hand *tai yang* which traverses the shoulders and the neck.

[15]Ma Shi explains in *Ling Shu Zhu Zheng Fa Wei (An Annotated Exposition on the Intricacies of the Spiritual Pivot)*, "For pain in the submandibular region, it is necessary to take the foot *yang ming* stomach channel, needling the point Jawbone (*Jia Che*, St 6). This point is located at the tip of the mandibular curve below the auricle. Because there is a pulsating vessel encircling this area, the place is called curved surround."

Because there is an artery at Man's Prognosis, one should push the artery aside in needling this point. This is what is meant by pressing the channel.

[16]Part 1 is derived from Chap. 24, Vol. 5, *Ling Shu*; Part 2 from Chap. 26, Vol. 5, *Ling Shu*; and Part 3 from the *Zhen Jiu Ming Tang Zhi Yao*.

[17]"The Sixtieth Difficulty" in the *Nan Jing* states, "(Heart pain) due to interference of the qi of the five viscera with each other is called inversion heart pain." In a commentary in the same passage, Yang Xuan-cao explains, "All the channels and network vessels are ascribed to the heart. Once one channel is diseased, its vessel will counterflow and the counterflow will overwhelm the heart. When the heart is overwhelmed, heart pain results and is, therefore, called inversion heart pain. This pain is caused by counterflow surging of the visceral qi rather than by the heart *per se*."

[18]Zhang Jing-yue in his *Lei Jing* explains, "Exuberant gatherings in the center are spoken of as tangible concretions or accumulations or blood which stagnates and gathers in the center. The disease lies in the viscera rather than the channel, and, therefore, (one) should not take the points of the channel. It is necessary to treat it by regulating the interior." One should note the Chinese term *shu* is rendered here as channel points but may specifically mean the transporting points. There is a question whether all acupoints are prohibited or only the transporting points are prohibited. In this context, it would seem that no points whatsoever can be needled, since the author first declares all needling to be prohibited.

[19]In the *Ling Shu* and *Tai Su*, "hand *shao yang*" is in place of "hand *shao yin*."

[20]This paragraph is omitted in the current Chinese versions, but it appears in the form of a quotation

attributed to the *Jia Yi Jing* in the *Qian Jin* and other classics.

[21]The three kinds of worms are pinworms, tapeworms, and roundworms.

[22]Heart *shan* refers to upper abdominal pain and peri-umbilical pain with inhibited voiding of urine, rumbling of the intestines, abdominal distention, and protrusion of the intestines. It may send qi surging upward into the heart, thus causing dizziness and, in the extreme, loss of consciousness.

[23]In some versions, this item is placed at the end of Part 2 above, and the correction has been made in accordance with the *Qian Jin*.

[24]Zhang Jing-yue explains in his *Lei Jing (A The Classified Classic)*, "If on examination, the pulse is found to be urgent, the disease is heart *shan*. (In this case,) there will be tangible masses in the lateral lower abdomen. One should prick the blood network vessels of the foot *tai yin* and foot *jue yin* because both channels gather in the lateral lower abdomen. Removal of the blood in the network vessels dissipates the evils there."

[25]Part 1 is derived from Chap. 20, Vol. 5, *Ling Shu*; Part 2 from Chap. 38, *Su Wen*; Part 3 from Chap. 75, Vol. 11, *Ling Shu*; and Part 4 from the *Zhen Jiu Ming Tang Zhi Yao*.

[26]*I.e.*, points like Cloud Gate (*Yun Men*, Lu 2), Central Treasury (*Zhong Fu*, Lu 1), and Lung Shu (*Fei Shu*, Bl 13).

[27]Although Empty Basin (*Que Pen*, St 12) is a point on the foot *yang ming*, the hand *tai yin* lung channel also ascends to and emerges here. For that reason, Empty Basin should be chosen to dissipate lung evil. One should not, however, insert the needle too deeply or this will give rise to counterflow dyspnea.

[28]There are two kinds of cold evils implied, one from the exterior which strikes the skin and hair first and the other contained in food and drink which enters the stomach first. Zhang Jing-yue explains in the *Lei Jing*, "The lung channel begins in the middle burner, following the opening of the stomach, penetrating above the diaphragm, and homing to the lung. For that reason, the cold in food and drink in the stomach follows the lung vessel up into the lung. This paragraph offers a good explanation for the statement that cold food and cold drink damage the lung." In other words, lung cough is a product of the combination of two colds.

[29]Concerning the first sentence, most scholars of Chinese medicine agree with Zhang Jing-yue who explains in his *Lei Jing*, "The liver, for example, should be subject to disease in spring because it is its prevailing season. There are, however, seasons when wood does not prevail. The reason why the liver is diseased in those seasons is that the lung is first afflicted by disease and is capable of transmitting it to (the liver). This explains the subjection of any viscus to disease in its nonprevailing seasons. It follows that all the five viscera and six bowels may have a cough, and, without exception, the lung should be held responsible." According to him, the first sentence can be paraphrased as "Each of the five viscera and the six bowels can contract cough, and they do it in their own prevalent seasons. When they contract cough in other seasons, the disease is transmitted from the lung."

There is, however, another plausible interpretation. The following several paragraphs deal with transmission of cough around the five viscera and six bowels, and the author in the last sentence of this paragraph repeatedly says that this or that viscus is the first to be subject to disease in this or that season. This, of course, suggests that in a certain season another viscus may be affected in its wake.

The consummate yin is long summer.

[30]Fecal qi means flatulence.

[31]The unknown editor(s) is right.

[32]Ma Shi explains in his *Su Wen Zhu Zheng Fa Wei (An Annotated Exposition on the Intricacies of the Basic Questions)*, "Coughs of the five viscera and six bowels produce different manifestations. (The evil,) however, concentrates in the stomach in all these cases because the stomach is the ruler of the viscera and bowels. Cough involves the lung because it is the first to be subjected to evils, and only afterward does it transmit the disease to other viscera and bowels. Copious snivel and sputum, and puffy swelling of the face are all impugned to qi counterflow. All these are the manifestations common among the coughs of the five viscera and six bowels."

[33]If one is affected by dampness in winter when cold water prevails, the dampness and cold water will conspire. What is more, in winter, the lung qi is at a low ebb. These factors combined, the lung is overwhelmed, giving rise to cough.

[34]Dusting means to realize an effect in no time as easily and quickly as removing dust by dusting.

Since the *Jiu Juan* was written long after the death of the Yellow Emperor, it is impossible for him to raise questions by referring to it. The *Jiu Juan* might be mistaken for the *Needling Strategies*, another classic, long lost.

In Chap. 5, Vol. 22, the *Tai Su*, there is an explanation of the external channels. It says, "Those parts of the twelve channel vessels that enter the viscera and bowels are regarded as the internal channels, while those that travel in the limbs and the skin are regarded as the external channels." Qi Bo defines yang disease below.

[35]There are two different interpretations regarding the blood in the last sentence. On the one hand, it may be interpreted as complexion, since the Chinese often use *xue se* (blood color) to express complexion. On the other hand, some interpret it as the circulation of blood. In that case, the subordinate clause should be rendered "until the vessels are coursed."

The word *li* may be synonymous with *cun*. This has been regarded as an error since the Ming dynasty, but it is not, in fact, erroneous at all. It is often seen in acupuncture texts and means *cun*. For example, we have *Zu San Li* (Foot Three Li, St 36) which means point three *cun* below the knee.

[36]This paragraph has been so truncated that it has been eliminated in many versions of the *Jia Yi Jing*, but appears here in accordance with the *Wai Tai*.

[37]According to the *Wai Tai* and *Yi Xin Fang*, the unknown editor was correct.

[38]All the signs and symptoms after the phrase "sudden internal counterflow...the liver" are ascribed to the counterflow and transmission.

[39]*I.e.*, Yin Cleft (*Yin Xi*, Ht 6)

[40]Part 1 is derived from Chap. 20, Vol. 5, *Ling Shu*; Part 2 a combination of parts of Chap. 59, Vol. 9 and Chap. 26, Vol. 5, *Ling Shu*; and Part 3 from the *Zhen Jiu Ming Tang Zho Yao*.

[41]Since this is a disease involving the liver, the blood vessels to be pricked should be those along the liver channel and the vessels around the auricles should be those belonging to the foot *shao yang* which is associated with the liver channel.

[42]The subordinate clause of the second sentence here rendered literally as "Since the accumulated stale qi has no constant dwelling place" also implies that the qi fails to circulate where it should. The rendering that appears in the text has been chosen in light of the responses given below.

[43]*I.e.*, Ridge Spring (*Lian Quan*, CV 23)

[44]*I.e.*, Camphorwood Gate (*Zhang Men*, Liv 13)

[45]This refers to inserting one needle vertically with two others inserted at an angle on either side.

[46]There is no consensus as to the precise location of the depression of the bosom. Chest Center (*Dan Zhong*, CV 17), Breast Window (*Ying Chuang*, St 16) and Roof (*Wu Yi*, St 15) are among the most probable points. This is the case with the pulsating vessel as well. Ma Shi thinks it is Chest Center (*Dan Zhong*, CV 17), while Zhang Jing-jue believes it to be Central Treasury (*Zhong Fu*, Lu 1).

[47]Reflux retching and vomiting means that food is ejected immediately after consumption.

[48]*I.e.*, Surging Qi (*Qi Chong*, St 30)

[49]There is another interpretation which would render the sentence, "For not daring to take a deep breath which will produce pain in the chest..." This discrepancy in understanding arises out of the ambiguity of the term *da qi* (great qi). Chinese often say *da qi bu gan chu* (not daring to emit great qi) as an expression of inability to take a deep breath, but this usage is a modern one.

[50]Part 1 is derived from Chap. 47, *Su Wen*; Part 2 from Chap. 26, Vol. 5, *Ling Shu*; Part 3 from the *Zhen Jiu Ming Tang Zhi Yao*; and Part 4 is a combination of parts of Chap. 20, Vol. 5, Chap. 4, Vol. 1, and Chap. 19, Vol. 4, *Ling Shu*.

[51]*I.e.*, Sun & Moon (*Ri Yue*, GB 24), the alarm point, and Gallbladder Shu (*Dan Shu*, Bl 19), the associated point

[52]This is an ancient medical classic, long lost, which is believed to be a classic on acupuncture therapeutics.

The first sentence in the emperor's question is not found in the *Tai Su*, but is present in the *Su Wen*. Some scholars, such as Quan Yuan-qi, suspect that it was inserted by mistake.

[53]Cardiac *bi* is characterized by oppression, shortage of qi, dyspnea and dry throat. It develops from vascular *bi*.

[54]As before, *shu* here simply refers to the (pertinent) channel.

[55]The next to last sentence implies that the points of the foot *shao yang* should be needled and moxaed.

[56]Part 1 is derived from Chap. 29, *Su Wen*; Part 2 from the *Zhen Jiu Ming Tang Zhi Yao*.

[57]Zhang Jing-jue explains in his *Lei Jing*, "As to the (seasons) ruled by the five viscera, liver wood, for example, rules the spring and is monarch in the east. Heart fire rules the summer and is monarch in the south. Lung metal rules autumn and is

monarch in the west. Kidney water rules the winter and is monarch in the north. The only exception is the spleen which is ascribed to earth, raising and nourishing everything. Therefore, it is located in the center. It borrows eighteen days from each of the other four viscera to reign then. Being the leader of the other four viscera, it is not in a position to rule one entire season. In reference to the calendar, ...in the four seasons, prior to the Beginning of Spring, Beginning of Summer, Beginning of Autumn, and Beginning of Winter, earth is monarch then, managing eighteen days, totalling seventy-two days in a year."

[58]There is no duct between the spleen and the stomach. However, the spleen is, nonetheless, said to circulate fluid and humor on behalf of the stomach. This is because the *tai yin* channel, the channel of the spleen, does it instead. Circulating stomach qi or fluid and humor to the three yang is the work of the *yang ming*. It is, however, associated with the *tai yin*, and, therefore, the *tai yin* should also be credited with the circulation in the three yang. The *yang ming* in "Through the *yang ming*..." should be understood as the stomach. However, some of the essential points in this passage may be interpreted differently. In light of this interpretation, the relevant lines should read as follows. "The foot *yang ming* stands in an exterior/interior relationship with the *tai yin*, and it is the sea of all the viscera and bowels. Therefore, it also takes the responsibility of circulating fluid and humor on behalf of the stomach, but only to the three yang channels. Thus the five viscera and six bowels receive qi from the stomach through their own channels respectively, which are linked with the *tai yin* and the *yang ming*." The lines beginning "The limbs cannot receive..." to the end of this paragraph are a repetition of the relevant lines in the first paragraph of this chapter, and, as such, are suspected to be an erroneous addition. These lines are, however, present in the *Su Wen*.

[59]Part 1 is derived from Chap. 20, Vol. 5, *Ling Shu*; Part 2 a combination of parts of Chap. 19, Vol. 4 and Chap. 4, Vol. 1, *Ling Shu*; Part 3 from Chap. 26, Vol. 5, *Ling Shu*; Part 4 from Chap. 28, *Su Wen*; and Part 5 from the *Zhen Jiu Ming Tang Zhi Yao*.

[60]A surplus of yang qi combined with an insufficiency of yin qi is indicative of a yang evil penetrating the bowel, i.e., the stomach. This locates the disease in the *yang ming*, giving rise to internal heat which disperses food quickly. An insufficiency of yang qi combined with a surplus of yin qi is indicative of a yin evil penetrating the viscus, i.e., the spleen. This locates the disease in the *tai yin*, giving rise to internal cold. If the yang qi and yin qi are both in a state of surplus, this is reflects exuberance of the evils in both the bowel and vis-

cus. If they are both insufficient, this is reflects an insufficiency of the righteous qi of both the spleen and the stomach.

[61]Because the upper venter and lower venter are also point names, needling the points Upper Venter (*Shang Wan*, CV 13) and Lower Venter (*Xia Wan*, CV 10) is implied.

[62]*I.e.*, Sea of Qi (*Qi Hai*, CV 6)

[63]Anomalies imply any disorder.

[64]*I.e.*, points such as Huang Shu (*Huang Shu*, Ki 12) of the foot *shao yin* and Celestial Pivot (*Tian Shu*, St 25) of the foot *yang ming*

[65]*I.e.*, Kidney Shu (*Shen Shu*, Bl 23)

[66]This refers to both hand and foot *tai yang* channels. Quite a number of places in this paragraph may be interpreted in a different way. These are paraphrased below.

For sudden abdominal fullness which cannot be relieved by pressure, one should prick the blood veins of the hand *tai yang* (in the *Su Wen* "hand" is explicit) and then relief will be realized. In addition, one should needle five points in the neighborhood of Kidney Shu (*Shen Shu*, Bl 23) which are located three *cun* bilateral to the spine. Then relief will be effected soon. This multipoint needling can be performed only when the evil is found to pass the yang channel.

The following paragraph is a paraphrase of the passage in question as it appears in the current edition of the *Su Wen*.

For sudden fullness of the abdomen taut enough to resist pressure, take the network vessels of the hand *tai yang* channel, which are points where the stomach qi concentrates, and the foot *shao yin* associated back point, which is located one and a half *cun* bilateral to the spine, needling five times with the sharp-round needle.

[67]*I.e.*, Camphorwood Gate (*Zhang Men*, Liv 13)

[68]There are two kinds of wind inversion. One is characterized by susceptibility to fright, backache, frequent belching, and yawning. This is a disease involving the *tai yang* and the *jue yin*. Another is characterized by generalized fever with sweating and vexation which is unrelieved by diaphoresis.

[69]The point above the medial malleolus may be Three Yin Intersection (*San Yin Jiao*, Sp 6), but the last sentence is too abstruse not to provoke suspicion of a transcription error. In the *Wai Tai*, it reads "For abdominal distention with relieving qi

which radiates to the elbows and region of the free rib, this point is also the ruling point."

In our source edition, "rumbling of the abdomen" appears in place of "rumbling of the intestines" and "lateral malleolus" in place of "medial malleolus."

[70]*Xia xia* (groaning) in Chinese means talkativeness.

[71]The symptoms of both patterns reflect disharmonies of the sinew characterized by a loss of nourishment by the fluid and humor. Sinew Support (*Cheng Jin*, Bl 56) is the point of choice for sinew disharmonies. The meaning of the last sentence is obtuse at best and the translators can shed no light on it. In the next chapter of the present volume, there is a similar paragraph, which is often recommended as a reference. It reads as follows:

The meeting yin vessel (*hui yin zhi mai*) causes people pain in the lumbus with soaking perspiration during the attack of the pain, desire for drinks after the sweat is dried, and desire to walk after drinking. Prick the straight yang vessel (*zhi yang zhi mai*), three holes at the transversely lying vessel which is located three *cun* above the (yang) motility vessel and (three *cun*) below the cleft, letting out blood of the vessel found exuberant.

[72]Part 1 is derived from Chap. 20, Vol. 5, *Ling Shu*; Part 2 from Chap. 19, Vol. 4, *Ling Shu*; Part 3 from Chap. 4, Vol. 1, *Ling Shu*; Part 4 from Chap. 46, *Su Wen*; Part 5 from Chap. 41, *Su Wen*; and Part 6 from the *Zhen Jiu Ming Tang Zhi Yao*.

[73]Yin *bi* is a disease caused by yin evils, such as cold dampness, striking the kidney. This syndrome involves the urinary bladder channel as well as the kidney. Therefore, points on the foot *shao yin* and *tai yang* should be needled, and, if prominent blood vessels on the two channels are found, these should all be bled as well.

[74]*I.e.*, Sea of Qi (*Qi Hai*, CV 6)

[75]This syndrome is apparently small intestinal *shan*. Sea of Qi (*Qi Hai*, CV 6) is the point of choice for treating periumbilical region with cold qi and all other qi problems, such as insufficiency of the true qi. Usually it is moxaed. The small intestine is associated with the point Lower Great Hollow (*Xia Ju Xu*, St 39) and is, therefore, effective in conducting evil qi in the small intestine. Because the problem involves the lung and liver, their associated channels, the hand *tai yin* and the foot *jue yin*, should be treated as well.

[76]Awkward feeling of the posterior implies an urgent and uncomfortable desire to evacuate the stools.

[77]The pulse should be deep in the winter, and the kidney is deep as well. This is normal. A pulse image contrary to this is pathological and reflects a disease of the kidney. A superficial pulse is a lung pulse, and the lung is involved in this case. In the *Su Wen* the second and third sentences are combined together and read more smoothly as "The pulse on the left should indicate disease in the kidney with the lung...." Because the lumbus is the abode of the kidney, when the kidney is diseased, the lumbus must be affected.

[78]About the close relationship between the kidney and the lung because of the foot *shao yin* channel, refer to Chap. 1 (Part 1), Book 7, present work.

[79]The point to be needled is Bend Middle (*Wei Zhong*, Bl 40). It is a point where the foot *tai yang* channel submerges and is, therefore, called the cleft point. It is also the point where the primary branch of the foot *tai yang* passes and, therefore, is referred to as the primary for short. The kidney and the urinary bladder stand in a interior/exterior relationship. The kidney reigns in the winter, while in the spring it is diminished. In spring, bloodletting may inflict a dual reduction of the kidney. This is why bloodletting is prohibited at this time.

[80]The liver stands in an interior/exterior relationship with the gallbladder. In spring, the liver reigns, while in summer it is diminished. Therefore, the foot *tai yang* should not be bled in the summer.

[81]The three points are Leg Three Li (*Zu San Li*, St 36), Upper Great Hollow (*Shang Ju Xu*, St 37), and Lower Great Hollow (*Xia Ju Xu*, St 39). The second to the last sentence may be understood to read "Prick the foot *yang ming* at *Zu San Li* three times, and prick the points *Shang Ju Xu* and *Xia Ju Xu* to harmonize below and above."

Zhang ZhiBcong explains in his *Su Wen Ji Zhu* (*Condensed Annotations on the Basic Questions*), "When the blood vessels are in harmony, essence and spirit enjoy a peaceful life, for the spirit is the essence qi from the grains. If the *yang ming* vessel is diseased, the spirit and qi become vacuous. The essence and spirit become vacuous and chaotic, and one sees weird things. Insufficiency of the spirit results in sorrow." This approach explains the common presence of mental disorders in diseases of the stomach and the *yang ming* channels. Wang Bing explains the last sentence, by saying, "The *yang ming* is associated with the spleen, and the spleen reigns in long summer. Since earth is at a low ebb in autumn, bloodletting should not be performed in this season."

[82]*I.e.*, Recover Flow (*Fu Liu*, Ki 7)

[83]The point to be needled is Woodworm Canal (*Li Gou*, Liv 5). The fish belly in this context refers to the calf.

In our source edition, before the word "silent" there is the word "*shan*" which may mean constant(ly). With this word retained, the sentence should be interpreted as follows: "The disease makes the patient talkative, silent..." However, this is a contradiction. Our correction is made in accordance with the *Tai Su*. One should note that the current editions of the *Su Wen* are identical to our source edition of the *Jia Yi Jing* on this point.

[84]Wang Bing explains in a note in the *Su Wen*, "The unraveled vessel is a vessel which travels in a scattered way and is spoken of as not uniting with but instead deviating from the path of the main pathway. This is (a branch of) the foot *tai yang* channel starting from the inner canthi, travelling onto the forehead, joining at the vertex, going along the shoulder and scapula, passing by the spine, arriving in the lumbus, emerging at the paravertebral sinews, connecting with the kidney, homing to the urinary bladder, and proceeding down to enter the hollow of the knee. This route accounts for the manifestations of this disease. Furthermore, its ramification deviates at the inner border of the scapula, penetrating down the paravertebral muscles, travelling via the outer border of the thigh to join the former at the hollow of the knee below. These two vessels are like two unraveled strands of rope and, therefore, called the unraveled vessel."

The place to be pricked is the area around Bend Yang (*Wei Yang*, Bl 39), where the prominent vessels should be bled. One should note that point names often refer to an area in which blood vessels should be pricked.

[85]Wang Bing explains the merging-into-yin vessel in a note to the *Su Wen* where he says, "(This is) a deviating connecting vessel of the foot *shao yang*, travelling together with the *shao yang* channel deviating to the (foot) *jue yin* at five *cun* above the lateral malleolus, proceeding together with the channel to connect with the insteps of the feet below. This is why it is called the merging-into-yin vessel." The point described as lying at the end of the severed bone is Yang Assistance (*Yang Fu*, GB 38).

[86]Quan Yuan-qi (471-556), mistakenly named Jin Yuan-qi and Quan Yuan-yue in some history books, was the first scholar in history to present comprehensive and trustworthy annotations to the *Su Wen*.

[87]Since the Chinese word *zhe* can be understood as breaking or bending, therefore "often bent" can be changed to "(the lumbus) often (feels) as if it will break."

[88]The point suggested is Mountain Support (*Cheng Shan*, Bl 57). The yang linking vessel starts from Metal Gate (*Jin Men*, Bl 63) which is a meeting point for all the foot yang channels, and proceeds upward along the lateral aspect of the leg meeting the foot *tai yang* in the hollow of the knee and finally arriving at the head.

[89]There is no consensus as to which points should be pricked here. Wang Bing holds that one is Bend Yang (*Wei Yang*, Bl 39). This is located at the lateral border of the popliteal fossa. The other is Gate of Abundance (*Yin Men*, Bl 37), located one *chi* above the popliteal fossa. But Lou Ying, of the *Ming* dynasty argues in his *Yi Xue Gang Mu* (*Systematically Arranged Medical Work*) that the author is actually referring to two prominent blood vessels rather than two acupoints. According to him, the lower one is located between sinews at the lateral border of the popliteal fossa and the upper one is found several *cun* above the fossa.

[90]According to Zhang Zhi-cong, the meeting-yin vessel is simply the conception vessel, while the straight yang vessel is the governing vessel, but many other scholars disagree. One different interpretation is that the meeting-yin-vessel is the governing vessel while the straight yang is the foot *tai yang* channel. Another says that both the vessels are essentially one and the same vessel, that being the conception vessel.

The yang motility vessel means the point Extending Vessel (*Shen Mai*, Bl 62), and the Cleft is Bend Middle (*Wei Zhong*, Bl 40). Therapy consists of pricking the prominent blood vessels lying transversely between Extending Vessel and Bend Middle, pricking a single vessel either three times or pricking three separate points once.

[91]There is no consensus regarding this vessel, although Wang Bing believes it to be the yin linking vessel which originates and travels together with the foot *shao yin* from the border of the calf five *cun* above the medial malleolus.

In the *Tai Su*, it is said to be the divergent channel of the foot *tai yang* which deviates to the foot *shao yin* at seven *cun* above the lateral malleolus.

Ni Wa Yuan-jian, in the *Su Wen Shi* (*Conceptual Knowledge about the Basic Questions*) argues against both of the above two opinions, believing it to be the point Woodworm Canal (*Li Gou*, Liv 5).

[92]The glorious yang vessel is Recover Flow (*Fu Liu*, Ki 7), a point on the kidney channel. The foot *shao yin* channel proceeds from the kidney, penetrating the diaphragm, entering the lung, passing through the throat, and visiting the root of the tongue. One of its branches starts from the lung, connecting the heart, and pouring into the chest. The pathway of this channel accounts for symptoms of the syndrome.

[93]The dispersing vessel is the divergent connecting vessel of the foot *tai yin*. It travels upward in a dispersed manner, passing through the inner aspect of the thigh to submerge in the abdomen, binding at the cavity between the lower back and the ilium. The pathway of this channel accounts for the symptoms of this syndrome.

The description of the point location is puzzling and, therefore, has provoked a great deal of contention. Wang Bing believes it to be Earth Mechanism (*Di Ji*, Sp 8) which is located below the knee at the medial aspect of the lower leg, while Lou Ying believes it to be in the knee joint at the lateral aspect above Leg Three Li (*Zu San Li*, St 36) and Yang Mound Spring (*Yang Ling Quan*, GB 34).

[94]The interior flesh vessel is difficult to identify. According to Wang Bing, it is a vessel generated by the (foot) *shao yang* which originates or is produced at the yang linking vessel. This is vague in itself. The point to be needled may be Yang Assistance (*Yang Fu*, GB 38).

[95]The point to be pricked is Bend Middle (*Wei Zhong*, Bl 40).

[96]The point to be needled is Lower Bone Hole (*Xia Liao*, Bl 34). There are four points in the sacral foramina, all of which are called meeting points because the foot *tai yin*, *jue yin*, and *shao yang* meet at the sacrum.

With the moon waxing, the qi in the human body grows exuberant. With the moon waning, the qi in the human body diminishes. For that reason, in the former situation, the amount of needling should increase each day, while in the latter circumstance, the amount should decrease each day. The maximum number of punctures which may be made is fifteen and the minimum is, of course, one.

[97]Zhang Jing-yue provides an explanation of this paragraph in a note in the *Lei Jing*. It is paraphrased as follows. In the case of cold, needling the yang channel removes the yin evil from the yang phase. In the case of heat, needling the *jue yin* removes wind heat from the yin phase. The *shao yang* vessel travels along the sides of the body,

and this is why it is needled in the case of inability to bend either forward or backward. The *shao yin* governs water and, in a water disease, nothing can restrain fire, resulting in heat in the center. Since the *shao yin* vessel penetrates the liver and enters the lung, the case is manifested by dyspnea. Therefore, the foot *shao yin* should be needled, and Gushing Spring (*Yong Quan*, Ki 1) and Large Goblet (*Da Zhong*, Ki 4) are both ruling points.

There is another interpretation as to the place where cold or heat arise. This asserts that cold or heat occur at the place of pain in the lower back rather than in the upper part of the body. Both interpretations center on how the character *shang* is to be read. It may be rendered either as "on", making cold or heat occur "on" the place of pain, or it may be read as "above" or "upper", placing the cold in the upper part of the body. Since the author here explicitly mentions the location of cold or heat in contrast to the "center", we believe that it is preferable to interpret the place where cold and heat arise as the upper body. However, in a similar context but without the contrast to the center, such as in the following passage, it should be rendered simply as the place of pain.

[98]I.e., Long Strong (*Chang Qiang*, GV 1)

[99]Upper Bone Hole (*Shang Liao*, Bl 31), Second Bone Hole (*Ci Liao*, Bl 32), Central Bone Hole (*Zhong Liao*, Bl 33), and Lower Bone Hole (*Xia Liao*, Bl 34)

[100]Part 1 is derived from Chap. 19, Vol. 4, *Ling Shu*; Part 2 from Chap. 4, Vol. 1, *Ling Shu*; Part 3 a combination of parts of Chap. 55, *Su Wen* and Chap. 26, Vol. 5, *Ling Shu*; and Part 4 from the *Zhen Jiu Ming Tang Zhi Yao*.

[101]I.e., Beng Yang (*Wei Yang*, Bl 39)

[102]The triple burner functions as a sluice to ensure the flow of water, and it links with the urinary bladder. For that reason, when there is a water problem, one should treat the foot *tai yang*.

[103]This is the divergent connecting vessel of the foot *tai yang*.

[104]The prominent blood vessels around Bend Yang (*Wei Yang*, Bl 53) should be pricked. These are located at the lateral border of the hollow of the knee, between the foot *tai yang* and *shao yang*.

[105]Because of the ambiguity of the word *pian* (偏), "swelling and pain throughout the lower abdomen" can also be rendered as "lower abdominal swelling and pain on one side."

[106]The word "foot" may have been inserted by some

unknown editor(s), since Huang-fu Mi was in the habit of omitting such words wherever possible.

[107] A.k.a. *Cheng Fu.*

[108] Part 1 is derived from Chap. 22, Vol. 22, *Ling Shu*; Part 2 from the *Zhen Jiu Ming Tang Zhi Yao.*

[109] The following points on the channels can be selected: Gushing Spring (*Yong Quan*, Ki 1), Guest House (*Zhu Bin*, Ki 9), Bend Yang (*Wei Yang*, Bl 39), Flying Yang (*Fei Yang*, Bl 58), Kneeling Visitor (*Pu Can*, Bl 61), and Metal Gate (*Jin Men*, Bl 63).

[110] I.e., Long Strong (*Chang Qiang*, GV 1)

[111] I.e., Hidden White (*Yin Bai*, Sp 1), Offspring of Duke (*Gong Sun*, Sp 4), Leg Three Li (*Zu San Li*, St 36), and Ravine Divide (*Jie Xi*, St 41)

[112] I.e., Recover Flow (*Fu Liu*, Ki 7) and Ravine Divide (*Jie Xi*, St 41)

[113] Part 1 is derived from Chap. 75, Vol. 11, *Ling Shu*; Part 2 from Chap. 47, *Su Wen*; and Part 3 from the *Zhen Jiu Ming Tang Zhi Yao.*

[114] The *Ci Jie (Needling Strategies)* is a long lost classic. Undressing has two meanings. One use describes rapid or immediate effect. The other, as used in this chapter, describes a perceptible, powerful effect as undressing exposes the bare body.

[115] The syndrome of a swollen, enlarged scrotum affecting movement, etc. is a species of *tui shan.* It is due to water accumulating in the testicles caused by dietary irregularities and inordinate joy and anger. When water gathers in the scrotum, qi circulation comes to a standstill and urination becomes inhibited. In this case, a sword needle should be administered to the network vessels at the joints. Thus water swelling will soon disappear. In Chap. 1 (Part 1), Book 7, the term disrobing is encountered which is synonymous with undressing. The *Ling Shu* uses the term "divesting claws" in the same context.

[116] A repellence-like disorder in the neck and bosom implies congestion and obstruction in the throat and chest as if something has become stuck in them. The *tai yin* pulse means the hand *tai yin* pulse, i.e., the *cun kou* pulse.

[117] Fivefold surplus is characterized by a generalized fever that is as hot as a charcoal fire. It is a repellence-like disorder in the neck and bosom with an agitated and exuberant *ren ying* pulse, dyspneic breathing, and qi counterflow. Dual insufficiency is dribbling urinary block with voiding of urine many tens of times a day with the *tai yin* pulse faint and fine like a hair.

[118] One should note the differences in the wording in the discussion of surplus and insufficiency. This insufficiency does not refer to some inadequacy of the diseased qi itself; rather it refers to an overall state of diminished righteous qi.

[119] Since yin *shan* is characterized by swelling and pain of the external genitals, the term might also be rendered as genital *shan.*

[120] Intermittent fullness and relief in the abdomen with pain is called qi *shan.*

[121] Qi blockage is caused by vacuity of the spleen and kidney and heat in the urinary bladder. It is divided into repletion and vacuity types. Aside from the signs mentioned above, the repletion type is characterized by intense abdominal pain, while the vacuity type is characterized by weakness in voiding.

[122] Portal here refers to the urethra.

[123] This whole chapter is derived from the *Zhen Jiu Ming Tang Zhi Yao.*

[124] The anterior yin is the external genitals, while the posterior yin is the anus.

[125] For bone erosion, cf. Chap. 10, Book 11, present work

[126] A.k.a. *Cheng Fu*

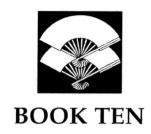

BOOK TEN

Chapter One

The Contraction of Disease by Yin Causing *Bi* (Part 1)[1]

(1)

The Yellow Emperor asked:

Global *bi* (*zhou bi*) travels around the body upward and downward, following the (affected) channel up and down. (It attacks) the left and right sides at the corresponding places with no intermission. I would like to learn where this pain lies, in the blood vessel or in the partings of the flesh, and how it comes about in this way. It moves (so swiftly) that there is no time for one to insert the needle, and the time it takes for the pain to build up is (so brief) that it has come to an (abrupt) stop before a treatment is decided upon. What causes it to behave in such a way?

Qi Bo answered:

This is multiple *bi* (*zhong bi*, 众痹) rather than circulatory *bi*. (The pains) are fixed in location, alternately erupting and then ceasing in succession, with the left responding to the right and the right responding to the left. However, (the *bi*) is incapable of moving, only starting and stopping (in a fixed location). To needle this, treat the painful place even once the pain there has ceased in order to prevent it from recurring.[2]

The Yellow Emperor asked:

What is circulatory *bi* like?

Qi Bo answered:

Global *bi* lies within the blood vessels, following the vessels up and following the vessels down, but it does not travel from the left to the right or vice versa, nor does it have a fixed location. For the pain travelling from above to below, one must first needle points below to thwart it and then needle points above to eliminate it. As for the pain travelling from below to above, one must first needle points above to thwart it and then needle points below to eliminate it.[3]

The Yellow Emperor asked:

How is this disease engendered and why is it so named?

Qi Bo answered:

When the qi of wind, cold, and dampness have intruded upon the partings of the flesh, (fluid and humor) are oppressed and condensed into foam. When this foam contacts cold, it gathers and, while gathering, it presses and separates the partings of the flesh. This separation produces pain. This pain invokes the spirit and, when the spirit is invoked, this results in heat. With this heat, the pain is resolved, but when the pain is resolved, this produces inversion and inversion causes *bi* in another place. So it goes (on and on) in this manner. This (problem) lies neither internally in the viscera, nor does it develop externally in the skin. Rather it lodges solely in the partings of the flesh.

Since the true qi cannot circulate, it acquires the name circulatory *bi*.[4]

In needling *bi*, one must first palpate the grand channels above and below to identify vacuity and repletion, to locate the blood bind and congestion in the major network vessels, and to detect the vacuous vessels, (*i.e.,*) sunken and empty vessels. Then one must perform a regulating (therapy) and ironing to free the flow (of the channel qi). In the case of tugging and tension (in the muscles), one must perform cultivation of qi and massage to promote circulation.

(2)

The Yellow Emperor asked:

What are the indicators of those with a tendency to contract diseases of *bi*?

Shao Yu answered:

Those with coarse (skin) texture and weak muscles have a tendency to contract diseases of *bi*. In order to tell whether it is high or low, it is necessary to study the three regions.[5]

(3)

The Yellow Emperor asked:

(I understand that) there are three variations in needling, but what are they?

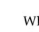

Bo Gao answered:

One is needling the constructive, another is needling the defensive, and the last is needling cold *bi* that lodges within the channels. Needling the constructive lets out blood, needling the defensive lets out qi, and needling cold *bi* admits heat into the body.[6]

The Yellow Emperor asked:

What are the characteristics of diseases of the constructive, defensive, and cold *bi* respectively?

Bo Gao answered:

Disease generated in the constructive is characterized by cold and heat, diminished qi, and (undisciplined) flow of blood up and down. Disease generated in the defensive is characterized by qi pain that intermittently comes and goes, oppression and fullness, and furious rumbling (of the intestines. All this is due to) wind cold intruding upon the stomach and intestines. Cold *bi* disease is characterized by persistence with intermittent pain and insensitivity of the skin.

The Yellow Emperor asked:

In needling cold *bi*, by what means can heat be admitted (into the body)?

Bo Gao answered:

In needling a cheaply clad person, fire can be used, but in needling the nobility, drug-ironing is recommendable. The formula consists of twenty *sheng* of good wine, one *sheng* of Fructus Zanthoxyli Bungeani (*Shu Jiao*), one *sheng* of dry Rhizoma Zingiberis (*Gan Jiang*), and one *sheng* of Ramulus Cinnamomi (*Gui Zhi*). The above ingredients, sliced thin, are dipped into the clear wine together with one *jin*[7] of silk fiber and four *zhang* and two *chi* of fine, white cloth. Tightly sealed lest its qi should escape, the pot of wine is put over a slow fire made of horse's droppings for five days and nights. (The sealed ingredients) are then removed and the fiber and cloth are dried in the sun. After that, they are dipped once again into the mixture to absorb more of the liquid. Each dipping must last for one day and night, and the fiber and cloth must dry up before the next dipping. Once (the liquid is completely absorbed and) the fiber and cloth are dried up, the cloth is to be cut into six pieces, each six or seven *chi* long. They are to be made into six bags in which the fiber and the drug dregs are wrapped. After heating over a mulberry charcoal fire, a bag is placed on the part overwhelmed by cold *bi* and the heat should be allowed to penetrate to the level of the illness. When cooled, the bag can be heated over the fire again. This ironing should be repeated thirty times until sweat appears (on the patient). Then heat the bag again and rub the body (of the patient) with it. This rubbing should be repeated thirty times. At this point, the patient is instructed to walk around in (an airtight) room without being exposed to wind. Each needling treatment should be followed by ironing, and the disease will be cured in due time. This is what is referred to as admitting heat.[8]

(4)

The Yellow Emperor asked:

How does *bi* develop?

Qi Bo answered:

The three qi of wind, cold, and damp all arrive in miscellaneous ways and combine to produce *bi*. When wind qi prevails, this is migratory *bi* (*xing bi*, 行痹). When cold qi prevails, this is painful *bi*. And when damp qi prevails, this is fixed *bi*.

The Yellow Emperor asked:

What are the five types (of *bi*)?

Qi Bo answered:

When (the above three qi) are met within winter, this is bone *bi*. When they are met within spring, this is sinew *bi*. When they are met within summer, this is vessel *bi*. When they are met within the consummate yin, this is muscle *bi*.[9] And when they are met within autumn this is skin *bi*.

The Yellow Emperor asked:

What kind of qi allows (*bi*) to lodge internally within the five viscera and six bowels?

Qi Bo answered:

Each of the five viscera has its associate (in the exterior). A disease (in the exterior), if it persists, will enter and lodge in the associate. It follows that bone *bi*, if left uncured and affected by a new

evil, will enter and lodge in the kidney. Sinew *bi*, if left uncured and affected by a new evil, will enter and lodge in the liver. Vessel *bi*, if left uncured and affected by a new evil, will enter and lodge in the heart. Muscle *bi*, if left uncured and affected by a new evil, will enter and lodge in the spleen. And skin *bi*, if left uncured and affected by a new evil, will enter and lodge in the lung. What are referred to here as *bi* are all due to a seasonal contraction of wind, cold, and damp qi.

All the types of *bi* develop inward if left uncured. *Bi* in which wind qi prevails is easy to overcome.

The Yellow Emperor asked:

Why does (*bi*) sometimes lead to death or result in chronic pain and yet may (sometimes) be cured easily?

Qi Bo answered:

When it has entered the viscus it is fatal. When it becomes lodged in the sinews and bones, it results in chronic pain. When it becomes lodged in the skin it is easily cured.

The Yellow Emperor asked:

How does it intrude upon the six bowels?

Qi Bo answered:

In this case, diet and living environment are also at the root of this disease. Each of the six bowels has its associated point. If wind, cold, and damp qi strike the associated point and this is (complicated by some harmful) dietary factor, (the evil qi) will enter into a certain bowel via its associated point.[10]

The Yellow Emperor asked:

Then how can this be treated by needling?

Qi Bo answered:

The five viscera have rapids, while the six bowels have confluences. These points are all located along and supplied by their (associated) channels. If that which is at fault is treated through them, the disease will be effaced.[11]

The Yellow Emperor asked:

Can constructive or defensive qi also cause people to suffer from *bi*?

Qi Bo answered:

The constructive is the essence qi from water and grain, harmonizing and regulating the five viscera and spraying the six bowels before it enters the vessels. Therefore, it follows the vessels up and down, permeating the five viscera and connecting with the six bowels. The defensive is the impetuous qi from water and grain. Because it is fierce, swift, slippery, and volatile, it cannot enter the vessels. Consequently, it travels in the skin and runs in the partings of the flesh, fumigating the *huang* and membranes, and gathering ["disperses" in the *Su Wen* {later editor}] in the chest and abdomen. When there is counterflow (of constructive and defensive) qi, this causes disease, but when these qi are normalized, recovery ensues. They never conspire with wind, cold, and damp qi and, therefore, they do not cause *bi*.[12]

Chapter One

The Contraction of Disease by Yin Causing *Bi* (Part 2)[13]

(1)

The Yellow Emperor asked:

Why may *bi* be painful, painless, or insensitive (*i.e.*, numb), cold or hot, dry or wet?

Qi Bo answered:

Painful (*bi*)) is due to prevalence of cold qi. If there is cold, there will be pain. Painless and insensitive (*bi*) are due to the chronicity and deep penetration of the disease. Stagnation in the cir-

culation of the constructive and defensive together with constant destitution of the channels and network vessels is the cause of painlessness, while malnutrition of the skin is the cause of insensitivity. Cold (*bi*) is due to diminished yang qi and an abundance of yin qi. These conditions promote diseases of a similar nature, and this accounts for cold. Hot *bi* is due to an abundance of yang qi and diminished yin qi. As a result of the prevalence of the diseased qi, yang overwhelms yin, thus producing heat. (*Bi*) with abundant cold and perspiration that (constantly) wet the clothing is due to its coming in contact with a prevailing damp (evil). When the yang qi is diminished and the yin qi is exuberant, two (evil) qi interact upon each other, and, therefore, this results in cold and perspiration that (constantly) wet the clothes.[14]

Bi that lies within the bone causes heaviness. If it lies in the vessels, it causes congelation and failure of blood flow. If it lies in the sinews, it results in the ability to contract but inability to stretch. If it lies in the flesh, it causes insensitivity. If it lies in the skin, it causes cold. In the case of any of these five patterns, there is no pain. Any type of *bi* may give rise to hypertonicity when coming in contact with cold, and to slackness when coming in contact with heat.

(2)

The Yellow Emperor asked:

A single vessel may generate tens of diseases with pain or *yong*, heat or cold, itching or *bi*, or insensitivity, the variations of which are endless. What is the cause?

Qi Bo answered:

All of them are generated by an evil qi.

The Yellow Emperor asked:

Humans have true qi, correct qi, and evil qi. What are they?

Qi Bo answered:

The true qi is that which is received from heaven and joins the qi from water and grain in replenishing the body. The correct qi is the correct wind blowing from a certain direction, as opposed to a vacuity wind ["disastrous wind" in the *Tai Su* {later editor}]. An evil qi is a vacuity wind. When bandit vacuity wind injures people, it strikes a person deeply and will not depart on its own. The correct wind strikes people shallowly and departs of its own accord. Because its qi is soft and tender, doing no harm to the true qi, it leaves the body of its own accord (later).[15]

When a vacuity evil strikes a person, it causes shivering which shakes the form, stands the hair on end, and forces open the interstices. It may penetrate deeply. When it hits the bone, this results in bone *bi*. When it hits the sinews, this results in hypertonicity of the sinews. When it hits within the vessels, blood is blocked and does not flow resulting in *yong*. When it hits within the muscles, it wrestles with the defensive qi and, if yang overwhelms, heat results, while if yin overwhelms, cold results. Cold makes the true qi depart, and when the true qi departs, there is vacuity. When there is vacuity, cold is generated. If a vacuity evil hits the skin, its qi (tends to) effuse outward, forcing open the interstices and shaking the fine hair. If the qi ["the sapping qi" in a variant version {later editor}] circulates in a gentle way, itching results. If the qi lingers on, *bi* is caused. When the defensive qi fails to circulate, this results in insensitivity.

(3)

When the disease lies in the bone, the bones become heavy and cannot be lifted, along with aching pain in the bone marrow and the arrival of cold qi. This disease is called bone *bi*. While it must be inserted deeply, the needle must not damage the vessels or muscles. The pathway (for the penetration of the needle) is found in the partings of the large and small flesh. When the bone feels hot, the disease is relieved.[16]

When the disease lies in the sinews, the sinews become hypertonic. There is pain in the joints and inability to walk. This disease is called sinew *bi*.

One must needle the sinew. To do this, (the needle) should be inserted through the borders of the flesh but must not strike the bone. When the affected sinew feels warm, the disease is checked.

When the disease lies in the muscles and skin, the muscles and skin throughout the body become painful. This disease is called muscle *bi*. It is due to damage done by cold and dampness. Needle at the partings of the small and large flesh with as many needles as possible and insert them deeply. The key is (to induce) heat. (Care should be taken) not to injure the sinews and bones. If the sinews and bones are injured, *yong* may develop, but only in the case of (pathological) transmutation. When all the affected partings of the flesh feel warm, the disease is checked.

(4)

The Yellow Emperor asked:

When people are not cold as a result of (thin) clothing, nor do they suffer from cold qi in the center of the body, from where within (the body) is this cold generated?[17]

Qi Bo answered:

These people must be subject to a great deal of *bi*. Because the yang qi is diminished and the yin qi is abundant, the body feels cold as if it has just emerged from (cold) water.[18]

The Yellow Emperor asked:

Some people are just generally cold. Neither soups nor fires are capable of heating them up, nor is thick clothing able to warm them, yet they never shiver as if freezing (cold). What kind of disease is this?

Qi Bo answered:

These people must have overwhelming kidney qi. Those involved with water in their pursuits have debilitated *tai yang* qi and desiccated kidney grease (*shen zhi*) which ceases to grow. The kidney is water and governs the bones. Once the bones are no longer generated, the marrow cannot be filled. For this reason, the cold is severe and reaches (as deep as) the bones. The reason one does not shiver from freezing (cold) is that the liver is one yang, the heart is a second yang, while the kidney is a solitary (yin) viscus. Since a single water cannot overwhelm two fires, freezing cold cannot produce shivering. This disease is called bone *bi* and the patient ought to suffer from hypertonicity of the joints as well.[19]

Fixed *bi* that is not eliminated and is characterized by unrelieved and long-lasting cold may develop into lower leg bone *bi*.

(5)

For bone *bi* with pain and the loss of use of all the joints of the body, downpour sweating, and vexation of the heart, take the three yin channels and supplement them.

For inversion *bi* with inversion qi ascending into the abdomen, take the network vessels of the yin or the yang. Depending on which (channel) is primarily diseased, (one should) drain the yang and supplement the yin channel.[20]

Wind *bi* outpour disease (*feng bi zhu bing*, 风痹注病) ["aching and weakness" replaces "outpour disease" in the *Ling Shu* {later editor}] becomes incurable, when characterized by feet that are as (cold) as if walking on ice but may occasionally be (hot) as if in hot water.

(There will also be) aching and weakness of the lower leg bones, vexation of the heart, headache, intermittent retching, intermittent oppression, visual dizziness that occurs when (oppression) has become chronic but is relieved with perspiration, sorrow, joy, and anger (*i.e.*, capricious moods), shortage of qi, and melancholy. In no more than three years, (this condition) is fatal.[21]

For feet and thighs which cannot be lifted, with the patient lying on his side, take the center of the hip joint[22] using a round-sharp needle. A large needle cannot be used.

For pain in the knees, take Calf's Nose (*Du Bi*, St

35) with a round-sharp needle, needling the point once every other day. The needle is as large as a yak hair, and so one may needle the knee without misgiving.

(6)

For insensitivity of the feet, needle Wind Mansion (*Feng Fu*, GV 16).[23]

For frigidity and insensitivity (radiating) from the lumbar region down through the feet with an inability to sit up or to lift the sacrococcygeal (region), Lumbar Shu (*Yao Shu*, GV 2) is the ruling point.

For *bi*, Meeting of Yin (*Hui Yin*, CV 1), Great Abyss (*Tai Yuan*, Lu 9), Dispersing Riverbed (*Xiao Luo*, TH 12), and Shining Sea (*Zhao Hai*, Ki 6) are the ruling points.[24]

For somnolence with inability to stir the body due to great warmth ["dampness" in a variant version {later editor}], Three Yang Connection (*San Yang Luo*, TH 8) is the ruling point.[25]

For bone *bi* with vexing fullness, Shang Hill (*Shang Qiu*, Sp 5) is the ruling point.

For heat in the soles of the feet, pain in the lower legs with inability to stand on one's feet for long, and damp *bi* with inability to walk, Three Yin Intersection (*San Yin Jiao*, Sp 6) is the ruling point.

For pain in the medial borders of the knees radiating to the kneecaps such that they cannot bend or stretch and involving the abdomen and radiating to the throat, Knee Joint (*Xi Guan*, Liv 7) is the ruling point.

For *bi* with swelling in the lower legs, debilitated insteps, and pain in the heels, the Lower Ridge of the Great Hollow (*Ju Xi Xia Lian*, St 39) is the ruling point.

For pain in the lower legs, flaccid feet in which one's shoes are often dropped, damp *bi*, heat in the soles of the feet, and inability to stand for a long time, Ribbon Opening (*Tiao Kou*, St 38) is the ruling point.

For chronic ["tormenting" in a variant version {later editor}] lower leg *bi* where the knees cannot be bent and stretched and one cannot walk, Beam Hill (*Liang Qiu*, St 34) is the ruling point.

For cold *bi* in the knee with insensitivity, atony, and inability to bend and stretch, Thigh Joint (*Bi Guan*, St 31) is the ruling point.

For pain, atony, and *bi* of the skin, Outer Hill (*Wai Qiu*, GB 36) is the ruling point.

For pain in the lateral aspects of the knees with inability to bend and stretch (the knees) and lower leg *bi* with insensitivity, Yang Pass (*Yang Guan*, GB 33) is the ruling point.

For upper thigh *bi* which radiates pain to the thigh and lateral aspect of the knee producing insensitivity and sinew tension, Yang Mound Spring (*Yang Ling Quan*, GB 34) is the ruling point.

For cold qi in the partings of the flesh which produces an attack of pain up and down and (causes) sinew *bi* with insensitivity, Central River (*Zhong Du*, Bl 32) is the ruling point.

For pain in the hip joints with inability to lift (the legs), use a filiform needle and, if there is cold, retain (the needle). The number of punctures is determined by the waxing and waning of the moon. Relief follows immediately. A long needle may also be used.

For dragging pain and tension between the lumbar region and the lateral costal region, tugging of the sinews of the upper thigh, lower leg pain that prevents bending or stretching, and *bi* with insensitivity, Jumping Round (*Huan Tiao*, GB 30) is the ruling point.

For wind cold beginning at the small toes of the feet and vessel *bi* moving up and down with migratory pain in the chest and the lateral costal regions, Reaching Yin (*Zhi Yin*, Bl 67) is the ruling point.

Trauma of the large toe of the foot due to bump-

ing it in the process of getting off a cart and trauma of the arch and the toes of the foot may develop into sinew *bi*. Ravine Divide (*Jie Xi*, St 41) is the ruling point.

Chapter Two

The Contraction of Disease by Yang Producing Wind (Part 1)[26]

(1)

The Yellow Emperor asked:

When wind injures people, it may give rise to cold and heat, heat in the center, cold in the center, pestilential wind, or hemilateral withering. Wind when developed is capable of differing diseases with (correspondingly) differing names, and it may penetrate as deeply as the five viscera and six bowels. I do not know how to explain this and would like to hear a lecture on it.

Qi Bo answered:

When wind qi is hidden in the skin, there is no internal communication nor is the exterior effused. The wind qi moves swiftly and changes capriciously. When the interstices are open, there is chilling ["quivering with cold" in the *Su Wen* {later editor}], and when the interstices shut, there is heat and oppression. This resulting cold reduces food intake, while the resulting heat wastes the muscles, causing languor and lassitude ["causing shuddering with cold" in the *Su Wen* {later editor}], oppression, and inability to take in food. This is called cold and heat.

The wind qi that has entered the stomach via the *yang ming* follows the vessel up to the inner canthi. In fat people, the wind qi cannot be drained outward, and this causes heat in the center with yellowing of the eyes. In thin people, (the yang qi) is drained outward (which generates) cold, and this causes cold in the center and tearing.[27]

Wind qi entering via the *tai yang* circulates

through the points of all the vessels, dispersing in the partings of the flesh. The defensive qi is impetuous. It is often interfered with by evil [the whole sentence is condensed into "often interfering with the defensive qi" in the *Su Wen*. {later editor}] When the passageways (of the defensive qi) become inhibited, this results in swelling and distention of the muscles and sores. Because the defensive qi is congealed and no longer circulates, the flesh becomes insensitive.

In the case of pestilential qi, the constructive qi heats up and decays. Because the (constructive) qi becomes turbid, the nose pillar is marred, its complexion spoils, and open sores break out on the skin. Wind cold that has intruded upon the vessels and persists is called pestilential qi or cold and heat.[28]

Wind damage inflicted on *jia* and *yi* days[29] in spring is liver wind. Wind damage inflicted on *bing* and *ding* days in summer is heart wind. Wind damage inflicted on *wu* and *ji* days in late summer is spleen wind. Wind damage inflicted on *geng* and *xin* days in autumn is lung wind. Wind damage inflicted on *ren* and *gui* days in winter is kidney wind.

Wind qi striking the points of the five viscera and six bowels may also develop into visceral and bowel wind. It enters through various gates and, where this wind strikes, it causes hemilateral wind.[30]

Wind qi travelling upward by way of the wind mansion may develop into brain wind. If (wind qi) enters and links to the head, it may develop into eye wind with cold in the eyes. Wind stroke (contracted) through drinking wine may develop into leaking wind. Wind stroke (contracted) through sweating during sexual intercourse may develop into the internal wind. Wind stroke (contracted) when washing the head may develop into head wind. Enduring wind entering the center may develop into an intestinal wind with swill diarrhea and, if it lodges externally in the interstices, it may develop into draining wind.[31]

Wind is the leader of all the hundreds of diseases.

Whenever it transforms, it may produce a disease of a different nature and follows no predictable law. Nevertheless, (it may always be identified) as wind qi.[32]

The symptoms of lung wind include copious sweating, aversion to wind, a light white complexion, and intermittent coughing with shortage of qi. By day, (the condition) improves, but by night, (the condition) is aggravated. It is diagnosed (in the region) above the eyebrows which will have a white complexion.[33]

The symptoms of heart wind include copious sweating, aversion to wind, anxiety, restlessness and irascibility, a red complexion and, when exacerbated, faltering speech. It is diagnosed at the mouth which will have a red complexion.[34]

The symptoms of liver wind include copious sweating, aversion to wind, a tendency toward sentimentality, a slightly greenish-blue complexion, dry throat, irascibility, and occasional hatred for women. It is diagnosed (in the region) below the eyes which will have a green-blue complexion.[35]

The symptoms of spleen wind include copious sweating, aversion to wind, fatigue and listlessness, disinclination to stir the four limbs, a thin, faintly yellowish complexion, and no desire for food. It is diagnosed on the nose which will have a yellow complexion.

The symptoms of kidney wind include copious sweating, aversion to wind, hideous, puffy swelling of the face, pain in the lumbar spine, inability to stand straight, a sooty complexion, and inhibited private affairs. It is diagnosed on the *yi* which will have a black complexion.[36]

The symptoms of stomach wind include copious sweating in the neck, aversion to wind, inability of food and drink to descend, diaphragmatic obstruction and stoppage, frequent abdominal fullness, abdominal distention arising with removal of clothing, and diarrhea arising when cold food (is taken in). It is diagnosed by emaciation of the form with an enlarged abdomen.[37]

The symptoms of head wind include copious sweating on the head and face, aversion to wind, and aggravation (of the condition) one day before the wind blows. There is a headache (so severe that it) prevents one from going outdoors, but on days when the wind blows, the condition is somewhat relieved.[38]

The symptoms of leaking wind include copious sweating on some occasions yet intolerance of thin clothing, perspiration when eating which, in severe cases, covers the entire body, dyspneic breathing, aversion to wind, one's clothes being constantly soaked (by sweat), a dry mouth with constant thirst, and inability to exert one's self.

The symptoms of draining wind include copious perspiration that wets one's clothing, dry throat ["mouth" in the *Su Wen* {later editor}], the upper (half of the body) soaked (with sweat), wind penetrating exertion (sic), and generalized pain with cold.[39]

(2)

The Yellow Emperor asked:

When evil exists in the channels, what kinds of disease does it cause in people and how are these treated?

Qi Bo answered:

In heaven there are constellations situated at specific degrees. On earth there are great waters. And in the body there are channels and vessels. When heaven and earth are temperate and harmonious, the great waters are quiet and tranquil. When the heaven is cold and earth frozen, the great waters become congealed and frozen. In summerheat when the earth is hot, the great waters boil and flood. When violent winds suddenly arise, the great waters surge ["billow" in the *Su Wen* {later editor}] and seethe.

Evil enters the vessels. If (the evil) is cold, the blood may congeal and freeze, and, in the case of summerheat, the qi may become overexuberant. A vacuity evil can then enter and intrude upon (the channels). Since the great waters are worked under the influence of wind, so the beating vessels of the channels, when they come, can also be seething. Although (blood) runs within the vessels at all times, when it reaches the *cun cou* and strikes the (palpating) hand, it may sometimes feel large and other times small. If (the pulse) is large, the evil has arrived, while if small, (the qi) is normal. (A vacuity evil) circulates with no fixed location, possibly in the yang and possibly in the yin, and in a quite unpredictable way. (It is necessary to) examine the three positions and the nine indicators one by one. Once (the vacuity evil) is detected, (one must) intercept its advance, as soon as (possible).[40]

The needle must be inserted with the inhalation lest the qi be disrupted and should be retained in tranquility lest the evil be spread. The needle should be twisted with the inhalation to obtain the qi. The needle must be drawn out with the exhalation before the end of the exhalation. (This manipulation) allows the great qi to be completely drawn out and is, therefore, called drainage.[41]

The Yellow Emperor asked:

How is supplementation applied in the case of insufficiency?

Qi Bo answered:

One must first palpate (the channel) and rub (the point), cutting (the place) so as to disperse (the qi), pushing, pressing, and flicking to enrage (the point). One then thrusts (the needle in with the left hand), extracting (the needle when the channel) is freed, and then shutting the gate to keep the spirit in. The needle should be inserted at the end of an exhalation and retained quietly until the qi arrives, as if one were waiting (patiently) for a distinguished guest heedless of the setting sun. When the qi arrives, it should be taken care of. The needle should be withdrawn with the inhalation so that the qi does not escape. (One should then) press and close the gate to preserve the true qi ["spiritual qi" in the *Su Wen* {later editor}]. (This manipulation is able to) hold back the great qi and is, therefore, known as supplementation.[42]

The Yellow Emperor asked:

How is the qi reflected?

Qi Bo answered:

Once an evil leaves the connecting vessel, the evil enters the channel and will lodge in the blood vessel. At this time, as its tendency to cold or heat is not yet certain, it is like a surging wave that has just arisen, sometimes coming and sometimes going. Therefore, it is not yet fixed in location. It is, therefore, said that when it has just come, one must suppress it to arrest (its advance), and once it is arrested, one must then exterminate it. (One should) not try to drain it in the face of ["to encounter headlong" in the *Su Wen* {later editor}] its surging.[43]

The true qi is the channel qi, (and) the channel qi is (in this case) extremely vacuous. This is the reason for the admonition that one must not encounter the qi ["the oncoming qi" in the *Su Wen* {later editor}] headlong.[44]

Therefore, it is said that if the evil is not attended to carefully and drainage is not performed until the great qi is passed, this will cause the true qi to desert and such a desertion cannot be restored. Then the evil qi returns, and the disease accumulates all the more. This is the reason for the admonition that one must not chase that which is already gone.[45]

What is referred to as not drawing the bow without letting the arrow fly implies insertion of the needle and draining at the very moment when the evil is arriving. (If one acts) earlier or later (than that), blood and qi are already vacuous, and, therefore, the disease will not be eliminated. Thus, it is said that one who knows when to take (the evil) is likened to one who (is skilled at) shooting with a bow, while one who does not know when to take (the evil) is likened to one who strikes a wooden spike. Therefore, it is said that those who know the mechanism (of shooting) will never draw a bow without letting the arrow fly, while those who do not know it can bend the bow full but never hit the target. This is the reason for the (above) admonition.[46]

The Yellow Emperor asked:

When the true and evil have combined and surging waves no longer arise, how then may this be diagnosed?

Qi Bo answered:

Examine, palpate, and touch the three positions and nine indicators to determine exuberance or vacuity and then regulate it. Those ignorant of the three positions are unable to tell yin from yang or to distinguish heaven from earth. The earth reflects earth, the heavens reflect heaven, and humanity reflects humankind. By referring to the central abodes, (the conditions of) the three positions are determined. In practicing needling, those who are ignorant of what is reflected by the three positions, the nine indicators, and the pathologic pulses cannot prevent (disease) when even an excessive abundance threatens to assail.[47]

Attacking and punishing the innocent is known as grand confusion which does nothing but plunge the grand channels into chaos, and, (consequently,) the true (qi) can never be restored. Treating repletion as vacuity or mistaking an evil for the correct ["the true" in the *Su Wen* {later editor}] is an unjustifiable needling (practice) and cannot help but be a qi bandit, robbing people of their correct qi, turning the favorable into the unfavorable, dissipating and deranging the constructive and defensive. Since the true qi is lost, the evil is left to take exclusive possession of the interior. This deprives people of their long lives causing them to suffer premature death or disaster.[48]

If one is ignorant of the three positions and nine indicators, (one's patients) cannot live a long life. Therefore, ignorance of how to make a combined analysis with reference to the dispositions of the four seasons, five phases, and the superimposition and inter-restraining relationships is as good as simply allowing the evil to attack the righteous to cut short a person's long life.[49]

When a recent evil has just arrived and intruded but has not yet settled in a fixed location, it may advance if pushed or establish itself if it is conducted. Or the disease may be eradicated instantly if drainage is applied to encounter (the evil) head on.[50]

(3)

The Yellow Emperor asked:

What are the indicators of those susceptible to wind disease with shivering with cold and sweating?

Qi Bo answered:

Those with weak flesh and sparse interstices are susceptible to wind disease.

The Yellow Emperor asked:

What is the indicator of weak flesh?

Qi Bo answered:

If the major muscular masses are not strong and without (distinct) partings of the flesh, the flesh is weak. Rough skin which is not compact indicates sparse interstices.

Chapter Two

The Contraction of Disease by Yang Producing Wind (Part 2)[51]

(1)

The Yellow Emperor asked:

It is well known that (the technique of) resolving confusion advanced in the *Ci Jie (Needling Strategies)* involves the regulation (and balance) of yin and yang and the supplementation of insufficiency and drainage of surplus to overcome the prevalence and dislocation (between yin and yang). Then how is the resolution carried out?[52]

Qi Bo answered:

When there is great wind within the body, the blood vessels are hemilaterally vacuous. Vacuity means insufficiency, while repletion means surplus. (Thus) heaviness and lightness lose their balance, bumping and falling, and there is no telling the east from the west and no telling the south from the north. (Problems may be seen) in the upper (part of the body) this moment but may be found in the lower the next, appearing and disappearing erratically with inextricable infatuation in an unpredictable way. These are more serious than confusion. Supplement the insufficiency and drain the repletion and the balance between yin and yang will be restored. Needling in this way works quicker than resolving a confusion.[53]

If a rampant evil visits one side of the body, it may penetrate deeply, lodging internally in the constructive and defensive. Once the constructive and defensive become even slightly debilitated, the true qi departs and the evil qi is left to lodge alone, causing hemilateral withering. If the evil qi penetrates shallowly, there will be hemilateral pain in the vessels.

(2)

Wind counterflow is characterized by sudden swelling of the four limbs, the body appearing as if water has accumulated within it, intermittent shivering with cold, vexation occurring when the stomach is empty, and restlessness occurring when the stomach is full. Take the hand *tai yin* and its exterior (associated channel) as well as the foot *shao yin* and *yang ming* channels. In case of frigid flesh, take their brook (points). In case of frigid bones, take their well and stream (points).[54]

(3)

Hemilateral withering is characterized by loss of use of, and pain on one side of the body in which the speech is unaffected and there is an absence of mental disturbance. This disease is located in the partings of the flesh. Made to lie in a warm place to promote perspiration, (the patient) should be treated with grand needling. However, insufficiency must be boosted and surplus reduced in order for him to recover.[55]

The disease of *fei* (痱) is characterized by an absence of pain in the body and loss of use of the four limbs. If the mental disturbance is not severe and speech remains at least somewhat lucid, the condition is curable. If these conditions are very severe, however, the disease cannot be cured.[56]

If a disease starts from the yang and then enters the yin, first take the yang and then take the yin. One must first examine the (evil) qi and determine whether it is up-floating or sinking qi before taking them.[57]

(4)

A great wind can cause the bony articulations to become heavy and one's eyebrows and beard to fall out. (This disease) is called great wind. One must needle the muscles to induce perspiration for one hundred days, and then needle the bone marrow to induce perspiration for another hundred days for a total of two hundred days. When the beard and eyebrows begin to grow again, the needling may be discontinued.[58]

(5)

The Yellow Emperor asked:

There is a disease which is characterized by generalized fever, fatigue and listlessness, perspiration so copious it is as if one were bathing, aversion to wind, and shortage of qi. What kind of disease is this?

Qi Bo answered:

It is known as wine wind. To treat it, prescribe 10 *fen* of Alismatis (*Ze Xie*), 10 *fen* of Rhizoma Atractylodes Macrocephalae (*Bai Zhu*), and 5 *fen* of Herba Ipomoeae Aquaticae (*Mi Xin*). Mix them together and take a three-fingered pinch after meals.

(6)

Bodily injury with copious bleeding followed by wind cold stroke or impact injuries such as in falls may lead to fatigue, listlessness, and debility of the four limbs. This is called body listlessness (*ti jie*). Take the triple-joining point below the umbilicus in the lower abdomen. The triple-joining point is where the foot *yang ming* and the *tai yin* ["*tai yang*" in a variant version {later editor}] join (the conception vessel) three *cun* below the umbilicus. It is the point Origin Pass (*Guan Yuan*, CV 4).[59]

(7)

For wind dizziness with frequent retching and vexing fullness, Spirit Court (*Shen Ting*, GV 24) is the ruling point. In the case of green-blue complexion at the forehead, Upper Star (*Shang Xing*, GV 23) is the ruling point. In taking Upper Star, first take Yi Xi (*Yi Xi*, Bl 45), and finally Celestial Window (*Tian You*, TH 16) and Wind Pool (*Feng Chi*, GB 20). In the case of headache and green-blue complexion at the forehead, Fontanel Meeting (*Xin Hui*, GV 22) is the ruling point.

For wind dizziness initiating pain in the submandibular region, Upper Star (*Shang Xing*, GV 23) is the ruling point. It is taken in the same way as described above.

For wind dizziness with heavy eyes, aversion to wind and cold, and a swollen red face, Before the Vertex (*Qian Ding*, GV 21) is the ruling point.

For pain in the vertex with wind heavy-headedness, eyes (so painful) it is as if they were about to burst (from their sockets), and inability to turn left or right, Hundred Convergences (*Bai Hui*, GV 20) is the ruling point.[60]

For wind dizziness with visual dizziness and pain at the top of the head, Behind to Vertex (*Hou Ding*, GV 19) is the ruling point.

For heavy-headedness, pain in the nape of the neck, dim vision, cold in the brain once exposed to wind, inability to get warm even with many clothes on, (spontaneous) sweating, and aversion of the head to wind, needle Brain's Door (*Nao Hu*, GV 17).

For headache, hypertonicity of the nape of the

neck with inability to turn around, visual dizziness, inability to breathe (through the nose), and rigidity of the tongue with difficult speaking, needle Wind Mansion (*Feng Fu*, GV 16).

For spinning of the head with pain in the eyes and hemilateral cold ["hemilateral cold and pain" in the *Qian Jin* {later editor}] in the head, Jade Pillow (*Yu Zhen*, Bl 9) is the ruling point.

For brain wind (*nao feng*) with heavy eyes and headache, (or for) wind dizziness with pain in the eyes, Brain Hollow (*Nao Kong*, GB 19) is the ruling point.

For stuffing fullness in the neck and submandibular region with pain radiating to the teeth, clenched jaw, and tension and pain (of the mouth) with inability to speak, Temporal Hairline Curve (*Qu Bin*, GB 7) is the ruling point.

For pain in the nape radiating to (the front of) the neck, Portal Yin (*Qiao Yin*, GB 11) is the ruling point.[61]

For wind in the head with pain (in the region) posterior to the auricles, vexation of the heart, debilitated feet with loss of the ability to stride, deviated mouth, shaking of and tugging pain in the head and the nape of the neck, and rigidity of the jaws, Completion Bone (*Wan Gu*, GB 12) is the ruling point.[62]

For dizziness, pain and heaviness of the head, eyes (so painful) it is as if they were about to burst (from their sockets, pain in) the nape of the neck as if it were being pulled up, manic attacks in which one claims to see ghosts, upturned eyes, stiffness of the nape of the neck with inability to turn round, sudden hypertonicity, inability of the feet to bear the body, and breaking pain, Celestial Pillar (*Tian Zhu*, Bl 10) is the ruling point.[63]

For rigidity of the lumbar spine with inability to bend either forward or backward, needle Spinal Center (*Ji Zhong*, GV 6).

For sweating in great wind, Diaphragm Shu (*Ge Shu*, Bl 17) is the ruling point. Yi Xi (*Yi Xi*, Bl 45) is also the ruling point. ["For sweating in a great wind, moxa Yi Xi" in the "*Gu Kong Lun* (The Treatise on Bone Cavities)", *Su Wen*.[64] {later editor}][65]

For dizziness and headache, needle Silk Bamboo Hole (*Si Zhu Kong*, TH 23) as the ruling point.

For deviated mouth, Cheek Bone Hole (*Quan Liao*, SI 18), Gum Intersection (*Yin Jiao*, GV 28), and Lower Pass (*Xia Guan*, St 7) are the ruling points.

For aversion of the face and eyes to wind and cold, swelling, pronounced swelling and pain in the suborbital region, trembling (of the limbs), and a fixed gaping, tugging and slackening, and deviated mouth, Great Bone Hole (*Ju Liao*, St 3) is the ruling point.

When the mouth cannot hold in liquid and deviates, Water Trough (*Shui Gou*, GV 26) is the ruling point.

For deviated mouth with clenched jaw, Outer Pass (*Wai Guan*, TH 5) is the ruling point.

For tugging and slackening with foaming at the mouth, Upper Pass (*Shang Guan*, GB 3) is the ruling point.

For hemilateral withering with loss of use of the four limbs and susceptibility to fright, Great Gigantic (*Da Ju*, St 27) is the ruling point.

For qi counterflow during great wind with much cold and sentimentality, Great Horizontal (*Da Heng*, Sp 15) is the ruling point.

For inability to lift the hands and arms to the head, Cubit Marsh (*Chi Ze*, Lu 5) is the ruling point.

For sweating (during the contraction of) wind, generalized swelling, dyspneic wheezing, copious sputum, trance and poor memory, and somnolence, Celestial Storehouse (*Tian Fu*, Lu 3) is the ruling point ["which is located three *cun* under the axilla, at the pulsating vessel in the inner aspect of the arm" {later editor}].[66]

For wind heat with irascibility, (unreasonable) joy and sorrow when the heart is struck, anxiety, (groundless) sobbing, and incessant laughing, Palace of Toil (*Lao Gong*, Per 8) is the ruling point.[67]

For hypertonicity of the hands with inability to stretch affecting the axillae (and for) hemilateral withering with insensitivity, tugging of the hands, and hypertonicity of the minor sinews (of the arm), Great Mound (*Da Ling*, Per 7) is the ruling point.[68]

For wind heat in the head and trunk with frequent retching and vomiting, apprehension, cold in the center, diminished qi, heat in the palms, hypertonicity of the elbows, and swelling of the axillae, Intermediary Courier (*Jian Shi*, Per 5) is the ruling point.

For debilitated feet with pain and inability to walk, Celestial Spring (*Tian Quan*, Per 2) is the ruling point.

For slack feet with loss of the ability to stride, Surging Yang (*Chong Yang*, St 42) is the ruling point.

For hypertonicity of the hands and arms, Spirit Gate (*Shen Men*, Ht 7) is the ruling point.

For *fei* and atony with loss of use of the arms and wrists and inability to contract the lips and corners of the mouth, Union Valley (*He Gu*, LI 4) is the ruling point.

For pain in the elbows such that one cannot dress oneself, spinning of the head on attempting to stand up, pain in the submandibular region, a black facial complexion, and pain in the shoulders and upper back with inability to turn round, Passage Hub (*Guan Chong*, TH 1) is the ruling point.

For swelling on the outside of the throat, pain in the elbows and arms, distorted hands, tugging of the five fingers with inability to contract or stretch, spinning of the head, and pain in the submandibular region, forehead, and the top of the head, Central Islet (*Zhong Zhu*, TH 3) is the ruling point.

For saber swollen lumps and fistulae, pain in the eyes, inability to lift the shoulders, heart pain and stuffing fullness, qi counterflow, sweating, and clenched jaw, Branch Trough (*Zhi Gou*, TH 6) is the ruling point.

For great wind with mutism, pain which cannot be located, somnolence, susceptibility to fright, and tugging and slackening, Celestial Well (*Tian Jing*, TH 10) is the ruling point.[69]

For hemilateral withering with pain in the arm and wrist, ability to contract but not to stretch (the elbow, and for) head wind with headache, tearing, pain in the shoulder, arm and neck, hypertonicity of the nape of the neck, vexing fullness, susceptibility to fright, tugging of the five fingers with inability to bend or stretch, and shuddering, Wrist Bone (*Wan Gu*, SI 4) is the ruling point.

For wind dizziness, susceptibility to fright, and pain in the wrists or for draining wind with sweating down to the waist, Yang Valley (*Yang Gu*, SI 5) is the ruling point ["contracted hands" instead of "pain in the wrists" in the *Qian Jin* {later editor}].

For wind counterflow with sudden swelling of the four limbs, dampness causing shivering with cold, vexation of the heart arising when the stomach is empty, and dizziness arising when the stomach is full, Great Metropolis (*Da Du*, Sp 2) is the ruling point.

For wind penetrating the abdomen with periumbilical tension, stuffing fullness in the chest and lateral costal regions, incessant nosebleeding, and pain in the tips of all the five toes preventing the feet from touching the ground, Gushing Spring (*Yong Quan*, Ki 1) is the ruling point.

For hemilateral withering with inability to walk, great wind with mutism, pain which cannot be located, seeing stars, yellowish urine, heat in the lower abdomen, and dry throat, Shining Sea

(*Zhao Hai*, Ki 6) is the ruling point. (It is necessary to) drain the yin motility vessel and the right (point of) the *shao yin*. First needle the yin motility and then the *shao yin* (point) which is located at the pubic bone.[70]

For wind counterflow with swelling of the four limbs, Recover Flow (*Fu Liu*, Ki 7) is the ruling point.

For wind (penetrating) from the head to the feet with red facial complexion and reddening of the eyes, pain in the mouth, and biting of the tongue, Ravine Divide (*Jie Xi*, St 41) is the ruling point.

For great wind with pain in the outer canthi, generalized fever with miliaria, and pain in the supraclavicular fossae, Overlooking Tears (*Lin Qi*, GB 41) is the ruling point.[71]

For frequent biting of the cheeks and hemilateral withering with pain in the lumbus and hip joints and constant shaking of the head, Capital Bone (*Jing Gu*, Bl 64) is the ruling point.

For great wind with profuse sweating on the head, lumbar, sacrococcygeal, and abdominal pain, swollen calves and heels, pain in the upper teeth, heaviness of the spine, back, and sacrococcygeal (region) with disinclination to stand up, (liking for) the smell of food, aversion to the voice of people, and draining wind from the head down to the feet, Kun Lun Mountain (*Kun Lun*, Bl 60) is the ruling point.[72]

For atonic inversion with wind heavy headedness, pain in the root of the nose, pain in the bones at the lateral aspect of the hip joints, thighs, and calves, tugging and slackening, insensitive *bi*, quivering with cold, intermittent fever, and inability to lift the four limbs, Give Yang (*Fu Yang*, Bl 59) is the ruling point.

For lumbar pain, pain in the nape and neck, sweating and loss of ability to stride in articular wind, cold, insensitivity of the abdomen, and pain in the calves, Flying Yang (*Fei Yang*, Bl 58) is the ruling point.[73]

Chapter Three

Contraction of Disease by the Eight Hollows Causing Hypertonicity[74]

(1)

The Yellow Emperor asked:

Humans have eight hollows. What are the indicators of each of them?

Qi Bo answered:

If there is evil in the lung and heart, their qi is retained in the elbows. If there is evil in the liver, its qi is retained in the armpits. If there is evil in the spleen, its qi is retained in the hip joints. If there is evil in the kidney, its qi is retained in the popliteal fossae. The eight hollow parts are all cavities of joints. The true qi passes through them and the blood network vessels flow across them. Therefore, evil qi and the foul blood find it easy to become lodged there, and, once they become lodged, they damage the sinews and the bones, prohibiting (the joints) from contracting and stretching. This results in hypertonicity.

(2)

For sudden hypertonicity, epilepsy, dizziness, and inability of the feet to carry the body, Celestial Pillar (*Tian Zhu*, Bl 10) is the ruling point.

(3)

For sudden hypertonicity of the armpits with sudden tense vessels initiating a pain in the lateral costal regions and sending a dragging (discomfort) to the heart and lung, Yi Xi (*Yi Xi*, Bl 45) is the ruling point. (And, at the same time, it is necessary to) needle all the tender points found in palpating parallel to the spine from the nape down to the twelfth (thoracic) vertebra.[75] Relief follows immediately.

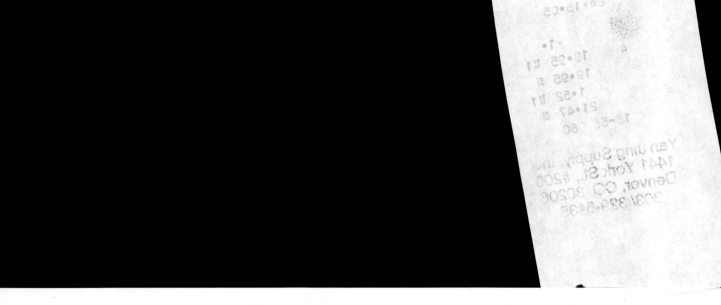

(4)

For cramps, needle with (the patient) standing and a cure will be effected on the spot. (To needle) in the case of atonic inversion, (the patient should be) made to lie supine, full stretched, and this will offer instant relief.

Chapter Four

Heat in the Five Viscera Causing Atony[76]

(1)

The Yellow Emperor asked:

Why can the five viscera cause people to suffer from atony?

Qi Bo answered:

The lung governs the body's skin and hair, the heart governs the body's blood vessels, the liver governs the body's sinew membranes, the spleen governs the body's muscles, and the kidney governs the body's bone marrow. For this reason, when the lung qi gets hot, the lobes of the lung will get parched, and, when they become parched, the skin and hair become weak, tense, and thin. Because (the heat qi) becomes fixed (to the lung), atonic limpness (*wei bi*) is generated.[77]

When the heart qi becomes hot, (the qi of) the lower vessels becomes inverted and ascends. When it ascends, the lower vessels become vacuous, and this vacuity generates vessel atony (with symptoms of) impairment and rigidity of the key joints, slack lower legs, and inability to stand on the ground.[78]

When the liver qi becomes hot, the gallbladder leaks, causing a bitter taste in the mouth and the sinew membranes become dry. When the sinew membranes are dry, the sinews become tense and hypertonic, causing sinew atony.

When the spleen qi becomes hot, the stomach becomes dry with thirst and insensitivity of the muscles, causing fleshy atony.

When the kidney qi becomes hot, this causes an inability to lift the lumbar spine, the bones dry out, and the marrow diminishes, causing bone atony.

The Yellow Emperor asked:

How do these things occur?

Qi Bo answered:

The lung is the leader of the viscera and the canopy of the heart. Frustrations and disappointments or being short of what is desired may cause the lung to ring. When it rings, the lung becomes hot and its lobes become parched, causing atonic limpness.[79]

If there is an excess of sorrow and sadness, the connecting vessel of the pericardium expires. When it expires, the yang qi stirs internally, causing (blood) to collapse below the heart with frequent hematuria. Therefore, the *Ben Bing (The Root of Disease)* concludes that emptiness and vacuity of the grand channels causes vessel *bi* which is (further) transmuted into vascular atony.[80]

Endless thought and aspiration, frustration of desires, preoccupation with external (beauty), and overindulgence in sexual intercourse cause the gathering sinew to slacken and wear out, causing sinew atony and white flux. Therefore, the *Xia Jing* concludes that sinew atony is generated in the liver due to labors of the bedroom.[81]

Gradual affliction by dampness and engagement in activities relating to water may cause dampness to lodge (in the body), and (damp) living environments may cause damage. (As a result,) the muscles become wet and soaked and contract *bi* characterized by insensitivity, thus causing fleshy atony. Therefore, the *Xia Jing* concludes that fleshy atony is generated on the damp ground.

Taxation fatigue during a long trip and during intensely hot weather causes thirst. In thirst, the yang qi attacks inward, and, in consequence, heat converges into ["lodges in" the, *Su Wen* {later editor}] the kidney. The kidney is the water viscus. Since this water (is disabled and) cannot restrain fire, the bones become dry and the marrow empty. This results in an inability of the feet to carry the body, causing bone atony. Therefore the *Xia Jing* concludes that bone atony is generated by intense heat.[82]

The Yellow Emperor asked:

How are (the various types of atony) differentiated?

Qi Bo answered:

Lung heat is (characterized by) a white complexion and withered hair. Heart heat is (characterized by) red complexion and inundated network vessels. Liver heat is (characterized by) green-blue complexion and desiccated nails. Spleen heat is (characterized by) yellow complexion and vermicular movement of the flesh. And kidney heat is (characterized by) black complexion and dried teeth.[83]

The Yellow Emperor asked:

To treat atony, why does one take only the *yang ming*?

Qi Bo answered:

The *yang ming* is the sea of the five viscera and six bowels and governs the moisturizing of the gathering sinews. These gathering sinews bind the bones and provide mobility to the joints. The penetrating vessel is the sea of all the channels and vessels and governs the percolation and irrigation of the ravines and valleys. It joins the *yang ming* at the gathering sinew. All the yin and yang (channels) converge at the gathering sinew, then meet at Qi Surge (*Qi Chong*, St 30), and the *yang ming* is the leader (of them all). They are all ascribed to the girdling vessel and connected to the governing vessel. Therefore, when the *yang*

ming is vacuous, the gathering sinew becomes slack and the girdling vessel is no longer able to contract (it), resulting in atony of the feet with loss of use. To treat this, (one should) supplement at the brook point and free the flow within the rapids point (of the involved channel), regulate vacuity and repletion, and harmonize the counterflow and normal flow. In this way, the sinews, the vessels, the bones, and the flesh will each recover from disease in their prevailing dates and months.[84]

(2)

For atonic inversion, bind up the four limbs and release them as soon as suppression is felt, twice a day. For (atony with) insensitivity, sensation is regained in ten days. If (the illness) is not terminated, (the treatment) should be continued until recovery.

(3)

For slack and debilitated mouth with inability to speak, and hand and foot atony with inability to walk, Earth Granary (*Di Cang*, St 4) is the ruling point.

For atony with no sensation ["generalized heaviness and bone atony with no sensation" in a variant version {later editor}], Supreme White (*Tai Bai*, Sp 3) is the ruling point.

For atonic inversion with generalized insensitivity and hemilateral hand and foot atrophy, first take Capital Bone (*Jing Gu*, Bl 64) and then take Mound Center (*Zhong Feng*, Liv 4) and Severed Bone (*Jue Gu*, GB 38),[85] draining at all these points.

For atonic inversion with cold and debility of the ankles, limpness, inability to stand up from a sitting posture, and pain in the hip joints and feet, Hill Ruins (*Qiu Xu*, GB 40) is the ruling point.

For vacuity resulting in atonic limpness with inability to stand up from a sitting posture, for repletion resulting in inversion, heat in the lower legs and pain in the knee, or for generalized insensitivity, hand and foot atrophy hemilaterally, and frequent biting of the cheeks, Bright Light (*Guang Ming*, GB 37) is the ruling point.

Chapter Five

Stirring in the Hand *Tai Yin*, *Yang Ming*, *Tai Yang*, & *Shao Yang* Vessels Causing Pain in the Shoulders, Upper Back, Region Anterior to the Shoulders, & Upper Arm, and the Shoulders Painful as if Being Pulled Up[86]

For pain in and inability to lift the shoulders, Celestial Countenance (*Tian Rong*, SI 17) and Grasping the Wind (*Bing Feng*, SI 12) are the ruling points.

For *bi* pain in the shoulders and upper back, inability to lift the arms, fever and chills, and shivering with cold, Shoulder Well (*Jian Jing*, GB 21) is the ruling point.

For swollen shoulder with inability to look around, Qi Abode (*Qi She*, St 11) is the ruling point.

For *bi* pain in the shoulders and upper back, inability to lift the arms, and blood stasis in the shoulders with inability to move them, Great Bone (*Ju Gu*, LI 16) is the ruling point.[87]

For heat in the shoulders and pain in the fingers and forearms, Shoulder Bone (*Jian Yu*, LI 15) is the ruling point.

For heaviness of, and inability to lift the shoulders and pain in the arms, Shoulder Bone Hole (*Jian Liao*, TH 14) is the ruling point.

For heaviness of the shoulders, and pain in and inability to lift the elbows and arms, Celestial Gathering (*Tian Zong*, SI 11) is the ruling point.

For pain in the scapulae with cold extending to the elbows, Outer Shoulder Shu (*Jian Wai Shu*, SI 14) is the ruling point.

For peripheral *bi* of the scapulae, Crooked Wall (*Qu Yuan*, SI 13) is the ruling point.

For pain in and inability to lift the shoulders radiating to the supraclavicular fossae, Cloud Gate (*Yun Men*, Lu 2) is the ruling point.

For pain in the elbow, Cubit Marsh (*Chi Ze*, Lu 5) is the ruling point.

For tugging of the arms affecting the mouth, aversion to cold, swelling of the suborbital regions, and pain in the shoulders radiating a dragging (discomfort) to the supraclavicular fossae, Shang Yang (*Shang Yang*, LI 1) is the ruling point.

For pain in the shoulders and elbows causing difficulty contracting and stretching, inability of the hands to lift weights and hypertonicity of the wrists, Pool at the Bend (*Qu Chi*, LI 11) is the ruling point.

For aching, heaviness, and *bi* pain of the shoulder and elbow joints with inability to contract or stretch them, Elbow Bone Hole (*Zhou Liao*, LI 12) is the ruling point.

For pain in and inability to lift the shoulders, lack of perspiration, and pain in the neck, Yang Pool (*Yang Chi*, TH 4) is the ruling point.

For fattened elbows, pain in the inner aspect of the arms, and inability to lift (the arms) to the head, Outer Pass (*Wai Guan*, TH 5) is the ruling point.[88]

For pain in the elbows radiating to the shoulders with inability to contract or stretch (the arms), shivering with cold, fever and chills, pain in the neck and nape, shoulders, and upper back, and atonic *bi* with insensitivity in the arms ["numbness of the medial borders of the shoulders" in the *Qian Jin* {later editor}], Celestial Well (*Tian Jing*, TH 10) is the ruling point.

For inability to lift the shoulders and to dress oneself, Clear Cold Abyss (*Qing Leng Yuan*, TH 11) is the ruling point.

For pain in the elbows, forearms, and wrists, swelling of and inability to turn the neck, tension and pain in the head and nape of the neck, dizziness, aching and weakness (of the limbs), and pain in the scapulae and small fingers, Front Valley (*Qian Gu*, SI 2) is the ruling point.

For pain in the shoulders causing inability to dress oneself and pain in the radial aspect of the arms and wrist with inability to lift (the arms), Yang Valley (*Yang Gu*, SI 5) is the ruling point.

For inability to lift the arms, pain in the nape of the neck, headache, and swollen throat preventing swallowing, Front Valley (*Qian Gu*) is the ruling point.

For breaking pain in the shoulders, excruciating pain in the upper arms, and inability to move the hands up or down, Nursing the Aged (*Yang Lao*, SI 6) is the ruling point.

For pain in the shoulders, upper back, and nape of the neck with intermittent dizziness, Gushing Spring (*Yong Quan*, Ki 1) is the ruling point.

Chapter Six

Water & Beverage Failing to Disperse Producing Rheum [89]

For spillage rheum with hardness and pain in the free rib regions, Central Venter (*Zhong Wan*, CV 12) is the ruling point.

For frigidity in the lumbus, rigidity of the spine, fatigue and listlessness of the four limbs, irascibility, coughing, diminished qi, depression, and inability to catch the breath, counterflow inversion, inability to lift the shoulders, saber fistula, and twitching (of the muscles) all over the body, Camphorwood Gate (*Zhang Men*, Liv 13) is the ruling point.

For spillage rheum, with blocked water passageways, yellowish urine, pain, lateral lower abdominal pain with urgency and swelling inside, out-

pour diarrhea, and pain in the upper thighs radiating a dragging (discomfort) to the back, Capital Bone (*Jing Gu*, Bl 64) is the ruling point.

For drinking unable to quench thirst, generalized pain, and copious sputum, Hidden White (*Yin Bai*, Sp 1) is the ruling point.

For (stagnant) qi in the interstices, Upper Arm Convergence (*Nao Hui*, TH 13) is the ruling point.[90]

Endnotes

[1] Part 1 is derived from Chap. 27, Vol. 5, *Ling Shu (Spiritual Pivot)*; Part 2 from Chap. 46, Vol. 7, *Ling Shu*; and Part 3 from Chap. 43, *Su Wen (Basic Questions)*.

[2] Multiple *bi* is characterized by pains that break out alternately on the right and the left but which do not move up and down, although it exists in the channel.

[3] Global *bi* is characterized by pains moving up and down along the affected channel that do not travel from one side to the other.

[4] Whenever there is pain, this catches our attention. In other words, the spirit is drawn toward the painful place. Then qi and blood are drawn toward it, too, giving rise to heat. Although this heat may resolve pain, a counterflow of qi or inversion arises. With the counterflow, cold qi gathers in another place to produce pain once again. This cold qi lodges in the partings of the flesh, obstructing the circulation of channel qi and, therefore, acquires the name of circulatory *bi*.

[5] The three regions are the upper, middle, and lower regions of the body.

[6] The constructive is ascribed to the blood; the defensive to qi.

[7] 1 *jin* = 2 kilo or one catty; four *zhang* = 12 meters (approximately); 10 *chi* = 1 *zhang*; 1 *chi* = 0.33 meters.

[8] In old times, cheaply clad people were all poor laborers who had tough muscles and good resistance to pain and drastic therapies. Therefore, red-hot needling or moxing was good for them. One should note that in ancient times, moxibustion was usually performed, unlike modern methods of moxibustion, directly on the skin, requiring good resistance to burning and pain.

[9]The consummate yin is long summer.

[10]Viscus and bowel associated points such as Spleen Shu (*Pi Shu*, Bl 20) and Gallbladder Shu (*Dan Shu*, Bl 19), lie on the back, and the back is vulnerable to attack by external evils.

[11]The rapids of the five viscera are Supreme Surge (*Tai Chong*, Liv 3), Great Mound (*Da Ling*, Per 7), Supreme White (*Tai Bai*, Sp 3), Great Abyss (*Tai Yuan*, Lu 9), and Great Ravine (*Tai Xi*, Ki 3). The confluences of the six bowels are Leg Three Li (*Zu San Li*, St 36), the confluence point of the stomach, Upper Great Hollow (*Shang Ju Xu*, St 37), the confluence point of the large intestine, Lower Great Hollow (*Xia Ju Xu*, St 39), the confluence point of the small intestine, Bend Yang (*Wei Yang*, Bl 39), the confluence point of the triple burner, Bend Middle (*Wei Zhong*, Bl 40), the confluence point of the urinary bladder, and Yang Mound Spring (*Yang Ling Quan*, GB 34), the confluence point of the gallbladder.

"That which is at fault" means the diseased channel or viscusBbowel.

[12]Any interstices between membranes are called *huang*, whether in the internal cavities or between the flesh in the exterior.

[13]Part 1 is derived from Chap. 43, *Su Wen*; Part 2 from Chap. 75, Vol. 11, *Ling Shu*; Part 3 from Chap. 55, *Su Wen*; Part 4 from Chap. 34, *Su Wen*; Part 5 is a combination of parts of Chap. 21, 24, 26, Vol. 5, *Ling Shu*; and Part 6 from the *Zhen Jiu Ming Tang Zhi Yao*.

[14]Cold causes pain. A chronic disease debilitates qi and blood, stagnating the flow of the defensive and the constructive, making the channels and network vessels empty, and, as a result, there is lack of nourishment. This causes painlessness and insensitivity. Pathological factors lead to disorders of a similar nature. For example, exuberant yang qi engenders heat problems which are a yang evil. This accounts for the genesis of hot or cold *bi*. The meaning of the phrase "diseased qi" depends on the context in which it is used, and in this paragraph, it implies an exuberance of yang qi. Wet *bi* is due to two evil qi, *i.e.*, dampness and exuberant yin qi or cold qi.

[15]The true qi is a combination of prenatal qi and the great qi or air in modern terms. In this context, the correct qi is the qi of wind which blows from a direction congruent to the season, for example, the east in spring and the west in autumn. This can be understood in a broad sense as a normal seasonal change. A vacuity wind is a wind blowing from a direction counter to its seasonal disposition. For example, spring is wood, and is associated with east. If a west wind blows in the spring, this wind is a vacuity wind, since west is metal and metal restrains wood.

[16]When cold qi penetrates the bones, bone *bi* develops. To treat this condition, the needle must be inserted to the bone, but one must be careful not to injure the vessels or muscles. The points to be needled are located in the partings of the flesh.

[17]Some people wear warm enough clothes to keep cold off the body, and have had no cold qi within in the past, but they may suffer from a cold disorder.

[18]*Bi* here simply means a blockage of qi which leads to a cessation of the flow of yang qi and accumulation of yin qi.

[19]The kidney qi is yin. Involvement in water in one's pursuits has two meanings: First, one's work puts them constantly in contact with cold water. Fishing might be an example of this. Secondly, this phrase also implies excessive sexual activity. The kidney grease mentioned in the text is a synonym for kidney essence. When the kidney essence is dried up and has stopped growing, the bone marrow will be empty, resulting in severe cold. Zhang Jing-yue discusses the reasons one does not quiver in the *Lei Jing*, "The liver is in possession of the ministerial fire of the *shao yang*, and the heart is the sovereign fire of the *shao yin*, while the kidney is water, a singular water. While this singular water is dried up, the two fires are still in existence. This means that the yin qi is already vacuous in the center, while the floating yang is solitarily overwhelming externally. This is why the cold inside the bones, however severe, does not produce shivering with cold."

[20]Inversion *bi* is cold qi that is blocked in the lower part of the body producing an upward counterflow in the three yang channels. This stops in the abdomen, unable to reach the head. Because this problem involves the abdomen, one should needle the network vessels of the foot *tai yin* spleen and the foot *yang ming* stomach channel. Since the *yang ming* generally has an abundance of qi and blood, one should apply drainage here, while one should supplement the foot *tai yin*. However, as the illness may manifest itself in a manner different than this, affecting channels other than the *yang ming* and the *tai yin*, one should administer therapies that are specific to the presenting condition.

[21]Wind *bi* is migratory *bi* due to wind. This has been discussed in the preceding chapter of this book. Wind *bi* outpour disease is the late stage of this condition.

[22]*I.e.*, Jumping Round (*Huan Tiao*, GB 30)

[23]Wind Mansion is the meeting point of the governing vessel, the foot *tai yang*, and the *yang wei* vessel. As such, it unblocks and regulates the yang and eliminates wind dampness to treat this condition.

[24]Meeting of Yin is the lowest point of the conception, governing, and penetrating vessels and regulates the qi and blood in these channels. Great Abyss assists the lungs in treating the skin and hair. Dispersing Riverbed regulates the three warmers and eliminates wind damp. And Shining Sea regulates blood stasis in the network vessels.

[25]Three Yang Connection harmonizes the yang qi and dissipates yin dampness.

[26]Part 1 is derived from Chap. 42, *Su Wen*; Part 2 from Chap. 27, *Su Wen*; and Part 3 from Chap. 46, Vol. 7, *Ling Shu*.

[27]There are two notes in the *Tai Su* that are quite to the point. They read "Because the people are fat, their interstices are compact, solid, and cannot be opened. Therefore, the wind qi is held up, unable to drain out, thus resulting in heat in the center." And, "In thin people, the interstices are thin and void, and, therefore, the warm qi is drained out, thus inviting wind qi in, which results in cold in the center. Because the foot *yang ming* vessel is vacuous and cold, the eyes (frequently) shed tears."

[28]Wang Bing explains in a note to the *Su Wen*, "The constructive circulates inside the vessels. Once wind enters the vessels, it attacks the blood and mixes with the constructive to generate heat, and then the blood decays. Turbidity of the qi is spoken of as chaos of the qi. Since the blood vessels become chaotic and the constructive is mingled with wind, all the yang vessels go up to the head. The nose is responsible for breathing. Therefore its pillar is marred..." Cold and heat usually is not regarded as pestilential qi. The author may be suggesting that cold and heat is the initial stage of pestilential wind.

[29]See note 18, Chap. 2, Book 1, present work.

[30]The gates referred to here are acupoints. If wind qi strikes a point or points on the left side, for example, then this causes left hemilateral wind. Hemilateral wind is hemilateral withering. However, the former term is preferred when talking about disease causation, while the latter is adopted in describing the symptoms involved.

[31]Head wind, leaking wind, and draining wind are discussed in the following passages. Internal wind is so named because wind qi directly strikes the interior. Since sexual intercourse consumes the yin essence, while sweating exhausts the yang qi, both yin and yang become debilitated. Intestinal wind is diarrhea of blood in the stools.

[32]Although a wide diversity of illnesses may arise out of wind, these problems invariably possess the properties of wind. Wind changes swiftly, travels from place to place, and comes and goes.

[33]During the day, the yang is in the exterior. Therefore the patient experiences relief. During the evening, the yang submerges into the interior and is influenced by the wind qi there. Therefore the condition deteriorates. The lung is metal which is white, and this accounts for white complexion.

[34]The heart governs the tongue. When the condition deteriorates, the tongue will become stiff, affecting speech.

[35]When the liver is diseased, the heart can no longer be supplied and becomes vacuous. As a result, unreasonable sorrow and sadness occur. Since the liver channel encircles the genitals, when it is in good order, one expresses sexual desire, but when it is debilitated, a hatred for women arises.

[36]Private affairs include sexual desire and functions of the reproductive organs. *Yi* is the area above and beside the chin and below and beside the angle of the mouth over the laterosuperior part of the jaw.

[37]The foot *yang ming* channel travels through the neck and Man's Prognosis (*Ren Ying*, St 9) is a key point there. Therefore, the neck often sweats when the stomach is affected. When one wears less clothes than necessary, external cold tends to strike, and, therefore, the abdomen becomes distended.

[38]Zhang Jing-yue explains in his *Lei Jing*, "In all cases, head wind may start and stop at any moment. The reason why wind qi is set off one day before wind blows is that the yang evil (*i.e.*, wind) is in the yang phase, and yang takes a lead and acts swiftly." Zhang Zhao-huang, son of Zhang Zhi-cong, supplements a note to his father's work, the *Su Wen Ji Zhu* (*Condensed Annotations on the Basic Questions*), saying, "When wind is about to blow, the wind lodging within the body is starting as well. Because the qi in the human body communicates with heaven, the condition deteriorates one day earlier."

Wang Bing explains in a note to the *Su Wen*, "Because the condition deteriorates earlier than the wind begins to blow, it abates earlier. For this reason, the condition is relieved on the day the wind blows."

[39]A note to the "*Feng Lun* (Treatise on Wind)" of the *Su*

Wen advances the opinion that draining wind should be replaced by internal wind. "Wind penetrating exertion..." is puzzling. The words "wind" may simply be redundant, and we should change the phrase to "incapability of exertion."

[40]One should note that when the author speaks of large and small pulses, he is defining them in a specific way. The three positions and the nine indications are discussed in Chap. 6, Book 4, of the present work. The last sentence tells us that one should administer treatment as early as possible to check the progression of the evil.

The words "strikes the hand" may be a redundancy, giving this sentence an awkward structure.

[41]Great qi here refers to the accumulated evil qi.

[42]Before needling, one should first feel along the involved channel, gently rubbing the points to be needled and marking or cutting with the nails of the fingers to smooth the qi of the channel and make it flow freely. Pushing, pressing, and flicking fill the channel or vessel with qi, and this is what is meant by enraging the qi. The needle is then inserted with the right hand while holding or pinching the skin of the point with the left hand. After extraction of the needle, the gate or the needle hole should be pressed shut immediately. This serves to preserve the accumulated true qi within "the gate." One should note the opposite meaning of the term great qi in the above two passages.

The passage "extracting (the needle when the channel) is freed" may be understood in a different way. According to this interpretation, it may be read as "to launch a charge at the evil when the channel qi is running smooth and steady."

[43]The second to last sentence may also be interpreted in another way. "Before the evil qi has settled, one must press the points to arrest (its advance) and then begin to attack it with the needle."

[44]When the evil runs wild, the true qi is so overwhelmed it cannot be drained. This is why we should not impose drainage in the face of a surging evil. Encountering the qi headlong in this context means drainage, and the qi, except where explicitly stated otherwise, refers to the evil qi.

[45]If drainage is performed in the face of a surging evil, this is malpractice, but neither must one delay in needling. Therefore, the application of drainage requires opportune timing.

[46]The author reiterates the importance of opportune needling. The opportune time for treatment should not be missed by so much as a hair's breadth.

[47]A knowledge of the three positions and nine indicators is very important in needling. If ignorant of them, one will not be able to determine the location of the evil, whether it is in the yin or in the yang, in the upper part of the body or in the lower. The earth position, *i.e.*, the lower, reflects problems in the lower body. The heaven position, *i.e.*, the upper, reflects problems in the upper body. And the human position, *i.e.*, the middle, reflects problems in the middle of the body. The central abodes refer to the internal organs, including the viscera and bowels together with their qi. Another interpretation defines the central abode merely as the stomach and its qi. Only when one has an understanding of the normal and abnormal conditions of the five viscera and six bowels as well as their qi can we determine the significance of the reflection by the three positions.

[48]The grand channels are simply the primary channels.

[49]One must make a comprehensive analysis of the reflections of the three positions and nine indicators with reference to many other factors. Superimposition and inter-restraining relationship refer to the five movements and six qi. The five movements are determined by the five phases, and, therefore, there is an interBrestraining relationship between them. The five movements have three categories: the ruling five movements, the middle or major five movements, and the guest five movements. Combining the three, we have a picture of the characters of the weather in a particular year. The six qi are wind, cold, summerheat, dampness, dryness, and fire. They are arranged in the order of the earthly branches, unlike the five movements which are in order of the heavenly stems. There are two categories of the six qi: the ruling qi and the guest qi. These two kinds of qi may superimpose each other to reveal abnormal weather change.

[50]To treat a recent disorder, one should not employ supplementation. This means pushing and conduction. Instead, one should use prompt drainage.

[51]Part 1 is derived from Chap. 75, Vol. 11, *Ling Shu*; Part 2 from Chap. 22, Vol. 5, *Ling Shu*; Part 3 from Chap. 23, Vol. 5, *Ling Shu*; Part 4 from Chap. 55, *Su Wen*; Part 5 from Chap. 46, *Su Wen*; Part 6 from Chap. 21, Vol. 5, *Ling Shu*; and Part 7 from the *Zhen Jiu Ming Tang Zhi Yao*.

[52]The last sentence is a pun. At one and the same time it is both a question of how the disorder called

confusion should be treated and also a request to further resolve the questioner's confusion.

[53]Great wind refers to a wind qi which is capable of causing serious disorders like wind stroke. The commonplace statement that "Vacuity means insufficiency, while repletion means surplus" is classically interpreted as "Vacuity is insufficiency of the righteous qi, while repletion is a surplus of the evil qi." When a person is struck by the great wind, one side of the body is heavy and the other is light, and, consequently the patient loses his balance in movement or even his sense of direction. This is a disorder known as confusion, but it is not the confusion one feels when, for example, struck by a blow, puzzled by some difficult question, or affected by some temporary mental disorder. However, if treated in a proper way, it will be resolved more quickly than finding the answer to a puzzle.

As to the phrase "bumping and falling", it may be understood quite differently as "unable to look round or turn over the body when lying down."

[54]According to Zhang Jing-yue, wind counterflow is an internal counterflow of inversion qi when there is an external contraction of wind. The exterior associated channel of the hand *tai yin* is the hand *yang ming.*

[55]Grand needling is also known as channel needling, *i.e.*, the method of needling the channel on the side contralateral to the problem. One should note that some TCM scholars mistake this for a type of needle, *i.e.*, a long and thick needle. In the English language literature, this is sometimes referred to by the French term, *grand picqure.*

[56]*Fei* is a type of wind stroke. The Chinese word *fei* means loss of use or debilitation. It differs from hemilateral withering in that it produces no pain and can affect one side or both sides. *Fei* may also be understood as the later stage of hemilateral withering.

[57]If the disease is first seen in the external or lateral aspect of the body, one should needle the yang channel and then the yin channel. The depth of the needle insertion depends on the location of the evil qi, whether at the surface or deep in the interior.

[58]Great wind qi may penetrate deep in the bone to impair the yin, causing depressive heat and debilitated yin essence. Consequently, this causes heaviness of the joints, etc. This illness is called great wind and is also known as pestilential wind or leprosy. The promotion of perspiration expels depressive heat, and, when the depressive heat is drained off, hair begins to grow and recovery is effected.

[59]Origin Pass (*Guan Yuan*, CV 4) is called a triple-joining point because the foot *yang ming* and the foot *tai yin* join the conception vessel there.

[60]Wind heavyBheadedness is heavy headedness arising from exposure to wind.

[61]Portal Yin is a meeting point of the foot *tai yang* and foot *shao yang* in the head.

[62]Completion Bone is a meeting point of the foot *tai yang* and foot *shao yang.*

[63]All of these symptoms are due to evil in the foot *tai yang* channel, hence the choice of Celestial Pillar.

[64]*I.e.*, Chap. 60, *Su Wen.*

[65]Great wind here means a serious external contraction of wind.

[66]This description of the location of the point Celestial Storehouse (*Tian Fu*) is included in our source text. However, this practice is incompatible with HuangBfu Mi's norm. Therefore, the translators have inserted the square brackets, indicating that this is likely the addition of some later editor.

[67]Depressive wind brews heat. This wind heat then affects the liver, resulting in irascibility. If it affects the heart, the heart becomes vacuous, resulting in a tendency to sentimentality. If the heart qi is replete, the patient suffers from incessant laughing.

[68]It is interesting to note that different punctuation of the original Chinese text may alter the meaning of this sentence very much. For instance, this line may be read as, "For...to stretch, which involves the axilla with withering and insensitivity at one side of the body, tugging of the hands, which are smaller than normal, and hypertonicity of the sinews (of the hands)."

[69]At the end, an unknown editor supplements a note, saying, "The *Qian Jin* gives, "sorrow, sadness, and melancholy." Because this is included in a previous section, Chap. 7, Book 7, of this present work, the note is redundant.

[70]*I.e.*, Shining Sea, (*Zhao Hai*, Ki 6) and Horizontal Bone (*Heng Gu*, Ki 11)

[71]Miliaria or prickly heat is an acute skin disease resulting from inflammation of the sweat glands most often resulting from exposure to heat. It is characterized by small, red or white eruptions.

[72]Draining wind implies profuse sweating in draining wind disease.

[73]Articular wind is also known as white tiger wind or painful wind. It is a disorder mainly affecting the joints with manifestations of pain and swelling of hip joints, loss of mobility, sweating, fever, etc.

[74]Part 1 is derived from Chap. 71, Vol. 10, *Ling Shu*; Part 2 from Chap. 21, Vol. 5, *Ling Shu*; Part 3 from the *Zhen Jiu Ming Tang Zhi Yao*; and Part 4 from Chap. 2, Vol. 1, *Ling Shu*.

[75]*I.e.*, points of the foot *tai yang* channel on the back

[76]Part 1 is derived from Chap. 44, *Su Wen*; Part 2 from Chap. 26, Vol. 5, *Ling Shu*; and Part 3 from the *Zhen Jiu Ming Tang Zhi Yao*.

[77]The membranes between any tissues are referred to as sinew membranes. Zhang Jing-yue provides the following definition in his *Lei Jing*, "Membranes are like canopies. The patches of thin sinew layers between the masses of the flesh or between the viscera or bowels are all called membranes. They serve to protect and screen the blood and qi. The sites of membranes are all places where vessels are divided and blood and qi concentrate."
Atonic limpness is atony of the feet with inability to walk or walking with lame steps.

[78]The key points refer to the ankles and knees.

[79]Ringing of the lung is a syndrome characterized by cough, dyspnea, gasping, and rough breathing. Since the lung is metal, it is reasonable to describe these symptoms as ringing of the lung. Frustration, etc. affect the heart, but the heart is linked with the lung. Therefore, the lung may become depressed by emotional disturbances and trigger the aboveBmentioned problems.

[80]Too much sorrow and sadness makes the heart ligation tense, obstructing the network vessels of the pericardium. Thus the yang qi, which can be thought of as the heart qi here, is depressed and stirs. This forces the blood to run wildly downward, causing hematuria. The *Ben Bing (The Root of Disease)* is a long lost classic.

[81]The liver is said to be the gathering of sinews, and the gathering sinew is the reproductive organ. White flux, also known as white turbidity, is characterized by whitish urine in males and whitish vaginal discharge in females. Labors of the bedroom refer to sexual intercourse. However, since the Chinese *nei* for boudoir also means internal, the term also implies an exhaustion of yin essence. The *Xia Jing (Lower Classic)* is a long lost medical classic.

[82]This kind of taxation fatigue damages fluid, causing thirst. Fluid is yin. When yin fluid is diminished, the yang qi is overwhelming and inevitably attacks the yin qi in the interior. Thus heat overwhelms the true yin, *i.e.*, the kidney.

[83]The author has apparently described two different sets of atony patterns. In the first passage, he ascribes the five types of atony to heat existing in the five viscera, while in the second passage, he analyzes different geneses of atony. The current passage is a continuation of the first passage.

[84]There are two kinds of gathering sinew discussed in this passage. One is located around the joint; the other is specific, referring to the anterior yin or genitals.

It is easy to see that the foot *yang ming* channel is much concerned with the sinews because it provides supplies for the five viscera and six bowels and moistens the sinews. The penetrating vessel is also closely connected with sinews and joints because it transports nourishment to the large and small cavities between bones, *i.e.*, the ravines and valleys. However, because it starts from Qi Thoroughfare, travelling together with the foot *shao yin*, it is closely related to the foot *yang ming* as well as the foot *shao yin*. Furthermore, since all the channels meet at the gathering sinew or the external genitals and then meet again at Qi Surge (*Qi Chong*, St 30) which is a point of the foot *yang ming*, the *yang ming* is the leader of the channels. The girdling vessel encircles the body at the waist, and all the channels that travel the trunk vertically must cross it. The governing vessel links with all the yang channels, hand and foot, because all the yang channels join at its point Great Hammer (*Da Zhui*, GV 14). From all this, it is clear that the *yang ming* is concerned with the sinews and joints most of all. Therefore, to treat any kind of atony, one should needle the *yang ming*. However, different kinds of atony involve different channels. Thus one should at the same time needle the involved channel besides the *yang ming*.

Prevalent dates and months are those of the phase ruled by the involved viscus, when a disease of the viscus is most likely to heal. Disease of the lung, for example, is easy to cure in autumn or on *geng* and *xin* days.

[85]A.k.a. *Yang Fu*

[86]This whole chapter is derived from the *Zhen Jiu Ming Tang Zhi Yao*.

[87]In combination with pain, *bi* may simply denote insensitivity.

[88]Fattened means swollen.

[89]This whole chapter is derived from the *Zhen Jiu Ming Tang Zhi Yao*.

[90]The implication here is that since water spills in the skin, the qi becomes stagnant in the interstices.

Upper Arm Convergence should be needled when the stagnated qi affects the arms or the elbows.

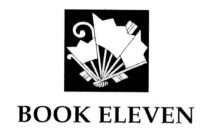

BOOK ELEVEN

Chapter One

Cold in the Chest Producing
a Regularly Interrupted Pulse[1]

For failure of an interrupted pulse to reach the *cun kou*, counterflow frigidity of the limbs, and a pulse that beats in an inhibited manner, Cloud Gate (*Yun Men*, Lu 2) is the ruling point.

For cold in the chest with resumption of the pulse following occasional long periods of interruption, heaviness above and lightness below, inability to stand steadily on one's feet, lower abdominal distention, (qi) surging up into the heart, stuffing fullness in the chest and lateral costal regions, and coughing and spitting of blood, Blazing Bone (*Ran Gu*, Ki 2) is the ruling point.[2]

Chapter Two

Yang Inversion & Great Fright
Producing Mania & Epilepsy[3]

(1)

The Yellow Emperor asked:

What is the cause of congenital madness?

Qi Bo answered:

It is contracted while in the abdomen of the mother. The mother has experienced a great fright on several occasions. Because her qi ascends without descending, her essence is subordinated to her qi, thus causing the child to develop madness.[4]

(2)

A disease of all the various yang vessels with cold or heat (in the channels) and cold or heat in the masses of flesh is called mania. One should needle until the vessels become vacuous and the masses of flesh all feel warm. By then, the disease will be relieved. The disease initially occurs once a year, but if left untreated, will occur once a month. If it is further left untreated, it will occur once every four or five days. This is known as madness. (One should) needle the places on the vessels and masses of the flesh that are especially cold with a supplementation needling (manipulation). [The *Su Wen* says, "(one should) perform regulation with the needle at the places found not to be cold on the vessels and the masses of flesh and continue it till recovery." {later editor}][5]

(3)

The Yellow Emperor asked:

In the case of a disease of manic rage, where does this disease lie?

Qi Bo answered:

It is generated within the yang.

The Yellow Emperor asked:

How can the yang cause people to suffer from mania?

Qi Bo answered:

Since it is difficult for yang qi to resolve sudden frustrations (that may arise), this may result in irascibility. This disease is called yang inversion.[6]

The Yellow Emperor asked:

How can one determine this?

Qi Bo answered:

The *yang ming* beats constantly, while the *tai yang* and *shao yang* remain still. When the still (channels) stir violently, this is the indicator.[7]

The Yellow Emperor asked:

How is this treated?

Qi Bo answered:

Reduce food intake and it will be relieved. Food enters the yin, whereas qi grows in the yang. For this reason, a reduction of food intake produces immediate relief. Administer iron dust to the patient following meals. Iron dust is capable of downbearing qi illnesses.[8]

(4)

Madness with a pulse that is forceful, large, and slippery will, over time, cure itself. However, madness with a small, hard, and urgent pulse is fatal and cannot be treated. [In a variant version it says, "a deep, small, urgent, and racing pulse is fatal and cannot be treated, while a small, firm, urgent pulse can be treated." {later editor}][9]

Madness with a vacuous pulse is curable, but is fatal if the pulse is replete. Inversion may develop into madness.[10]

Penetrating *ju* ["jaundice" in the *Su Wen* {later editor}], diseases of sudden inversion, madness, and mania are all generated by enduring counter-

flow, while disharmony of the five viscera is generated by the blockage and congestion of the six bowels.

(5)

For madness that is preceded by melancholy with a heavy and painful head, uprolled, reddened eyes, and vexation of the heart occurring both at the climax and at the end of an episode, look to the forehead. Take the hand *tai yang, yang ming,* and *tai yin.*[11] (The treatment) should continue till the blood changes to a normal (color).[12]

For madness that is characterized by arched-back rigidity at the outset of an episode and then pain in the spine, look to the foot *tai yang, yang ming, tai yin,* and the hand *tai yang* (to treat this condition. Therapy) should continue until the blood changes to a normal (color).[13]

For madness with deviated mouth, shouting and crying, dyspnea and palpitation at the onset of attack, look to the hand *yang ming* and *tai yang,* (selecting points to) attack the right side ["left side" in a variant version {later editor}] when the left side is rigid, and (points on) the left side ["right side" in a variant version {later editor}] when the right side is rigid. (Therapy) should continue till the blood changes to a normal (color).

To treat madness, (the practitioner must) take up residence with the patient to (best) locate the points that require needling. As an episode approaches, one must examine the most pertinent (vessels) and drain them immediately, allowing the blood to drain into a pot. As an episode occurs, the blood will appear to move on its own. If not, moxa with twenty cones at the end bone, *i.e.,* the tail bone.[14]

Bone madness is characterized by fullness at all the acupoints located in the partings of the flesh in the submandibular region and teeth (*i.e.,* gums), stiffness and rigidity of the bones, sweating, vexation, and oppression. If there is retching of a copious foamy substance and qi leakage below, it is incurable.[15]

Vessel madness is characterized by sudden collapse and distended and slackened vessels in all the four limbs. If the vessels are full, needle them all to let blood out. If they are not full, moxa the *tai yin* at the sides of the nape of the neck as well as the girdling vessel three *cun* anterior to the loin and the points of the various channels in the partings of the flesh. If there is retching of a copious foamy substance and qi leakage below, it is incurable.[16]

Sinew madness is characterized by curling up of the body, hypertonicity, and a large pulse. Needle Great Shuttle (*Da Zhu*, Bl 11) of the grand channel. If there is retching of a copious foamy substance and qi leakage below, it is incurable.[17]

Mania preceded by spontaneous sorrow, forgetfulness, irascibility, and susceptibility to fright is produced by worry and hunger. To treat it, first take the hand *tai yin* and *yang ming*.[18] (The therapy is continued) until the blood changes to a normal (color), and then one should take the foot *tai yin* and *yang ming*.[19]

Mania may be preceded by sleeplessness and lack of appetite and may be characterized by the delusion that one is a lofty sage, eloquent speaker, or respectable noble. One may be capable of all sorts of abusive words and be restless both day and night. To treat it, take the hand *yang ming*, *tai yang*, *tai yin*, the point below the tongue, and the (foot) *shao yin*, pricking all the exuberant vessels that can be found in them. (One should) let alone the other vessels.[20]

Mania with susceptibility to fright, constant laughing, a propensity for dancing and singing, and endless frenetic movement is produced by violent horror. To treat it, take the hand *yang ming*, *tai yang*, and *tai yin*.

Mania with confused vision and hearing and frequent shouting is a result of diminished qi. To treat it, take the hand *tai yang*, *tai yin*, and *yang ming*, and the foot *tai yin* as well as (the points) in the head and the submandibular region.[21]

Mania with large food intake, a propensity

toward claiming to witness apparitions, and a propensity toward laughter never in the presence of people is produced by overjoy. To treat it, take the foot *tai yin*, *yang ming*, and *tai yang*. Then take the hand *tai yin*, *yang ming*, and *tai yang*.

For newly developed mania without the presentations cited above, first take the pulsating vessels and the exuberant vessels by the point Spring at the Bend (*Qu Quan*, Liv 8) and bleed them. A cure is assured after about the time it takes to eat a meal. If not, treat as instructed above, and moxa the sacrum with twenty cones [the sacrum is the bend of the tail. {later editor}][22]

(6)

For madness with retching of foamy substance, Spirit Court (*Shen Ting*, GV 24), Extremity of the Mouth (*Dui Duan*, GV 27), and Sauce Receptacle (*Cheng Jiang*, CV 24) are the ruling points.

(For madness) without retching of foamy substance, Root Spirit (*Ben Shen*, GB 13), Hundred Convergences (*Bai Hui*, GV 20), Behind the Vertex (*Hou Ding*, GV 19), Jade Pillow (*Yu Zhen*, Bl 9), Celestial Surge (*Tian Chong*, GB 9), Great Shuttle (*Da Zhu*, Bl 11), Curved Bone (*Qu Gu*, CV 2), Cubit Marsh (*Chi Ze*, Lu 5), Yang Ravine (*Yang Xi*, LI 5), Outer Hill (*Wai Qiu*, GB 36), Open Valley (*Tong Gu*, Bl 66) ["five *fen* lateral to Upper Venter (*Shang Wan*, CV 13)" {later editor}], Metal Gate (*Jin Men*, Bl 63), Sinew Support (*Cheng Jin*, Bl 56), and Yang Union (*He Yang*, Bl 55) ["two *cun* under Bend Middle {*Wei Zhong*, Bl 40}" {later editor}]] are the ruling points.[23]

For madness, Upper Star (*Shang Xing*, GV 23) is the ruling point. Take first Yi Xi (*Yi Xi*, Bl 45) and finally Celestial Window (*Tian You*, TH 16) and Wind Pool (*Feng Chi*, GB 20).

For madness with retching of foamy substance, collapse on attempting to rise up, aversion to wind and cold, and swollen face with red complexion, Fontanel Meeting (*Xin Hui*, GV 22) is the ruling point.

For madness with wild running, tugging and

slackening, shaking of the head, deviated mouth, and rigidity of the neck, Unyielding Space (*Qiang Jian*, GV 18) is the ruling point.

For madness with tugging and slackening, wild running, stiffness of the neck and pain in the nape, Behind the Vertex (*Hou Ding*, GV 19) is the ruling point.

For madness, aching in the bones, dizziness, mania, tugging and slackening, clenched jaw, and sheep like bleating ["rale in the throat" in the *Qian Jin* {later editor}], Brain's Door (*Nao Hu*, GV 17) is the ruling point.[24]

For insanity (*kuang yi*) with endless talkativeness, wild running, desire for suicide, upturned eyes, and confused vision, needle Wind Mansion (*Feng Fu*, GV 16).[25]

For madness with collapse, confused vision, trance and melancholy, wild running, and tugging and slackening, Declining Connection (*Luo Que*, Bl 8) is the ruling point.

For madness with haggard emaciation, Brain Hollow (*Nao Kong*, GB 19) is the ruling point.

For madness with collapse or insanity, Completion Bone (*Wan Gu*, SI 4) and Wind Pool (*Feng Chi*, GB 20) are the ruling points.

For madness with tugging (of the limbs), Celestial Pillar (*Tian Zhu*, Bl 10) is the ruling point.

For madness with an angry desire to commit murder, Body Pillar (*Shen Zhu*, GV 12) is the ruling point ["tugging and slackening, generalized fever, wild running, ravings and claiming to see apparitions" added in the *Qian Jin* {later editor}].

For wild running in madness with rigidity of the spine and upturned eyes, Sinew Contraction (*Jin Suo*, GV 8) is the ruling point.

Madness that presents like mania with facial skin that is thickened is incurable. In the case of vacuity, the head is heavy, there is throughflux diarrhea, dribbling urinary blockage, piles, difficult

urination and defecation, the lumbar and sacrococcygeal areas feel heavy, and there is difficulty in attending upon oneself in daily life. Long Strong (*Chang Qiang*, GV 1) is the ruling point.[26]

For madness with abhorrence of wind, occasional shivering with cold, mutism, exacerbation of the condition with cold, generalized fever, wild running, desire for suicide, upturned eyes with confused vision, tugging and slackening, tearing, and deathlike coma, Lung Shu (*Fei Shu*, Bl 13) is the ruling point.

For madness, Diaphragm Shu (*Ge Shu*, Bl 17) and Liver Shu (*Gan Shu*, Bl 18) are the ruling points.

For madness with tugging (of the limbs), arched-back rigidity, upturned eyes, dizziness, wild running, insomnia and vexation of the heart, Bamboo Gathering (*Zan Zhu*, Bl 2) is the ruling point.[27]

For madness and mania with vexation and fullness, needle Silk Bamboo Hole (*Si Zhu Kong*, TH 23).[28]

For madness with tugging (of the limbs), Water Trough (*Shui Gou*, GV 26) and Gum Intersection (*Yin Jiao*, GV 28) are the ruling points.

For fright mania with tugging and slackening and dizziness and collapse, or madness with loss of voice and sheep-like bleating and foaming, Auditory Palace (*Ting Gong*, SI 19) is the ruling point.

For madness with tugging and slackening, deviated mouth, dyspnea and palpitation, Great Reception (*Da Ying*, St 5) is the ruling point, and (it is necessary to) take the *yang ming* and the *tai yin*[29] until the blood in the hands and feet changes to a normal (color).

For mania and madness with protrusion of the tongue, Supreme Unity (*Tai Yi*, St 23) and Slippery Flesh Gate (*Hua Rou Men*, St 24) are the ruling points.

For sighing, propensity toward sentimentality, heat in the lower abdomen, and desire to run about, Sun Moon (*Ri Yue*, GB 24) is the ruling point.

For insanity, Fish Border (*Yu Ji*, Lu 10), Union Valley (*He Gu*, LI 4), Wrist Bone (*Wan Gu*, SI 4), Branch to the Correct (*Zhi Zheng*, SI 7), Lesser Sea (*Xiao Hai*, Ki 6), and Kun Lun Mountain (*Kun Lun*, Bl 60) are the ruling points.

For maniac speech, Great Mound (*Da Ling*, Per 7) is the ruling point.

For the sensation that the heart is suspended as if in hunger, sentimentality, fright mania, a red facial complexion, and yellowing of the eyes, Intermediary Courier (*Jian Shi*, Per 5) is the ruling point.

For manic speech, propensity toward laughter, and claiming to see ghosts, take Yang Ravine (*Yang Xi*, LI 5) and besides, the hand and foot *yang ming* and *tai yang*.

For madness with talkativeness, ringing in the ears, deviated mouth, swollen cheeks, and, in the case of repletion, deafness, throat *bi* with inability to speak, tooth decay and ache, and runny snivel nosebleeding or, in the case of vacuity *bi* blockage, Veering Passageway (*Pian Li*, LI 6) is the ruling point.[30]

For madness with protrusion of the tongue, chattering of the jaws, manic speech, and claiming to see ghosts, Warm Dwelling (*Wen Liu*, LI 7) [located five *cun* distal to the wrist {later editor}] is the ruling point.[31]

For dim vision, hypertonicity of the wrist, generalized fever, fright mania, atonic limpness with *bi* heaviness, and tugging and slackening, Pool at the Bend (*Qu Chi*, LI 11) is the ruling point.

For madness with protrusion of the tongue, Pool at the Bend (*Qu Chi*, LI 11) is the ruling point.

For mania, Humor Gate (*Ye Men*, TH 2) is the ruling point. In addition Pinched Ravine (*Xia Xi*, GB 42), Hill Ruins (*Qiu Xu*, GB 40), and Bright Light (*Guang Ming*, GB 37) are ruling points as well.

For mania with tugging (at the limbs), headache, ringing in the ears, and eye pain, Central Islet (*Zhong Zhu*, Ki 15) is the ruling point.

For febrile disease with lack of perspiration, tugging (of the limbs), external swelling of the neck and throat, aching and heaviness of the shoulders and arms, tension and pain in the region of the ribs below the armpits, inability to lift the four limbs, scabbed scales, and inability to turn the neck, Branch Ditch (*Zhi Gou*, TH 6) is the ruling point.

For madness with protrusion of the tongue, foaming at the mouth, sheep-like bleating, and distorted neck, Celestial Well (*Tian Jing*, TH 10) is the ruling point ["which is located at the posterior side of the elbow" {later editor}].

For febrile disease with lack of perspiration, mania, tugging (at the limbs), madness, Front Valley (*Qian Gu*, SI 2) is the ruling point.

For mania with tugging (at the limbs) and frequent attack of madness, Back Ravine (*Hou Xi*, SI 3) is the ruling point.

For mania and madness, Yang Valley (*Yang Gu*, SI 5), Guest House (*Zhu Bin*, Ki 9), and Open Valley (*Tong Gu*, Bl 66) are the ruling points.

For madness and mania with large food intake, propensity to laughter but never in the presence of people, vexation of the heart, and thirst, Shang Hill (*Shang Qiu*, Sp 5) is the ruling point.

For madness with shortage of qi, retching of blood, and pain in the chest and upper back, Moving Between (*Xing Jian*, Liv 2) is the ruling point.

For atonic inversion with madness and through-flux diarrhea, Blazing Valley (*Ran Gu*, Ki 2) is the ruling point.

For mania with collapse, Warm Dwelling (*Wen Liu*, LI 7) is the ruling point.

For mania and withdrawal, Yin Valley (*Yin Gu*, Ki 10) is the ruling point.

For madness with fever and chills, yawning, vexing fullness, sorrow and tearing, Ravine Divide (*Jie Xi*, St 41) is the ruling point.

For mania with wild wandering and a propensity toward yawning, the Upper Ridge of the Great Hollow (*Ju Xu Shan Liang*, St 37) is the ruling point.

For insanity where one sees ghosts and fire, Ravine Divide (*Jie Xi*, St 41) is the ruling point.

For withdrawal and mania with tugging (of the limbs) and collapse, Extending Vessel (*Shen Mai*, Bl 62) is the ruling point. First take the yin motility vessel[32] and finally Capital Bone (*Jing Gu*, Bl 64) and the five columns in the head.[33] In the case of upturned eyes with redness and pain spreading from the inner canthi, treat the point half a *cun* below the malleolus[34] for three punctures. For problems at the left, choose the point on the right. For problems of the right, choose the point on the left.

For cold inversion madness with lockjaw, grinding of the teeth, tugging and slackening, and (for) fright mania, Yang Intersection (*Yang Jiao*, GB 35) is the ruling point.

For madness and mania with frenetic movement, and shivering with cold, Capital Bone (*Jing Gu*, Bl 64) is the ruling point.

For generalized pain, mania, a propensity toward walking, and madness, Bundle Bone (*Shu Gu*, Bl 65) is the ruling point.

For madness with collapse and cramping of the sinews, Kneeling Servant (*Pu Can*, Bl 61) is the ruling point.

For madness with blurred vision and runny snivel nosebleeding, Kun Lun Mountain (*Kun Lun*, Bl 60) is the ruling point.

For withdrawal and mania with generalized pain, Taking Flight (*Fei Yang*, Bl 58) is the ruling point.

For madness with arched-back rigidity, Bend Middle (*Wei Zhong*, Bl 40) is the ruling point.

For all cases of frequent sighing, no desire for food, much cold and heat, sweating, a propensity to retching at the start of attacks and abatement of the attack with the end of retching, take Offspring of Duke (*Gong Sun*, Sp 4) and the well point.[35]

For lancinating pain in the intestines, inversion, swollen head and face, vexation of the heart, mania, massive drinking and no desire to sleep in the case of repletion, and for inflating distention, great fullness of qi in the abdomen, burning pain, no desire for food, and choleraic disease in the case of vacuity, Offspring of Duke (*Gong Sun*, Sp 4) is the ruling point.

Chapter Three

Sagging of the Yang Vessel with the Yin Vessels Ascending in Contention Producing Cadaverous Inversion[36]

For cadaverous inversion characterized by death-like coma and a pulse that beats normally, Hidden White (*Yin Bai*, Sp 1) and Large Pile (*Da Dun*, Liv 1) are the ruling points.[37]

For trance (developing into) cadaverous inversion with (generalized) vexation and aching, Central Pole (*Zhong Ji*, CV 3) and Kneeling Servant (*Pu Can*, Bl 61) are the ruling points.

For cadaverous inversion with the appearance of real sudden death, Metal Gate (*Jin Men*, Bl 63) is the ruling point.

Chapter Four

Chaotic Qi in the Intestines & Stomach Producing Sudden Turmoil Resulting in Vomiting & Diarrhea[38]

(1)

For sudden turmoil (*huo luan*), needle (the point)

beside the associated point five (times) and needle the foot *yang ming* and (the point) above and lateral to it three (times).[39]

(2)

For retching and vomiting and vexing fullness, Po Door (*Po Hu*, Bl 37) is the ruling point.

For yang counterflow producing sudden turmoil, needle Man's Prognosis (*Ren Ying*, St 9), needling to a depth of four *fen*. This may unfortunately kill the patient.[40]

For sudden turmoil with fecal incontinence, first take Great Ravine (*Tai Xi*, Ki 3), and then take the source point of the great granary.[41]

For sudden turmoil, Great Tower Gate (*Ju Que*, CV 14), Passage Hub (*Guan Chong*, TH 1), Branch Ditch (*Zhi Gou*, TH 6), Offspring of Duke (*Gong Sun*, Sp 4), and Pinched Ravine (*Jie Xi*, St 41) are the ruling points. ["Yin Mound Spring (*Yin Ling Quan*, Sp 9)" is included in the *Qian Jin*. {later editor}]

For sudden turmoil with throughflux diarrhea, Cycle Gate (*Qi Men*, Liv 14) is the ruling point.

For counterflow inversion and sudden turmoil, Bowel Abode (*Fu She*, Sp 13) is the ruling point.

For counterflow of the stomach (qi) causing sudden turmoil, Fish Border (*Yu Ji*, Lu 10) is the ruling point.

For sudden turmoil with counterflow qi, Fish Border and Supreme White (*Tai Bai*, Sp 3) are the ruling points.

For sudden turmoil with fecal incontinence and fecal qi, Three Li (*San Li*, St 36) is the ruling point.[42]

For acute sudden turmoil, Kneeling Servant (*Pu Can*, Bl 61) is the ruling point.

For sudden turmoil causing cramping, Metal Gate (*Jin Men*, Bl 63), Kneeling Servant, Mountain Support (*Cheng Shan*, Bl 57), and Sinew Support (*Cheng Jin*, Bl 56) are the ruling points.[43]

For sudden turmoil with insensitive lower leg *bi*, Sinew Support is the ruling point. [The *Qian Jin* suggests this point for "tugging and slackening, and aching pain in the feet." {later editor}]

For cramps in the yang, rectify the yang. For cramps in the yin, rectify the yin. (These conditions require) needling without delay.[44]

Chapter Five

Vessel Disease of the Foot Tai Yin & Jue Yin Causing Duck-Stool Diarrhea & Dysentery[45]

(1)

Wind damage inflicted in spring will develop into swill diarrhea and intestinal *pi* in summer. Enduring wind develops into swill diarrhea. If swill diarrhea is accompanied by a small pulse and cold hands and feet, it is difficult to cure. However, if swill diarrhea is accompanied by a small pulse and warm hands and feet, it is easily cured.[46]

(2)

The Yellow Emperor asked:

What about intestinal *pi* with blood in the stools?[47]

Qi Bo answered:

Generalized fever foretells death, while (generalized) cold means survival.[48]

The Yellow Emperor asked:

What about intestinal *pi* with whitish, foamy stools?

Qi Bo answered:

A pulse that is deep means survival, while a superficial pulse foretells death.[49]

The Yellow Emperor asked:

What about intestinal *pi* with pus and blood in the stools?

Qi Bo answered:

A suspended and expiring (pulse) foretells death, while a slippery, large (pulse) means survival.[50]

The Yellow Emperor asked:

What about diseases whose nature is like intestinal *pi* where the pulse is not suspended or expiring?

Qi Bo answered:

A slippery, large pulse always means survival, while a suspended, choppy pulse always (means) death. The viscera decide the date of death.[51]

(3)

For swill diarrhea, apply supplementation at Three Yin Intersection (*San Yin Jiao*, Sp 6) and Yin Mound Spring (*Yin Ling Quan*, Sp 9) above it, retaining (the needle) until heat circulates through (the needled areas).

(4)

For diarrhea with blood in the stools, treat Spring at the Bend (*Qu Quan*, Liv 8) and Five Li (*Wu Li*, Liv 10).[52]

For cold in the abdomen with outpour diarrhea and intestinal *pi* with blood in the stools, Meeting of Yang (*Hui Yang*, Bl 35) is the ruling point.

For rumbling of the intestine, intestinal *pi*, and diarrhea, Lower Bone Hole (*Xia Liao*, Bl 34) is the ruling point.

For intestinal *pi* and diarrhea with lancinating pain (in the abdomen), Fourfold Fullness (*Si Man*, Ki 14) is the ruling point.

For pus and blood in the stools, cold in the center, untransformed food in the stool, and pain in the abdomen, Abdominal Lament (*Fu Ai*, Sp 16) is the ruling point.

For periumbilical pain, (qi) surging into the heart, cold in the knees, and diarrhea, Abdominal Bind (*Fu Jie*, Sp 14) is the ruling point.

For duck-stool diarrhea, conglomeration, pain in the abdomen, and visceral *bi*, Earth's Crux (*Di Ji*, Sp 8) is the ruling point.[53]

For swill diarrhea, Supreme Surge (*Tai Chong*, Liv 3) is the ruling point.

For duck-stool diarrhea with untransformed food due to immoderate accommodation to cold and heat, Yin Mound Spring (*Yin Ling Quan*, Sp 9) is the ruling point.

For intestinal *pi*, Central Cleft (*Zhong Xi*)[54] is the ruling point.

For swill diarrhea with pain in the large intestine, the Upper Ridge of the Great Hollow (*Ju Xu Shang Lian*, St 37)[55] is the ruling point.

Chapter Six

Spillage of Qi of the Five (Grains) CausingPure Heat Wasting Thirst & Jaundice[56]

(1)

The Yellow Emperor asked:

What are the indicators for those with propensity toward diseases of pure heat wasting thirst?

Qi Bo answered:

Those in whom all the five viscera are tender and weak have a propensity toward pure heat wasting thirst. Those with tender and weak (viscera) must be unyielding and obstinate, and people who are unyielding and obstinate will often become angry, thus subjecting their tender (viscera) to damage. These people have thin skins and firm and deeply sunken eyes with long, uplifted eyebrows. Because their hearts are unyielding, they often become angry, and this anger forces qi to counterflow upward. (Subsequently,) qi and blood accumulate in the chest where they counterflow and lodge ["lodge and accumulate" in the *Tai Su* {later editor}], causing the skin of the abdomen to become inflated and distended ["inflating the skins and distending the muscles" in the *Tai Su* {later editor}]. (Thus,) the blood vessels cease flowing and heat is generated. Since heat consumes the muscles, this results in pure heat wasting thirst. Thus it is said that the persons in question have unyielding and fiery tempers and have muscles that are weak.

(2)

A slightly yellow facial complexion, yellowish, grimy teeth, and yellowish nails are (indications of) jaundice. Somnolence, yellowish or dark-colored urine, and a small, choppy pulse (will be accompanied by) a lack of desire for food.

(3)

The Yellow Emperor asked:

There is a disease characterized by a sweet taste in the mouth. What is this disease called and what is its nature?

Qi Bo answered:

This is spillage of the qi of the five (grains) and is known as spleen pure heat. Once the five flavors have entered the mouth, they are stored in the stomach. The spleen transports the essential qi on behalf of (the stomach), and, if fluid lingers in the spleen, this causes a person to experience a sweet taste in the mouth. This arises out of fatty and refined food. These patients must often have had an enriched diet of sweets and fat. Fat produces internal heat in people, and sweets cause people

to suffer from fullness in the center. As a result, the qi spills upward, converting into pure heat wasting thirst. To treat it, administer Herba Eupatorii Fortunei (*Lan Cao*) which eliminates the stale qi.[57]

(4)

In terms of treatment, pure heat wasting thirst, sudden collapse, hemilateral withering, and counterflow and fullness of inversion qi are all illnesses resulting from the consumption of fatty meat and refined grains by those who are obese. Whereas blockage, obstruction, and congestion as well as (qi) flow stoppage above and below are illnesses due to violent (anger) and worries.[58]

Pure heat wasting thirst accompanied by a pulse that is replete and large is curable even if it is long-standing. However, if the pulse is suspended, expiring, small, and hard, and (the illness) is longstanding, then the (condition) is incurable.

(5)

The Yellow Emperor asked:

In the case of heat in the center and central wasting thirst one may not administer fatty meat, fine grains, fragrant (medicinal) herbs, and mineral drugs. Mineral drugs cause *ju* ["madness" in the *Su Wen* {later editor}] and fragrant medicinal herbs cause mania. Heat in the center and central wasting thirst are contracted only by the rich and noble, and the prohibition of fatty meat and fine grains is not to their liking, while the prohibition of fragrant medicinal herbs and mineral drugs itself does not cure the diseases. I would like to hear your views.[59]

Qi Bo answered:

The qi of fragrant medicinal herbs is pleasing and that of mineral medicinals is impetuous. The qi of these two materials is characterized by swiftness, violence, and ferocity. Therefore, they are not substances that relax the heart or bring harmony to the people. These two substances may not be administered (in such cases) because the heat qi is impetuous and aggressive, as is the qi of the medicinals. When these two qi come into contact with one another, there is a likelihood that the spleen will be damaged when the two kinds of qi join. The spleen is earth and, therefore, hates wood. If one administers these medicinals, (these conditions) deteriorate ["exacerbate" in the *Su Wen* {later editor}] on *jia* and *yi* days. Pure heat may develop into center wasting thirst.[60]

(6)

For jaundice [the *Qian Jin* states "abdominal heaviness with inability to move" {later editor}], needle Spinal Center (*Ji Zhong*, GV 6).[61]

For jaundice with a propensity toward yawning, fullness in the region of the free ribs, and desire to vomit ["generalized heaviness and reluctance to stir" in the *Qian Jin* {later editor}], Spleen Shu (*Pi Shu*, Bl 20) is the ruling point.

For pure heat wasting thirst with generalized fever and yellowing of the face and eyes, Reflection Abode (*Yi She*, Bl 44) is the ruling point.

For pure heat wasting thirst with (frequent) desire to drink, Sauce Receptacle (*Cheng Jiang*, CV 24) is the ruling point.

For jaundice with yellowing of the eyes, Palace of Toil (*Lao Gong*, Per 8) is the ruling point.

For somnolence, reluctance to stir the limbs, and generalized yellowing, moxa Arm Five Li (*Shou Wu Li*, LI 13). If the illness is on the left, chose the (point on) the right, and if the illness is on the right, choose the left.

For pure heat wasting thirst, Wrist Bone (*Wan Gu*, SI 4) is the ruling point.

For jaundice and heat in the center with constant thirst, Supreme Surge (*Tai Chong*, Liv 3) is the ruling point.

For generalized yellowing, intermittent slight fever, no desire for food, pain in the medial border of the knees and (in the regions) anterior to the medial malleolus, diminished qi, and generalized heaviness, Mound Center (*Zhong Feng*, Liv 4) is the ruling point.

For pure heat wasting thirst (with) frequent belching, (counterflow) qi penetrating the throat prohibiting speech, frigid hands and feet, yellowish urine, difficult defecation, swelling and pain in the throat, spitting of blood, heat in the mouth, and gluey sputum, Great Ravine (*Tai Xi*, Ki 3) is the ruling point.[62]

For pure heat wasting thirst and jaundice with cold in one foot but heat in the other, slack tongue, and vexation and fullness, Blazing Valley (*Ran Gu*, Ki 2) is the ruling point.

For insufficient yin qi (with) heat in the center, swift digestion of grains followed by (rapid) hungering, heat in the abdomen, generalized vexation, and manic speech, Three Li (*San Li*, St 36) is the ruling point.

Chapter Seven

Unwise Lifestyle Damaging the Internal & External Causing Profuse Bleeding in the Center, Static Blood, and Vomiting & Spitting of Blood[63]

(1)

The Yellow Emperor asked:

(Nowadays) people who are barely half a hundred years old become decrepit. Have people been forsaken (by the world)?

Qi Bo answered:

People today drink wine like water, view absurdities as normal routines, engage in sexual intercourse while drunk, consume their essence with lust, and disperse their true (qi) with prurience. They do not know how to hold a brimful container. They overtax their spirit as often as not simply to entertain their heart and lead an irregular life in defiance of laws ensuring a happy life. Because of all of this, they become decrepit in just half a hundred years. The sages teach that the form should not be taxed to the level of fatigue, so that the spirit and qi maintain their normalcy (*i.e.*, remain tranquil and in harmony. The sages also teach) that the eye should ward off taxation by beauty, and the heart should beware of becoming perplexed by perverse doctrines. (Following these teachings,) people, be they wise or silly, worthy or unworthy, will have nothing to fear, and hence they are in compliance with the requirements and principles for maintaining health. The reason that (people) even on the far side of a hundred years do not lose their agility is that they are completely virtuous. Therefore, nothing has endangered them.[64]

(2)

Prolonged inspection damages the eyesight. Lying down for a prolonged period of time damages the qi. Prolonged sitting damages the flesh. Prolonged standing damages the bones. Prolonged movement damages the sinews.

(3)

The Yellow Emperor asked:

There is a disease characterized by stuffy fullness in the chest and lateral costal regions affecting the appetite. Just before the onset of this illness, (the patient) will first experience a foul, fishy, and urine-like smell. He will then have clear, thin snivel, spitting of blood at the inception (of the illness), frigid limbs, visual dizziness, and frequent hemafecia and hematuria. How is this contracted?

Qi Bo answered:

This illness is called blood desiccation. It is contracted in youth, when there has been a great loss of blood, or when one has engaged in sexual intercourse while drunk. Because the qi in the center is exhausted and the liver is damaged, the menses diminish till they cease to come altogether. It is treated with Os Sepiae Seu Sepiellae (*Wu Zei Gu*) and Rubiae Cordifoliae (*Lu Ru*). They are mixed with sparrow eggs into pills the size of red beans, five pills (as a dose taken) with abalone

soup after meals. This assists (in treating) damage of the center and damage of the liver.[65]

(4)

The Yellow Emperor asked:

As for taxation wind, what is this disease like?

Qi Bo answered:

Taxation wind should lie below the lung. Once it has developed into a disease, it causes people to suffer from rigidity above, dim vision, saliva as sticky as snivel, aversion to wind, and shivering with cold. This is (so-called) taxation wind disease.[66]

The Yellow Emperor asked:

How is it treated?

Qi Bo answered:

(It is crucial to) facilitate forward and backward bending. If the *tai yang* is able to draw the essence, (relief is achieved) in three days. For an intermediate case (relief is achieved) in five days. But for a case of destitution of essence, seven days (are required). [The *Qian Jin* states, "if observation for three to five days fails to find bright essence, it can be diagnosed as such a pattern." {later editor}] Coughing and expectorating yellowish green-blue pus-like masses of mucus as big as pellets (should) be expelled through the mouth or the nose. If they (become stuck) and are not expelled, the lung is damaged, and if the lung is damaged, death ensues.[67]

(5)

For diminished qi, shivering with cold, a weakened and interrupted voice, aching of the bones, generalized heaviness, fatigue and lassitude, and inability to stir, supplement the foot *shao yin*.[68]

For shortness of breath, interrupted, shallow breathing, and gasping for breath with any movement, supplement the foot *shao yin* and remove the blood network vessels.

(6)

For cold in the tip of the penis in males with (qi) surging up into the heart giving a sensation of the heart being twisted, Convergence of Yin (*Hui Yin*, CV 1) is the ruling point.

For hypertonicity of the spine with red eyes in males, Branch Ditch (*Zhi Gou*, TH 6) is the ruling point.

For pain in the inner side of the spine, difficulty voiding urine, impotence, hypertonicity of the lower abdomen affecting the yin organ, and pain in the medial side of the feet, Yin Valley (*Yin Gu*, Ki 10) is the ruling point.

For those subject to frequent nightmares, Shang Hill (*Shang Qiu*, Sp 5) is the ruling point.

For loss of essence in males, Central Pole (*Zhong Ji*, CV 3) is the ruling point.[69]

For spillage of essence[70] with retracted testicles in males, Great Manifestation (*Da He*, Ki 12) is the ruling point.

For spillage of essence and aching of the lower legs with inability to stand for long periods of time in males, Blazing Valley (*Ran Gu*, Ki 2) is the ruling point.[71]

For insufficiency of essence in males, Supreme Surge (*Tai Chong*, Liv 3) is the ruling point.

For profuse bleeding in the center with migratory pain in the abdomen, Central Cleft (*Zhong Xi*, Liv 6) is the ruling point.

For stagnant blood in the chest with stuffy fullness in the chest and lateral costal regions, pain in the diaphragm, inability to stand for long, and atony of and cold in the knee, Three Li (*San Li*, St 36) is the ruling point.

For obstruction below the heart and retching of blood, Upper Venter (*Shang Wan*, CV 13) is the ruling point.

For retching of blood, shrugging of the shoulders to facilitate breathing, pain in the region of the free ribs, dry mouth, heart pain radiating to the upper back, and not daring to cough because the cough radiates to the kidney resulting in pain, Not Contained (*Bu Rong*, St 19) is the ruling point.

For spitting of blood, shivering with cold, and dry throat, Great Abyss (*Tai Yuan*, Lu 9) is the ruling point.

For retching of blood, Great Mound (*Da Ling*, Per 7) and Cleft Gate (*Xi Men*, Per 4) are the ruling points.

For retching of blood with qi ascension, Spirit Gate (*Shen Men*, Ht 7) is the ruling point.

For internal damage with insufficiency (of blood and qi), Three Yang Connection (*San Yang Luo*, TH 8) is the ruling point.

For internal damage with spitting of blood, insufficiency (of blood and qi), and an external lack of luster and sheen, needle Earth Fivefold Convergence (*Di Wu Hui*, GB 42). [The *Qian Jin* says "for any case with spitting of blood, drain at Fish Border (*Yu Ji*, Lu 10) and supplement at *Chi Ze* (Lu 5)." {later editor}][72]

Chapter Eight

Gathering of Evil Qi in the Lower Venter Producing Internal *Yong*[73]

(1)

The Yellow Emperor asked:

Qi may cause upper obstruction.[74] Upper obstruction is the vomiting of food immediately upon ingestion. With this I am acquainted. Worms may cause lower obstruction.[75] Lower obstruction is the vomiting of food a cycle of watches after ingestion. About this, however, I know little and would like to be instructed at length.[76]

Qi Bo answered:

In the case of inordinate joy and anger, dietary irregularities, and untimely cold and warmth, the cold juice may be retained in the intestines, and, when (cold) is retained, (any) worms (there might) become cold. When the worms become cold, they gather and accumulate, keeping to the lower venter. In keeping to the lower venter, the worms fill and dilate the stomach and intestines. (As a result,) the defensive qi fails to operate, and the evil qi (is provided a chance to) lodge. While people eat, the worms ascend for the food. When they ascend for food, the lower venter is left empty. When the lower venter is empty, the evil qi overwhelms that area. Overwhelming (the lower venter), it gathers and accumulates to lodge there. Once it becomes lodged, a *yong* develops. After *yong* has developed, the lower venter is constricted. The *yong* may be located (deep) within the venter, producing a deep-lying pain. (If this is) outside the venter, the *yong* is located externally, producing a superficial pain with heat in the skin over it.[77]

Press the *yong* gently to examine the tendency of its qi. First insert the needle shallowly by the side (of the *yong*). A while after, (insert it) a little deeper and then withdraw it for another insertion. (In a single treatment, this needling technique) should not be administered more than three times. The depth (of the insertion) is determined by the depth (of the *yong*), and each needling must be followed by ironing to induce the heat to penetrate. If heat is let in daily, the evil qi will gradually be diminished, and the *yong*, however great, will be crushed. This treatment should go together with observation of (dietary and living) prohibitions to eliminate (the evil) from the interior, and (the patient should) remain free from aspirations or anxieties, taking things easy to enable the qi to circulate (freely). Later on, when sour and bitter (medicinals) are administered, grains will be transformed and precipitated.[78]

(2)

The Yellow Emperor asked:

How can a disease of *yong* in the stomach venter be diagnosed?

Qi Bo answered:

To diagnose it, it is necessary to examine the stomach pulse. The pulse must be deep and choppy ["fine" in the *Su Wen* {later editor}]. With a deep and choppy pulse, qi must counterflow. When qi counterflows, the *ren ying* becomes extremely exuberant, and an extremely exuberant *ren ying* pulse (in turn indicates) heat. The *ren ying* is the stomach pulse. Counterflow and extreme exuberance of (the stomach qi) make heat concentrate and stagnate around the opening of the stomach. As a result, *yong* develop in the venter.[79]

(3)

Liver fullness, kidney fullness, or lung fullness are all repletion patterns that may result in (*yong*) swelling. Lung *yong* is characterized by dyspnea and fullness in the subaxillary regions. Liver *yong* is characterized by fullness in the region of the free ribs ["subaxillary regions" in the *Su Wen* {later editor}], susceptibility to fright when lying down (to sleep), and inability to void urine. Kidney *yong* is characterized by fullness from the subaxillary regions down ["from the feet up" in the *Su Wen* {later editor}] to the lateral lower abdomen, lower legs different in thickness, limpness of the hip joints and lower legs and tendency toward hemilateral withering.[80]

Chapter Nine

Cold Qi Intrudes Upon the Channels & network vessels Producing Yong & Ju; Wind Develops Producing Pestilential Wind & Infiltrating Sores (Part 1)[81]

The Yellow Emperor asked:

Once the stomach and intestines have received grain, the upper burner emanates qi to warm the partings of the flesh, nurture the bone joints, and free the interstices. The middle burner emanates qi as if spreading a mist, pouring upward into the ravines and valleys and percolating through the minute network vessels. (Under these conditions,) fluid and humor, which are in harmony and well balanced, are transformed red to produce blood. When blood is harmonious, the minute network vessels are the first to be filled. (Blood) then pours into the network vessels, and, once the network vessels are filled, it pours into the channels. Thus the yin and yang are impregnated and begin to circulate in synchrony with respiration. They circulate to the measure of the warp and weft and in accordance with the law, all in step with the (movement of) heaven, perpetually without cessation.[82]

To regulate them, palpate (the body carefully). In removing a repletion (component) from a vacuity (condition), drainage results in insufficiency and rapid (needling) reduces the qi. Therefore, (the needle) should be retained till the arrival (of the qi). In removing a vacuity (component) from a repletion (condition), supplementation results in surplus, and only when blood and qi are well regulated can the spirit qi be sustained.[83]

The Yellow Emperor asked:

I understand the balance and imbalance of blood and qi, yet I do not understand how *yong* and *ju* are engendered, when (these conditions) become critical, or the times of death or recovery. (The development of these illnesses) may be long or short and how is this determined?

Qi Bo answered:

The channels and vessels flow incessantly in synchrony with (the movement of) heaven and according to the measure of earth. When the constellations move out of synchrony, the sun and moon are eclipsed. When the great waters on earth run in an undisciplined way, water passageways will flood. (As a result,) auspicious plants fail to flourish, the five grains cannot grow, paths and roads are blocked, and people are unable to communicate with one another, becoming crowded in alleyways and townships and stranded in strange places.[84]

The case is the same with blood and qi. Please let me explain. The channels and vessels and the constructive and defensive which circulate incessantly correspond to the constellations above and the great waters in number below. When cold qi intrudes upon the channels and network vessels, the blood curdles. When blood curdles, it produces blockage. Where there is blockage, the defensive qi gathers, and is unable to flow away. Consequently, there is *yong* swelling. The cold qi may transform into heat. If the heat is overwhelming, the flesh becomes putrefied. Putrefied flesh produces pus. If the pus is not discharged, the sinews are eroded. Eroded sinews damage the bone. When the bone is damaged, the marrow is whittled away. If (the decay) is not located in the bone hollows, (the pus) cannot be discharged. Thus the sinews become dried and the bone hollowed. With drying and hollowing, the sinews and bones and muscles and flesh lose their mutual affinity, and the channels and vessels break down and leak with (the putrid qi) fuming the five viscera. When the viscera are damaged, death ensues.[85]

Chapter Nine

Cold Qi Intrudes Upon the Channels & network vessels Producing *Yong* & *Ju*; Wind Develops Producing Pestilential Wind & Infiltrating Sores (Part 2)[86]

(1)

The Yellow Emperor asked:

Disease begins with unexpected joy and anger and dietary irregularities. (Then) the yin qi becomes insufficient, there is a surplus of yang qi, and the constructive qi stops circulating. This produces *yong* and *ju*. Because the yin and yang qi cease to communicate, two kinds of heat conspire, transforming into pus. Is the small needle able to take it?[87]

Qi Bo answered:

Once the body is afflicted with *yong* and *ju* due to accumulation of putrefied blood, has not the condition strayed too far from the path already? The generation of *yong* and *ju*, and the maturity of putrefied blood are the product of a (long) accumulation of (seemingly) insignificant factors. Therefore, the sage treats them before they have taken shape, but fools (choose to) be afflicted with that which has already matured.[88]

The Yellow Emperor asked:

What will happen when (*yong* and *ju*) have taken shape and pus matures?

Qi Bo answered:

Once the pus matures, ten die and one lives.

The Yellow Emperor asked:

Can a small needle be used to treat (*yong* and *ju*) with mature pus and blood?

Qi Bo answered:

The use of a small (needle) to treat a small (*yong* or *ju*) achieves a minor effect. The use of a large (needle) to treat a big (*yong* or *ju*) achieves a major effect. The use of a small needle to treat a big (*yong* or *ju*) produces more harm (than good). Therefore, to take (*yong* and *ju*) with mature pus and blood, the only recourse is to apply a stone needle, sword needle, or sharp needle.

The Yellow Emperor asked:

If harm has been done (by inappropriate needling), can it not be mended?

Qi Bo answered:

It depends on the favorable or unfavorable (factors).

The Yellow Emperor asked:

I would like to learn what factors are favorable and what are unfavorable.

Qi Bo answered:

Suppose harm has already been done. A blackish, green-blue coloring of the whites of the eye with narrowing of the eye are the first unfavorable signs. Retching of medicine upon ingesting it is the second unfavorable sign. Abdominal pain with burning thirst is the third. Loss of flexibility of the shoulder and the nape of the neck is the fourth. And a hoarse voice with a desertion complexion is the fifth. Any (signs) other than the above five are considered favorable.[89]

(2)

When evil has penetrated the body deeply, cold and heat will contend. If allowed to persist long, they will lodge internally. If cold prevails over heat, there will be pain in the bones with desiccated flesh. (On the contrary,) if heat prevails over cold, the flesh becomes putrefied and the muscles decay, producing pus. If the bone is damaged internally, this results in bone erosion.

If there is a binding (in the sinews), the sinews contract but cannot stretch, and if (the evil) qi settles there without leaving, this results in sinew tumor.[90]

If there is binding where (the evil) qi gathers and the defensive qi is detained prohibiting its circulation, then fluid, when detained for long, will combine with (the evil qi) to engender intestinal *ju* ["sore" in a variant version {later editor}]. *Ju* due to long detention (of fluid) takes several years to develop, and feels soft when palpated.[91]

If there is binding, where (the evil) qi gathers and fluid is detained, once a (new) evil strikes, (the fluid) will congeal and grow bigger and bigger until (individual areas) coalesce to develop into an old tumor which feels hard when palpated.

If there is binding and the (evil) qi strikes deeply

into the bone, the (evil) qi will cling to the bone. This qi, coexisting with the bone, grows larger day by day to develop into bone *ju*.[92]

If there is binding and the (evil) qi strikes the flesh, the ancestral qi will gather there. If the evil lodges and will not depart, pus will be transformed if there is heat or flesh *ju* develops in the absence of heat.

While the qi (discussed above) have no fixed locations, they nevertheless have established names.

(3)

The Yellow Emperor asked:

What kind of disease is characterized by *yong* swelling with pain in the neck, fullness in the chest, and abdominal distention?

Qi Bo answered:

This disease is called counterflow inversion. Moxibustion in (this case) will produce loss of voice, while stone needling will result in mania. One must wait until the qi have combined, and only then can treatment be administered. Because the yang qi continues to ascend ["lodge in the upper" in a variant version {later editor}] with a resulting surplus above, moxibustion causes the yang qi to enter the yin, and this entry (damages the yin), causing loss of voice. Stone needling makes the yang qi vacuous, and this vacuity causes mania. One must wait until the qi have combined, and only then can treatment be administered.[93]

(4)

The Yellow Emperor asked:

The disease of *yong* in the neck can be treated with stone needling or acupuncture and moxibustion therapy and may be cured by either of them. What accounts for the (effect of) the treatments?

Qi Bo answered:

While these (*yong*) have the same name, they fall into different categories. *Yong* due to qi settling requires the use of a (metal) needle for opening and conducting to remove it. *Yong* due to exuberant qi and a gathering of blood requires the use of a stone needle to drain it. This is said to be treatment of the same disease with different methods.

(5)

The Yellow Emperor asked:

What gives rise to the various kinds of *yong*, hypertonicity of the sinews, and pain in the bone?

Qi Bo answered:

These are all swellings due to cold qi and are transmuted by the eight winds.

The Yellow Emperor asked:

How are they treated?

Qi Bo answered:

Since they are seasonal diseases, they may be treated through the points in accordance with the restraining interrelationships (of the five phases).[94]

(6)

For sudden *yong* with limp sinews and pain travelling along a specific channel, incessant *po* sweating,[95] and insufficient qi in the urinary bladder, treat the points of the (concerned) channel.

For axillary *yong* with intense heat, needle the foot *shao yang*[96] five times. If one needles and the heat does not cease, then needle the hand heart-governor channel,[97] the connecting vessel of the hand *tai yin* channel,[98] and the meeting point of the big bone[99] three times.

(7)

One must not let *yong* or *ju* turn inward for a moment. If one cannot locate the *yong* and nothing can be determined by palpation, and (the pain) is sometimes present and sometimes absent, then one must needle the points lateral to the hand *tai yin*[100] three times and the points by the vessel of the throat knot[101] twice.

To treat *yong* swelling one must needle directly into the *yong*, needling in a manner appropriate to its size and depth. For a large *yong*, one must use many (needles and insert them) deeply. In thrusting the needle, one must hold (the needle) upright and only once one has reached an appropriate depth may one stop. [The last two sentences in the *Su Wen* read "A large (*yong*) requires a great deal of bleeding while a small (*yong*) requires deep insertion. In thrusting the needle, one must hold (the needle) upright and only once one has reached an appropriate depth may one stop." {later editor}]

(8)

For swelling in the neck accompanied by an inability to bend it either forward or backward and swelling in the cheek affecting the ear, Completion Bone (*Wan Gu*, GB 12) is the ruling point.

For swollen throat with difficulty in speaking, Celestial Pillar (*Tian Zhu*, Bl 10) is the ruling point.

For swelling in the suborbital region and *yong* in the lip, Cheek Bone Hole (*Quan Liao*, SI 18) is the ruling point.

For swelling and pain in the cheek, Celestial Window (*Tian Chuang*, SI 18) is the ruling point.

For *yong* swelling in the neck with inability to speak, Celestial Countenence (*Tian Rong*, SI 17) is the ruling point.

For generalized swelling, Pass Gate (*Guan Men*, St 22) is the ruling point.

For fullness and pain in the region below the chest and swelling in the breast, Breast Root (*Ru Gen*, St 18) is the ruling point.

For saber swelling and fistula, Armpit Abyss (*Yuan Ye*, GB 22), Camphorwood Gate (*Zhang Men*, Liv 13), and Branch Ditch (*Zhi Gou*, TH 6) are the ruling points.

For swollen face and *yong* swelling of the eye, needle Sunken Valley (*Xian Gu*, St 43) and cure is effected as soon as blood is let out.

For swelling in the calf's nose, needle directly on (the swelling). However, if (the swelling) is hard, do not attack it (by needling) for attacking may cause death.

For *yong* and *ju*, Portal Yin (*Qiao Yin*, GB 44) is the ruling point.

(9)

For pestilential wind, one must needle the swollen place. After needling, suck at the place and then press out the malignant blood. Stop once the swelling is alleviated. (The patient) should eat only common foods and never consume anything unusual.

Wind in the vessels may develop into pestilential wind.

(10)

For pestilential wind due to tubular *ju*,[102] Portal Yin (*Qiao Yin*, GB 44) is the ruling point.

For an enlarged head with infiltrating sores, Intermediary Courier (*Jian Shi*, Per 5) is the ruling point.

For tubular *ju*, Shang Hill (*Shang Qui*, Sp 5) is the ruling point.

For stagnant scratching[103] and desire to vomit, Great Mound (*Da Ling*, Per 7) is the ruling point.

For itchy scabs, Yang Ravine (*Yang Xi*, LI 5) is the ruling point.

(11)

The Yellow Emperor asked:

I would like to learn in detail about the manifestations of *yong* and *ju* and the days on which they may cause death.

Qi Bo answered:

Yong arising in the throat is called fiendish *ju*. If it is not treated promptly, it will produce pus. If not discharged, the pus will choke the throat and cause death in half a day. Once the pus is transformed and drained, the patient should be made to hold hog's lard in his mouth and be advised not to take cold food. (Treated in this way,) he will recover in three days.

(*Yong*) arising in the neck is called fatal *ju* and is large and reddish-black. If it is not treated immediately, the heat qi will spread to the Armpit Abyss (*Yuan Ye*, GB 22), damaging the conception vessel in the front and steaming the liver and the lung in the interior. If it does steam (these areas), death occurs in a little more than ten days.

A major development of yang qi[104] results in dispersion of the brain and a spreading (of *yong*) in the nape. (This is) known as brain smelting (*nao shuo*, 脑烁). It is characterized by an unhealthy complexion and pricking pain in the nape. If there is vexation of the heart, the case is fatal and cannot be cured.

(*Yong*) developing in the shoulder and the upper arm is called blemished *ju* and looks blackish-red. Prompt treatment must be performed to induce (generalized) sweating extending down to the feet so that no harm will come to the five viscera. If the *yong* is four to five days old, one must employ counterflow ignition.[105]

(*Yong*) developing under the armpit which is red and hard is called cinnabar *ju*. It should be treated with a stone needle which should be thin and long. The pricking should be performed on as few points as possible. Hog's lard should be applied to the places that are pricked. In six days

there will be a cure. Do not bandage (the punctures). *Yong* which is hard and does not open is (called) saber (lump) or pearl-string lump and requires prompt treatment.

(*Yong*) developing in the bosom is called well *ju*. It is shaped like the soybean and matures in three to four days. If not treated early, it will descend and enter the abdomen. If left untreated, it will cause death in seven days.

(*Yong*) developing in the breast is called sweet *ju*. It is green-blue, shaped like a Fructus Broussentiae Papyriferae or Fructus Trichosanthes Kirilowii. (The patient) is usually tormented by fever and chills. It requires prompt treatment to clear the cold and heat. If it is not treated promptly, death occurs in ten years. Death occurs once (the *yong*) suppurates.

(*Yong*) developing in the lateral costal region is called decaying blemish. It is said to be a disorder occuring in females. In a long-standing case it can be very large with suppurative *yong* (abscesses) from which fleshy enlargements grow as large as red beans. Treatment consists of one *sheng* each of the root of Fructus Forsythiae and Radix Pinii Japonicae boiled with one *dou* and six *sheng* of water (and cooked) down to three *sheng*. After drinking the solution while still hot, the patient is made to sit over a basin of hot water with thick clothes on to induce perspiration (all over the body) down to the feet.

(*Yong*) developing in the thigh and shin is called thigh and shin desertion *ju*. The complexion has not significantly changed, but the abscess infiltrates as deep as the bone. It requires prompt treatment. If it is not treated promptly, death occurs in thirty days.

(*Yong*) developing in the sacrococcygeal region is called sharp *ju*. It is extensive, red, and hard and requires prompt treatment. If it is not treated, death occurs in thirty days.

(*Yong*) developing in the yin (*i.e.*, medial) aspect of the thigh is called red slackness. If it is not treated, death occurs in sixty days. If it occurs in the inner sides of both thighs and remains untreated, death occurs in ten days.

(*Yong*) developing in the knee is called blemished *ju*. There is a major abcess but the (overlying skin) complexion remains unchanged. If there is cold and heat and (the *yong*) is hard, do not (needle with) stone or this will cause death. Once the *yong* has turned an abnormal color and softened, stone (needling) will provide a cure.

Any *yong* that occur in the joints which correspond to one another cannot be cured.[106]

(*Yong*) arising in the yang[107] causes death in one hundred days, while (*yong*) arising in the yin causes death in forty days.

(*Yong*) developing in the lower leg is called rabbit biting. It is shaped like a red bean and penetrates to the bone. It requires prompt treatment. If not treated promptly, it is fatal.

(*Yong*) developing in the medial malleolus is called walking restriction. The complexion of the (skin overlying) the abcess is unchanged. If one uses a stone needle at many points (around the *yong*) and can check the cold and heat, the (the patient) will not die.

(*Yong*) developing in the upper and lower part of the foot is called quadruple excessiveness and manifests as a major abscess. If it is not treated promptly, death occurs in one hundred days.

(*Yong*) developing in the lateral aspect of the foot is called pestilential *yong*. It is not large in size and starts from the small toe. It requires prompt treatment to remove the blackened (tissue). If it continues to grow despite treatment, the condition is incurable, and death occurs in one hundred days.

(*Yong*) developing in the toe is called desertion *ju*. If it is blackish-red, it is fatal and incurable, but if it is not blackish-red, it is not fatal. If treatment is ineffective, promptly cut off (the entire toe). If one does not cut off (the toe), then the patient will die.

The Yellow Emperor asked:

What is *yong*?

Qi Bo answered:

When the constructive qi accumulates and lodges in the channels and the network vessels, the blood congeals and fails to circulate. This lack of circulation arrests the defensive qi, producing a lack of flow. In creating a blockage and, failing to circulate, it generates heat. As this great heat increases and is not arrested, this heat prevails, decaying the flesh. Decayed flesh produces pus. However, it does not penetrate as deeply as the bone marrow. Therefore, the marrow does not become parched or dried and the five viscera are not damaged. (The condition) is therefore called *yong*.[108]

The Yellow Emperor asked:

What is *ju*?

Qi Bo answered:

When heat qi becomes extremely effulgent it penetrates through the muscles, skin, sinews, marrow, bones, and flesh into the five viscera in the interior. It exhausts the blood and qi such that no healthy sinew, bone, or flesh is left beneath the abcess. Therefore, the disorder is called *ju*.[109] *Ju* is characterized by its hardness and the lusterless complexion of the skin in the affected area which is like the hide of an ox's neck. On the other hand, *yong* is characterized by the skin (in the affected area) being thin and shiny. These are reflections (which differentiate *yong* and *ju*).

The Yellow Emperor asked:

What causes the death when one has *ju*?

Qi Bo answered:

There are five (critical) parts in the body. The crouching rabbit is the first, the calf is the second, the upper back is the third, the transport points of the five viscera are the fourth, and the nape of the neck is the fifth. If any of these points contract *ju*, then death results.

(12)

The Yellow Emperor asked:

How does bodily form correspond to the nine districts?[110]

Qi Bo answered:

Please let me tell you about the correspondence of the body form to the nine districts. The left foot corresponds to the Beginning of Spring and its corresonding days are *wu yin* and *ji chou*.[111] The left side of the chest ["left lateral costal region" in a variant version {later editor}] corresponds to the Spring Equinox and its corresponding day is *yi mou*. The left hand corresponds to the Beginning of Summer and its corresponding days are *wu chen* and *ji si*. The breast, throat, and head correspond to the Summer Solstice and their corresponding day is *bing wu*. The right hand corresponds to the Beginning of Autumn and its corresponding days are *wu shen* and *si wei*. The right side of the chest ["right lateral costal region" in a variant version {later editor}] corresponds to the Autumn Equinox and its corresponding day is *xin you*. The right foot corresponds to the Beginning of Winter and its corresponding days are *wu xu* and *si hai*. The lumbar region, sacrum, coccyx, and lower portals[12] correspond to the Solstice of Winter and its corresponding day is *ren zi*. The six bowels and the three viscera below the diaphragm correspond to the central district and their corresponding days are the forbidden days.[113] They are the moving days of *tai yi*[114] as well as all the *wu* and *ji* days.

Equipped with an understanding of these nine districts, one will become skilled at locating the eight corresponding parts of the body once they are affected by *yong* swelling be it located on the left or right or the upper or lower (aspects of the body). If one desires to treat *yong* swelling, one should not try to cure it on the corresponding days, which are called heaven forbidden days.

The midnight watch (11 p.m. to 1 a.m.) of the five *zi* days,

The cock-crow watch (1 to 3 a.m.) of the five *chou* days; The calm-dawn watch (3 to 5 a.m.) of the five *yin* days; The sun-rise watch (5 to 7 a.m.) of the five *mao* days; The breakfast watch (7 to 9 a.m.) of the five *chen* days; The outlying region watch (9 to 11 a.m.) of the five *si* days; The mid-day watch (11 a.m. to 1 p.m.) of the five *wu* days; The sun's descent watch (1 to 3 p.m.) of the five *wei* days; The late afternoon watch (3 to 5 p.m.) of the five *shen* days; The sundown watch (5 to 7 p.m.) of the five *you* days; The dusk watch (7 to 9 p.m.) of the five *xu* days; The serenity watch (9 to 11 p.m.) of the five *hai* days.

Yong swelling erupting on these days cannot be cured.

Endnotes

[1]This entire chapter is derived from the *Zhen Jiu Ming Tang Zhi Yao* (*Acupuncture & Moxibustion Treatment Essentials of the Enlightening Hall*).

[2]Heaviness above refers to a sense of heaviness in the head, and lightness below means a sense of lightness in the legs.

[3]Part 1 is derived from Chap. 47, *Su Wen* (*Basic Questions*); Part 2 from Chap. 55, *Su Wen*; Part 3 from Chap. 46, *Su Wen*; Part 4 from Chap. 28, *Su Wen*; Part 5 from Chap. 22, Vol.5, *Ling Shu* (*Spiritual Pivot*); and Part 6 from the *Zhen Jiu Ming Tang Zhi Yao*.

[4]Zhang Jing-yue explains in his *Lei Jing* (*A The Classified Classic*), "Fright plunges qi into chaos and counterflow, and, as a result, qi ascends without descending. When qi becomes chaotic, essence follows suit. Consequently, essence and qi together affect the fetus, causing madness in the child." Based on another understanding, we might as well put the part "her essence . . . her qi" as follows, "her (chaotic) essence and qi dwell together (in the uterus)." We have reluctantly rendered *dian ji* as madness to maintain a uniform translation of this term. However, this Chinese term may, in fact, also mean epilepsy and, more often, madness *and* epilepsy. The reader should keep both possibilities in mind when reading this chapter.

[5]Zhang Jing-yue explains in his *Lei Jing*, "When yang overwhelms, this causes mania. In all cases of disease in the yang phase with cold or heat in the channels and masses of flesh, the yang evil upsets the blood and qi, and, when heat goes to the extreme, cold is generated." He continues,

"Needling until the vessels become vacuous means draining and transforming the exuberant into the vacuous. When the various masses of flesh being needled are found to have become hot, the qi is shown to have arrived and the evil to have retreated. By now the disease is already relieved and (the needling) can be stopped."

[6]It is clear that yang inversion in this context is simply madness. A note by Wang Bing to the *Su Wen* explains, "This (passage) discusses frustration and depression of yang qi. The patient is constantly angry because the sudden frustration (of yang qi) also results in the impeded flow of heart (qi). In such cases, all the problems are caused by the counterflow and extreme agitation of the yang (qi). For that reason, this disease is called yang inversion."

The first sentence may also be rendered in the following manner: "It is difficult for the yang qi to flow freely when it is frustrated,..."

[7]Ma Shi explains in his *Su Wen Zhu Zheng Fa Wei (An Annotated Exposition on the Intricacies of the Basic Questions)*, "...at all the points (including) Surging Yang (*Chong Yang*, St 42), Earth Granary (*Di Cang*, St 4), Great Reception (*Da Ying*, St 5), Lower Pass (*Xia Guan*, St 7), Man's Prognosis (*Ren Ying*, St 9), Surging Qi (*Qi Chong*, St 30), etc., there are pulsating vessels, and Surging Qi pulsates in a particularly conspicuous manner. On the contrary, the foot *tai yang* urinary bladder channel and foot *shao yang* gallbladder channel remain still. Although (there are pulsating vessels around) Celestial Window (*Tian Chuan*, SI 16), Bend Middle (*Wei Zhong*, Bl 40), and Kun Lun Mountain (*Kun Lun*, Bl 60) of the urinary bladder channel, and Celestial Countenance (*Tian Rong*, SI 17), Suspended Bell (*Xuan Zhong*, GB 39), and Auditory Convergence (*Ting Hui*, GB 2) of the gallbladder channel, they beat less (strongly) than those along the stomach channel."

[8]Zhang Jing-yue explains in his *Lei Jing*, "After the five flavors have entered through the mouth, they are transformed in the spleen. (This is what is meant by) food entering the yin. They are stored in the stomach to nourish the qi of the five viscera. (This is what is meant by) growing qi in the yang. Less food intake results in diminished qi. Therefore, when food intake is reduced or one abstains completely, the fire in the stomach cannot assist the yang evil. Thus yang inversion with rage and mania is relieved."

[9]Madness is a yang disease, while a small pulse is a yin pulse. This incompatibility between the pattern and the pulse quality indicates that the condition is fatal.

[10]Zhang Jing-yue explains in his *Lei Jing*, "A vacuous (pulse) is soft and slow. It indicates that the evil qi is slight and, therefore, the patient will survive. A replete (pulse) is wiry and urgent, indicating that the evil qi is exuberant and, therefore, the condition is fatal." A close study reveals a contradiction in the statements of this and the last paragraphs, and there is reason to suspect that there may be some corruption in the text.

Inversion may present as an incessant ascending counterflow of qi. It then causes repletion above and vacuity below, resulting in sudden spinning collapse. Such a condition is more a case of epilepsy than madness.

[11]The points involved are Branch to the Correct (*Zhi Zheng*, SI 7), Lesser Sea (*Xiao Hai*, SI 8), Veering Passageway (*Pian Li*, LI 6), Warm Dwelling (*Wen Liu*, LI 7), Great Abyss (*Tai Yuan*, Lu 9), and Broken Sequence (*Lie Que*, Lu 7). Note that bleeding therapy is implied.

[12]Looking to the forehead implies observing a redness in the region above the eyes and inquiring about heaviness and pain in the forehead. Clearly the points are to be bled.

[13]Although the characters and sentence structure in this passage are the same as the above, here *hou zhi* implies that one should "look to" the channels in question for treatment rather than as a means of diagnosing the condition.

This paragraph does not appear in our source edition and has been included in accordance with its appearance in the *Su Wen, Tai Su (Essentials)*, and *Qian Jin (Thousand Gold)*.

[14]The end bone is Long Strong (*Chang Qiang*, GV 1). Moxibustion at this point facilitates the drainage of blood when administering this therapy.

[15]Bone madness is a species of epilepsy in which the evil qi lies deeply in the bones and is characterized by symptoms involving the bones. This is an illness of the kidney. Terms like vessel madness below may be understood in a similar way.

[16]The points on the nape are Celestial Pillar (*Tian Zhu*, Bl 10) and Great Shuttle (*Da Shu*, Bl 11). The girdling vessel refers specifically to Girdling Vessel (*Dai Mai*, GB 26). Only the points of the various channels where the vessels are distended and slack are recommended for needling.

[17]The grand channel is the foot *tai yang* because it is the longest channel.

[18]*I.e.*, Great Abyss (*Tai Yuan*, Lu 9), Broken Sequence

(*Lie Que*, Lu 7), Veering Passageway (*Pian Li*, LI 6), and Warm Dwelling (*Wen Liu*, LI 7)

[19]*I.e.*, Hidden White (*Yin Bai*, Sp 1), Yellow Emperor (*Gong Sun*, Sp 4), Leg Three Li (*Zu San Li*, St 36), and Pinched Ravine (*Jie Xi*, St 41)

A note in the *Tai Su* states, "Madness in people is first ascribed to severe depression and binding which remains unresolved and persists in the heart, and then is ascribed to hunger vacuity. They result in an inability of the spirit and orientation to maintain their abode."

[20]The meaning of the phrase, "the point below the tongue and the *shao yin*" is ambiguous. It is possible that Ridge Spring (*Lian Quan*, CV 23), Spirit Gate (*Shen Men*, Ht 7), and Lesser Surge (*Shao Chong*, Ht 9) are suggested. However, it is also possible that only the point on the foot *shao yin* below the tongue is suggested.

[21]Confused vision and hearing imply visual and auditory distortions and hallucinations.

[22]Spring at the Bend (*Qu Quan*, Liv 8) is located at the medial border of the popliteal fossa where there is no pulsating vessel. Exuberant vessels refer to petechiae and varicosities.

[23]Root Spirit (*Ben Shen*, GB 13), Celestial Surge (*Tian Chong*, GB 9), and Outer Hill (*Wai Qiu*, GB 36) resolve depression. Hundred Convergences (*Bai Hui*, GV 20), and Behind the Vertex (*Hou Ding*, GV 19) clear the brain. Jade Pillow (*Yu Zhen*, Bl 9), Great Shuttle (*Da Zhu*, Bl 11), Metal Gate (*Jin Men*, Bl 63), Sinew Support (*Cheng Jin*, Bl 56), and Yang Union (*He Yang*, Bl 55) promote free flow of yang and soften the sinew. Cubit Marsh (*Chi Ze*, Lu 5) and Yang Ravine (*Yang Xi*, LI 5) regulate the lungs. While Open Valley (*Tong Gu*, Bl 66) and Curved Bone (*Qu Gu*, CV 2) downbear surging qi in the penetrating and conception vessels.

The first pair of square brackets are inserted by the translators. In our source edition, this passage is erroneously placed before Open Valley (*Tong Gu*, Bl 66).

[24]Brain's Door (*Nao Hu*, GV 17) is a meeting point of the governing vessel and the foot *tai yang*.

[25]Wind Mansion (*Feng Fu*, GV 16) is a meeting point of the governing and yang linking vessels.

[26]Long Strong (*Chang Qiang*, GV 1) is the connecting point of the governing vessel.

[27]This passage has been deleted from our source edition. It is included here in accordance with the *Wai Tai* and *Qian Jin*.

[28]This passage has been deleted from our source edition. It is included here in accordance with the *Qian Jin* and *Wai Tai*.

[29]The hand and foot channels are both included. The points Leg Three Li (*Zu San Li*, St 36), Pinched Ravine (*Jie Xi*, St 41), Veering Passageway (*Pian Li*, LI 6), Warm Passageway (*Wen Liu*, LI 7), Hidden White (*Yin Bai*, Sp 1), Offspring of Duke (*Gong Sun*, Sp 4), Great Abyss (*Tai Yuan*, Lu 9), and Broken Sequence (*Lie Que*, Lu 7) are recommended.

[30]*Bi* blockage is blockage caused by cold qi. The last part of the sentence is distorted by some unknown editor(s) as "...in the case of vacuity, *bi*, Diaphragm Shu (*Ge Shu*, Bl 17) and Veering Passageway (*Pian Li*, LI 6) are the ruling points."

[31]These square brackets do not appear in our source text. They have been inserted by the translators since such a location in these lists of points is uncharacteristic of Huang-fu Mi and thus are, in all likelihood, a later interpolation.

[32]*I.e.*, Shining Sea (*Zhao Hai*, Ki 6)

[33]*I.e.*, the three channels on the head.

[34]*I.e.*, Extending Vessel (*Shen Mai*, Bl 62)

[35] *I.e.*, Hidden White (*Tai Bai*, Sp 1)

[36]This entire chapter is derived from the *Zhen Jiu Ming Tang Zhi Yao*. Note that the qi in the yang channels is referred to as the yang vessel, while the qi in the yin channels is referred to as the yin vessel.

[37]The pulse beats normally because the qi of the yang vessels suddenly collapses as the qi of the yin vessels simultaneously counterflows upward. They essentially switch places. The selection of the well points of both the foot *tai yin* and *jue yin* channels serves to normalize the qi of both the yin and yang channels.

[38]Part 1 is derived from Chap. 28, *Su Wen*; Part 2 from the *Zhen Jiu Ming Tang Zhi Yao*; and Part 3 from Chap. 19, Vol. 4, *Ling Shu*.

[39]The reader should first note that the translators have inserted the word "(times)" merely to facilitate the readability of the passage. However, the numbers five and three may well refer to something other than the number of times the respective points are to be needled.

Zhang Jing-yue explains in his *Lei Jing*, "When evil exists in the middle burner, this causes vomiting and diarrhea, the visceral qi come and go (in disarray), and there is deranged spirit and orientation. Therefore, this is called sudden turmoil." In the *"Wu Luan Pian* (On Five Types of Chaos)", Chap. 34, Vol. 6, of the *Ling Shu*, sudden turmoil is described as "the clear qi in the yin, the turbid qi in the yang, the constructive qi following the vessels, the defensive qi flowing counter to the vessels, mutual interference of the clear and the turbid." This condition is defined as "chaotic (qi) in the stomach and intestines."

The associated point referred to is probably Kidney Shu (*Shen Shu*, Bl 23), and, if this assumption is correct, the point beside it would be Will Chamber (*Zhi Shi*, Bl 52). The author may, therefore, be instructing that Will Chamber is to be needled five times. Another interpretation is that one must needle five points beside Kidney Shu.

The phrase beginning with "the foot *yang ming*" may be interpreted in several different ways, and hence there are as many different translations. As to the three points in question, one commentary to the *Su Wen* interprets this passage as indicating three separate points Stomach Shu (*Wei Shu*, Bl 21) relating to the foot *yang ming*, and Kidney Shu (*Shen Shu*, Bl 23) and Stomach Granary (*Wei Cang*, Bl 50). Ma Shi contends that the points Stomach Granary and Reflection Abode (*Yi She*, Bl 49) and *Yi She* (Bl 49) are each to be punctured thrice. Zhang JieBbin, on the other hand, asserts that the points Stomach Shu (*Wei Shu*, Bl 21) and Reflexion Abode are each to be punctured thrice. Finally Zhang Zhi-cong holds the position that the number three indicates that the associated point of the *yang ming* Stomach Shu (*Wei Shu*, Bl 21) is to be needled to three different depths. He explains, "The number three implies that it is necessary first to needle shallowly through the skin to drive out the yang evil, then a little deeper to drive out the yin evil, and finally extremely deep into the border of the flesh to reach the grain qi."

[40]If one mistakenly punctures the artery in needling this point, the result is fatal.

[41]*I.e.*, Surging Yang (*Chong Yang*, St 42)

[42]Fecal qi means flatulence.

[43]This condition refers to muscle cramping due to dehydration in choleraBlike diseases.

[44]The yang here means the lateral aspect of the limbs, while the yin means their medial aspect.

[45]Part 1 is derived from Chap. 74, Vol. 11, *Ling Shu*; Part 2 from Chap. 28, *Su Wen*; Part 3 from Chap. 19, Vol. 4, *Ling Shu*; and Part 4 from the *Zhen Jiu Ming Tang Zhi Yao*.

[46]This is a case of a deep-lying evil manifesting at some time later than when it was originally contracted. Wind damage inflicted in the spring and enduring wind refer to wind evil injuring the liver. If allowed to persist through the following summer, this liver evil will be transferred to the spleen and stomach, impairing the transformation and transportation of grains. This results in swill diarrhea or dysentery. The presence of warm hands and feet indicates that the spleen qi remains essentially intact, thus the condition is easily cured.

[47]Intestinal *pi* is stagnation in the intestines characterized by frequent but difficult evacuation of the stools. Intestinal *pi* with blood in the stools is also known as red dysentery. That with whitish foamy substance is known as white dysentery. And that with pus and blood in the stools, is known as red and white dysentery.

[48]The presence of generalized fever indicates that the yang has overwhelmed the yin. This is a fatal condition. Generalized cold, on the other hand, indicates that the constructive qi has not been damaged, and, therefore, the patient will live. Care must be taken to discriminate between a generalized experience of cold and heat in the body from a more localized sensation of heat or cold in the hands and feet.

[49]Cold diarrhea with a deep pulse means that the pulse remains rooted, indicating that the patient will survive. While a floating pulse is not rooted and indicates a fatal vacuity of qi and blood.

[50]A suspended and expiring pulse is a pulse that is superficial, faint, and sometimes impalpable. It indicates the departure of the righteous qi or absence of the stomach qi. In any case, this is a fatal sign. A slippery and large pulse, on the other hand, reflects the presence of stomach qi.

[51]From the point of view of five phase theory, death usually comes on the day of the restrained phase of the involved viscus. *Jia* (S1) and *yi* (S2) days are ascribed to wood which restrains earth. If intestinal *pi* involves the spleen which is earth, death may come on *jia* and *yi* days.

[52]In the *Wai Tai Mi Yao* (Secret [Medical] Essentials of a Provincial Governor) and *Yi Xin Fang* (The Heart of Medicine Formulary), "five viscera" is substituted for "*Wu Li*" and is placed at the beginning of the next passage.

[53]Visceral *bi* is blockage or obstruction within the viscera.

[54]This is usually called Central River (*Zhong Du*, Liv 6).

[55]This is usually called Upper Great Hollow (*Shang Ju Xu*, St 37).

[56]Part 1 is derived from Chap. 46, Vol. 7, *Ling Shu*; Part 2 from Chap. 74, Vol. 11, *Ling Shu*; Part 3 from Chap. 47, *Su Wen*; Part 4 from Chap. 28, *Su Wen*; Part 5 a combination of Chap. 40 and 17, *Su Wen*; and Part 6 from the *Zhen Jiu Ming Tang Zhi Yao*.

[57]This is the initial stage of pure heat wasting thirst and is due to dampness and heat depressing the spleen. Herba Eupatorii Fortunei (*Lan Cao*) is pungent and aromatic and diffuses the spleen in eliminating dampness and heat. Its clinical use for pure heat wasting thirst is based upon this classical reference.

[58]Sudden collapse often refers to sudden wind stroke, while counterflow and fullness often suggest distressed rapid dyspneic breathing.

[59]Heat in the center is characterized by frequent drinking and frequent voiding of urine, while center wasting thirst is characterized by large food intake and frequent voiding of urine.

[60]Pleasing may be understood as synonymous with penetrating. Heat in the center, etc. is caused by heat qi which is impetuous and aggressive. If it joins forces with the qi of the same nature inherent in the drugs, this yang qi will overwhelm yin, and the consummate yin is the spleen. *Jia* (S1) and *yi* (S2) are wood which boosts fire and heat and restrain spleen earth. Therefore, these days promote the advancement of this disease.

[61]In actuality, the *Qian Jin* reads, "abdominal fullness with inability to ingest food."

[62]Our source edition reads "dyspnea" in place of "belching." This correction made in accordance with the *Wai Tai* and the *Yi Xin Fang*.

[63]Part 1 is derived from Chap. 1, *Su Wen*; Part 2 from Chap. 23, *Su Wen*; Part 3 from Chap. 40, *Su Wen*; Part 4 from Chap. 33, *Su Wen*; Part 5 from Chap. 22, Vol. 5, *Su Wen*; and Part 6 from the *Zhen Jiu Ming Tang Zhi Yao*.

[64]For the maintenance of health, in addition to the avoidance of overwork, Chinese medicine lays heavy emphasis on abstention from personal desires, especially licentiousness. One is commonly admonished to care for one's physique as mindfully as one would hold a cup filled to the rim with wine. Zhang Jing-yue explains in his *Lei Jing*, "One should not yield oneself up to lust. Overindulgence leads to exhaustion of the essence. ..Exhaustion of the essence leads to dispersion of the true qi. The essence generates qi, while the qi in turn generates the spirit... One must value the essence. When the essence is plentiful, the qi becomes exuberant. When qi is exuberant, the spirit is sound. When the spirit is sound, the physique is strong. And when the physique is strong, there is less disease. Strong spirit and qi and (therefore) remaining vigorous at an advanced age are both rooted in essence." One should note that essence in this context is often understood specifically as semen.

[65]The liver stores blood. Therefore, great loss of blood brings damage to the liver. The consumption of wine makes the blood vessels exuberant, thus generating internal heat. If one engages in sexual intercourse while drunk, the bone marrow and the fluid and humor will all be discharged, thus exhausting the kidney qi. This results in diminished essence manifesting as an insufficiency of semen in males and diminished or even cessation of menstrual flow in females.

The lung governs qi, and its smell is fishy, while the liver governs blood, and its smell is of urine. The lung qi, which is metal, fails to restrain the liver, which is wood. Both the lung qi and liver qi counterflow upward, emitting a smell of fish and urine. Running of clear snivel and vomiting of blood are also disorders involving the lung and liver.

The formula prescribed is effective not only for amenorrhea or diminished menstrual flow in females, but for lack of semen and blood or impotence in males.

Our source edition reads "in the intestines" in place of "damage of the center." This correction is made in accordance with the *Su Wen*.

[66]Taxation wind is also known as taxation of the center. It implies taxation of the kidney plus wind stroke or rather intrusion of wind. According to a note by Wang Bing in the *Su Wen*, the first sentence in Qi Bo's reply means, "The kidney channel starts from the kidney, penetrating upward through the liver and the diaphragm, entering the lung. Therefore, when a taxation wind is generated within the kidney, it may be located as far up in the body as the region just below the lung." Rigidity above means rigidity of the head and nape of the neck with inability to bend the body either forward or backward. This is a result of the influence of the urinary bladder channel which must be affected when the kidney qi is damaged.

[67]In facilitating range of movement in spinal flexion and extension, one assists the kidney and lung, since, as explained above, this symptom primarily involves these two viscera. There are a number of different understandings about the nature of this pattern. Ma Yuan-tai describes it as a taxation pattern, and Ye Wen-ling regards it as a tetany pattern. Wang Hua-gu considers it as a species of lung atony. The phrase "facilitate forward and

backward bending" may be interpreted as "cure dyspnea." You Zai-jing explains this position when he says, "The lung governs qi and takes the responsibility of breathing. When there is wind heat in the lung, the fluid must be bound and the qi congested. For this reason, (breathing) is inhibited both in the prone and supine postures (*fu yang*, the same term in Chinese for forward and backward bending—tr.). It follows that it is necessary to facilitate *fu yang*. The facilitation of *fu yang* disinhibits the lung qi and disperses evil qi." This is supported by Zhang Wan-lin, who says, "To facilitating *fu yang* disinhibits the qi duct, thus freeing breathing." There is another contrary interpretation which asserts that since this disease is caused by taxation, it is important to relieve taxation by avoiding bending the body forward or backward as much as possible.

As to the second sentence, our rendering is supported by Wu Kun, who says, "The great yang and the *shao yang* kidney (channels) stand in an exterior/interior relationship. The kidney is the abode of the essence, and the essence is an entity of yin which is unable to move by itself but is conducted by the qi of the great yang. When the great yang is said to conduct the essence, this refers to young and strong people, where water is still abundant enough to match fire. For this reason, a cure can be effected in three days. Middle-aged people, though their essence is not yet exhausted, are weaker than young and strong people. Therefore, they will recover in five days. Aged people have exhausted their *tian gui* or heavenly water, and are, therefore, said to be destitute of essence. Destitution of essence is debility and collapse of the true yin which is no longer a match for fire. Hence it takes seven days to cure them."

It is possible to render this sentence in another way, and this is paraphrased as follows: The kidney is associated with the urinary bladder whose vessel starts from the inner canthi, submerging and deviating down the nape of the neck. Now that the kidney is taxed and its essence is depleted, it is no longer able to follow the *tai yang* vessel to nurture the head and nape of the neck. As a result, there arise rigidity above with dim vision and inability to bend either forward or backward. It follows that the treatment method is to conduct the kidney essence to help the *tai yang*. If the kidney essence arrives upon appealing, a cure can be effected in three to five days. If the essence is slow in coming, one can only expect the patient to recover in seven days.

[68]It is true that diminished qi may involve the lung qi, but its root may be in the kidney. It should be understood that lack of or diminished essence may lead to diminished qi. Therefore, the kidney is sometimes treated rather than the lung.

[69]As explained previously, essence is often referred to as semen. Therefore, loss of essence can be understood as too frequent sexual intercourse resulting in diminished essence.

[70]*I.e.,* slippery spermatorrhea

[71]In our source edition, this item is omitted. It is supplemented here in accordance with a version recently unearthed from a Tang dynasty tomb and the *Wai Tai*.

[72]In our source edition, the square bracketed text is originally arranged as an independent item and the brackets have been added by the translators. However, in a version copied in the Ming dynasty, the arrangement is identical to our English edition. Our practice is supported by the *Qian Jin*, where this item is absent from a pertinent quotation from the *Jia Yi Jing*.

[73]Part 1 is derived from Chap. 68, Vol. 10, *Ling Shu*; Part 2 from Chap. 46, *Su Wen*; and Part 3 from Chap. 48, *Su Wen*.

[74]Wiseman translates this as vomiting from above the diaphragm.

[75]Wiseman translates this as vomiting from below the diaphragm.

[76]Upper obstruction is impugned to qi. However, in relation to qi, there are vacuity and repletion, both of which may cause upper obstruction. In the case of qi repletion, the qi is depressed, leaving no room for food. In the case of vacuity, the qi is cold and unable to transform food.

A cycle of watches is twelve watches or a day and a night.

[77]There is no consensus as to the nature of this pattern. It appears to be a complication of lower esophageal constriction with worms and internal *yong*.
A word about the term venter, which may not be the most precise word for the Chinese *wan*. *Wan* means the cavity inside the stomach, and the triple *wan*, i.e., the upper, middle, and lower *wan*, are all located inside the stomach. This is unlike the English word venter, a synonym with the abdomen which covers a larger area. The upper venter is the upper opening of the stomach, and the lower is the lower opening.

[78]The *Tai Su* explains the "to examine the tendency of qi" as having three aspects. These include the extent and degree of the *yong* qi, its depth, and determination of the needling point(s) and manipulation.

[79]In the normal state, the stomach pulse at the *cun kou* should be strong. Here it is deep and choppy. This indicates that the stomach qi counterflows. When the stomach qi counterflows upward, it creates an exuberance of the stomach pulse in the *ren ying* pulse above. One should note that when the author mentions pulse, he includes vessels, and that exuberant pulse, therefore, may equally mean exuberant vessel or exuberant channel qi. It is because of the counterflowing and exuberant stomach qi that *yong* develops. As to what this kind of *yong* is, the *Sheng Ji Zong Lu (The Complete Records of Life Securing [Medical Classics])* provides an explanation. It says, "When qi counterflows and is obstructed, it is retained and bound to develop into *yong*. *Yong* in the venter is due to cold qi obstructing the yang (qi). As heat gathers in the stomach opening, there arises abnormal changes in cold and heat, decaying the flesh there...It causes people to suffer from malariaBlike cold and heat... coughing or retching or spitting pus and blood."

[80]In the *Lei Jing*, Zhang Jing-yue explains, "Fullness is congestion and stagnation of the evil qi causing distention and fullness. It is implied here that any one of the channels of the liver, kidney, or lung can be full, and, if the pulse is replete, there should be water swelling." In liver *yong*, susceptibility to fright develops because the liver governs the emotions of fright and scare, and inability to void can be explained by the fact that the liver channel encircles the genitals. In kidney *yong*, the group of signs are explainable by the route of the kidney channel.

[81]This entire chapter is derived from Chap. 81, Vol. 12, *Ling Shu*.

[82]In the *Lei Jing*, Zhang Jing-yue explains, "The qi emanated from the upper burner is the ancestral qi. The ancestral qi exits through the throat, facilitating respiration, to warm the partings of the flesh, nurture the bone joints and free the interstices. It is from the ancestral qi that the defensive qi is transformed."

That which emanates from the middle burner is the constructive qi, which may be in the form of fluid and humor to nourish the whole body, as rain and dew moistens every living thing. And the most valuable substance, blood, is transformed from the fluid and humor. Yin and yang are understood as the constructive and defensive, qi and blood, and the yin and yang channels.

It was believed that the heavenly bodies, including the sun and the moon, moved at a fixed tempo in the sky which was divided by warp and weft into certain areas, and that the circulation of the constructive and defensive was carried on around the body at a rate corresponding to these heavenly bodies. In this context, the term *dao li* simply means the laws by which yin and yang travel around the body.

[83]Drainage is inappropriate in eliminating an element of repletion from an overall vacuity condition. This is especially true of rapid drainage since this may exacerbate the vacuity and jeopardize the righteous qi. In this condition, one should retain the needle until it is reached by the qi. Conversely, supplementation is inappropriate in eliminating an element of vacuity from an overall repletion pattern because it may exacerbate the repletion. In such cases, the therapy of choice is a balanced regulation of qi and blood to restore them to harmonization.

Nearly each phrase of this paragraph may be understood in quite a different manner. It is summarized as follows:

One should be very concentrated in regulating them. To treat repletion, one should carry out drainage, which may diminish the evil qi. However, excessively drastic drainage may damage the righteous qi. In performing drainage, one should extract the needle quickly and in such a way that the evil qi may be made weakened. To supplement, the needle should be retained and held steady all the time. To treat vacuity, supplementation is necessary, but drastic supplementation may help the repletion evil turn stronger, although it may at the same time replenish the righteous qi. On this account, treatment calls for focus of attention. When qi and blood are well balanced, the spirit qi is stabilized.

[84]The Chinese word for auspicious plants is *cao ming* (grass pod). This is an unidentifiable botanical. Zhang Jing-yue provides the following description in the *Lei Jing*. He says, "...an auspicious grass. In the times of Yao (first legendary king in China—tr.), it grew in the courtyard. It thrived and withered in line with the waxing and waning of the moon. One day after *shuo* (the first day of the lunar calendar—tr.) it grew pods, and one day after *wang* (the fifteenth day of the lunar calendar—tr.) the pods fell." Here we can regard it as a collective term for plants indicative of good luck.

[85]In this context the bone hollows refer to the cavities in the joints between the bones rather than the cavity within the bone itself.

[86]Part 1 is derived from Chap. 60, Vol. 9, *Ling Shu*; Part 2 from Chap. 75, Vol. 11, *Ling Shu*; Part 3 from Chap. 40, *Su Wen*; Part 4 from Chap. 46, *Su Wen*; Part 5 from Chap. 17, *Su Wen*; Part 6 from Chap. 28, *Su Wen*; Part 7 from Chap. 55, *Su Wen*; Part 8 from the *Zhen Jiu Ming Tang Zhi Yao*; Part 9 a combination of parts of Chap. 19, Vol. 4, *Ling Shu* and Chap. 17, *Su Wen*; Part 10 from *Zhen Jiu Ming Tang Zhi Yao*; Part 11 from Chap. 81, Vol. 12, *Ling Shu*; and Part 12 from Chap. 78, Vol. 12, *Ling Shu*.

[87]Zhang Jing-yue explains in the *Lei Jing*, "In the case of unexpected joy and anger, qi counterflows. In the case of dietary irregularities, the visceral qi may be damaged. When the yin qi becomes insufficient, the constructive qi stops circulating. When the surplus of yang qi develops, heat is generated and gathers. All this is enough to give rise to *yong* and *ju*. The two kinds of heat mentioned in the text are the heat produced by surplus yang qi caused by overjoy, etc., and the heat generated by depressed or stagnated constructive qi."

[88]This last sentence might be understood as "fools choose to encounter that which is matured."

[89]An explanation put forth by Zhang Zhi-cong in his *Ling Shu Ji Zhu* about the unfavorable signs, though somewhat farfetched, is of some referential value. The first unfavorable sign is ascribed to collapse of the liver, the second to that of the stomach, the third to that of the spleen, the fourth to that of the yang channels, and the fifth to that of the heart.

[90]Binding refers to a gathering of evils.

[91]Intestinal *ju* is probably an intestinal tumor. It is referred to as such in the *Ling Shu*, but there are no other sources available to corroborate this reading in this context.

[92]Bone *ju* most likely refers to a bony tumor.

[93]The problem lies in the upper and middle burner and is due to upward counterflow of qi from below. Therefore, it is referred to as counterflow inversion. This is a case of a surplus of yang above. This is a localized repletion of yang qi. Moxibustion promotes the yang, thus it is prohibited. Stone needling is a drastic draining therapy, and it may excessively drain the yang qi. Thus the yin and yang are both made vacuous. As a result, the spirit can no longer keep to its abode, causing mania. To treat this condition, one should wait for the separated yin and yang qi to communicate with each other. The text is unclear on how this is done.

[94]The four (or five) seasons have correspondences with the five viscera and the five phases. If a *yong* is contracted in spring, which is liver wood, then we should choose the metal channel, *i.e.*, the lung/large intestine channel, to cure it. There is another way of understanding the practical implications of this line which may be explained in the following way. Take the above example again, but the *yong* may be due to wind from the south which is fire. One should then select points on the kidney/urinary bladder channels since these are water and, therefore, can restrain fire.

The translators believe in general that Huang-fu Mi focuses his emphasis on the selection of the channel rather than the individual point. There is a common saying that the selection of points should be subordinated to that of the channels. It must be admitted, however, that we are not aware of any commentary pertaining particularly to this passage that validates this point of view.

[95]Perspiration due to a lung disorder is called *po* (corporeal soul) perspiration.

[96]Ma Shi believes that the point needled is Armpit Abyss (*Yuan Ye*, GB 22), while Zhang Jing-yue thinks that two points, Armpit Abyss together with Sinew Rut (*Ze Jin*, GV 23), are indicated.

[97]*I.e.*, Celestial Pool (*Tian Chi*, Per 1)

[98]*I.e.*, Broken Sequence (*Lie Que*, Lu 7)

[99]*I.e.*, True Shoulder (*Jian Zhen*, SI 9)

[100]The reference to the hand *tai yin* refers specifically to Central Treasury (*Zhong Fu*, Lu 1) and the points located near it are Qi Door (*Qi Hu*, St 13) and Storeroom (*Ku Fang*, St 14).

[101]*I.e.*, Water Prominence (*Shui Tu*, St 10) and Qi Abode (*Qi She*, St 11)

[102]*Ju* in the nasal cavities is characterized by ulceration and deformation of the bridge of the nose.

[103]Stagnant scratching (*zhu yang*) is a condition characterized by tendency to scratch at itchy, hardened swellings.

[104]This refers specifically to a heat toxin.

[105]The recommendation to employ "counterflow ignition" implies the administration of moxibustion using drainage techniques.

[106]An example of joints which correspond to one another are the elbows and knees or the wrists and ankles, etc. These relationships may be from upper body to lower body, from left to right, or may even be contralateral relationships, such as left elbow to right knee.

[107]Yin and yang may be interpreted here in several ways. The anterior and medial aspects are yin, while the other aspects are yang. The viscera are yin, while the bowels are yang. The genitals in males are yang, while those in females are yin.

[108]In ancient Chinese, the word *yong* could mean jamming, crowding, or being held up.

[109]In ancient Chinese, the word *ju* could mean stoppage or thwarting.

[110]The nine districts refer to the nine palaces which is the core of an entire system of correspondences among the five phases, the calendar with the days, months, and seasons included, the orientations, the constellations, the ten heavenly stems and twelve earthly branches, etc. Note that although the nine districts are ostensibly the topic of discussion, they are scarcely mentioned. This is because of the established corrspondences between all of the factors involved. One need only mention a single factor, for instance the heavenly stems, and all of its associated seasons, orientations, and phases are determined.

[111]The matching of the ten heavenly stems and the twelve earthly branches yields sixty pairs, each of which represents a day in a sixtyBday cycle. With the earthly branches as the signposts we have: *Jia-Zi, Bing-Zi, Wu-Zi, Geng-Zi,* and *Ren-Zi; Yi-Chou, Ding-Chou, Si-Chou, Xin-Chou,* and *Gui-Chou;ia-Yin, Bing-Yin, Wu-Yin, Geng-Yin,* and *Ren-Yin; Yi-Mao, Ding-Mao, Ji-Mao, Xin-Mao,* and *Gui-Mao. Jia-Chen, Bing-Chen, Wu-Chen, Geng-Chen,* and *Ren-Chen; Yi-Si, Ding-Si, Ji-Si, Xin-Si,* and *Gui-Si; Jia-Wu, Bing-Wu, Wu-Wu, Geng-Wu,* and *Ren-Wu; Yi-Wei, Ding-Wei, Si-Wei, Xin-Wei,* and *Gui-Wei; Jia-Shen, Bing-Shen, Wu-Shen, Geng-Shen,* and *Ren-Shen; Yi-You, Ding-You, Si-You, Xin-You,* and *Gui-You; Jia-Xu, Bing-Xu, Wu-Xu, Geng-Xu,* and *Ren-Xu; Yi-Hai, Ding-Hai, Si-Hai, Xin-Hai,* and *Gui-Hai.*

[112]This is a reference to the external genitals and the anus.

[113]These are days when needling is prohibited.

[114]*Tai Yi* was a god in ancient Chinese mythology but his identity is not certain. Many scholars consider him to be the Heavenly Emperor. He was said to reside in each of his heavenly palaces in turn for fortyBfive or forty-six days.

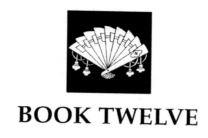

BOOK TWELVE

Chapter One

Yawning, Retching, Sobbing, Shivering with Cold, Belching, Sneezing, Drooping, Tearing, Sighing, Drooling, Ringing in the Ears, Tongue-Biting, Poor Memory, & Constant Hunger[1]

(1)

The Yellow Emperor asked:

What kind of qi makes people yawn?

Qi Bo answered:

The defensive qi circulates within the yang by day and within the yin by night. Yin governs the night, and night in turn governs sleep. The yang governs above while the yin governs below. Therefore, while the yin qi accumulates below and the yang qi is nearly exhausted, yang is making its way upward and the yin is making its way downward. The mutual attraction between yin and yang results in frequent yawning. When the yang qi is exhausted and the yin qi is just becoming exuberant, the eyes are shut. On the other hand, when the yin qi is exhausted and the yang qi is just becoming exuberant, there is wakefulness. Since the kidney governs yawning, one must drain the foot *shao yin* and simultaneously supplement the foot *tai yang* (to treat it).[2]

The Yellow Emperor asked:

What causes people to retch?

Qi Bo answered:

Once grain has entered the stomach, the stomach qi ascends and pours into the lung. If long-standing cold qi combines with fresh grain qi in returning to the stomach, then these two qi will interfere with one another. (In other words,) the true and evil (qi) will come into conflict. Thus these two qi mix together to cause counterflow which must exit via the stomach resulting in retching. Since the lung is responsible for retching, one must supplement the hand *tai yin* and drain the foot *tai yin* (to treat it). Retching can also be checked immediately by pricking the nose with straw to provoke sneezing or by arresting one's breath (on the exhale) and then abruptly drawing in the breath. Giving the patient a fright may also be used.[3]

The Yellow Emperor asked:

What causes people to sob?

Qi Bo answered:

This is due to an exuberance of yin qi and a vacuity of yang qi. The yin qi acts swiftly, while the yang qi acts sluggishly. The exuberance of the yin qi with expiry of the yang qi results in sobbing. Because sobbing is due to exuberance of yin and expiry of yang, (one must) supplement the foot *tai yang* and drain the foot *shao yin*.[4]

The Yellow Emperor asked:

What causes people to shiver with cold?

Qi Bo answered:

When cold qi intrudes upon the skin, the yin qi becomes exuberant, while the yang qi becomes vacuous. As a result, there is shivering and quivering with cold. (One should) supplement the various yang.[5]

The Yellow Emperor asked:

What causes people to belch?

Qi Bo answered:

When cold qi intrudes upon the stomach, it counterflows from below, spreading upward. When it comes out of the stomach again, it causes belching. (One must) supplement the foot tai yin and the foot yang ming ["supplement at the root of the eyebrow" in a variant version {later editor}].[6]

The Yellow Emperor asked:

What causes people to sneeze?

Qi Bo answered:

When the yang qi is in harmony and flows freely, it fills the heart and exits through the nose and this results in sneezing. (One should) supplement at the spring (point) of the foot *tai yang* and the root of the eyebrow.[7]

The Yellow Emperor asked:

What causes people to suffer from drooping?

Qi Bo answered:

When the stomach is not replete, the various vessels become vacuous, and when the various vessels are vacuous, the sinew vessels become listless and inert. When exertion is made in performance of yin affairs, qi cannot be restored. This results in drooping. (One should) supplement at the border of the flesh involved.[8]

The Yellow Emperor asked:

What is the cause of tearing and snivelling when people lament?

Qi Bo answered:

The heart is the ruler over the five viscera and six bowels. The eyes are the converging place of the gathering vessels and the passageway for the ascension of fluid. The mouth and nose are the gateways of qi. Sorrow, sadness, worry, or depression stir the heart. When the heart is stirred, the five viscera and six bowels are upset, and when they are upset, the gathering vessels are affected. When they are affected, the passageway of fluid is opened, and when it is open, tears and snivel issue forth. Fluid is that which irrigates essence to moisten the hollow cavities. It follows that once the passageways for the ascension of fluid are open, there is tearing, and when the tearing is incessant, fluid becomes exhausted. When the fluid is exhausted, essence cannot be irrigated and, when the essence is not irrigated, the eyes lose their sight. For this reason, this is called deprivation of essence (*duo jing*. One must) supplement at the channel (point) Celestial Pillar (*Tian Zhu*, Bl 10) which is located at the sides of the neck near the midline of the head.[9]

(2)

The Yellow Emperor asked:

In crying, tears may fail to emerge or (tears) may be accompanied by scanty snivel. I wonder where this water is generated and from where this snivel exits.[10]

Qi Bo answered:

The heart among the five viscera is in charge of essence. The eyes are its portals and an efflorescent (facial) complexion is the expression of its luxuriance. It follows that when people make gains, their harmonious qi is reflected in their eyes, and when they are frustrated and worried, these are made known in their (facial) complexion. It follows that in sorrow and sadness, tears run down, and this running of tears is a product of water. All kinds of essence ["sources of water" in the *Su Wen* {later editor}] derive from accumulated water, and accumulated water is the consummate yin, which is the kidney essence. The reason why the water of the ancestral essence cannot emerge is that the (ancestral) essence confines it. The essence contains and wraps it, so it is prevented from flowing (wantonly). Related to the transformation of qi, the essence of water forms will, and that of fire forms spirit. When water and fire interact on each other, both will and spirit may become sorrowful. Thus water is produced in the eyes.[11]

As the proverb goes, sorrow in the heart is the name of sorrow in the will. Because will and the heart both converge their essence in the eyes, when they both become sorrowful, the spirit qi is transferred to the heart. Whereas, essence ascends and is not transferred to the will, leaving the will alone in sorrow. Thus tears emerge. Snivel in crying is ascribed to the brain. The brain is yin and marrow fills the bones. That which leaks from the brain is snivel. The will is the governor of the bones. That snivel follows suit when water runs out is because they are of a kind. Tears and snivel are like brothers. In an urgent situation, they both perish, and, (if one) lives, they both live. [For the second clause, the *Tai Su* reads "they both come to their end when they come out." {later editor}] When the will is rocked by sorrow, snivel and tears both emerge, following one another because they are of a kind.[12]

The Yellow Emperor asked:

How is it that people may cry without shedding tears or that one may shed a few tears, yet snivel does not follow it out?

Qi Bo answered:

A failure to shed tears means that one's crying lacks sorrow. A lack of tears means that the spirit lacks compassion. When the spirit lacks compassion, the will lacks sorrow. While yin and yang are at a stalemate, how can tears flow alone? Sorrowful will gives rise to woe, and woe surges

into the yin. When there is a surge into the yin, the will departs from the eyes, and when the will has departed from the eyes, the spirit is no longer able to hold the essence back. Since the spirit and essence have departed from the eyes, tears and snivel are shed.[13]

The classics explain that inversion causes the eyes lose their sight. [The part from "tears and snivel can be compared to brothers" down to "the eyes lose their sight" is absent from the original version and is now appended with reference to the *Su Wen* and the *Ling Shu*. {later editor}][14]

When a person suffers from inversion, the yang qi is merged above and the yin qi is merged below. When yang is merged above, fire alone glows brightly. When yin is merged below, the feet become cold. If the feet are cold, there will be distention. Since a single water is unable to prevail over five fires, the eyes become diseased. Therefore, qi surging due to wind causes incessant tearing. When wind strikes the eyes, the yang qi catches hold of essence in the interior. In other words, the fire qi scorches the eyes. This is the reason why tears flow when the eyes are exposed to wind. Some people compare this to (the fact) that unless strong wind breaks out ["unless fire is effulgent and wind breaks out" in the *Su Wen* {later editor}], rain is an impossibility. The situations are quite similar. [The *Jiu Juan* focuses on the form, while the *Su Wen* on the emotions. They shed light on each other. {later editor}][15]

(3)

The Yellow Emperor asked:

What causes people to sigh?

Qi Bo answered:

Worry and thought causes the heart ligation to become tense. When the heart ligation becomes tense, the qi tracts become constrained, and this constraint causes (the qi tracts) to become inhibited. Therefore, one sighs deeply so as to draw out (the depressed qi. One must) supplement the heart-governor (channel) of the hand *shao yin* and the foot *shao yang* with retention (of the needle).[16]

The Yellow Emperor asked:

What causes people to drool?

Qi Bo answered:

Food and drink all enter the stomach. If there is heat in the stomach, this heat will cause worms to stir. When worms stir, the stomach becomes slack. With a slack stomach, the ridge spring is open, and consequently drool runs down. (One must) supplement the foot *shao yin*.[17]

The Yellow Emperor asked:

What causes people to suffer from ringing in the ears?

Qi Bo answered:

The ears are a converging place of the gathering vessels. When the stomach is empty, the gathering vessels become vacuous. Because of the vacuity, (their qi) slides down and the vessels become exhausted. This results in ringing of the ears. (One must) supplement at Guest Host Person (*Ke Zhu Ren*),[18] and (the point) at the junction between the nail and the flesh in the thumb.[19]

The Yellow Emperor asked:

What causes people to bite their own tongue?

Qi Bo answered:

This is because inversion (qi) counterflows upward, and all kinds of vessel qi arrive there. If the qi of the *shao yin* arrives there, (people) bite their own tongues. If the qi of the *shao yang* arrives, (people) bite their own cheeks. If the qi of the *yang ming* arrives, (people) bite their own lips. (One should) supplement the (channel) which rules the disorder.[20]

(4)

The Yellow Emperor asked:

What causes people to suffer from forgetfulness? Qi Bo answered:

The qi above is insufficient and there is a surplus of qi below. The stomach and the intestines are replete and the heart and lung are vacuous. With the vacuity (of the heart and the lung), the constructive and defensive are detained below and are unable to ascend in a timely fashion. Thus, poor memory results.[21]

The Yellow Emperor asked:

What causes people to (quickly become) hungry yet possess no desire for food?

Qi Bo answered:

When essence and qi are both merged in the spleen, heat is detained in the stomach. This stomach heat disperses grain (swiftly). Because grain is dispersed (swiftly), one (quickly) becomes hungry. (However,) since the stomach qi counterflows upward, this causes the openings of the stomach (*wei wan*, 胃脘) to become congested, and when the stomach openings are congested, there is no desire for food.[22]

(To treat) forgetfulness and rapid hungering, (one must) first examine the viscera and bowels, attack their insubstantial fault, and then regulate their qi. In the case of exuberance, perform drainage. In the case of vacuity, perform supplementation.[23]

(5)

The above fourteen evils are all unusual evils that penetrate the hollow portals. Wherever there is an evil, there is vacuity. It follows that since the qi above is insufficient, the brain is not replenished, the ears tend to ring, the head is inclined, and the eyes are heavy. If the center qi is insufficient, there is change in urination and defecation and the intestines tend to rumble. When the qi below is insufficient, there is atonic inversion and oppression of the heart. (One must) supplement at (the point) below the lateral malleolus[24] and retain (the needle). Also immediately needle (the point) two *cun* above the big toe[25] and retain (the needle). Some say supplement (the point) under the lateral malleolus and retain (the needle).

Chapter Two

Intrusion of Cold Qi Upon the Epiglottis Producing Loss of Voice & Inability to Speak[26]

(1)

The Yellow Emperor asked:

When people suddenly become worried and indignant and lose their voice, what kind of qi has ceased to circulate?

Shao Shi answered:

The pharynx is the passageway for water and grain. The larynx is (the passage) for qi to ascend and descend. The epiglottis is the door of the voice. The lips and the mouth are the door leaves of the voice. The tongue is the reed of the voice. And the uvula is the pass of the voice. The nasopharynx separates qi for the purpose of discharging, while the transverse bone is at the service of the spirit and qi and governs the movement of the tongue.[27]

It follows that when people have nasal hollowing (*bi dong*, 鼻洞) with endless running of mucus, the nasopharynx is not shut and fails to separate the qi. If the glottis is small and thin, it starts out swiftly, for it opens and closes with facility and draws out qi with ease. Whereas, if it is large and thick, it opens and closes with difficulty and is slow in drawing out qi, thus giving rise to repetition of words. So-called stammering is the counterflow (of qi) in speaking which causes (words to be) repeated. Sudden loss of voice is due to cold qi intruding into the glottis. As a result, the mobility of the glottis is disabled, and even once it becomes mobile, it cannot reach the reed and door leaves. Since the reed and door leaves are inhibited in their opening and closure, there is no voice. The vessel of the foot *shao yin* links upward with the root of the tongue, connecting to the transverse bone and terminating in the glottis. (One must) twice drain the blood vessel (of the channel) and the turbid qi will be purged. Because the vessel of the epiglottis connects with the conception vessel above, (one must) additionally take Celestial Prominence (*Tian Tu*, CV 22). This will produce (mobility) in the glottis.[28]

(2)

For sudden loss of voice and qi choking, prick Protuberance Assistance (*Fu Tu*, LI 18) and the root of the tongue[29] to let blood out.

(3)

For loss of voice with inability to speak, needle Brain's Door (*Nao Hu*, GV 17).

For sudden loss of voice with inability to speak and sore throat, needle Wind Mansion (*Feng Fu*, GV 16).

For a slack tongue and loss of voice with inability to speak, needle Loss of Voice Gate (*Yin Men*).[30]

For sore throat and loss of voice with inability to speak, Celestial Window (*Tian Chuang*, SI 16) is the ruling point.[31]

For sudden loss of voice with qi choking, throat *bi* and swollen larynx, difficult breathing, and inability to swallow food and drink, Celestial Tripod (*Tian Ding*, LI 17) is the ruling point.

For frequent retching upon ingestion and inability to speak, Open Valley (*Tong Gu*, Ki 20) is the ruling point.

For loss of voice with inability to speak, Cycle Gate (*Qi Men*, Liv 14) is the ruling point.

For sudden loss of voice with inability to speak, Branch Ditch (*Zhi Gou*, TH 6) is the ruling point.

For loss of voice with inability to speak, Union

Valley (*He Gu*, LI 4), Gushing Spring (*Yong Quan*, Ki 1), and Yang Intersection (*Yang Jiao*, GB 35) are the ruling points.

Chapter Three

Insomnia, Loss of Eyesight, Somnolence, Disturbed Sleep, Inability to Lie Supine, Torpidity of the Flesh, Noise in Breathing, & Dyspnea[32]

(1)

The Yellow Emperor asked:

Why is it that, once evil qi has intruded upon people, it may cause them to suffer from insomnia?

Bo Gao answered:

Once the five grains have entered the stomach, their wastes, fluid, and ancestral qi are separated into three canals. The ancestral qi accumulates in the chest, coming out through the throat, to permeate the heart and lung so as to operate respiration. The constructive qi distills fluid and humor and pours them into the vessels where they are transformed into blood to nourish the four extremities (externally) and pours them internally into the five viscera and six bowels. The circulation (of blood) is in accordance with the watches. The defensive qi issues (from the upper burner) as a swift and fierce impetuous qi. It is fierce and first circulates in the four extremities, the partings of the flesh, and the skin. Its course is uninterrupted, circulating in the yang by day and in the yin by night, submerging into the yin as a rule from the foot *shao yin* which serves as a dividing line and then circulating among the five viscera and six bowels.[33]

If an evil qi has intruded upon the five viscera, the defensive qi must single-handedly defend the exterior. It circulates in the yang, unable to enter the yin. Its circulation (solely) in the yang results

in an exuberance of yang qi, and this exuberance of yang qi (in turn) causes the yang motility (vessel) to become filled up. Its inability to enter the yin produces a vacuity of the yin qi, and this results in insomnia.

To treat it, (one must) supplement the insufficiency and drain the surplus to regulate vacuity and repletion. This will open the passageways (between the constructive and defensive) to remove the evil. Drink a single dose of *Ban Xia Tang* (Pinellia Decoction), yin and yang will be freed, and sleep will come in no time. This is likened to dredging the river to break up congestions and blockages. The channels and the network vessels are unblocked completely and the yin and yang are restored to harmony. The decoction is prepared as follows. Fetch eight *sheng* of water that has run over a thousand *li*, stir it ten thousand times, and then scoop out five *sheng* of the clear part, and boil it over a reed fire. When it is boiling, put in one *sheng* of glutinous millet and five *he* of processed Rhizoma Pinelliae Ternatae (*Ban Xia*). Continue to boil over a slow fire till (the mixture) is boiled down to one and a half *sheng* and then clear away the dregs. Drink a small cup of this juice three times daily. (The dosage) may be increased little by little as determined by the degree (of improvement). If the illness is recent, tip up one cup and lie down. Once one perspires, recovery is already effected. If the condition is chronic, one must drink it three times to effect a recovery.[34]

(2)

The Yellow Emperor asked:

What is the cause of heavy eyes and loss of sight?[35]

Bo Gao answered:

The defensive qi circulates (solely) within the yin and cannot enter the yang. Its circulation (exclusively) within the yin results in an exuberance of yin qi, and this exuberance of yin qi (in turn) causes the yin motility to become filled up. Inability to enter the yang causes a vacuity of the yang qi making the eyes close. [The *Jiu Juan* uses "lodges" instead of "circulates" and "circulate" instead of "enter." {later editor}]

The Yellow Emperor asked:

What causes people to suffer from somnolence?

Bo Gao answered:

These people have enlarged intestines and stomachs and rough ["damp" in the *Jiu Juan*; same hereafter {later editor}] skin. Rough skin allows no freedom in the partings of the flesh, and enlarged intestines and stomachs detain the circulation of the defensive qi. When the skin is rough and the partings of the flesh are not free, (the defensive qi) is slow in circulating. The defensive qi generally circulates in the yang by day and in the yin by night. So when the yang qi runs out, (people) lie down, but when the yin qi runs out, (people) wake up. With large stomach and large intestines, the circulation of the defensive qi is detained. When the skin is rough and the partings of the flesh are not free, it is slow in circulating. Thus it remains in the yin for a long period of time and the qi is not smart ["clear" in a variant version {later editor}]. As a result, the eyes are inclined to close and sleep is plentiful. When the stomach and intestines are small, the skin is slippery and slack and the partings of the flesh are free and uninhibited. Thus the defensive qi remains in the yang for a long period of time. As a result, there is less sleep.

The Yellow Emperor asked:

What is the cause of sudden (development of) somnolence in those having seldom experienced it?

Bo Gao answered:

If evil qi lodges in the upper burner, the upper burner becomes shut and blocked. After taking in food or drinking soups, the defensive qi will be detained in the yin and fail to circulate, resulting in sudden somnolence.

The Yellow Emperor asked:

How are all these evils treated?

Bo Gao answered:

First examine the viscera and bowels, attack the insubstantial fault, and then regulate the qi, draining that which is exuberant and supplementing that which is vacuous. It is necessary to acquire a clear knowledge of the afflictions and distractions in connection with the form and orientation before (one) can determine (a modality) and take on (the evil).[36]

(3)

The Yellow Emperor asked:

Some people have disturbed sleep, why?

Bo Gao answered:

When the viscera are somehow damaged and one's emotions become obsessive, sleep is not restful. ["When the essence has somewhere to rely on, sleep is freed from disturbance" in the *Su Wen*; "If (one's) essence has become obsessed, (sleep) is disturbed" in the *Tai Su*. {later editor}] Therefore, people are unable to suspend their disease.

The Yellow Emperor asked:

What causes people to suffer from an inability to lie supine?

Bo Gao answered:

The lung is the canopy of the viscera. When the lung qi is exuberant, the vessels become enlarged, and enlarged vessels make it impossible to lie supine (quietly).

(4)

The Yellow Emperor asked:

What causes people to suffer from torpidity of the flesh (*rou ke*, 肉苛)? What kind of disease is this?

Bo Gao answered:

The constructive qi is vacuous, and the defensive qi is replete. Vacuity of the constructive qi results in insensitivity. Vacuity of the defensive qi results in loss of use. If both the constructive and defensive are vacuous, this results in insensitivity as well as loss of use, (i.e.,) torpidity visiting the flesh. If the formal body and the orientations are not congruous, death will occur in thirty days.[37]

The Yellow Emperor asked:

Some people who experience a counterflow of qi are unable to lie down, and make sounds when breathing. Some are unable to lie down but emit no sound when breathing. Some carry on daily life in a normal way but make sounds in breathing. Some are able to lie down and move around but suffer from dyspnea. Some can neither lie down nor move around and suffer from dyspnea. And some are unable to lie down, or suffer from dyspnea when lying down. Which viscus is responsible?

Bo Gao answered:

Inability to lie down and the production of sounds while breathing is caused by counterflow of the (foot) *yang ming*. The three foot yang (channels) should travel downward, but now (the *yang ming*) counterflows upward. Therefore, breathing produces a sound. The *yang ming* is the vessel of the stomach, and the stomach is the sea of the six bowels. Its qi ought to circulate downward as well. If the *yang ming* counterflows, deviating from its normal course, this results in an inability to lie down. [The *Xia Jing*[38] states, "When the stomach is in disharmony, sleep becomes disturbed." {later editor}] This is an example of what is explained by it. Normal daily life (accompanied by) sounds emitted in breathing is caused by the counterflow of the connecting vessel of the lung. Since it fails to follow the channel up and down, (its qi) is detained in the channel and does not circulate. The connecting vessel afflicts people with only a mild malady, and, therefore, (the patients) carry on normal daily life except for the sound produced in

breathing. Inability to lie down or dyspnea resulting from lying down is caused by intruding water qi. Water qi is that which flows with fluid and humor, and the kidney, the water viscus, governs fluid and humor and (hence) governs lying down and dyspnea.[39]

(5)

For insomnia due to fright, propensity toward bruxism, and water qi moving up and down which is the wandering qi of the five viscera, Yin Intersection (*Yin Jiao*, CV 7) is the ruling point.[40]

For inability to lie down, Superficial Cleft (*Fu Xi*, Bl 52) is the ruling point.

For generalized swelling, pain in the skin exacerbated by even the lightest touch of clothes, aching and weakness (of the limbs) with tugging and slackening, and, in long-lasting cases, insensitivity, Roof (*Wu Yi*, St 15) is the ruling point.

Chapter Four

Stirring in the Vessels of the Foot *Tai Yang*, *Yang Ming*, & the Hand *Shao Yang* Producing Eye Disorders[41]

(1)

The Yellow Emperor asked:

Once I climbed a platform high up in the green-blue clouds. Halfway up the steps, I looked round and then had to crawl on. I felt curious and puzzled. Dazzled, I closed my eyes to calm down my heart and settle my qi. (The dizziness, however,) remained unresolved. Loosing my hair, I knelt down for some time and then tried to look down again. (The dizziness) was still not recovered for long. (Somehow,) it was suddenly relieved of itself (later). What kind of qi caused this?

Qi Bo answered:

The essence qi from the five viscera and six bowels all ascend and pour into the eyes to transform into essence. The wrapper ["socket" in the *Ling Shu* {later editor}] of the essence is the oculi. The essence of the bone forms the pupils. The essence of the sinews form the dark of the oculi ["dark of the eyes" in the *Ling Shu* {later editor}]. The essence of blood forms the network vessels. The essence of qi forms the white of the oculi ["white of the eyes" in the *Ling Shu* {later editor}]. And the essence of the muscles form the eyelids. (The eyelids) wrap and bind the essences of the sinews, bones, blood, and qi and join the vessels to form the ocular ligation. This homes to the brain above and emerges from the nape of the neck behind.[42]

Once an evil has struck the (nape of the neck, and moved into) the head and eye, if the body is vacuous, it will penetrate deeply, following the ocular ligation into the brain. As a result, the brain spins, and when it spins, the brain draws and tenses the ocular ligation. When the ocular ligation becomes tense, the eyes become dizzy and (feel as if they were) spinning. If the evil strikes (some of) the essences (of the eyes), the essence struck will be out of proportion, and this disproportion causes the essences to disperse. When the essences are dispersed, this causes double vision or, in other words, seeing two things (where there is only one).[43]

The eyes are (formed of) the essences of the five viscera and six bowels, are nurtured by the constructive and defensive, the corporeal and ethereal souls, and are given birth to by the spirit qi. For that reason, when the spirit is taxed, the corporeal and ethereal souls are dispersed and will-reflection becomes chaotic. The pupils and the dark of the eyes obey the laws of yin, while the white of the eyes and the red vessels in them obey the laws of yang. On this account, when yin and yang are in balance and equilibrium, the essence is bright. The eyes are at the service of the heart, and the heart is the dwelling place of the spirit. Therefore, when the spirit is distracted, the essence is chaotic and (the yin and yang) are out of equilibrium. If (one) unexpectedly looks upon some uncommon place, the essence and spirit, the corporeal and ethereal souls will be dispersed and out of balance. This is, therefore, called confusion.

The Yellow Emperor asked:

I am doubtful (of your explanation). I have never been to the Eastern Hunting Park but I have been confused, and I have recovered after I have left it. Can I have my spirit taxed by nothing but the park? How odd it is!

Qi Bo answered:

This is not (odd). The heart may have something to delight in, and the spirit may have something to take aversion to. When (the two emotions) suddenly react upon each other, the essence qi becomes chaotic with mistaken vision resulting in confusion. When the spirit is distracted (away from this situation), recovery follows. A mild (case) is known as puzzling (*mi*, 迷) and a serious one as confusion.

(2)

The canthi pointing to the lateral sides of the face are called the sharp canthi, while of those near to the nose, the upper one is known as the outer canthus and the lower one as the inner canthus.[44]

(3)

If the color of the eyes is red the disease is in the heart. If the color is white, the disease is in the lung. If the color is green-blue, the disease is in the liver. If the color is yellow, the disease is in the spleen. If the color is black, the disease is in the kidney. And if the color is a nondescript yellow, the disease is in the chest.[45]

(4)

In examining pain in the eyes, a red vessel extending from above to below indicates disease of the *tai yang*. (A red vessel) from below to above, indicates disease of the *yang ming*, and that from the outer to the inner (eye), disease of the *shao yang*.[46]

The gallbladder transmits heat to the brain, giving rise to pungent nose nasal hollowing characterized by incessant running of turbid snivel which can be transmuted into nosebleeding of filthy blood and heavy eyes. This is a result of inversion qi.

(5)

That aspect of the foot *yang ming* which travels bilaterally to the nose, entering the face is called suspended skull. It homes to the mouth, going straight to submerge into the eye, connecting with its root. Take it for headache affecting the submandibular region. For faults (in the area), take it, reducing surplus and supplementing insufficiency. Contrary (treatment) will only aggravate (the condition).[47]

That part of the foot *tai yang* which enters the brain via the nape of the neck and directly homes to the root of the eye is called the ocular ligation. For tormenting pain in the head and eye, take (the point) between the two sinews in the middle of the nape. Upon submerging into the brain, (the channel) diverges into the yin motility and yang motility (channels). The yin and yang (motility) cross each other, the yang (qi) submerging and the yin (qi) emerging. They cross at the sharp canthus. While the yang qi is exuberant, the eyes are open, and while the yin qi is exuberant, the eyes are closed.[48]

(6)

For reddening and pain in the eye spreading from the inner canthus, take the yin motility.[49]

(7)

For pain in the eye with inability to look, Upper Star (*Shang Xing*, GV 23) is the ruling point. First take Yi Xi (*Yi Xi*, Bl 45) and finally Celestial Casement (*Tian You*, TH 16) and Wind Pool (*Feng Chi*, GB 20).

For clear-eyed blindness and poor eyesight for distant objects, Light Guard (*Cheng Guang*, Bl 6) is the ruling point.[50]

For heavy eyes and blurred vision for distant objects, Eye Window (*Mu Chuang*, GB 16) is the ruling point.

For blurred vision and reddening of and pain in the eye, Celestial Pillar (*Tian Zhu*, Bl 10) is the ruling point.

For visual dizziness with inability to see and hemilateral headache dragging and tensing the outer canthus, Mandibular Movement (*Han Yan*, GB 4) is the ruling point.

For dim vision, aversion to wind, tearing eyes with an abhorrence of cold, headache and visual dizziness, reddening of and pain in the inner canthus, blurred vision, itching and pain in the canthus, excessive (moisture) of the skin (of the eyelid), and white screen, Bright Eyes (*Jing Ming*, Bl 1) is the ruling point.

For clear-eyed blindness, blurred vision for distant objects, excessive (moisture) in the skin (of the eyelid), and white screen covering the pupil, Eye Window (*Mu Chuang*, GB 16) is the ruling point.[51]

For dim vision, tearing, visual dizziness with head spinning, itching of the pupil, blurred vision for distant objects, night blindness, eye twitching radiating to the mouth and nape of the neck, and deviated mouth with inability to speak, needle Tear Container (*Cheng Qi*, St 1).

For pain in the eye, deviated mouth, tearing, and dim vision, Four Whites (*Si Bai*, St 2) is the ruling point.

For reddening or yellowing of the eye, Cheek Bone Hole (*Quan Liao*, SI 18) is the ruling point.

For squinting eyes, Water Trough (*Shui Gou*, GV 26) is the ruling point.

For pain in the eye and dim vision, Gum Intersection (*Yin Jiao*, GV 28) is the ruling point.

For heavy eye and generalized sweating, Sauce Receptacle (*Cheng Jiang*, CV 24) is the ruling point. For clear-eyed blindness, ocular disorders, and aversion of the eyes to wind and cold, Upper Pass (*Shang Guan*, GB 3) is the ruling point.

For clear-eyed blindness, Shang Yang (*Shang Yang*, LI 1) is the ruling point.

For ocular disorders and blurred vision, Veering Passageway (*Pian Li*, LI 6) is the ruling point.
For pain in the eye, Lower Ridge (*Xia Lian*, LI 8) is the ruling point.

For ocular disorders, blurred vision, and diminished qi, moxa Five Li (*Wu Li*, LI 13). For afflictions on the left side, treat the right, and for afflictions on the right side, treat the left.

For white screen in the eye, pain in the eye with tearing, and, in serious cases, (the eye painful) as if about to burst from the sockets, Front Valley (*Qian Gu*, SI 2) is the ruling point.

For white screen covering the eyeball and hiding the pupil with loss of eyesight, Ravine Divide (*Jie Xi*, St 41) is the ruling point.

Chapter Five

Stirring of the Hand *Tai Yang* & *Shao Yang* Causing Disorders of the Ear[52]

(1)

Sudden inversion may cause deafness, as may congestion and blockage in one ear. All are ascribed to sudden assault of internal qi. This disease is not a case of wind stroke due to either internal or external causes. (The patient) must be thin and bony.

Headache, ringing in the ear, and inhibition of the nine portals are all (disorders) produced by the stomach and intestines.

(2)

The Yellow Emperor asked:

The *Ci Jie (Needling Strategies)* states that acuity-imparting (*fa meng*, 發蒙) is needling the points of the bowels to rid the bowels of disease. (Specifically,) which point is efficacious?

Qi Bo answered:

In needling, (one) must needle Auditory Palace (*Ting Gong*, SI 19) at midday, hitting the pupil of the eye (with qi). Then sounds from the outside can be heard. This is the point.[53]

The Yellow Emperor asked:

What is meant by the statement that sounds from the outside can be heard?

Qi Bo answered:

After having inserted the needle, firmly press (the patient's) two nostrils and instruct him to immediately arrest his breath. A sound must occur in the ears in response.[54]

(3)

For ringing in the ear, take the pulsating vessel in front of the auricle.[55]

Pain in the ear may not be needled if there is pus in the ear or wax in the ear producing loss of hearing.

For deafness, take (the points) on the hand and foot at the junction between the nail and the flesh on the ring finger and the fourth toe.[56] First take (the point on) the hand and then (that on) the foot.

For ringing in the ear, take (the point) at the nail of the middle finger.[57] For (afflictions on) the left side, treat the right. For (afflictions on the) right side, treat the left. First take (the point on) the hand, and then (that on) the foot.[58]

For deafness with an absence of pain (in the ear), take the foot *shao yang*. For deafness with pain (in the ear), take the hand *yang ming*.

(4)

For ringing in the ear, Hundred Convergence (*Bai Hui*, GV 20), Mandibular Movement (*Han Yan*, GB 4), Skull Rest (*Lu Xi*, TH 19), Celestial Window (*Tian Chuang*, SI 16), Great Mound (*Da Ling*, Per 7), Veering Passageway (*Pian Li*, LI 6),

Front Valley (*Qian Gu*, SI 2), and Back Ravine (*Hou Xi*, SI 3) are the ruling points.

For ear pain, ringing in the ear, and deafness, Upper Pass (*Shang Guan*, GB 3) is the ruling point. The needle may not be inserted deeply.

For deafness and ringing in the ear, Lower Pass (*Xia Guan*, St 7), Yang Ravine (*Yang Xi*, LI 5), Passage Hub (*Guan Chong*, TH 1), Armpit Gate (*Ye Men*, TH 2), and Yang Valley (*Yang Gu*, SI 5) are the ruling points.

For deafness, ringing in the ear, headache, and pain in the submandibular region, Ear Gate (*Er Men*, TH 21) is the ruling point.

For heavy-headedness and pain in the sub-mandibular region radiating to the ear with a buzzing noise, Harmony Bone Hole (*He Liao*, TH 22) is the ruling point.

For deafness accompanied by a noise like wind blowing in the ear, Auditory Convergence (*Ting Hui*, GB 2) is the ruling point.

For deafness with rumbling noise in the ear or loss of hearing accompanied by a buzzing noise in the ear like the chirping of a cicada or quail, Auditory Palace (*Ting Gong*, SI 19) is the ruling point. With the mandible lowered, if the point emits a cracking sound, insert the needle here. ["This is the so-called acuity-imparting point" in the *Jiu Juan*. {later editor}]

For deafness, Wind Screen (*Yi Feng*, TH 17), Convergence and Gathering (*Hui Zong*, TH 7), and Lower Pass (*Xia Guan*, St 7) are the ruling points.

For deafness, Celestial Window (*Tian Chuang*, SI 16) is the ruling point.

For deafness with a buzzing noise such that one cannot hear, Celestial Countenance (*Tian Rong*, SI 17) is the ruling point.

For ringing in the ear with loss of hearing, Shoulder True (*Jian Zhen*, SI 9) and Wrist Bone (*Wan Gu*, SI 4) are the ruling points.

For a sound in the ear like blowing wind and intermittent loss of hearing, Shang Yang (*Shang Yang*, LI 1) is the ruling point.

For deafness and blockage in the ear, Union Valley (*He Gu*, LI 4) is the ruling point.

For deafness and pain in the temples, Central Islet (*Zhong Zhu*, TH 3) is the ruling point.

For a dim din in the ear with loss of hearing, Outer Pass (*Wai Guan*, TH 5) is the ruling point.

For sudden deafness due to qi (blockage), Four Rivers (*Si Du*, TH 9) is the ruling point.

Chapter Six

Stirring in the Vessels of the Hand & Foot *Yang Ming* Producing Oral & Dental Disorders[59]

(1)

In examining tooth decay and pain, (one must) palpate the vessels of the *yang ming*. If there is a fault, there is a single (vessel) that is hot. If (the evil) is on the left, the left (vessel) is hot. If it is on the right, the right (vessel) is hot. If (the evil) is in the upper (part of the face), the upper (vessel) is hot. And if it is in the lower (part of the face), the lower (vessel) is hot.[60]

(2)

That aspect of the arm *yang ming* that enters the suborbital region and runs throughout the teeth is called Great Reception (*Da Ying*, St 5). For decay of the lower teeth, take (the *yang ming*) of the arm. In the case of aversion to cold, perform supplementation ["take it" in a variant version {later editor}]. In the case of an absence of aversion (to cold), perform drainage. [The *Ling Shu* names this part of the *yang ming* Grain Bone Hole (*He Liao*, LI 19) or Great Reception. Because it is known that Great Reception (*Da Ying*) originates with the vessel qi of the *yang ming* vessel, so it is only reasonable to name it Grain Bone Hole. For decay of the lower teeth, however, it is necessary to take both Grain Bone Hole and Great Reception of the foot *yang ming*. Try them and (you will) understand. {later editor}][61]

That aspect of the hand *tai yang* that submerges into the suborbital region and runs throughout the teeth is called Angle Vertex (*Jiao Sun*, TH 20). For decay of the upper teeth, take the points around the nose and those anterior to the suborbital region. In attacks (of pain), the vessel must be exuberant. If the vessel is exuberant, perform drainage, and if (the vessel) is vacuous, perform supplementation. It is also stated that (the points) outside the nose must be taken. In attacks (of pain), the exuberant (vessel requires) drainage, and the vacuous, supplementation.[62]

(3)

For toothache, take the foot *yang ming* in the absence of an aversion to cold drinks, but take the hand *yang ming* if there is an aversion to cold drinks.

For a slack tongue with drooling and vexation and oppression, take the foot *shao yin*.

For double tongue, prick the tongue pillar[63] with a sword needle.

(4)

For decay and swelling of the upper teeth, Eye Window (*Mu Chuang*, GB 16) is the ruling point.[64]

For decay and pain of the upper teeth with aversion to wind and cold, Upright Nutrition (*Zheng Ying*, GB 17) is the ruling point.[65]

For decay and pain of the front and back teeth, Floating White (*Fu Bai*, GB 10) and Completion Bone (*Wan Gu*, GB 12) are the ruling points.

For toothache, Cheek Bone Hole (*Quan Liao*, SI 18) and Second Space (*Er Jian*, LI 2) are the ruling points.

For decay of the upper teeth, Extremity of the Mouth (*Dui Duan*, GV 27) and Ear Gate (*Er Men*, TH 21) are the ruling points.

For gum bleeding due to damage by sourness and pain in the tooth bed with inability to open the mouth affecting the nose, Gum Intersection (*Yin Jiao*, GV 28) is the ruling point.[66]

For swollen cheek, rigidity of the mouth, pain in the jawbone, and inability of the teeth to chew, Jawbone (*Jia Che*, St 6) is the ruling point.

For inversion, deviated mouth with inability to yawn, pain in the lower teeth, swollen cheek with aversion to cold, inability to contract the mouth, inability of the tongue to enunciate, and inability to chew, Great Reception (*Da Ying*, St 5) is the ruling point.[67]

For decay and pain in the upper teeth and deviated mouth with clenched teeth, Upper Pass (*Shang Guan*, GB 3) is the ruling point.

For inability to yawn, decay of the lower teeth, pain in the lower teeth, and swelling of the suborbital region, Lower Pass (*Xia Guan*, St 7) is the ruling point.

For decay and pain in the teeth, Auditory Convergence (*Ting Hui*, GB 2) and Surging Yang (*Chong Yang*, St 42) are the ruling points.[68]

For inability of the teeth to chew and swollen gums, Angle Vertex (*Jiao Sun*, TH 20) is the ruling point.

For deviated mouth, inability to yawn, dislocation of the jaw, and clenched teeth, Wind Screen (*Yi Feng*, TH 17) is the ruling point.

For swelling under the tongue, difficult speech, protrusion of the tongue, and twisted (mouth), Open Valley (*Tong Gu*, Bl 66) is the ruling point.

For swelling under the tongue, difficult speech, protrusion of the tongue, and drooling, Ridge Spring (*Lian Guan*, CV 23) is the ruling point.

For deviated mouth, needle Great Abyss (*Tai Yuan*, Lu 9) to conduct (the evil) downward.

For swelling and fishy smell in the mouth, Palace of Toil (*Lao Gong*, Per 8) is the ruling point.

For a dry mouth, pain in the lower teeth with aversion to cold, and swelling of the suborbital region, Shang Yang (*Shang Yang*, LI 1) is the ruling point.

For tooth decay and pain with aversion to coolness, Third Space (*San Jian*, LI 3) is the ruling point.

For a deviated mouth, Veering Passageway (*Pian Li*, LI 6) is the ruling point.

For pain in the mouth and teeth, Warm Dwelling (*Wen Liu*, LI 7) is the ruling point.

For decay of the lower teeth and pain in the upper teeth, Humor Gate (*Ye Men*, TH 2) is the ruling point.

For toothache, Four Rivers (*Si Du*, TH 9) is the ruling point.

For decay and pain in the upper teeth, Yang Valley (*Yang Gu*, SI 5) ["yang connecting vessel" in a variant version {later editor}] is the ruling point.

For decay and pain in the teeth, Union Valley (*He Gu*, LI 4) is the ruling point.

For decay and ache in the teeth, Small Sea (*Xiao Hai*, SI 8) is the ruling point.

For protrusion of the tongue, drooling, and vexation and oppression, Yin Valley (*Yin Gu*, Ki 10) is the ruling point.

Chapter Seven

Blood Spillage Producing Nosebleed[69] (With Appendices on Runny Snivel Disorders and Polyp)

(1)

When there is a sudden counterflow of pure heat in the interior, the liver and the lung are persecuted, and blood spills into the nose and mouth. Take the Celestial Storehouse (*Tian Fu*, Lu 3) which is one of a quintet (*wu bu*) of grand points of the stomach. [In regards to this quintet, the *Ling Shu* states, "For yang counterflow headache and fullness in the chest with inability to catch one's breath, take Man's Prognosis {*Ren Ying*, St 9}. For sudden loss of voice and qi choking, prick Protuberance Assistant {*Fu Tu*, LI 18} and the root of the tongue to let blood out. For sudden deafness and qi clouding, loss of acuity of hearing and vision, take Celestial Casement {*Tian You*, TH 16}. For sudden hypertonicity, epilepsy, tetany and inability of the feet to carry the body, take Celestial Pillar {*Tian Zhu*, Bl 10}. For sudden pure heat counterflow in the internal, persecution of the liver and the lung, and blood spillage in the nose and the mouth, take Celestial Storehouse. This is the quintet of the five grand points of the stomach." Now Shi-an breaks up and arranges them in different chapters. Celestial Storehouse is just one member of this quintet. {later editor}]

(2)

For nosebleed with an absence of coagulated blood where the blood flows (incessantly), take the foot *tai yang*. For massive nosebleed with coagulated blood, take the hand *tai yang*. If this does not staunch (the bleeding), needle (the point) below the wrist bone (*i.e., Wan Gu*, SI 4). If this still does not staunch (the bleeding), prick the center of the popliteal fossa to let blood out.

(3)

For runny snivel nosebleeding, Upper Star (*Shang Xing*, GV 23) is the ruling point. First take Yi Xi (*Yi*

Xi, Bl 45) and finally Celestial Window (*Tian You*, TH 19) and Wind Pool (*Feng Chi*, GB 20).

For nasotubular *ju*[70] producing pestilential wind nose, Brain Hollow (*Nao Kong*, GB 19) is the ruling point.

For runny snivel disorder inhibiting (nasal respiration), nasal congestion and stoppage of qi, deviated mouth, copious nasal mucus, and runny snivel nosebleeding with *yong* (in the nose), Welcome Fragrance (*Ying Xiang*, LI 20) is the ruling point.

For runny snivel nosebleeding with discharge of mucus, suspended *yong* and polyp in the nose, nasal congestion, and inability to detect fragrance or fetor, White Bone Hole (*Si Liao*, GV 25) is the ruling point.

For nasal congestion, deviated mouth, incessant discharge of clear nasal mucus, and runny snivel nosebleeding with *yong* (in the nose), Grain Bone Hole (*He Liao*, LI 19) is the ruling point.

For polyp in the nose inhibiting respiration, pain in the tip and root of the nose, and erosive sores in the nose, Gum Intersection (*Yin Jiao*, GV 28) is the ruling point.

For runny snivel disorder with inability to catch the breath, inability to control the discharge of mucus, inability to detect fragrance or fetor, and incessant nosebleeding, Water Trough (*Shui Gou*, GV 26) is the ruling point.

For incessant nosebleeding, Sauce Receptacle (*Cheng Jiang*, CV 24) and Bend Middle (*Wei Zhong*, Bl 40) are the ruling points.

For inhibited nasal (respiration), Front Valley (*Qian Gu*, SI 2) is the ruling point.

For nosebleed, Wrist Bone (*Wan Gu*, SI 4) is the ruling point.

Chapter Eight

Stirring in the Vessels of the Hand & Foot *Yang Ming* & *Shao Yang* Producing Throat *Bi* & Sore Throat[71]

(1)

For throat *bi* with inability to speak, take the foot *yang ming*, (but for throat *bi*) with ability to speak, take the hand *yang ming*.[72]

(2)

For throat *bi*, Completion Bone (*Wan Gu*, GB 12), Celestial Countenance (*Tian Rong*, SI 17), Qi Abode (*Qi She*, St 11), Celestial Tripod (*Tian Ding*, LI 17), Cubit Marsh (*Chi Ze*, Lu 5), Union Valley (*He Gu*, LI 4), Shang Yang (*Shang Yang*, LI 1), Yang Valley (*Yang Xi*, LI 5), Central Islet (*Zhong Zhu*, TH 3), Front Valley (*Qian Gu*, SI 2), Shang Hill (*Shang Qiu*, Sp 5), Blazing Valley (*Ran Gu*, Ki 2), and Yang Intersection (*Yang Jiao*, GB 35) are all the ruling points.

For throat *bi* and swollen larynx where even fluids cannot be ingested, Jade Pivot (*Xuan Ji*, CV 21) is the ruling point.

For throat *bi* where food cannot be ingested, Turtledove Tail (*Jiu Wei*, CV 15) is the ruling point.

For throat *bi* with a sensation of a lump in the larynx, Third Space (*San Jian*, LI 3) is the ruling point.

For throat *bi* with inability to speak, Warm Dwelling (*Wen Liu*, LI 7) and Pool at the Bend (*Qu Chi*, LI 11) are the ruling points.

For throat *bi* with qi counterflow, deviated mouth, and a sensation as if the throat were being strangled, Moving Between (*Xing Jian*, Liv 2) ["Intermediary Courier (*Jian Shi*, Per 5)" in the *Qian Jin* {later editor}] is the ruling point.

For sore throat with inability to ingest food,

Gushing Spring (*Yong Quan*, Ki 1) is the ruling point.

Chapter Nine

Qi Binding Producing Tumor & Goiter[73]

For goiters, Celestial Window (*Tian Chuang*, SI 16) ["Celestial Countenance {*Tian Rong*, SI 17}" in a variant version, and Celestial Storehouse {*Tian Fu*, Lu 3} in the *Qian Jin* {later editor}] and Brain's Door (*Nao Hui*, TH 13) are the ruling points.[16]

For tumors, Qi Abode (*Qi She*, St 11) is the ruling point.

Chapter Ten

Miscellaneous Disorders in Females[75]

(1)

The Yellow Emperor asked:

Some women who have carried double bodies for nine months lose their voice. What kind of disease is this?[76]

Qi Bo answered:

The connecting vessel of the uterus is interrupted. The uterine connecting vessel links with the kidney, and the vessel of the *shao yin* penetrates the kidney, linking with the tongue root. This accounts for the loss of voice. It does not require treatment since (the voice) will recover in the tenth month. The *Ci Fa* (*Needling Techniques*) states that one must not reduce insufficiency, nor must one boost a surplus lest one become guilty (of mistreatment) ["be inflicted with papules" in the *Su Wen* {later editor}]. The statement that one must not reduce insufficiency is an admonition against administration of needles to an emaciated body. That one must not boost a surplus is an admonition against administering drainage to those with form in their abdomen. If drainage is

applied, essence will emerge, and the illness will take exclusive possession of the center. This is called becoming guilty (of mistreatment).[77]

(2)

The Yellow Emperor asked:

How can pregnancy and childbirth be determined?

Qi Bo answered:

The body is ill but there is no evil pulse.[78]

In examining women, if the pulse of the hand *shao yin* beats energetically, a child is gestated. Breast-feeding heat disease (乳子而病热) with a small, suspended pulse is survived if the hands and feet are warm, but ends in death if they are cold.[79]

Breast-feeding wind stroke is a disease of fever, dyspnea, thirst ["dyspneic rale" in the *Su Wen* {later editor}], and shrugging of the shoulders to facilitate breathing with a pulse that is replete and large. A moderate (pulse indicates) survival, an urgent (one portends) death.[80]

(3)

For red and white vaginal discharge while breast-feeding, Lumbar Shu (*Yao Shu*, GV 2) is the ruling point.

For females with infertility, vaginal protrusion, and dribbling white vaginal discharge, Upper Bone Hole (*Shang Liao*, Bl 31) is the ruling point.

For females with dribbling red and white vaginal discharge and accumulation and distention in the region below the heart, Second Bone Hole (*Ci Liao*, Bl 32) is the ruling point. [The *Qian Jin* says, "For lumbar pain with inability to bend either forward or backward, Second Bone Hole (*Ci Liao*) is the ruling point." {later editor}] Take first Empty Basin (*Que Pen*, St 12) and finally the tail bone[81] and the eight bone holes.[82]

For females with red flux with intermittent white

vaginal discharge, dribbling urinary qi block, and scanty menses, Central Bone Hole (*Zhong Liao*, Bl 33) is the ruling point.

For a greenish, thin vaginal discharge or incessant dribbling red vaginal discharge and itching and pain in the genitals radiating to the upper and lower abdomen with inability to bend (the body) either forward or backward, Lower Bone Hole (*Xia Liao*, Bl 34) is the ruling point. In needling the paravertebral muscles at the lumbar and sacrococcygeal joints,[83] the number of the holes is determined by the days of waning and waxing of the moon. With the (extraction) of the needle, the effect occurs immediately.

For rumbling in the intestines and outpour diarrhea, Lower Bone Hole (*Xia Liao*, Bl 34) is the ruling point.[84]

For women with breast-feeding disorders, Huang Gate (*Huang Men*, Bl 46) is the ruling point.

For mammary *yong* with fever and chills, diminished qi and agitated sleep, Breast Window (*Ying Chuang*, St 16) is the ruling point.

For mammary *yong* with shivering, cold and heat, and pain in the nipple exacerbated by the slightest pressure, Breast Root (*Ru Gen*, St 18) is the ruling point.

For infertility, moxibustion at Center of the Navel (*Qi Zhong*)[85] promises pregnancy.

For females with hypertonicity of the hands and feet, abdominal fullness, *shan*, absence of menses, breast-feeding disorders, infertility, and genital itching, Yin Intersection (*Yin Jiao*, CV 7) is the ruling point.

For abdominal fullness, *shan* accumulation, breast-feeding disorders, infertility and genital itching, needle Stone Gate (*Shi Men*, CV 5). [The *Qian Jin* says, "For running piglet ascending with chest distension, pain and harness in the lower abdomen radiating down to the genitals, and inability to void urine, needle Yin Intersection to a depth of eight *fen*." {later editor}]

For females with infertility and coagulated blood in (the abdomen) which will not descend, Origin Pass (*Guan Yuan*, CV 4) is the ruling point. [The *Qian Jin* says, "For shifting of the womb prohibiting urination, lower abdominal fullness, and painful stone water, needle Origin Pass, and moxibustion is appropriate as well." {later editor}]

For females with forbidden center, abdominal heat and pain, breast-feeding disorders, infertility due to internal insufficiency, inclined infant's gate, tormenting cold in the lower abdomen, itching and pain in the genitals, absence of menses, and inhibited urination, Central Pole (*Zhong Ji*, CV 3) is the ruling point.[86]

For females with red and white vaginal discharge, dryness and pain in the genitals, aversion to sexual intercourse, distention and hardness in the lower abdomen, and urinary blockage, Curved Bone (*Qu Gu*, CV 2) is the ruling point.

For females with blood stoppage, Meeting of Yin (*Hui Yin*, CV 1) is the ruling point.[87]

For women with foul blood in the child's viscus and internal counterflow fullness and pain, Stone Pass (*Shi Guan*, Ki 18) is the ruling point.[88]

For menstrual stoppage and running piglet with its draining qi moving up and down, producing pain in the lumbar spine, Qi Point (*Qi Xue*, Ki 13) is the ruling point.[89]

For red flux in females, Great Manifestation (*Da He*, Ki 12) is the ruling point.

For females with pain in the uterus and menstruation that does not cease in a timely fashion, Celestial Pivot (*Tian Shu*, St 25) is the ruling point. [The *Qian Jin* says, "For abdominal fullness, rumbling intestines, and qi surging up into the chest, needle Celestial Pivot." {later editor}]

For lower abdominal distention, fullness and pain radiating to the genitals, ache in the lumbar spine occurring with menstruation, conglomeration in the uterus, and cold in the infant's gate radiating to the knee caps and thighs, Waterway

(*Shui Dao*, St 28) is the ruling point. [The *Qian Jin* says, "For... inability to urinate or defecate, needle Waterway." {later editor}]

For females with cold in the genitals, Return (*Gui Lai*, St 29) is the ruling point.

Females may experience inhibited menstruation or sudden menstrual blockage, abdominal distention and fullness, dribbling urinary block, aching and weakness (of the limbs) and generalized fever, and gripping abdominal pain. (They may also suffer from) *tui shan*, swollen genitals, difficult lactation, fetal (qi) surging up into the heart, or retention of the placenta with chaos in all the (channel) qi, abdominal fullness with inability to turn over, and forced supine posture with one knee bent and the other stretched (sic), together with Surging Qi (*Qi Chong*, St 30). The needle should be inserted upward to a depth of three *cun*, and when the qi arrives, administer drainage.[90]

For women with infertility and lower abdominal pain, needle Qi Surge (*Qi Chong*, St 30).

For women with postpartum disorders, such as inability to ingest food or drink, stuffing fullness in the chest and lateral costal region, visual dizziness, cold feet, difficult urination, lancinating heart pain, frequent retching, sour foul smell, *bi* aching (of the limbs), and abdominal fullness which is more conspicuous in the lower abdomen, Cycle Gate (*Qi Men*, Liv 14) is the ruling point.[91]

For women with lower abdominal hardness and pain and menstrual stoppage, Girdling Vessel (*Dai Mai*, GB 28) is the ruling point.[92]

For women with red and white vaginal discharge, urgency in the interior (of the abdomen), and tugging and slackening, Fifth Pivot (*Wu Shu*, GB 27) is the ruling point.

For grudging milk (*du ru*, 妒乳) ["pain in the bosom" in the *Qian Jin* {later editor}], Great Abyss (*Tai Yuan*, Lu 9) is the ruling point.[93]

For infertility, Shang Hill (*Shang Qiu*, Sp 5) is the ruling point. ["This point is located in a depression anterior to the medial malleolus." {later editor}][94]

For women with *shan* conglomeration producing heat that feels as if one were scalded by boiling water and which radiates down along the inside (of the thighs) to the knees, and swill diarrhea, moxa and needle Spring at the Bend (*Qu Quan*, Liv 8).

For women with pain in the genitals and lower abdominal hardness, urgency, and pain, Yin Mound Spring (*Yin Ling Quan*, Sp 9) is the ruling point.

For women with dribbling uterine bleeding, absence of menses, and qi counterflow abdominal distention, Sea of Blood (*Xue Hai*, Sp 10) is the ruling point.[95]

For inhibited menstruation, bleeding leading to abortion, and cold genitals, Moving Between (*Xing Jian*, Liv 2) is the ruling point.

For difficult lactation, Supreme Surge (*Tai Chong*, Liv 3) and Recover Flow (*Fu Liu*, Ki 7) are the ruling points.[96]

For females with *shan*, lower abdominal swelling, duck-stool diarrhea, dribbling urinary block, enuresis, pain in the genitals, sooty, black facial complexion, and pain in the lower eyelid, Supreme Surge is the ruling point.[97]

For females with enlarged lower abdomen, difficult lactation, dry throat and desire to drink, Mound Center (*Zhong Feng*, Liv 4) is the ruling point.[98]

For females with dribbling uterine bleeding, Supreme Surge is the ruling point.[99]

For females with periumbilical *shan*, Mound Center is the ruling point.

For major *shan* causing infertility, Guest House (*Zhu Bin*, Ki 9) is the ruling point.[100]

For females with *shan*, lower abdominal swelling, and red and white flux of irregular amounts, Woodworm Canal (*Li Gou*, Liv 5) is the ruling point.

For females with *shan* and conglomeration with a sensation as if their thighs were being scalded by boiling water, lower abdominal swelling, vaginal protrusion with pain, genital swelling or itching, a green-blue, vegetable soup-like discharge during menstruation, infertility due to menstrual blockage, and no desire for food, Spring at the Bend (*Qu Quan*, Liv 8) is the ruling point.[101]

For women who are sterile or have never been able to give birth, Yin Corner (*Yin Lian*, Liv 11) is the ruling point, ["which is located one *cun* under the groin. Insert the needle to a depth of eight *fen*." {later editor}][102]

For women with infertility, Gushing Spring (*Yong Quan*, Ki 1) is the ruling point.[103]

For females with sterility, sudden vaginal protrusion, and dribbling uterine bleeding, Blazing Valley (*Ran Gu*, Ki 2) is the ruling point.[104]

For females in whom the menses do not descend, Shining Sea (*Zhao Hai*, Ki 6) is the ruling point. [The *Qian Jin* says, "For *bi*, susceptibility to fright, sentimentality, melancholy, sensation of falling, and lack of perspiration, needle Shining Sea (*Zhao Hai*)." {later editor"][105]

For women with dribbling uterine bleeding, vaginal protrusion, aching and weakness of the four limbs, and oppression of the heart, Shining Sea is the ruling point.

For failure of the menses to arrive and blockage of the menses, pain below the heart, blurred vision for distant objects, Water Spring (*Shui Quan*, Ki 4) is the ruling point.

For women with dribbling uterine bleeding, abdominal distention and fullness with inability to catch the breath, and yellowish urine, Yin Valley (*Yin Gu*, Ki 10) is the ruling point. [The *Qian Jin* says "For dribbling uterine bleeding, lower abdominal block-like distention and full-ness, generalized fever and chills, and abdominal swelling at one side, needle Yin Valley." {later editor}]

For breast (-feeding) *yong* with heat, Three Li (*San Li*, St 36) is the ruling point.

For breast (-feeding) *yong*, susceptibility to fright, *bi*, heavy lower legs, debilitated insteps, and pain in heels, Lower Ridge of the Great Hollow (*Ju Xu Xia Lian*)[106] is the ruling point.

For inhibited menstruation, uterine bleeding leading to abortion, and swollen nipples, Overlooking Tears (*Lin Qi*, GB 41) is the ruling point.

For females in whom delivery is difficult or in whom the placenta is retained, Kun Lun Mountain (*Kun Lun*, Bl 60) is the ruling point.

Chapter Eleven

Miscellaneous Disorders in Children[107]

(1)

Diseased infants whose head hair stands up on end will die.[108]

Prominent green-blue veins around the auricles in infants indicate tugging and abdominal pain. Rotten milk-like green-blue stool with swill diarrhea, large pulses, and cold hands and feet, is difficult to cure. Swill diarrhea with small pulses and warm hands and feet, is easy to cure.

(2)

Five vessels are needled (to treat) fright epilepsy. Needle the hand and the foot *tai yin* with five (punctures) each. Needle the channels and the *tai yang*, five (punctures) each. Needle the by-branched connecting vessel of the hand *shao yin* channel, one (puncture) and the foot *yang ming*, one (puncture. Needle a point) located five *cun* above the malleolus, needling three times.[51]

(3)

For infantile fright epilepsy, Root Spirit (*Ben Shen*, GB 13), Before the Vertex (*Qian Ding*, GV 21), Fontanel Meeting (*Xin Hui*, GV 22), and Celestial Pillar (*Tian Zhu*, Bl 10) are the ruling points. In the case of upturned eyes, Overlooking Tears (*Lin Qi*, GB 15) is the ruling point.

For infantile fright epilepsy with tugging and slackening, rigidity of the spine, and uprolled eyes, Sinew Contraction (*Jin Suo*, GV 8) is the ruling point.

For infantile fright epilepsy with tugging and slackening, rigidity of the spine, and dragging (of limbs), Long Strong (*Chang Qiang*, GV 1) is the ruling point.

For infantile food gauntness (*xiao er shi hui*, 小儿食晦) with headache, Yi Xi (*Yi Xi*, Bl 45) is the ruling point.[110]

For attack of epilepsy with upturned eyes, Bamboo Gathering (*Zan Zhu*, Bl 2) is the ruling point.

For infant's umbilical wind with upturned eyes, needle Silk Bamboo Hole (*Si Zhu Kong*, TH 23).[111]

For infantile epilepsy with tugging, retching and vomiting, outpour diarrhea, susceptibility to fright, apprehension, loss of brightness (of the eyes) with dim vision, and gum in the eyes, Spasm Vessel (*Chi Mai*, TH 18) is the ruling point.[112]

For infantile epilepsy with gasping for breath, Skull (*Lu Xin*, TH 19) is the ruling point.

For infantile fright epilepsy with confused vision, Broken Sequence (*Lie Que*, Lu 7) is the ruling point. Take the connecting vessel of the *yang ming*[113] at the same time.

For a fishy, foul smell in the mouth and stuffing fullness in the chest and lateral costal region in children, Palace of Toil (*Lao Gong*, Per 8) is the ruling point.

For infantile goat epilepsy, the point below

Convergence and Gathering (*Hui Zhong*, TH 7) is the ruling point.[114]

For coughing, diarrhea and no desire for food in children, Shang Hill (*Shang Qiu*, Sp 5) is the ruling point.

For infantile epilepsy with tugging, agitated hands and feet, clouded vision, clenched jaw, and yellowish urine, Shang Hill is the ruling point.

For infantile epilepsy with tugging, enuresis of clear urine, and, in the case of vacuity, conglomerations and *tui* of various categories, or, in the case of repletion, dribbling urinary block, heat in the lower abdomen and somnolence, Great Pile (*Da Dun*, Liv 1) is the ruling point.

For infantile umbilical wind with clenched jaw and susceptibility to fright, Blazing Valley (*Ran Gu*, Ki 2) is the ruling point.

For abdominal fullness and inability to take in food or drink in children, Suspended Bell (*Xuan Zhong*, GB 39) is the ruling point.

For infantile horse epilepsy, Kneeling Servant (*Pu Can*, Bl 61) and Metal Gate (*Jin Men*, Bl 63) are the ruling points.

For wind penetrating from head to foot (manifested by) epilepsy with tugging, clenched jaw, sudden pressure-resisting abdominal fullness arising in defecation, belching, sadness and dyspnea, Kun Lun Mountain (*Kun Lun*, Bl 60) is the ruling point.

Endnotes

[1]Part 1 is derived from Chap. 28, Vol. 5, *Ling Shu* (*Spiritual Pivot*); Part 2 from Chap. 81, *Su Wen* (*Basic Questions*); Part 3 from Chap. 28, Vol. 5, *Ling Shu*; Part 4 from Chap. 80, Vol. 12, *Ling Shu*; and Part 5 from Chap. 28, Vol. 5, *Ling Shu*.

[2]In the *Lei Jing* (*The Classified Classic*), Zhang Jing-yue explains, "Yawning means that one opens the mouth as wide as possible to facilitate inhalation, possibly with the arms and the lumbus stretched. It arises because of the mutual drawing between yin and yang... Yawning invariably comes before

people go to bed because the yang is on the verge of submerging into the yin phase. (At this time,) yin is accumulating below, while yang has not yet calmed down. Therefore, yang tends to draw itself toward ascension, while yin draws itself toward descent. This upward and downward drawing produces yawning. There are people whose spirit is tired and are afflicted by taxation fatigue so as to cause yawning. This is a pattern of yang failing to restrain yin."

Ma Shi explains in his *Ling Shu Zhu Zheng Fa Wei* (*Annotations & Commentaries on the Intricacies of the Spiritual Pivot*), "Because there is an evil in the foot *shao ying* kidney channel, (people) are unable to fall asleep. It requires drainage at the point Shining Sea (*Zhao Hai*, Ki 6). Frequent yawning resulting from the vacuity of the yang motility requires supplementation at the Extending Vessel (*Shen Mai*, Bl 62) of the foot *tai yang* urinary bladder channel."

[3]Retching is unproductive vomiting. This may also be understood as the vomiting of "qi." In the *Lei Jing*, Zhang Jing-yue explains, "Retching is previously said to issue from the stomach, but now it is said to be governed by the lung. The reason for this is the upward counterflow of the cold qi that causes retching. That is to say, it is qi that causes trouble in the stomach and qi is governed by the lung." According to this explanation, it is quite reasonable to needle the hand *tai yin* to treat retching. Usually, one should needle Great Abyss (*Tai Yuan*, Lu 9) to supplement the lung with a view toward boosting and normalizing the lung qi so as to check qi counterflow. Then one must needle Great Metropolis (*Da Du*, Sp 2) and Supreme White (*Tai Bai*, Sp 3) to drain the spleen to downbear the turbid qi in the stomach.

[4]*I.e.*, Shining Sea (*Zhao Hai*, Ki 6) and Extending Vessel (*Shen Mai*, Bl 62) respectively

[5]In the *Lei Jing*, Zhang Jing-yue explains, "The source and confluence points of all the hand and foot yang channels and the point of the yang motility are among the choices."

[6]There are various causes for belching. Food accumulation is one. This requires drainage. Depressive phlegm fire is another. It calls for clearing fire and transforming phlegm. This paragraph deals only with cold qi in the spleen/stomach.

[7]*I.e.*, Valley Passage (*Tong Gu*, Bl 66) and Bamboo Gathering (*Zan Zhu*, Bl 2) respectively

Pathological sneezing is not associated with harmonious qi. Because of this, we suspect that there is an error in this passage.

[8]Drooping is a descriptive term. It is characterized by weak, languid, and listless muscles and flesh, often accompanied by drooping of the head. It may affect the limbs and other parts of the body. This condition requires supplementation of the spleen/stomach and invigoration of the kidney yang. The performance of yin affairs refers to sexual intercourse.

[9]The eyes are said to be the converging place of the gathering vessels because the essence qi of all the five viscera and six bowels pours into them to produce brightness.

[10]This whole section is derived from Chap. 81, of the *Su Wen* where the questions are raised by Lei Gong and the answers are provided by the Yellow Emperor. The Chinese editions fail to make this explicit. However, because the author declares in his instructions in the preliminary part of the work that, if there is no mention of the interlocutors, the same interlocutors as in the preceding section or chapter must be assumed, we respect the design of the author.

[11]Because qi is often used in both ancient and modern Chinese to denote temper, mood, etc., harmonious qi in this context is an alternative expression for delight, happiness, or joy, and complexion or color often means facial expression.

Ancestral essence means the kidney essence. Since all the five fluids have their common source in the kidney, it acquires the title ancestral. The ancestral qi or essence, as explained in the text, is in control of all fluids, including tearing and snivelling. This is the key in appreciating the meaning of the following abstruse paragraph.

[12]The reader should first note that will, water, and kidney and fire, spirit, and heart are interchangeable terms. When will, for example, is mentioned, the kidney may be implied. This is often the case with the ancient classics. When sorrow affects both the will, *i.e.*, the kidney, and the spirit, *i.e.*, the heart, the spirit qi is passed to the heart, and the essence qi ascends rather than descends to the kidney as it ought to. As a result, the kidney loses control of fluid, and tears run out. In sobbing, snivel may run too. This is ascribed to the brain. The marrow is that which replenishes the bone cavities and is stored in the brain. Since the nose is linked with the brain, marrow may leak from the brain in lamentation. Snivel is simply what leaks from the brain. Water, *i.e.*, tears, and marrow, *i.e.*, snivel, are both governed by the kidney and are in fact of one kind in that they are essentially fluid.

[13]The will or kidney is yin and the spirit or heart is yang. When both of them remain unaffected,

431

there can be no tears. If, however, great agony arises, surging into the yin (which as explained in the above text means the brain), a sequence of changes occurs to produce tears and snivel.

[14]The supplemented part is quoted from the *Su Wen*. It is absent from the *Ling Shu*. This supplementation was made in the Song dynasty and has been criticized as an example of wanton adulteration.

[15]In inversion, the yang qi concentrates above, while the yin qi is retained below. Thus fire blazes above, while cold is exuberant below. As they become separated, the yin and yang qi cease to circulate, resulting in distention. In the eyes, the kidney essence, the single water, and the fire or hyperactive yang from the five viscera come into conflict. Since the kidney essence is no match for the fires from the five viscera, the eyes become scorched. Once wind strikes them, the fire is fanned even brighter, causing tears to be shed.

[16]The heart-governor channel of the hand *shao yin* referred to is actually the hand *jue yin* channel, and the point implied is Inner Pass (*Nei Guan*, Per 6). On the foot *shao yang*, Pinched Ravine (*Xia Xi*, GB 43), Hill Ruins (*Qiu Xu*, GB 40), etc. are recommended. In the *Lei Jing*, Zhang Jing-yue explains, "Assisting the viscera of wood and fire soothes the yang qi and resolves depression. Therefore, supplementation with needle retention is indicated."

[17]A note in the *Tai Su* explains, "The ridge spring is the pores beneath the tongue that are passageways for saliva. If a person's spirit attends to its duty, these passageways are shut. Once affected by an inviting smell, the spirit lessens its duty. Then the pores open and saliva issues forth. There are also occasions that the ridge spring is open and saliva exudes because the stomach is hot and worms stir." Ridge Spring also denotes the acupuncture point *Lian Quan* (CV 23).

In the *Lei Jing*, Zhang JingByue explains, "The kidney serves as the pass for the stomach, and its vessel links with the tongue. For this reason, it should be supplemented to invigorate water to restrain fire. This way, the fluid is brought under the control of its ruler and drooling is checked."

[18]A.k.a. Upper Gate (*Shang Guan*, GB 3)

[19]*I.e.*, Lesser Shang (*Shao Shang*, Lu 11)

The ears are said to be a converging place of vessels because the network vessels of hand and foot *shao yang* and *tai yang* and the hand *yang ming* all enter them.

[20]In the *Lei Jing*, Zhang Jing-yue explains, "When inversion qi counterflows upward, blood surges and qi steams, resulting in the development of unusual maladies. (The channel qi) each visit a specific area. For example, the vessel of the *shao yin* travels the root of the tongue. The vessel of the *shao yang* goes along the cheek anterior to the ear. The vessel of the *yang ming* encircles the lips. They may produce swelling and distention or an exotic itching at the places where they are. It is not the tongue alone but all these places that are also subject to biting."

[21]Heart and lung vacuity and insufficient qi above mean the same thing, and a surplus of qi below refers to repletion of the stomach and intestines. Zhang Jing-yue explains in his *Lei Jing*, "The lower qi superabundance is spoken of in contrast to the upper qi insufficiency. It does not really mean that the lower is truly replete." He continues to say, "The heart and lung manifest themselves as vacuous above, so the constructive and defensive are retained below (*i.e.*, in the stomach/intestines). As a result, the spirit and qi are no longer able to circulate. Thus poor memory results, a sign of debilitated yang above."

[22]When the essence and qi are both concentrated in the spleen, the yin qi in the stomach becomes insufficient and, consequently, the yang becomes exuberant, generating heat.

[23]The insubstantial fault is the branch symptom or sign. The regulation of the qi means that one must treat the root.

[24]*I.e.*, Kun Lun Mountain (*Kun Lun*, Bl 60)

[25]*I.e.*, Supreme Surge (*Tai Chong*, Liv 3)

[26]Part 1 is from Chap. 69, Vol. 10, *Ling Shu*; Part 2 from Chap. 21, Vol. 5, *Ling Shu*; and Part 3 from the *Zhen Jiu Ming Tang Zhi Yao* (*The Acupuncture & Moxibustion Treatment Essentials of the Enlightening Hall*).

[27]The transverse bone is the hyoid bone.

[28]In Chinese, nasal hollowing may be pronounced *bi yuan* or *bi dong* which is known in modern terms as nasosinusitis. Repetition of words is a kind expression for stammering.

The glottis is most likely the epiglottis.

[29]*I.e.*, Ridge Spring (*Lian Quan*, CV 23)

[30]A.k.a. Mute's Gate (*Ya Men*, GV 15)

[31]In our source edition, Celestial Window (*Tian Tu*, CV 22) is prescribed. This correction is made in accor-

dance with the *Wai Tai Mi Yao (Secret [Medical] Essentials of a Provincial Governor)* and *Yi Xin Fang (The Heart of Medicine Formulary)*.

[32]Part 1 is derived from Chap. 71, Vol. 10, *Ling Shu*; Part 2 from Chap. 80, Vol. 12, *Ling Shu*; Part 3 from Chap. 46, *Su Wen*; Part 4 from Chap. 34, *Su Wen*; and Part 5 from the *Zhen Jiu Ming Tang Zhi Yao*.

[33]In ancient times, a day and night were divided into one hundred watches. See Chap. 9, Book 1, present work.

[34]Here the yin qi is insufficient, while there is a surplus of yang. Therefore, one must supplement Shining Sea (*Zhao Hai*, Ki 6) of the foot *shao yin* and drain Extending Vessel (*Shen Mai*, Bl 62) of the foot *tai yang*. The water referred to in this passage is known as distantBrunning water. In *Nei Jing Zhi Yao (Essential Knowledge of the Inner Classic)*, Li Nian-wo explains that "Water that has run a thousand *li* is used because of its long course and distant source. It is significant because it courses and dredges and thus is able to reach down." Water stirred is called worked water. It is believed able to harmonize yin and yang. Reeds have hollow stems producing a fire that is swift and vigorous. Glutinous millet, sweet, moderately cold, and nontoxic, is effective for the treatment of insomnia due to yang exuberance and yin vacuity.

[35]In this and the next sections, the questions are raised by the emperor and the answers are made by Qi Bo in the *Ling Shu* and the *Su Wen*, where these sections are derived. As the author does not make this known, we must assume the interlocutors are the same as those in the preceding section in compliance to the author's arrangement of the materials.

[36]Affliction is interpreted as taxation in any form, mental or physical, including emotional disturbances such as worry. While distraction is understood as pleasureBseeking of any form. In the *Ling Shu Ji Zhu (Condensed Annotations on the Spiritual Pivot)*, Zhang Zhi-cong explains, "Orientation is referred to as essence, spirit, corporeal soul, ethereal soul, will, and reflection. Form is that which is nurtured by the constructive and defensive, blood and qi. Affliction in orientation impairs spirit, while taxation of the form impairs essence qi." In the *Lei Jing*, Zhang Jing-yue explains "Affliction, meaning worry and taxation, most often damages the yang (qi) of the heart and lung. Pleasure seekers are licentious and libertine and most often damage the yin (qi) of the spleen and kidney."

[37]The first sentence may be erroneous since the author proceeds with a discussion of vacuity and never deals with the issue of a repletion of defensive qi.

[38](The) *Lower Classic*, an ancient medical classic, long lost

[39]Zhang Jing-yue gives an explanation of the last pattern in his *Lei Jing*, saying, "Water disease is rooted in the kidney and has its branch in the lung. Therefore, inability to lie down or dyspnea resulting from lying down is a disease of both the root and the branch."

[40]In *Zhu Bing Yuan Hou Lun (Treatise on Origins & Symptoms of Various Diseases)*, Chao Yuan-fang explains "When the five viscera are in disharmony, the triple burner will be full of qi, and when it is full, qi will wander about in the interior without dissipating, thus resulting in the diseases of vexation, fullness and vacuity distention."

[41]Part 1 is derived from Chap. 80, Vol. 12, *Ling Shu*; Part 2 from Chap. 22, Vol. 5, *Ling Shu*; Part 3 from Chap. 74, Vol. 11, *Ling Shu*; Part 4 from Chap. 37, *Su Wen*; Part 5 from Chap. 21, Vol. 5, *Ling Shu*; Part 6 from Chap. 23, Vol. 5, *Ling Shu*; and Part 7 from the *Zhen Jiu Ming Tang Zhi Yao*.

[42]Therefore, the first essence means the bright essence or the function of sight. *Jing* in Chinese has many meanings and may be interpreted as acute, sharp, and clever, as well as essence.

The verb *wei* generally means to be/form/become. However, many scholars of Chinese medicine prefer to interpret it in this context as "pours into." In that case, the passage should then read, "The essence of the sinews pour into the dark of the oculi".... etc. The modern Chinese translation of this section provided in our source text (edited by Shandong TCM College, published by the People's Hygiene & Health Press in 1979) supplies an example of this kind of interpretation.

In most cases, the Chinese word *mu* and *jing* both mean eye, but from the text, it appears that *mu* is used in a narrower sense, perhaps meaning eyeball, while *jing* (rendered here as oculi) is used in a wider sense and is better understood as the whole of the eye, including the socket.

[43]As explained above, the eyes are composed of various essences. If an evil strikes just one or two kinds of essence there, the essence(s) grow(s) out of proportion to the unaffected essences. This leads to double vision. Since the word *jing* has meanings other than essence, this passage may be interpreted in a different way: "If an evil strikes the eyes, (the object that) the eyes strike will be out of proportion. This disproportion disperses

the essence, and dispersed essence gives rise to double vision."

[44]This sentence is interpreted by some scholars of Chinese medicine as follows: "The upper eyelid belongs to the outer canthus, while the lower eyelid to the inner canthus." It appears that the paragraph has become terribly garbled.

[45]In the *Ling Shu Ji Zhu*, Zhang Zhi-cong explains, "Nondescript yellowing is a yellow coloring that encompasses the colors black, white, greenBblue, and red. It indicates disease in the chest because the qi of the five viscera issue forth through the diaphragm to present such a (blended) color."

[46]In the *Lei Jing*, Zhang Jing-yue explains, "The foot *tai yang* channel forms the upper eyelid, so a red vessel extending from above to below indicates disease of the *tai yang*. The foot *yang ming* forms the lower eyelid, so a red vessel extending from below to above indicates disease of the *yang ming*. The foot *shao yang* travels behind the sharp (outer) canthus, so a red vessel extending from the outer to the inner indicates disease of the *shao yang*.?

[47]A note in the *Tai Su* explains, "The major channel of the foot *yang ming* starts from the nose, crossing at the nasion, descending outside the nose, entering the upper teeth, submerging again to encircle the mouth, crossing at Sauce Receptacle (*Cheng Jiang*, CV 24), travelling across the jowl, passing Great Reception (*Da Ying*, St 5), ascending to the area anterior to the ear, going along the hairline. Its qi starts at the point Suspended Skull (*Xuan Lu*, GB 5)." According to this, Suspended Skull is a point on the foot *yang ming*. In modern times, however, it is thought of as a point on the foot *shao yang*. This is supported by many classics and *Ma Shi*, for example, is of the latter view.

[48]A note in the *Tai Su* explains, "The foot *tai yang* starts at the inner canthus, travelling across the forehead, its two routes crossing each other at the top of the head. The straight (branch) starts from the top of the head to submerge, connecting the brain, emerging again, deviating down the nape of the neck, with a connecting vessel homing to the root of the eye named the ocular ligation."

In *Ling Shu Zhu Zheng Fa Wei*, Ma Shi explains, "A part of the foot *tai yang* urinary bladder channel enters the brain via the nape of the neck (at the point) named Jade Pillow (*Yu Zhen*, Bl 9). This part directly homes to the root of the eye, where the ligations of the two eyes are both linked. Therefore, it is called the ocular ligation...The vessel submerges into the brain through (the point Jade Pillow) between two sinews in the nape of the neck and

deviates from the yin and yang motility."

The yin and yang motility cross each other at the point of Bright Eyes (*Jing Ming*, Bl 1) in the inner canthus. When the qi emerges externally, the yang motility is filled up and the yang qi becomes exuberant. When the yang qi submerges internally, the yin motility is filled up and the yin qi becomes exuberant.

[49]*I.e.*, Shining Sea (*Zhao Hai*, Ki 6)

[50]Clear-eyed blindness refers to impaired vision in the absence of any visible pathological changes in the eye itself.

[51]Modern scholars of Chinese medicine believe this paragraph contains a typographical error and that this paragraph should read, "excessive (moisture) of the skin (of the eyelid) with white screen, Pupil Bone Hole (*Tong Zi Liao*, GB 1) and Great Bone Hole (*Ju Liao*, St 3) are the ruling points."

[52]Part 1 is derived from Chap. 28, *Su Wen*; Part 2 from Chap. 75, Vol. 11, *Ling Shu*; Part 3 is a combination of parts of Chap. 24 and 26, Vol. 5, *Ling Shu*; and Part 4 from the *Zhen Jiu Ming Tang Zhi Yao*.

[53]This passage deals with poor eyesight and dull hearing or blindness and deafness. A note in the *Tai Su* explains, "A branch of the hand *tai yang* vessel reaches the sharp canthus and then returns backward into the ear. The branches of the hand and foot *shao yang* vessels enter the ear from behind the ear and then submerge, travelling before the ear to reach the sharp canthus. Therefore, the three vessels all meet at Auditory Palace (*Ting Gong*) in the ear and all link with the pupil of the eye." Since the point Auditory Palace (*Ting Gong*) is linked with the pupil, one can reach the pupil even when needling Auditory Palace.

Because the Chinese word *shu* for point can also mean transport, the last sentence also carries the connotation that "there is a transporting action here."

This passage is sometimes incorrectly interpreted as "...if we have reached the pupil with qi, then the patient's hearing is restored..." The following passages make it clear that this interpretation is erroneous.

[54]This provides us with a method of needling in combination with mobilizing the qi in the patient. In the *Ling Shu* and *Tai Su* (*Essentials*), the last clause is "...and a sound must find response in the needle."

[55]*I.e.*, Ear Gate (*Er Men*, TH 21)

[56]*I.e.*, Passage Hub (*Guan Chong*, TH 1) and Foot Portal Yin (*Zu Qiao Yin*, GB 44)

[57]*I.e.*, Central Hub (*Zhong Chong*, Per 9)

[58]Since no point on the foot is mentioned here, this last sentence makes little sense.

[59]Part 1 is derived from Chap. 74, Vol. 11, *Ling Shu*; Part 2 from Chap. 21, Vol. 5, *Ling Shu*; Part 3 a combination of parts of Chap. 26 and 21, Vol. 5 and Chap. 9, Vol. 2, *Ling Shu*; and Part 4 from the *Zhen Jiu Ming Tang Zhi Yao*.

[60]When there is trouble in either the upper or lower teeth, a vessel in a corresponding region of the face becomes hot or exuberant. The word single is likely a redundancy.

[61]In the *Ling Shu Zhu Zheng Fa Wei*, Ma Shi explains, "On the hand *yang ming* vessel, a branch starts from the supraclavicular fossa, travelling up the neck, passing Celestial Tripod (*Tian Ding*, LI 17) and Protuberance Assistant (*Fu Tu*, LI 18), travelling upward across the cheek, submerging into the gums of the lower teeth, and emerging again to encircle the mouth. Its two routes cross each other at Human Center (*Ren Zhong*, GV 26), proceed collaterally, travelling upward by the nostril, passing Grain Bone Hole (*He Liao*, LI 19) and Welcome Fragrance (*Ying Xiang*, LI 20) to meet the foot *yang ming* (at Great Reception [*Da Ying*, St 5])...This accounts for naming (that branch of the hand *yang ming*) Great Reception. Any disorders characterized by toothache are called tooth decay. For decay of the lower teeth, it is necessary to take the points of the arm *yang ming*. Aversion to cold food and drink reflect a vacuity condition, requiring supplementation. An absence of aversion to cold food and drink reflects a repletion condition requiring drainage."

The comments in the notes by the unknown editor(s) in the text are apparently incorrect in their ascription of the points, since they do not correspond to the current versions of the *Ling Shu*.

[62]In his *Ling Shu Zhu Zheng Fa Wei*, Ma Shi explains, "The point where the foot *tai yang* vessel submerges ...is Angle Vertex (*Jiao Sun*, TH 20) of the hand *shao yang* triple burner channel. In the case of decay in the upper teeth, where the vessel qi of the foot *yang ming* stomach channel passes, the points to be taken at the nose and anterior to the suborbital region are Earth Granary (*Di Cang*, St 4) and Great Bone Hole (*Ju Liao*, GB 29)....The points to be taken outside the nose are Grain Bone Hole (*He Liao*) and Welcome Fragrance (*Ying Xiang*, LI 20) of the (hand *tai yang*) channel."

In both the *Ling Shu* and *Tai Su*, foot *tai yang* is substituted for hand *tai yang*, and modern versions of the *Jia Yi Jing* mistakenly follow these texts on this point.

[63]*I.e.*, the vessel under the tongue

[64]Eye Window (*Mu Chuang*, GB 16) is a meeting point of the yang linking vessel.

[65]Upright Nutrition (*Zheng Ying*, GB 17) is a meeting point of the yang linking vessel.

[66]Tooth bed refers to the roots of the teeth.

[67]These symptoms are due to wind evil invading the *yang ming* vessel.

This paragraph is placed after the next one in our source edition and has been rearranged here in accordance with a version transcribed during the Ming dynasty.

[68]This paragraph does not appear in our source edition and has been included here in accordance with a version copied in the Ming dynasty and the *Wai Tai* and *Yi Xin Fang*.

[69]Part 1 is derived from Chap. 21, Vol. 5, *Ling Shu*; Part 2 from Chap. 26, Vol. 5, *Ling Shu*; and Part 3 from the *Zhen Jiu Ming Tang Zhi Yao*.

[70]This is an abscess in the bridge of the nose due to fumigating and steaming of lung fire. At the initial stage, it is a red patch, which is numb and hot with a pulsating pain. Later it becomes soft and suppurates.

[71]Part 1 is derived from Chap. 26, Vol. 5, *Ling Shu*; Part 2 from the *Zhen Jiu Ming Tang Zhi Yao*.

[72]In *Ling Shu Ji Zhu* by Zhang Zhi-cong, "Throat *bi* is a congestion of evil in the throat with swelling and pain. The vessel of the foot *yang ming* travels along either side of the throat knot when passing through the throat. Therefore, when an evil congests the throat, this produces an inability to speak. Then it is necessary to take the foot *yang ming*. The vessel of the hand *yang ming* passes farther from the throat knot. Therefore, ability to speak requires that one take the hand *yang ming*."

[73]This entire chapter is derived from the *Zhen Jiu Ming Tang Zhi Yao*.

[74]The word *ying* for a goiter or tumor growing in the neck originally meant cherry neck. In his *Zhu Bing Yuan Hou Lun* (*Treatise on Origins & Symptoms of Various Diseases*), Chao Yuan-fang explains, "Goiter is produced by qi bind due to worry and indignation. It may also be due to

drinking sandy water. Sand follows the qi into the vessels and gathers in the neck to develop into goiter. At the initial stage, it is the size of a cherry kernel, growing in the lower part of the neck, and the overlying skin is loose like a pendant. Goiter resulting from binding indignation qi is a pendant kernel without vessels in it, while goiter due to drinking sandy water has several kernels, is rootless, and floats inside the skin. It is also said that there are three categories of goiter: blood goiter, which is treated by breaking it; polyp goiter, which is treated by removing it; and qi goiter, which is treated by needling... In the mountain areas where springs issue from black soil, (people) cannot live long, for drinking the water over a prolonged period causes people to suffer from goiters..." He continues, " A tumor is sudden swelling in the skin and flesh. It is plum-sized at first and grows little by little. It is painless and does not itch, nor does it become hard. Because it lodges without dispersing, it is called a tumor..." In Chinese, tumor (liu) is a homonym with retention/ stay/ lodging, etc.

[75]Part 1 is derived from Chap. 47, Su Wen; Part 2 is a combination of parts of Chap. 40, 18, and 28, Su Wen; and Part 3 from the Zhen Jiu Ming Tang Zhi Yao.

[76]The term double bodies (chong shen) is a euphemism for pregnancy.

[77]Zhang Zhi-cong explains in his Ling Shu Ji Zhu, "In the ninth month of pregnancy, the fetus has grown to its full, easily presenting an obstacle to the uterine connecting vessel, interrupting and stopping its flow."

Administering drainage with needles to those with form in their abdomen (i.e., those who are pregnant), drains the essence and damages the fetal qi such that evil qi produced by the obstruction alone remains in the uterus.

In our source edition, Zhi Fa (Treatment Strategies) is in place of Ci Fa (Needling Strategies), a long lost medical classic.

[78]In his Lei Jing, Zhang Jing-yue explains, "That the body is ill refers to symptoms such as the interruption of menstruation and morning sickness. When the body is ill, the pulse should also reflect illness. Interrupted and irregular or wiry, choppy, thin, and rapid pulses are all evil pulses, indicating a true illness. If the six pulses are in harmony and slippery but the body suffers from afflictions, this is without a doubt fetal qi."

[79]Wiseman's rendering of ru zi er bing re as suckling heat disease is rather ambiguous since it is a dis-

ease of the mother in which a fever develops while nursing. Although the pulse lacks strength, it indicates that the illness is still in the exterior and has entered the yin vessel. Warmth in the hands and feet indicate that the original yang has not been severed. Cold hands and feet indicate that the evil has entered the viscera, destroying the original yang and this is a fatal condition.

In his Lei Jing, Zhang Jing-yue explains, "The pulse of the hand shao yin, which is located in the depression distal to the wrist, is the pulse aligned with the small finger of the feeling hand. It is referred to as the vessel of the heart channel, i.e., the point of Spirit Gate (Shen Men, Ht 7). This explanation is quite right. According to my experience, however, the left cun (pulse) responds, too."

[80]In his Su Wen Jing Zhu Jie Jie, Ma Shi explains "This is due to the subjection of the lung to wind cold where the qi floats and stirs. When the pulse is replete, large, and strong, this is an externally contracted repletion pattern. However replete and large, the pulse qi should also be moderate. This is an indication of the presence of stomach qi and excludes some unexpected danger. If the pulse is not moderate but urgent, (qi) is ascending without descending, and when the true visceral qi appears, death is a certainty."

[81]I.e., Long Strong (Chang Qiang, GV 1)

[82]I.e., Upper Bone Hole (Shang Liao, Bl 31), Second Bone Hole (Ci Liao, Bl 32), Central Bone Hole (Zhong Liao, Bl 33), and Lower Bone Hole (Xia Liao, Bl 34).

In our source edition, the signpost phrase, "The Qian Jin says," is dropped, and hence, what is in the brackets is incorporated into the text. This correction has been made in accordance with a version copied in the Ming dynasty, the Qian Jin, and Wai Tai.

[83]I.e., the so-called eight bone holes; see the above note.

[84]This item is irrelevant to female disorders and also appears in Chap. 5, Book 11, present work.

[85]A.k.a. Spirit Gate (Shen Que, CV 8)

[86]Forbidden center refers to an aversion to, or incapacity for sexual intercourse.

In our source edition, the word "itching" appears before "forbidden center" (in which case forbidden center simply refers to the genitals—tr.) However, it has been deleted here in accordance with the Wai Tai.

Some sources define the infant's gate as the cervix, others as the vagina. Actually, the term "inclined infant's gate" is a general reference to any sort of structural deviation of the womb.

[87]This is a reference to amenorrhea.

[88]The child's viscus is another name for the uterus.

[89]The word draining may well be a redundancy, but according to the *Tong Ren Jing (The Classic of the Bronze Statue)* by Wang Wei-yi of the Song dynasty, the relevant passage should be understood as "...diarrhea, qi moving up and down..."

[90]The above passage is structured in Huang-fu Mi's typical pattern with the exception of "together with Surging Qi (*Qi Chong*)." If his usual format were adhered to, the line would read, "Surging Qi is the ruling point." It seems to us that the words "together with" suggests the possibility that a second point name may have been dropped. If this suspicion is reasonable, then the description of the posture should be understood as the requirement for needling this point. This assertion, however, remains to be proved.

[91]This pattern is due to a disharmony of the liver and spleen.

[92]This pattern is due to blood stasis.

[93]Grudging milk is characterized by swelling, hardening, and pain in the nipple due to accumulated milk. It is ascribed to heat which boils down the breast milk and can be unbearably painful. In some cases, small sores grow in the nipple, producing pain and itching. Scratching will cause a yellow exudate to flow.

[94]In our source edition, the text in the brackets is incorporated in the main text. The translators have added the brackets in accordance with the *Yi Xue Gang Mu* by Lou Ying of the Ming dynasty.

[95]This pattern is due to blood vacuity.

[96]This symptom is due to postpartum blood vacuity.

[97]This pattern is due to the liver invading the spleen. The spleen is unable to control water and so the qi of the liver and kidney counterflows.

[98]This pattern is due to a great exuberance of wind fire in the liver channel.

[99]This pattern is due to the agitation of wind fire resulting in the failure of the liver to store the blood.

[100]Guest House (*Zhu Bin*, Ki 9) is the cleft point of the yin linking vessel.

[101]All of the above symptoms are due to vacuity of qi and blood and a failure of the liver's capacity for orderly reaching.

[102]In our source edition, the text in brackets is part of the main text. The brackets have been added by the translators in accordance with the *Yi Xue Gang Mu.*

[103]This is infertility due to vacuity cold in the lower source.

[104]Blazing Valley may be moxaed for this condition.

[105]This pattern is due to a vacuity of kidney yang and cold in the uterus. Moxa may be applied to Shining Sea.

[106]A.k.a. Lower Great Hollow (*Xia Ju Xu*, St 39)

[107]Part 1 is derived from Chap. 74, Vol. 11, *Ling Shu*; Part 2 from Chap. 28, *Su Wen*; and Part 3 from the *Zhen Jiu Ming Tang Zhi Yao.*

[108]In his *Lei Jing*, Zhang Jing-yue explains, "While infants are growing, water is their root, and the hair is the luxuriance of the kidney. When the head hair stands on end, water is insufficient. Thus the hair is dry and parched like desiccated grass..."

[109]As we have explained previously, a puncture refers to the number of points to be needled or the time of treatment. In this context, a number of punctures most likely refers to the number of needling treatments. Wu Kun explains, "When only a channel is mentioned without specifying the point(s) (to be needled), any (appropriate) point(s) of this channel can be chosen." This, too, has bearing on the phrase in the text "needle the channels."

Many outstanding scholars of Chinese medicine have given their own interpretations of this passage, but there has been no consensus in regard to the points to be needled. In general which points of the hand or foot *tai yang* are indicated has not been determined. The by-branched connecting vessel of the hand *shao yin* is also challenge. Wu Kun asserts, "When by-branch is spoken of, then no channel per se or (specific) point is meant, and it is necessary to prick the minute connecting vessel." Zhang Jing-yue asserts that the by-branch connecting vessel is Intelligence Tower (*Ling Tai*, GV 10). However, he may be referring to Intelligence Path (*Ling Dao*, Ht 4) beside the connecting vessel point Connecting Li (*Tong Li*, Ht 5). Wang Bing argues for Branch to the Correct (*Zhi Zheng*, SI 7). On the foot *yang ming*, the point suggested is Ravine Divide (*Jie Xi*, St 41). The point five *cun* above the malleolus may be Bright Light, (*Guang Ming*, GB 37), located above the lateral malleolus, or Guest House (*Zhu Bin*, Ki 9) located above the medial malleolus. According to some of the scholars, there are more than five channels to be needled.

[110]Food gauntness is a pattern of thinness despite large food intake.

[111]Umbilical wind usually occurs in infants under ten days old. It is an acute condition characterized by lockjaw, arched back, facial deviation, and generalized hypertonicity.

[112]In our source text, besides Spasm Vessel, Long

Strong (*Chang Qiang*, GV 1) is prescribed. It is omitted in accordance with the *Wai Tai*.

[113]*I.e.*, Veering Passageway (*Pian Li*, Lu 6)

[114]The point below Convergence and Gathering (*Hui Zong*, TH 7) may be Branch Ditch (*Zhi Gou*, TH 6).

Epilepsy is classified as goat epilepsy, ox epilepsy, horse epilepsy, etc., reflecting the particular moaning sound made by the patient during an attack.

General Index

A

B

Point Number Index

Pin Yin Point Name Index

English Point Name Index

A

Abdominal Bend (Sp 14), 97
Abdominal Bind (Sp 14), 97, 390
Abdominal Lament (Sp 16), 97, 390
Angle Vertex (TH 20), 59, 87, 423, 435,
Armpit Abyss (GB 22), 51, 54-55, 92, 161, 332, 399-400, 409
Armpit Gate (St 27), 96, 103, 228, 249, 269, 299, 334, 422
Assuming Fullness (St 20), 95, 337
Attached Branch (Bl 41), 84
Auditory Convergence (GB 2), 87, 187, 279, 316, 403, 422-423
Auditory Palace (SI 19), 74, 76, 87, 386, 421-422, 434

B

Back Ravine (SI 3), 104, 253, 268, 279, 299, 387, 422
Bamboo Gathering (Bl 2), 85, 251, 290, 347, 386, 430-431
Beam Gate (St 21), 95, 333
Beam Hill (St 34), 109, 334, 363
Before the Vertex (GV 21), 78, 279, 368, 430
Beginning of Light (Bl 2), 85
Behind the Vertex (GV 19), 78, 279, 385-386, 404
Bend Middle (Bl 40), 112, 138, 185, 235, 248, 255, 270, 279, 286, 289-290, 343-344, 346-347, 352-354, 376, 385, 388, 403, 425
Bend Yang (Bl 39), 112, 138, 152, 343, 347, 353-355, 376
Bending Joint (Ht 3), 101
Big Plume (GV 18), 78

B

Bladder Huang (Bl 53), 84, 322, 342
Blazing Bone (Ki 2), 383
Blazing Valley (Ki 2), 160, 168, 225, 297, 346, 387, 392, 394, 425, 429-430
Body Pillar (GV 12), 386, 81, 256
Bountiful Bulge (St 40), 50, 61, 109, 117, 226, 254, 278-279, 282, 285
Bowel Abode (Sp 13), 97, 306, 389
Brain Cover (Bl 8), 79
Brain Hollow (GB 19), 79, 249, 279, 369, 386, 425
Branch Ditch (TH 6), 61, 103-104, 331, 387, 389, 394, 399, 415, 438
Branch to the Correct (SI 7), 50, 61, 105, 253, 269, 387, 403, 437
Breast Center (St 17), 91-92, 160
Breast Root (St 18), 91, 399, 427
Breast Window (St 16), 91, 350, 427
Bright Eyes (Bl 1), 59, 85, 420, 434
Bright Light (GB 37), 50, 61, 85, 110, 261, 374, 387, 437
Broken Sequence (Lu 7), 49, 99, 251, 268, 289, 299, 308, 315, 317, 403-404, 409, 430
Bundle Bone (Bl 65), 111, 228, 255, 262, 269, 279, 282, 296, 300, 388
Burning Valley (Ki 2), 107, 167, 170, 185, 254, 261, 281, 285, 310, 326, 334

C

Calf Intestine (Bl 56), 112
Camphorwood Gate (Liv 13), 76, 97, 253, 281, 285, 306, 308, 310, 338, 342, 350-351, 375, 399
Capital Bone (Bl 64), 61, 67, 111, 117, 255, 262, 268, 290, 300, 326, 371, 373, 375, 388

D

E

T

OTHER BOOKS ON CHINESE MEDICINE
AVAILABLE FROM:

BLUE POPPY PRESS

5441 Western, Suite 2, Boulder, CO 80301

For ordering 1-800-487-9296 PH. 303\447-8372 FAX 303\245-8362

Email: info@bluepoppy.com Website: www.bluepoppy.com

ACUPOINT POCKET REFERENCE
by Bob Flaws
ISBN 0-936185-93-7

ACUPUNCTURE & IVF
by Lifang Liang
ISBN 0-891845-24-1

ACUPUNCTURE AND MOXIBUSTION FORMULAS &
TREATMENTS
by Cheng Dan-an, trans. by Wu Ming
ISBN 0-936185-68-6

ACUPUNCTURE PHYSICAL MEDICINE: An Acupuncture
Touchpoint Approach to the Treatment of Chronic Pain,
Fatigue, and Stress Disorders
by Mark Seem
ISBN 1-891845-13-6

AGING & BLOOD STASIS:
A New Approach to TCM Geriatrics
by Yan De-xin
ISBN 0-936185-63-5

BETTER BREAST HEALTH NATURALLY
with CHINESE MEDICINE
by Honora Lee Wolfe & Bob Flaws
ISBN 0-936185-90-2

THE BOOK OF JOOK: Chinese Medicinal Porridges
by B. Flaws
ISBN 0-936185-60-0

CHANNEL DIVERGENCES: Deeper Pathways of the Web
by Miki Shima and Charles Chase
ISBN 1-891845-15-2

CHINESE MEDICAL PALMISTRY:
Your Health in Your Hand
by Zong Xiao-fan & Gary Liscum
ISBN 0-936185-64-3

CHINESE MEDICAL PSYCHIATRY
A Textbook and Clinical Manual
by Bob Flaws and James Lake, MD
ISBN 1-845891-17-9

CHINESE MEDICINAL TEAS:
Simple, Proven, Folk Formulas for
Common Diseases & Promoting Health
by Zong Xiao-fan & Gary Liscum
ISBN 0-936185-76-7

CHINESE MEDICINAL WINES & ELIXIRS
by Bob Flaws
ISBN 0-936185-58-9

CHINESE PEDIATRIC MASSAGE THERAPY: A Parent's &
Practitioner's Guide to the Prevention & Treatment of
Childhood Illness
by Fan Ya-li
ISBN 0-936185-54-6

CHINESE SELF-MASSAGE THERAPY:
The Easy Way to Health
by Fan Ya-li
ISBN 0-936185-74-0

CLINICAL NEPHROLOGY IN CHINESE MEDICINE
by Wei Li & David Frierman,
with Ben Luna & Bob Flaws
ISBN 1-891845-23-3

CONTROLLING DIABETES NATURALLY WITH CHINESE
MEDICINE
by Lynn Kuchinski
ISBN 0-936185-06-3

CURING ARTHRITIS NATURALLY WITH CHINESE
MEDICINE
by Douglas Frank & Bob Flaws
ISBN 0-936185-87-2

THE HEART & ESSENCE OF DAN-XI'S METHODS
OF TREATMENT
by Xu Dan-xi, trans. by Yang Shou-zhong
ISBN 0-926185-49-X

THE HEART TRANSMISSION OF MEDICINE
by Liu Yi-ren, trans. by Yang Shou-zhong
ISBN 0-936185-83-X

HERB TOXICITIES & DRUG INTERACTIONS:
A Formula Approach
by Fred Jennes with Bob Flaws
ISBN 1-891845-26-8

HIGHLIGHTS OF ANCIENT
ACUPUNCTURE PRESCRIPTIONS
trans. by Honora Lee Wolfe & Rose Crescenz
ISBN 0-936185-23-6

IMPERIAL SECRETS OF HEALTH & LONGEVITY
by Bob Flaws
ISBN 0-936185-51-1

INSIGHTS OF A SENIOR ACUPUNCTURIST
by Miriam Lee
ISBN 0-936185-33-3

INTRODUCTION TO THE USE OF
PROCESSED CHINESE MEDICINALS
by Philippe Sionneau
ISBN 0-936185-62-7

KEEPING YOUR CHILD HEALTHY WITH CHINESE
MEDICINE
by Bob Flaws
ISBN 0-936185-71-6

MASTER TONG'S ACUPUNCTURE
by Miriam Lee
ISBN 0-926185-37-6

THE MEDICAL I CHING: Oracle of the Healer Within
by Miki Shima
ISBN 0-936185-38-4

MANAGING MENOPAUSE NATURALLY with
Chinese Medicine
by Honora Lee Wolfe
ISBN 0-936185-98-8

A NEW AMERICAN ACUPUNTURE
By Mark Seem
ISBN 0-936185-44-9

PATH OF PREGNANCY, VOL. I,
Gestational Disorders
by Bob Flaws
ISBN 0-936185-39-2

PATH OF PREGNANCY, Vol. II,
Postpartum Diseases
by Bob Flaws
ISBN 0-936185-42-2

POINTS FOR PROFIT: The Essential Guide to Practice
Success for Acupuncturists
by Honora Wolfe, Eric Strand & Marilyn Allen
ISBN 1-891845-25-X

THE PULSE CLASSIC: A Translation of the Mai Jing
by Wang Shu-he, trans. by Yang Shou-zhong
ISBN 0-936185-75-9

RECENT TCM RESEARCH FROM CHINA
by Bob Flaws and Charles Chase
ISBN 0-936185-56-2

SEVENTY ESSENTIAL CHINESE HERBAL FORMULAS
by Bob Flaws
ISBN 0-936185-59-7

SHAOLIN SECRET FORMULAS for Treatment of
External Injuries
by De Chan, trans. by Zhang Ting-liang &
Bob Flaws
ISBN 0-936185-08-2

STATEMENTS OF FACT IN TRADITIONAL
CHINESE MEDICINE
by Bob Flaws
ISBN 0-936185-52-X

STICKING TO THE POINT 1:
A Rational Methodology for the Step by
Step Formulation & Administration of
an Acupuncture Treatment
by Bob Flaws
ISBN 0-936185-17-1

STICKING TO THE POINT 2:
A Study of Acupuncture & Moxibustion Formulas
and Strategies
by Bob Flaws
ISBN 0-936185-97-X

A STUDY OF DAOIST ACUPUNCTURE
by Liu Zheng-cai
ISBN 1-891845-08-X

TEACH YOURSELF TO READ MODERN
MEDICAL CHINESE
by Bob Flaws
ISBN 0-936185-99-6

THE SYSTEMATIC CLASSIC OF ACUPUNCTURE &
MOXIBUSTION A translation of the Jia Yi Jing
by Huang-fu Mi, trans. by Yang Shou-zhong & Charles Chace
ISBN 0-936185-29-5

THE TAO OF HEALTHY EATING
ACCORDING TO CHINESE MEDICINE
by Bob Flaws
ISBN 0-936185-92-9

THE TREATMENT OF DISEASE IN TCM, Vol. 1: Diseases of the Head & Face, Including Mental & Emotional Disorders
by Philippe Sionneau & Lü Gang
ISBN 0-936185-69-4

THE TREATMENT OF DISEASE IN TCM, Vol. II:
Diseases of the Eyes, Ears, Nose, & Throat
by Sionneau & Lü
ISBN 0-936185-69-4

THE TREATMENT OF DISEASE, Vol. III: Diseases of the Mouth, Lips, Tongue, Teeth & Gums
by Sionneau & Lü
ISBN 0-936185-79-1

THE TREATMENT OF DISEASE, Vol IV: Diseases of the Neck, Shoulders, Back, & Limbs
by Philippe Sionneau & Lü Gang
ISBN 0-936185-89-9

THE TREATMENT OF DISEASE, Vol V: Diseases of the Chest & Abdomen
by Philippe Sionneau & Lü Gang
ISBN 1-891845-02-0

THE TREATMENT OF DISEASE, Vol VI: Diseases of the Urogential System & Proctology
by Philippe Sionneau & Lü Gang
ISBN 1-891845-05-5

THE TREATMENT OF DISEASE, Vol VII:
General Symptoms
by Philippe Sionneau & Lü Gang
ISBN 1-891845-14-4

THE TREATMENT OF EXTERNAL DISEASES
WITH ACUPUNCTURE & MOXIBUSTION
by Yan Cui-lan and Zhu Yun-long, trans. by Yang Shou-zhong
ISBN 0-936185-80-5

THE TREATMENT OF MODERN WESTERN
MEDICAL DISEASES WITH CHINESE MEDICINE
by Bob Flaws & Philippe Sionneau
ISBN 1-891845-20-9

THE TREATMENT OF DIABETES MELLITUS
WITH CHINESE MEDICINE
by Bob Flaws, Lynn Kuchinski
& Robert Casañas, MD
ISBN 1-891845-21-7

160 ESSENTIAL CHINESE HERBAL PATENT
MEDICINES
by Bob Flaws
ISBN 1-891945-12-8

630 QUESTIONS & ANSWERS ABOUT CHINESE
HERBAL MEDICINE:
A Workbook & Study Guide
by Bob Flaws
ISBN 1-891845-04-7

230 ESSENTIAL CHINESE MEDICINALS
by Bob Flaws
ISBN 1-891845-03-9

750 QUESTIONS & ANSWERS ABOUT
ACUPUNCTURE
Exam Preparation & Study Guide
by Fred Jennes
ISBN 1-891845-22